HESI

Comprehensive Review for the

NCLEX-PN®

Examination

Edition 7

HESI

Comprehensive Review for the
NCLEX-PN®
Examination

EDITOR

Denise M. Korniewicz, PhD, RN, FAAN

School of Nursing
Interim Dean and Professor
Northeastern University
Bouvé College of Health Sciences
Boston, Massachusetts

ELSEVIER

Elsevier
3251 Riverport Lane
St. Louis, Missouri 63043

Content Strategist: Heather Bays-Petrovic
Content Development Specialist: Andrew Schubert
Publishing Services Manager: Deepthi Unni
Senior Project Manager: Kamatchi Madhavan
Design Direction: Bridget Hoette

Printed in India

Last digit is the print number: 9 8 7 6 5 4 3 2 1

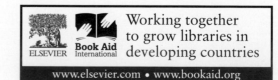

CONTRIBUTORS AND REVIEWERS

CONTRIBUTORS

Carol Patton, DrPH, FNP-BC, CRNP, CNE
Clinical Associate Professor
Northeastern University
Bouve College of Health Sciences
School of Nursing
Boston, Massachusetts

Charlene Romer, PhD, RN, CNE, CNEcl
BSN Faculty Nursing
Herzing University
Menomonee Falls, Wisconsin

Maridee Shogren, DNP, CNM, CLC
Clinical Professor
College of Nursing and Professional
    Disciplines;
Interim Dean, College of Health and
    Nursing
University of North Dakota;
Don't Quit the Quit-PI
Grand Forks, North Dakota

James J. Weidel, PhD, FNP-BC, PMHNP-BC
Adjunct Professor
Nicole Wertheim College of Nursing and
    Health Sciences
Florida International University
Miami, Florida

Mary Wyckoff, PhD, RN, NNP-BC, ACNP-BC, FNP-BC, CCNS, CCRN, FAANP
Neonatal Nurse Practitioner, Family Nurse
    Practitioner, Acute Care Nurse
    Practitioner & Neonatology Nurse
    Practitioner
University of California, Davis;
Professor Nursing
Samuel Merritt University
Sacramento, California

REVIEWER

Monica Lopez Surace, LVN, AS
Sacramento, California

Congratulations! This outstanding review manual with the companion Evolve site is designed to prepare practical nursing students for the most important examination they will ever take—the *Next Generation NCLEX-PN (NGN)* Licensing Examination. *HESI Comprehensive Review for the NCLEX-PN Next Generation Examination* allows the nursing student to prepare for the NCLEX-PN (NGN) Next Generation licensure examination in a systematic and structured way. This outstanding review manual with the companion Evolve website prepares PN students with the knowledge required to pass tests and perform safely and successfully in the clinical area. HESI Comprehensive Review for the *NCLEX-PN Examination* assists students in preparing for the NCLEX-PN license exam by challenging their critical thinking and application skills by using real-life clinical situations.

If you attended an accredited school for your LPN/LVN education, studied hard during each of your classes, and did well in your clinical rotations you have been prepared to take the NCLEX-PN License. The purpose of the exam is to let the public know that you are capable of providing safe and effective care for patients who are assigned to you. Your basic education provided a foundation and general knowledge about the principles of practical nursing. The NCLEX-PN test offers you the confidence to provide safe patient care and apply the knowledge and skills learned in your professional education.

The **HESI Comprehensive Review for the NCLEX-PN exam** helps students prepare for the NCLEX-PN licensure exam in a systematic structured way. The review offers you the ability to:

- Organize basic nursing knowledge previously learned.
- Review content learned during basic nursing curriculum.
- Identify weaknesses in content knowledge so that study efforts can be focused on systems versus single concepts.
- Develop test-taking skills so application of safe nursing practice from knowledge can be demonstrated.
- Reduce anxiety levels by increasing ability to correctly answer NCLEX-type questions.
- Boost test-taking confidence by being well prepared and knowing what to expect.

ORGANIZATION AND PREPARATION TO TAKE THE TEST

Chapter 1, *Introduction to Testing and the NCLEX-PN Examination* The NGN-NCLEX-PN exam uses a clinical decision model that measures clinical judgment by effectively measuring LPN/VN entry-level nursing and clinical-decision making skills (https://www.ncsbn.org/NGN_Fall20_Eng_03_FINAL.pdf). For the Next Generation NGN-NCLEX-PN EXAM (2020) it will be beneficial to use your critical thinking skills to systematically prepare for the exam.

Chapter 2, *Leadership and Management: Legal Aspects of Nursing*, reviews the legal aspects of nursing, leadership, and management, along with disaster nursing. Critical thinking is a vital component of every decision a nurse leader/nurse manager makes in every situation, regardless of the simplicity or complexity level of the required decision.

Chapter 3, *Advanced Clinical Concepts*, presents nursing assessment (data collection), analysis (nursing diagnosis), planning, and intervention at the practical nurse level. Respiratory failure, shock, disseminated intravascular coagulation (DIC), resuscitation, fluid and electrolyte balance, acid-base balance, electrocardiography (ECG), perioperative care, HIV, pain, and death and grief are reviewed. One of the most important areas that will be discussed includes the clinical judgment model. Discussion includes the six cognitive processes related to the clinical judgment model. These include: recognize cues, analyze cues, prioritize hypothesis, generate solutions, take action, and evaluate outcomes.

Chapters 4 through 8, *Medical-Surgical Nursing, Pediatric Nursing, Maternity Nursing, Psychiatric Nursing*, and *Gerontologic Nursing*, are presented in traditional clinical areas.

Each clinical area is divided into physiologic components, but essential knowledge about basic anatomy, medications, nutrition, communication, client and family education, acute and chronic care, leadership and management, and clinical decision-making is integrated throughout the different components. There are review questions for each of the content areas to prepare you for the essential content that may be on the NCLEX-PN Next Generation Examination. At the end of each chapter is a "bowtie" item that will test your conceptual knowledge of the essential content.

For each chapter, there are a group of questions that are used to expand your knowledge about the content area. These items are important because they offer you a comprehensive approach to the content area. Several learning opportunities are used to assist you in preparing for the exam. These strategies include:

- Reading the manual
- Discussing content with others
- Answering the review items
- Practicing the "bowtie" items to get used to the type of new items.

NEXT-GENERATION NCLEX® AND CLINICAL JUDGMENT

These learning experiences are all different ways that students should use to prepare for the Next-Generation NCLEX (NGN)-PN examination. The purpose of the questions appearing at the end of the chapter is not a focused practice session on managing NGN PN-style questions but rather a learning approach that allows for critical thinking about specific topics in the chapter. The use of the "bowtie"-style questions allows you to begin to make decisions based on the evidence presented in the cases at the end of each chapter. Multiple-choice questions alone cannot provide the essential analysis needed to know how to process nursing content that may be complicated. In addition, the questions presented at the end of the chapter provide a summary experience that helps students focus on the main topics that were covered in the chapter. Teachers use open-ended questions to stimulate the critical-thinking process, and *HESI Comprehensive Review for the NCLEX-PN Examination* facilitates the critical-thinking process by posing the same type of questions the teacher might ask.

When students need to practice multiple-choice questions, the online study exams on Evolve offer extensive opportunities for practice and skill building to improve their test-taking abilities. The online study exams include six content-specific exams (Medical-Surgical Nursing, Pharmacology, Pediatrics, Fundamentals, Maternity, and Psychiatric-Mental Health Nursing) and two comprehensive exams patterned after categories on the *Next-Generation NCLEX (NGN)-PN (NGN) Examination*. The online study exams on Evolve can be accessed as many times as necessary, and the questions from one study exam are not contained on another study exam. For instance, the Medical-Surgical study exam does not contain questions that are on the Pediatrics study exam.

The purpose of the study exams is to provide practice and exposure to the critical thinking—style questions that students will encounter on the Next-Generation NCLEX-PN examination. However, the study exams should not be used to predict performance on the actual Next-Generation NCLEX-PN examination. Only the HESI Exit Exam, a secure, computerized exam that simulates the Next-Generation NCLEX-PN examination has evidence-based results from numerous research studies indicating a high level of accuracy in predicting Next-Generation NCLEX-PN examination success, is offered as a true predictor exam. Students are allowed unlimited practice on each online study exam so that they can be sure to have the opportunity to review all of the rationales for the questions.

Here is a plan for a student to use with the online study exam:

1. Organize your knowledge.
2. Identify weaknesses in content knowledge to help focus your study time.
3. Review need-to-know content learned in nursing school.
4. Develop strong test-taking skills to demonstrate your knowledge.
5. Reduce your level of anxiety by dissecting test questions and using your foundational knowledge to arrive at the correct answer.

6. Know what to expect. Remember that knowledge is power. You are powerful when you are well prepared and know what to expect.
7. Take the PN study exam without studying for it to see your strengths and weaknesses.
8. After going over the content that relates to the study questions in a particular clinical area (e.g., Pediatrics, Medical-Surgical, or Maternity), review that section of the manual and take the test again to determine whether you have been able to improve your scores.
9. Purposely miss every question on the exam so that you can view the rationales for every question.
10. Take the exam again under timed conditions at the pace that you would have to progress.
11. Put the exam away for a while and continue review and remediation with other textbooks, resources, and results of any HESI secure exams that you have taken at your school. Then, take the study exams again to see if your performance improves after in-depth study and following a few weeks' break from these questions

Here is a plan for students to use the companion Evolve site:

• Trial 1: Take the PN Practice Exam without studying for it to determine your areas of strengths and weaknesses.
• Trial 2: After going over the content that relates to the practice questions on a particular practice test (for instance, Pediatrics, Medical-Surgical, Maternity), review that section of the manual and take the test again to determine whether you have been able to improve your scores.
• Trial 3: Purposely miss every question on the exam so that you can view rationales for every question.
• Trial 4: Take the exam again under timed conditions at the pace that you would have to progress to complete the NCLEX in the time allowed (approximately 1 minute per question). Find out whether being placed under timing constraints affects your performance.
• Trial 5: Put the exam away for a while and continue review and remediation with other textbook resources, results of any secure exams that you are taking at your school, and other study aids. Take the practice exams again after this study period to see whether your performance improves with in-depth study and a few weeks' break from the questions.

Trial 5 represents a good activity in preparation for the HESI Exit Exam presented in your final semester of the program, especially if you have not used the Evolve question site for several weeks. Repeated exposure to the questions, however, will make them less useful over time because students tend to memorize the answers. For this reason, these tests are useful only for practice and are not a prediction of NCLEX-PN success. The tendency to memorize the questions after viewing them multiple times falsely elevates the student's scores on the study exams.

Additional assistance for students to study for the NCLEX-PN examination can be obtained from a variety of products in the Elsevier family. Many nursing schools have also adopted the following resources:

- HESI Examinations—a comprehensive set of examinations designed to prepare PN nursing students for the NCLEX exam. These enable customized remediation from Elsevier textbooks that saves time for faculty and students. Each student is given an individualized report detailing exam results and is allowed to view questions and rationales for items that were answered incorrectly. The electronic remediation, a complimentary feature of the HESI specialty and exit exams, can be obtained on the subject matter in which the student did not answer a question correctly.
- HESI-PN Practice Test—a test that provides an introduction to real-world client situations with critical-thinking questions. These questions cover nursing care for clients with a wide range of physiologic and psychosocial alterations and a related coordination of client care, pharmacology, and nursing concepts.
- HESI Complete PN Case Study Collection—prepares students to manage complex patient conditions and make sound clinical judgments. These online case studies cover a broad range of physiologic and psychosocial alterations,

in addition to related coordination of care, pharmacology, and therapeutic concepts.

- HESI Live Review—a Live Review Course presented by an expert faculty member who has received training by the Manager of Review Courses for Elsevier Review and Testing. Students are presented with a workbook and practice NCLEX-style questions that are used during the course.
- eBooks—online versions of Elsevier textbooks used in the student's nursing curriculum. Search across titles, highlight, make notes, and more—all on your computer.
- Elsevier Simulations—using virtual clinical cases, standardized simulation scenarios, and electronic documentation software, Elsevier Simulations allow students to practice and apply skills in a controlled, monitored environment.

The National Council of State Boards of Nursing (NCSBN) is currently planning for the Next Generation NCLEX-PN, which at the time of this book's printing was scheduled for launch in 2023 at the earliest. More information can be found at https://www.ncsbn.org/next-generation-nclex.htm. Be sure to visit the site for updates and for more information about the clinical judgment model.

CONTENTS

1 Introduction to Testing and the NCLEX-PN® Examination, 1
- The NCLEX-PN Licensing Examination, 1
- Test-Taking Strategies, 1
- The NCLEX-PN Examination, 4
- NCLEX-PN Computer Adaptive Testing, 5
- General Priniciples to Remember, 6
- References and Bibliography, 6

2 Leadership and Management: Legal Aspects of Nursing, 7
- Leadership and Management, 7
- Maintaining a Safe, Effective Work Environment, 10
- Legal and Ethical Issues Influencing Practical Nursing, 11
- Psychiatric Nursing, 12
- Patient Identification, 13
- Disaster Nursing and Crisis Intervention, 15
- References and Bibliography, 19

3 Advanced Clinical Concepts, 21
- Respiratory Failure, 21
- Shock, 24
- Disseminated Intravascular Coagaulation, 28
- Resuscitation, 29
- Fluid and Electrolyte Balance, 35
- Intravenous Therapy, 38
- Electrocardiogram, 42
- Perioperative Care, 44
- HIV Infection, 47
- Pediatric Human Immunodeficiency Virus Infection, 55
- Pain, 56
- Death and Grief, 58
- References and Bibliography, 60

4 Medical-Surgical Nursing, 63
- Caring and Nursing, 63
- Cultural Diversity, 63
- Spiritual Assessment, 64
- Respiratory System, 64
- Renal System, 77
- Cardiovascular System, 83
- Gastrointestinal System, 98
- Endocrine System, 108
- Musculoskeletal System, 116
- Neurosensory System, 122
- Neurologic System, 126
- Hematology/Oncology, 137
- Reproductive System, 141
- Burns, 148
- References and Bibliography, 152

5 Pediatric Nursing, 155
- Growth and Development, 155
- Pain Assessment and Management in the Pediatric Client, 159
- Child Health Promotion, 160
- Diarrhea, 162
- Respiratory Disorders, 169
- Cardiovascular Disorders, 173
- Neuromuscular Disorders, 181
- Gastrointestinal Disorders, 193
- Hematologic Disorders, 197
- Metabolic and Endocrine Disorders, 200
- Skeletal Disorders, 203
- References and Bibliography, 208

6 Maternity Nursing, 209
- The Menstrual Cycle, 209
- Maternal Physiologic Changes During Pregnancy, 211
- Psychosocial Responses to Pregnancy, 215
- Antepartum Nursing Care, 216
- Antepartum Fetal and Maternal Assessments, 218
- Antepartum Complications, 220
- Hypertensive Disorders of Pregnancy, 223
- Other Vaginal Infections, 228
- Intrapartum Nursing Care, 230
- Labor and Delivery Preparation, 239
- Labor and Birth Complications, 246
- Postpartum Complications, 256
- The Normal Newborn, 259
- Newborn Complications, 267
- References and Bibliography, 272

7 Psychiatric Nursing, 273
- Safety, 273
- Structure, 273
- Support, 274
- Self-Management, 274
- Therapeutic Modalities, 274
- Common Mental Health Treatments and Interventions, 275
- Psychiatric Assessment Strategies for Inpatients: Resources with a Purpose, 276
- Alcohol Withdrawal Syndrome, 280
- Opioid Withdrawal, 280
- References and Bibliography, 283

8 Gerontologic Nursing, 285
- Aging and the Older Adult, 285
- Communication, 285
- Clinical Judgment Measures, 286
- Aging and its Effect on Body Systems, 286
- References and Bibliography, 303

Appendix A Normal Values, 305
Appendix B Answers to Review Questions, 311
Index, 325

Introduction to Testing and the NCLEX-PN® Examination

THE NCLEX-PN LICENSING EXAMINATION

In February 2020, the National Council of State Boards of Nursing (NCSBN) hosted the first Next-Generation NCLEX (NGN) item writing panel for Licensed Practical Nurses (LPN) and Licensed Vocational Nurses (LVN). This was a major event that launched the development of a variety of test items that would measure the student's ability to critically think and make critical decisions when caring for patients. As a result of this meeting, the NGN for LPN/LVNs was launched (https://www. ncsbn.org/NGN_Fall20_Eng_03_FINAL.pdf). Additionally, the items would test the candidate's ability to provide for safe and effective nursing practice by measuring current, entry-level practical nursing behavior.

Job Analysis Studies

A. The essential knowledge on the NCLEX-PN test is determined by practice analysis studies.
B. Practical nurses (PNs or vocational nurses VNs) submit statements about the frequency of nursing activities and the impact on patient safety.

> **HESI HINT** For the Next Generation NCLEX (NGN)-PNomit Examination (2020) it would be beneficial to use your critical thinking skills to systematically prepare for the exam.

C. Since you have successfully completed a basic LPN/VN nursing program and are well acquainted with your test-taking skills and ability to apply your clinical knowledge, you already have the basic knowledge required to pass the licensing examination.

Throughout your nursing education, you have learned that there is a systematic way of thinking to solve clinical problems and make clinical decisions. The problem-solving process has used a "scientific, clinical reasoning approach to patient care that has included assessment, analysis, implementation and evaluation" (NCSBN, 2018, p. 5). As a result, you have learned to organize your thoughts and systematically approach a client problem. These skills will help to set priorities and ensure your success in passing the NCLEX-PN Examination (2020).

D. Following these general guidelines will help ensure your success.
1. Organize your knowledge.
2. Identify weaknesses in content knowledge to help focus your study time.
3. Review need-to-know content learned in nursing school.
4. Develop strong test-taking skills to demonstrate your knowledge.
5. Reduce your level of anxiety by dissecting test questions and using your foundational knowledge to arrive at the correct answer.
6. Know what to expect. Remember that knowledge is power. You are powerful when you are well prepared and know what to expect.

Examination Formats

A. There are several different types of items presented on the NCLEX-PN Examination
1. The use of multiple-choice response. Items require you to select one or more responses from five to seven choices.
2. Extended drag-and-drop items.
3. Close or drop-down items.
4. Enhanced hot spot (highlighting).
5. Matrix/Grid items.
B. There is no set percentage of alternate items on the NCLEX-PN Examination. All examinations are scored based on the type of item versus partial or full score.

TEST-TAKING STRATEGIES

The test-taking strategies help you focus your study so that you can concentrate on what the exam questions are asking instead of being distracted by extraneous information that is not needed to answer the questions

A. The NCLEX-PN Examination (2020) aims to assess your overall readiness for practice. The NCSBN (2020) encompasses ways to measure your clinical judgment. This will assist you in being able to meet the nursing practice demands and clinical decisions that impact on patient outcomes. The NCSBN Clinical Judgement Model (Fig. 1.1) (CJMM, Betts et al., 2019) provides a framework to assess your clinical judgment when providing safe client care. The CJMM model helps you to develop your critical thinking, decision making, and clinical judgment skills. Based on the CJMM framework several core concepts will be included such as recognizing cues, analyzing cues, prioritizing hypothesis, generating solutions, taking action, and evaluating client outcomes. For example, a question may appear to be a medical-surgical or pediatric question, but the question can also cover such topics as communication, nutrition, growth and development, medication, client and family education, and safety.

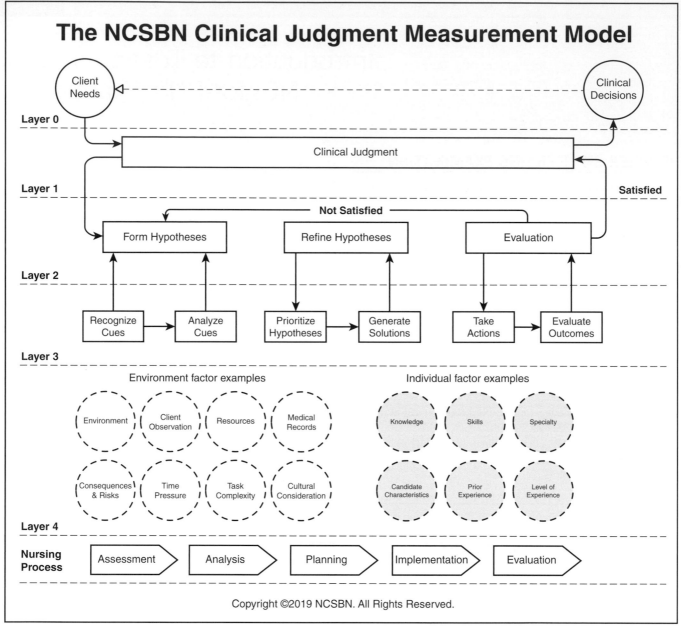

Fig. 1.1 Clinical Judgement Measurement Model. (© National Council of State Boards of Nursing.)

HESI HINT The NCLEX-PN Examination uses a clinical decision model that measures clinical judgment by effectively measuring LPN/VN entry-level nursing and clinical decision making skills (https://www.ncsbn.org/NGN_Fall20_Eng_03_FINAL.pdf).

HESI HINT Most questions are written in a positive style.

B. Understand the question.
1. Determine whether the question is written in a positive or negative style.
   a. A *positive* style question may ask what the nurse should do or ask for the best or first nursing intervention to implement.
   b. A *negative* style question may ask what the nurse should avoid, which prescription the nurse should question, or which behavior indicates the need for reteaching the client.

HESI HINT Negative style questions contain key words that denote the negative style.

Examples

A. "Which response indicates to the nurse a need to *reteach* the client about heart disease?" (Which information or understanding by the client is incorrect?)

B. "Which medication order should the nurse *question*?" (Which prescription is unsafe, not beneficial, inappropriate to this client situation?)

C. Identify key words.
   1. Ask yourself which words or phrases provide the critical information.
   2. This information may include the age of the client, the setting, the timing, a set of symptoms or behaviors, or any number of other factors.
      a. For example, the nursing actions for a 10-year-old postop client are different from those for a 70-year-old postop client.

D. Rephrase the question.
   1. Rephrasing the question helps eliminate nonessential information in the question to help you determine the correct answer.
      a. Ask yourself, "What is this question *really* asking?"
      b. While keeping the options covered, rephrase the question in your own words.

E. Rule out options.
   1. Based on your knowledge, you can most likely identify one or two options that are clearly incorrect.
   2. Physically mark through those options on the test booklet if allowed. Mentally mark through those options in your head if using a computer.
   3. Differentiate between the remaining options, considering your knowledge of the subject and related nursing principles, such as roles of the nurse, nursing

process, ABCs (airway, breathing, circulation), CAB (circulation, airway, breathing for cardiopulmonary resuscitation [CPR]), and Maslow's hierarchy of needs (Table 1.1).

F. Implement these guidelines.
   1. Consider the content of the question and what specifically the question is asking.
   2. Generally, an assessment of the client occurs before an action is taken, except in the case of an emergency; for example, if a client is bleeding profusely, stop the bleeding. Or, if a client is having difficulty breathing, open the airway then assess the client.
   3. Identify the least invasive intervention before taking action.
   4. Gather all the necessary information and complete the necessary assessments before calling the health care provider.
   5. Determine which client to assess first (e.g., most at risk, most physiologically unstable).
   6. Identify opposites in the answers.
      a. Example: prone versus supine; elevated versus decreased.
      b. Read *VERY* carefully; one opposite is likely to be the answer, but not always.
      c. If you do not know the answer, choose the most likely of the "opposites" and move on.
   7. Consider a client's lifestyle, culture, and spiritual beliefs when answering a question.

G. Use your critical thinking skills.
   1. Respond to questions based on
      a. Client safety
      b. ABCs

TABLE 1.1	Maslow's Hierarchy of Needs	
Need	**Definition**	**Nursing Implications**
Physiologic	Biologic needs for food, shelter, water, sleep, oxygen, sexual expression	The priority biologic need is breathing—that is, an open airway. If you were asked to identify the *most important* action, you would identify needs associated with physiologic integrity—for example, providing an open airway—as the *most important* nursing action
Safety	Avoiding harm; attaining security, order, and physical safety	Ensuring that the client's environment is SAFE is a priority—for example, teaching an older client to remove throw rugs that pose a safety hazard when ambulating would have a greater priority than teaching him/her how to use a walker—*first* priority is *SAFETY*, family safety, health, safe living arrangements are all safety issues (including self-harm)
Love and Belonging	Giving and receiving affection; companionship; and identification with a group; family, friendship, sexual intimacy	Although these needs are important, they are less important than physiologic or safety needs. For example, it is more important for a client to have an open airway and a safe environment for ambulating than it is to assist him/her to become part of a support group. However, assisting the client in becoming a part of a support group would have higher priority than assisting him/her in developing self-esteem. The sense of belonging would come *first*, and such a sense might help in developing self-esteem
Esteem and Recognition	Self-esteem and respect of others; respect by others, success in work; prestige	
Self-Actualization	Fulfillment of unique potential	It is important to understand that in Maslow's Hierarchy, self-actualization is associated with Health Promotion and Maintenance such as continued growth and development and self-care, as well as those associated with Psychosocial Integrity. However, you will probably not be asked to prioritize needs at this level. Remember, it is the goal of the NCSBN to ensure SAFE nursing practice, and such practice does not usually deal with the client's need for self-actualization unless it relates to a psychological need that is threatened (e.g., suicidal behavior)

c. CAB for CPR
d. Caring
e. Incorporation of culture and spiritual practices
f. Scientific, behavioral, and sociologic principles
g. Communication (spoken and written [documentation]) with client, family, colleagues, and other members of the health care team
h. Principles of teaching and learning
i. Maslow's hierarchy of needs
j. Nursing Clinical Judgment
k. Focus on what information is in the stem. Do not focus on information not included in the question. Do not read more into the question than is already there.

> **HESI HINT** The most essential element of nursing care is patient safety.

2. Do not respond to questions based on
   a. YOUR past client care experiences or your employer's policies
   b. A familiar phrase or term
   c. "Of course, I would have already"
   d. What you think is realistic; perceptions of realism are subjective
   e. Your children, pregnancies, parents, personal response to a drug, etc.
   f. The "what-ifs"
H. Keep memorization to a minimum.
   1. Don't try to memorize all the material found in your textbooks because it isn't possible. Only memorize core concepts.
      a. Growth and developmental milestones
      b. Death and dying stages
      c. Crisis intervention
      d. Immunization schedules
      e. Principles of teaching and learning
      f. Stages of pregnancy and fetal growth
      g. Nurse Practice Act: Standards of Practice and Delegation
      h. Ethical practices and standards
      i. Commonly used laboratory test values:
         1) Review Appendix A.
         2) Hemoglobin and hematocrit (H&H)
         3) White blood cells (WBCs), red blood cells (RBCs), platelets
         4) Electrolytes: K^+, Na^+, Ca^{++}, Mg^{++}, Cl^-, PO_4^-
         5) Blood urea nitrogen (BUN) and creatinine
         6) Relationship of Ca^{++} and PO_4^-
         7) Arterial blood gases (ABGs)
         8) simple blood test (SED) rate, erythrocyte sedimentation rate (ESR), prothrombin time (PT), international normalized ratio (INR), partial thromboplastin time (PTT), activated partial thromboplastin time (aPTT)

> **HESI HINT** Remember not to confuse PT, PTT, and aPTT.

   j. Nutrition
      1) High or low Na^+
      2) High or low K^+
      3) High PO_4^-
      4) Iron
      5) Vitamin K
      6) Proteins
      7) Carbohydrates
      8) Fats
   k. Foods and diets related to
      1) Body system disturbances (cardiac, endocrine, gastrointestinal)
      2) Chemotherapy, radiation, surgery
      3) Pregnancy and fetal growth needs
      4) Dialysis
      5) Buns
   l. Nutrition concepts
      1) Introduce one food at a time for infants and clients with allergies.
      2) Progression to "as tolerated" foods and diets
I. Understand medication administration.
   1. Safe medication administration requires more than knowing the name, classification, and action of the medication.
      a. The Six Rights, including techniques of skill execution
      b. Drug interactions
      c. Vulnerable organs to medication effects
         1) Know what to assess (kidney function, vital signs).
         2) Know which laboratory values relate to specific organs and their functions.
      d. Client allergies
      e. Presence of infections and superinfections
      f. Concepts of peak and trough levels
      g. How you would know if
         1) The drug is working.
         2) There is a problem.
      h. Nursing actions
      i. Client education
         1) Safety
         2) Empowerment
         3) Compliance

THE NCLEX-PN EXAMINATION

A. The main reason that the NCLEX-PN Examination is given is to protect the public.
B. Next Generation NCLEX-PN Examination
   1. Was developed by the NCSBN (NCSBN, 2019)
   2. Is administered by the State Board of Nurse Examiners
   3. Is designed to test candidates':
      a. Capabilities for safe and effective nursing practice

b. Essential entry-level nursing knowledge
c. Ability to problem solve by applying critical thinking skills
d. Proficiency in measuring your clinical judgment skills

> **HESI HINT** The NCSBN wants to ensure that the licensing examination measures current entry-level nursing behaviors. For this reason, job analysis studies are conducted every 3 years. These studies determine how frequently various types of nursing activities are performed, how often they are delegated, and how critical they are to client safety, with criticality given more value than frequency.

NCLEX-PN COMPUTER ADAPTIVE TESTING

A. Computer adaptive testing (CAT) is used for implementation of the NCLEX-PN Examination
B. The CAT is administered at a testing center selected by the NCSBN.
C. Pearson VUE is responsible for adapting the NCLEX-PN Examination to the CAT format, processing candidate applications, and transmitting test results to its data center for scoring.
D. The testing centers are located throughout the United States.
E. The NCSBN generates the NCLEX-PN Examination questions.

> **HESI HINT** Answering NCLEX-PN Examination questions often depends on setting priorities, making judgments about priorities, and analyzing the data and formulating a decision about care based on priorities. Using Maslow's hierarchy of needs can help you set nursing priorities (see Table 1.1).

How Computer Adaptive Testing Works

A. The candidate is presented with a variety of test items and possible answers.
B. Clinical Judgment will be measured two ways on the NCLEX-PN Examination, *Case Studies:* real world nursing scenario accompanied by multiple test items.
   Standalone Items: Individual items not part of the case. All items will be presented on a computer screen.
C. The NCLEX-PN Examination Test Design includes length of exam, type of items, and total score needed to pass the exam.
D. The NCLEX-PN Examination Test Design compared to the NCLEX-PN Examination will take 5 hours, however the items may be different, and the test may be shorter.
E. Scoring for the NCLEX-PN Examination may include partially correct answers and receive partial credit, for example, points possible: 0,1,2,3,4, etc. This is a new approach to scoring; therefore, you will need to be able to differentiate between clinical symptoms and clinical judgment.

F. Partial credit scoring allows for more complex item types and allows for more precise measurement. Additionally, having multiple ways to assign partial credit reduces the impact of random guessing.
G. The first optional break is offered after 2 hours of testing. The second optional break is offered after 3.5 hours of testing. The computer will automatically tell candidates when these scheduled breaks begin.
   1. All breaks count against testing time.
   2. When candidates take breaks, they must leave the testing room, and they will be required to provide a palm vein scan before and after the breaks.
H. A specific passing score is recommended by the NCSBN. All states require the same score to pass, so that if you pass in one state, you are eligible to practice nursing in any other state. However, states do differ in their requirements regarding the number of times a candidate can take the NCLEX-PN Examination.
I. Although the NCSBN can determine a candidate's score at the time of completion of the examination, it has been decided that it would be best for candidates to receive their scores from their individual Board of Nurse Examiners. The NCSBN does not want the testing center to be in a position of having to deal with candidates' reactions to scores, nor does the NCSBN want those waiting to take their examinations to be influenced by such reactions.
J. The candidate must answer each question to proceed. You cannot omit a question or return to an item presented earlier. There is no going back; this works in your favor!
K. The examination is written at a tenth grade reading level.

> **HESI HINT** Results are not given at the testing centers. Official results are mailed to the candidate by the boards of nursing about 1 month after taking the examination. The testing center staff does not have access to test results. The NCSBN does not want the testing center staff to be in a position of managing candidates' reactions to scores, nor does it want those waiting to take their examinations to be influenced by such reactions.

General Examination Formats

A. Several different types of examination items are presented on Next Generation NCLEX-EXAM. Many of the questions are multiple-choice items with four answer choices from which the candidate is asked to choose one correct answer. There are seven alternate-format item types of questions.
   1. Multiple-response items require the candidate to select one or more responses. The item will instruct the candidate to select all that apply.
   2. Fill-in-the-blank questions require the candidate to calculate the answer and type in numbers. A drop-down calculator is provided.
   3. Hot-spot items require the candidate to identify an area on a picture or graph and click on the area.

4. Chart or exhibit formats present a chart or exhibit that the candidate must read to be able to solve the problem.
5. Drag-and-drop items require a candidate to rank order or move options to provide the correct order of actions or events.
6. Audio format items require the candidate to listen to an audio clip using headphones and then select the correct option that applies to the audio clip.
7. Graphic format items require the candidate to choose the correct graphic option in response to the question.
8. Bow-Tie items include all six functions of clinical judgement in one item (recognize cues, analyze cues, generate solutions, prioritize hypotheses, take action and evaluate outcomes).

After a scenario is presented, the student will:
1. Select if the findings are normal or abnormal (recognizing cues).
2. Recognize any problems or medical issues the patient may be experiencing (analyzing cues).
3. Characterize any possible explanations that may address the patient's needs (generating solutions)
4. Decide what may be the cause of the patient's issues (prioritizing hypotheses).
5. Choose the proper actions to take (taking action).
6. Indicate which factors to monitor once interventions have been started (evaluating outcomes).

GENERAL PRINICIPLES TO REMEMBER

A. Be sure to take care of yourself. If you don't, you may be susceptible to illness that can cause you to miss the exam.
B. Eat well. Consume lots of fresh fruits, vegetables, and lean protein, and avoid high-fat foods and sugars. Processed sugar can cause blood sugar levels to spike and then plummet, which can cause brain fogginess.
C. Get enough sleep. This includes getting enough sleep the week of, not just the night before, the exam. The week of the exam is not the time to cram or to party.
D. Eliminate alcohol and other mind-altering drugs. These substances can inhibit your performance on the examination.
E. Schedule study times. During the weeks leading up to the examination, review nursing content, focusing on areas that you have identified as your weakest areas. Use a study schedule to block out the time needed for study.
F. Be prepared. Assemble all necessary materials the night before the examination (admission ticket, directions to the testing center, identification, money for lunch, glasses or contacts).
G. Bring the necessary items to the exam. Candidates are only allowed to bring a form of identification into the testing room. Watches, candy, chewing gum, food, drinks, purses, wallets, pens, pencils, beepers, cellular phones, post-It notes, study materials or aids, and calculators are not permitted. A

test administrator will provide each candidate with an erasable note board that may be replaced as needed while testing. Candidates may not take their own note boards, scratch paper, or writing instruments into the examination. A calculator on the computer screen will be available for use.
H. Arrive early. Allow plenty of time to eat breakfast and travel to the testing center. It is better to be early than late. Allow for traffic jams and so forth. The candidate may consider spending the night in a hotel or motel near the testing center the night before the examination.
I. Dress comfortably. Dress in layers so that you can put on or take off a sweater or jacket as needed.
J. Avoid negative people. During the weeks leading up to the examination, stay away from those who share their anxieties with you or project their insecurities onto you. Sometimes this is a fellow classmate or even your best friend. The person will still be there when the examination is over. Stay focused and positive.
K. Do not discuss the exam.
L. Avoid distractions. Take earplugs with you and use them if you find that those around you are distracting you.
M. Think positively. Use the affirmation, "I am successful." Obtain a relaxation and affirmation recording and use it during rest periods or any time you feel the need to boost your confidence. Think, "I have the knowledge to successfully complete the NCLEX-PN Examination."

HESI HINT The night before the NCLEX-PN Examination, allow only 30 min of study time. This 30 min period should be designated for review of test-taking strategies only. Practice these strategies with various practice test items if you wish (for 30 min only; do not take an entire test). Spend the night before the examination doing something that you enjoy.

REFERENCES AND BIBLIOGRAPHY

Betts, J., Muntean, W., Kim, D., Jorion, N., & Dickison, P. (2019). Building a method for writing clinical judgment items for entry-level nursing exams. *Journal of Applied Testing Technology, 20*(S2), 21—36.

Maslow, A. H. (1943). A theory of human motivation. *Psychological Review, 50*(4), 370—396. http://psycnet.apa.org/record/1943-03751-001.

National Council of State Boards of Nursing (NCSBN). (2018). *NCSBN clinical measurement model.* Retrieved from https://www.ncsbn.org/14798.htm.

National Council of State Boards of Nursing (NCSBN). (2019). *Report of findings from the 2018 LPN/VN practice analysis: Linking the NCLEX-PN®.* Retrieved from: https://www.ncsbn.org/2020_NCLEXPN_TESTPLAN.htm.

National Council of State Boards of Nursing (NCSBN). (Fall, 2020). *NCLEX-PN® Examination for Licensed Practical Nurses/Vocational Nurses.* Retrieved from https://www.ncsbn.org/NGN_Fall20_Eng_03_FINAL.pdf.

Leadership and Management: Legal Aspects of Nursing

Every practical nurse (PN), regardless of whether they want to be a PN leader or not, has to have some leadership and management skills, especially when providing patient care. For example, due to the rapidly changing technology, political processes, reimbursement, and regulatory changes within the health care delivery system, it is important that the nursing profession be aware of the decision-making processes that impact on safe patient outcomes. There are four major content areas that every PN should become familiar with since these concepts are within the nursing profession. These include:

1. General understanding of leadership and management within the scope of practical nursing
2. Maintaining a safe, effective work environment
3. Legal and ethical issues influencing nursing
4. Disaster nursing and crisis intervention

> **HESI HINT** Every nurse must know about and apply general leadership and management concepts to clinical practice when caring for individual patients, populations, or systems.

LEADERSHIP AND MANAGEMENT

Leadership and management are not synonymous terms. Managers maintain the general operations of a unit while leaders set a direction with expected follow-up and outcomes. Leaders motivate, inspire, and provide resources that motivate and enable others to meet organizational goals for organizational success.

Leaders Versus Managers

Registered and practical nurses desire and prefer to be led and not managed (Roussel et al., 2020, p. 25). Leaders inspire constituents through respecting one's dignity, autonomy, and self-esteem (Morriss et al., 2014). Good leaders inspire and motivate others in health care settings to foster and promote worker satisfaction and take pride in meeting organizational goals and strategic plans. Not every PN wants or aspires to be a formal nurse leader in a health care setting; however, there will be opportunities where one may have the required leadership knowledge, skills, and competencies to lead especially when providing patient care. For example, we can always improve our patient care by accepting opportunities that provide better patient care.

Essential Characteristics of a Practical Nurse Leader

1. Encourage, foster, and promote positive working relationships between and among members of the health care team
2. Create a work environment facilitating and role modeling open communication and collaboration
3. Serve as a role model to prevent and resolve conflict
4. Coach and mentor other members of the health care teams involving creative, evidence-based problem solving related to patient care
5. Prevent behaviors leading to hostile work environments and have a zero tolerance for incivility in the workplace
6. The role of the Registered Nurse (RN) and the role of the PN have been clearly differentiated in each State's Nurse Practice laws (Table 2.1).

Provider of Care

1. Assist in determining health status and health needs of patients based on interpretation of health-related data and preventive health practices in collaboration with other members of the health care team.
2. Assist in the formulation of goals/outcomes and a plan of care in collaboration with the patient and their families, and interdisciplinary health care team members.
3. Implement plan of care within legal and ethical parameters, including scope of practice and education, in collaboration with the patient and interdisciplinary health care team members.
4. Implement or reinforce teaching plan for patient with common health problems and well-defined learning needs.
5. Assist in the evaluation of the patient's responses and outcomes to therapeutic interventions.
6. Provide direct basic care to the assigned multiple patients in structured settings.
7. Use problem solving approach as the basis for decision making in practice.

Coordinator of Care

1. Assist in the coordination of human and material resources for the provision of care for assigned patients.
2. Collaborate with patients and the interdisciplinary health care team to provide direct care to assigned patients.
3. Participate in the identification of client needs for referral to resources that facilitate continuity of care.
4. Participate in activities that support organizational framework of structured health care settings.

TABLE 2.1	Comparison Between Roles of Practical Nurse and Registered Nurse
PN	**RN**
• Data collection	• Perform initial assessment
• Focused assessment	• Perform comprehensive assessments
• Participate in planning nursing care needs	• Determine nursing diagnoses
• Participate in modifying nursing care plan	• Formulate nursing care plan
• Implement care within scope of practice rather than legal, ethical, and educational parameters	• Implement nursing care
• Implement teaching plan for common health problems and well-defined learning needs	• Develop and implement teaching plans rather than promotion, maintenance, and restoration of health
• Provide direct basic care to assigned multiple clients in structured settings	• Provide for care of multiple clients either through direct care or assignment and/or delegation of care to other members of the health care team
• Assist in evaluation of client's responses and outcomes to therapeutic interventions	• Evaluate client's responses and outcomes to therapeutic interventions
• Use a problem-solving approach as the basis for decision making in practice	• Use critical thinking approach to analyze clinical data and current literature as a basis for decision making in nursing practice
	• Evaluate effects of care
	• Make independent decisions
	• Communicate and consult with other health care team members
Coordinator of Care—PN	**Coordinator of Care—RN**
• Assign specific tasks, activities, and functions	• Make assignments to licensed staff (PNs, RNs)
• Maintain appropriate supervision of licensed and unlicensed personnel in compliance with current state Board of Nursing rules in structured health settings for clients with predictable health care needs in accordance with designated job descriptions and/or job duties	• Delegate to unlicensed staff in compliance with current Board of Nurse Examiners rules in both structured and unstructured health settings for clients with predictable as well as unpredictable health needs

PN, Practical nurse; *RN*, registered nurse.

Member of a Profession

1. Demonstrate accountability for own nursing practice.
2. Participate as an advocate in activities that focus on improving the health care of patients.
3. Demonstrate behaviors that promote the development and practice of vocational nursing.

APPLICATION: LEADERSHIP CASE Jamie was a new graduate nurse who just received her PN license. She was employed as a medical surgical nurse on a very busy 40-bed telemetry unit. She was delighted to be on the unit, though it did seem understaffed. But because she was new to the facility she did not want to question the charge nurse or supervisor.

After 3 months working on the unit, one afternoon when she reported to work she was told that she would have to have an extra patient load because they could not get an extra nurse to cover, thus she would have five instead of four patients. Because the telemetry unit was always staffed with a 4:1 ratio this load was a little more than normal. During the 12-hour shift, three of Jamie's patients experienced chest pain, one had a full code and subsequently died, and the other two patients were stable.

Jamie discussed the short staffing problem with the charge nurse on duty, however, he did not think that it was an issue.

Managers

Managers are individuals who work to accomplish the goals of the organization. Nurse managers are RNs who act to achieve the goals of safe, effective patient care within the overall goals of a health care facility (Table 2.2). Registered nurse managers provide skills such as delegation, supervision, critical thinking, and evaluation of the overall outcomes of patients as an aggregate. They are responsible for knowing the skills that PNs have regarding patient care. PNs work within their state's scope of practice.

Delegation

The registered nurse has authority, accountability, and responsibility for safe delegation. Delegation for PNs is based on the State Nurse Practice Act, standards of professional nursing practice, policies of the health care organization, and ethical-legal models of behavior.

Delegation is not a simple matter of asking someone else on the health care team to help you out. Delegation involves legal components and is typically governed by state nurse practice acts. For example, PN nurse practice acts typically to identify to whom tasks PNs may delegate to others. The PN must be certain the delegation of tasks are within the scope of PN practice and that there is accountability and documentation that the task was delegated and performed in a timely, safe, and effective manner.

Delegation is a complex critical decision that requires critical thinking by the nurse. Delegation is an important responsibility and must be based on a firm scientific basis (Caputti, 2020, p. 79). Delegating consists of transferring responsibility for performing a task that you would do yourself to another member of the health care team. The PN may delegate to other PNs as well as ancillary and unlicensed assistive personnel (UAP) under certain conditions. The person delegated to perform the task must be competent in performing the task, legally able to perform the task within the health care system, and be accountable and competent for performing and completing the

TABLE 2.2 Skills, Characteristics of the Skill, and Characteristics of the Nurse Manager, and Evaluation

Skills of the Nurse Manager	Characteristics of the Skills	Characteristics of the Nurse Manager	Evaluation
Organization	Plan evidence-based strategies to address the individual, group, or organizational issue or problem	Accountability	Provides feedback to other health care providers about quality patient care
Supervision	Oversee, supervise care, and assess outcomes of care provided by other members of the health care team	Leadership	Prepares reports when off-boarding patients to next shift
Evaluation	Provide timely qualitative and quantitative feedback to other members of the health care team who are direct reports	Leadership	Requires staff to sign up and meet for work evaluations
Delegation	Identify members of the health care team to whom one can legally and ethically delegate components of care according to roles and responsibilities	Responsibility	Knowledgeable about each member of the health care team and delegates responsively
Communication	Serve as a liaison between individuals and/or groups internal and external to the organization when issues or gaps in communication or processes occur. Apply concepts and processes for written and verbal conflict management and resolution.	Authority	Requires staff to adhere to healthy workforce environments, counsels staff for poor behavior when needed; resolves employee conflicts.
Critical Thinking	Serve as a role model and resource for other members of the health care delivery team. Seek credible evidence-based sources to guide decisions.	Leadership	Arranges for continuing education for staff to promote quality patient care.

TABLE 2.3 Terms and Definition of Delegation

Term	Definition Delegation
Delegation	Delegating consists of transferring responsibility for performing a task yourself to another member of the health care team.
Responsibility	The obligation to complete the task or assignment delegated
Authority	The right to act or command actions of others
Accountability	Ability and willingness to assume responsibility for actions and related consequences according to the five rights of delegation as defined by the PN Council of State Boards of Nursing (NCSBN)

TABLE 2.4 The Five Rights and Associated Questions for Delegation by the Practical Nurse

Right	Associated Questions
1. Right Task	Is this a task that can be delegated by the PN?
2. Right Circumstance	Considering the setting and available resources, should this delegation take place?
3. Right Person	Is the task being delegated by the right person?
4. Right Direction/ Communication	Is the PN providing a clear, concise description of the task, including limits and expectations?
5. Right Supervision	Once the task has been delegated, is appropriate supervision maintained?

task safely, efficiently, and effectively. The RN maintains ultimate responsibility, accountability, and supervision when assignments or tasks are delegated. Table 2.3 depicts key terms associated with delegation by the nurse to another member of the health care team.

When the PN delegates a task or assignment to another person on the health care team, the PN must make certain the five rights of delegation as defined by the National Council of State Boards of Nursing (NCSBN) are met. The act of delegation requires a great deal of critical thinking based on foundational knowledge known as the five rights of delegation (Table 2.4). Individual accountability is a major component of delegation for nurse leaders. Individual accountability refers to the individual nurse's ability to explain their actions and the results of their actions as measured against standards (Yoder-Wise, 2019, p. 309).

Delegation is a high-level skill that requires a high degree of critical thinking and decision making. Delegation is based on several key components and considerations that include assessment, planning, assignment, supervision, and follow-up evaluation (Caputi, 2020, p. 77). Critical thinking in delegation requires the PN to think about what may/can happen when you delegate a task to another person. Think also about what might go wrong or happen in the context of when you delegate a task to another person or persons. Box 2.1 provides the Dos and Don'ts of delegation.

HESI HINT Delegating to the right person requires the nurse be aware of the qualifications and job description of the person delegated to perform the task. For example, the nurse must be certain the person to whom they are delegating the task has the requisite documented education, training, knowledge, skills, experience, and competencies to complete the delegated task. UAPs generally are not allowed or permitted by the state nurse practice act to perform sterile procedures or invasive procedures.

HESI HINT Some tasks may not be delegated to UAP. For example, delegated activities fall within the implementation phase of the nursing process and may not be delegated to UAPs. Any activity or task requiring nursing judgment cannot be delegated to a UAP.

HESI HINT The PN has the legal authority to delegate certain tasks or activities to a designated (delegate), competent individual but the PN is responsible for making certain the person to whom a task or activity is delegated is competent and duly supervised.

The PN is ultimately responsible for the outcome of the activities delegated to others.

The PN who delegates to the delegated must assess and evaluate the outcome(s) of the task(s) that have been delegated.

BOX 2.1 Delegation Dos and Don'ts

Do's
- Always use the five Rights of Delegation
- Provide adequate supervision of delegated tasks
- Guidance and direction
- Evaluation and monitoring
- Follow-up
- Understand the qualifications of each delegatee
- Appropriate education
- Training
- Experience
- Skills
- Demonstrated and documented competence

Don'ts
- Delegate tasks that require *nursing* judgment
- Assessment
- Diagnosis
- Planning
- Evaluation
- Delegate invasive or sterile procedures

☑ REVIEW OF LEADERSHIP AND MANAGEMENT

1. Which aspect of supervision is the PN performing?
   A. Checks on the staff after making assignments
   B. Carefully explains details of an assignment
   C. Suggests an improvement in a technique to UAP after completing a task
2. What are the five rights of delegation?
3. Which of these tasks can be delegated to an UAP?
   A. Insert a Foley catheter
   B. Measure and record urine output from a Foley catheter
   C. Teach a client how to perform self-care for a urinary catheter
   D. Assess for symptoms of a urinary tract infection (UTI)
4. What systematic problem-solving method in nursing is used for critical thinking?
5. Which assignment should be appropriate for the PN to delegate to a UAP? Select all that apply.
   A. Explain the side effects of chemotherapy to the client
   B. Feed a client who is 2 days postop
   C. Calculate the intake and output (I&O) on the client who is on total parenteral nutrition (TPN)
   D. Hang intravenous piggyback (IVPB) antibiotics
   E. Assist a client who is 2 days postop to the bathroom

See Answer Key at the end of this text for suggested responses.

MAINTAINING A SAFE, EFFECTIVE WORK ENVIRONMENT

A. Nurse managers are responsible for addressing
   1. Workplace violence
   2. Nursing staff substance abuse

3. Incivility and bullying
   a. Incivility and bullying includes actions taken and not taken.
   b. Example: Refusing to share pertinent information with another nurse regarding a client's status, thus jeopardizing the client's safety.
   c. Example: Deliberately withholding information pertinent to the client's well-being and safety, such as not telling a nurse that the HCP requested that a client's medication should be held.
B. The role of the PN is to maintain a safe practice environment:
   1. Assess, monitor, and observe the patient: PN practice requires the necessary skills and knowledge to properly monitor and implement safe practices to assure that the patient remains stable.
   2. Plan care: by maintaining and updating a written plan for nursing care based on the patient's status.
   3. Implement nursing care: according to the plan, advocate for the patient, intervene to prevent harm, and follow up as needed.
   4. Implement specific nursing actions: by responding to the patient, reinforcing educational information provided to the patient, and adequately supervising nursing care provided by others.
   5. Evaluate nursing care: PNs must document the patient's baseline and current status and report any changes. The patient's medical record must be accurate, current, and complete.
   6. Work within your scope of practice: perform only those nursing activities outlined in your job description and within your agency policies and procedures.

LEGAL AND ETHICAL ISSUES INFLUENCING PRACTICAL NURSING

Laws that impact practical nursing are divided into two large groups: criminal (public) and civil (private). Criminal laws are crimes against the country, state, or local government (Table 2.5).

Constitutional, administrative, and criminal are the three types of criminal law. Civil law involves disputes between individuals in areas such as contract and tort law. Tort law is further divided into intentional and unintentional torts.

Unintentional Torts: Negligence and Malpractice

A. **Negligence:** performing an act that a reasonable and prudent person would not perform. The measure of negligence is "reasonable" (i.e., would a reasonable and prudent nurse act in the same manner under the same circumstances?) That is, the PN provided the care that did not meet the standard. Negligence includes:
   1. Lack of skill
   2. Errors
   3. Professional misconduct
   4. Failure to act.
B. **Malpractice:** a negligent act performed by an individual in a professional role resulting in an injury. Four elements are necessary to prove malpractice: if any one element is missing, malpractice cannot be proved. The plaintiff must prove all of the following elements to prove malpractice:
   1. Duty: obligation to use due care (what a reasonable, prudent nurse would do); failure to care for and/or protect others against unreasonable risks. The nurse must anticipate foreseeable risk and use due care (what a reasonable, prudent nurse would do). Failure to care for and/or protect others against unreasonable risks violates duty. For example, if there is a puddle of water on the floor, the nurse is responsible for anticipating the risk of a client fall.
   2. Breach of duty: failure to maintain the nursing standard. A reasonable and prudent nurse in the same situation would not have performed this act or performed it in this manner. This is a failure to perform according to the established standard of conduct in providing nursing care.
   3. Injury/damages: a failure to meet the standard of care, which causes actual injury or damage to the client (physical injury). Neither emotional nor mental injury is enough to prove malpractice.
   4. Causation: the breach of duty caused the harm, and the nurse's action or lack of action caused harm to the plaintiff. A connection exists between conduct and the resulting injury, referred to as *proximate cause or remoteness of damage* (Table 2.6).

Intentional Torts: Assault and Battery

A. Assault and battery
   1. Assault: Mental or physical threat (e.g., forcing [without touching] a client to take a medication or treatment)
   2. Battery: Actual and intentional touching of one another, with or without the intent to do harm (e.g., hitting or striking a client). If a mentally competent adult is forced to have a treatment he or she has refused, battery occurs.
B. Invasion of privacy: Encroachment or trespassing on another's body or personality
   1. False imprisonment: Confinement without authorization
   2. Exposure of a person:
      a. Body: After death, a client has the right to be unobserved, excluded from unwarranted operations, and protected from unauthorized touching of the body.

TABLE 2.5	**Organization of Law**		
Courts	**Types of Law**	**Description**	**Example**
Criminal (public)	Constitutional	Constitutional and amendments	Right to free speech
		Government operation	Right to vote
	Administrative	Creates government and official agencies	Control of nursing through boards of nursing
			Nurse Practice Act
	Criminal	Misdemeanors and felonies	Theft
			Partner abuse
Civil (private)	Contract	Legally binding agreement between two or more individuals or groups	Hospital hires an agency nurse
			Buying/selling a car
	Tort	Unintentional	Heat application extending beyond time limit imposed by hospital policy
		Negligence	
		Malpractice	Amputating the wrong limb
		Intentional	Threatening to withhold pain medication
		Assault	Performing CPR on a client with a DNR order
		Battery	Intentionally making damaging verbal or written statements about a client's physician
		Defamation	
		False imprisonment	Unauthorized use of restraints
		Fraud	Providing false documents on an employment application
		Invasion of privacy	Releasing test results to the parents of an emancipated minor

CPR, Cardiopulmonary resuscitation; *DNR,* do not resuscitate.

TABLE 2.6 **Comparison of Nursing Negligence and Malpractice**	
Nursing Negligence	**Nursing Malpractice**
Leaving a heating pad on a client's skin without damage against institutional policy	Burning a client's skin as a result of leaving a heating pad on against institutional policy
Failing to assess a restrained client as required in institutional policy	Failing to assess a restrained client as required by institutional policy, resulting in a head injury occurring when the client tries to climb out of bed
Failing to notice the warning signs of a myocardial infarction (MI)	Failing to notice the warning signs of an MI, resulting in an acute MI
Forgetting to administer antianginal medication	Forgetting to administer antianginal medication, resulting in an acute MI

b. Personality: Exposure or discussion of a client's case or revealing personal information or identity.
3. Defamation: Divulgence of privileged information or communication (e.g., through charts, conversations, or observations)

C. Fraud: Illegal activity, willful and purposeful misrepresentation that could cause, or has caused, loss or harm to a person or property. Examples of fraud include
   1. Presenting false credentials for the purpose of entering nursing school, obtaining a license, or obtaining employment (e.g., falsification of records).
   2. Describing a myth regarding a treatment (e.g., telling a client that a placebo has no side effects and will cure the disease, or telling a client that a treatment or diagnostic test will not hurt, when indeed pain is involved in the procedure).

Crime

A. An act contrary to a criminal statute. Crimes are wrongs punishable by the state and committed against the state, with intent usually present. The PN remains bound by all criminal laws.
B. Commission of a crime involves the following behaviors:
   1. A person commits a deed contrary to criminal law.
   2. A person omits an act when there is a legal obligation to perform such an act (e.g., refusing to assist with the birth of a child if such a refusal results in injury to the child).
   3. Criminal conspiracy occurs when two or more persons agree to commit a crime.
   4. Assisting or giving aid to a person in the commission of a crime makes that person equally guilty of the offense (awareness must be present that the crime is being committed).
   5. Ignoring a law is not usually an adequate defense against the commission of a crime (e.g., a nurse who sees another nurse taking narcotics from the unit supply and ignores this observation is not adequately defended against committing a crime).
   6. Assault is justified for self-defense. However, to be justified, only enough force can be used to maintain self-protection.
   7. Search warrants are required before searching a person's property.
   8. It is a crime *not* to report suspected child abuse.

> **HESI HINT** The nurse has a legal responsibility to report suspected child abuse.

PSYCHIATRIC NURSING

A. **Civil procedures**: Methods used to protect the rights of psychiatric clients
B. **Voluntary admission:** The client admits himself or herself to an institution for treatment and retains civil rights.
C. **Involuntary admission:** Someone other than the client applies for the client's admission to an institution.
   1. This requires certification by a health care provider that the person is a danger to self or others. (Depending on the state, one or two health care provider certifications are required.)
   2. Individuals have the right to a legal hearing within a certain number of hours or days.
   3. Most states limit commitment to 90 days.
   4. Extended commitment is usually no longer than 1 year.
D. **Emergency admission:** Any adult may apply for emergency detention of another. However, medical or judicial approval is required to detain anyone beyond 24 hours.
   1. A person held against his or her will can file a writ of habeas corpus to try to get the court to hear the case and release the person.
   2. The court determines the sanity and alleged unlawful restraint of a person.
E. Legal and civil rights of hospitalized clients
   1. The right to wear their own clothes and to keep personal items and a reasonable amount of cash for small purchases
   2. The right to have individual storage space for one's own use
   3. The right to see visitors daily
   4. The right to have reasonable access to a telephone and the opportunity to have private conversations by telephone
   5. The right to receive and send mail (unopened)
   6. The right to refuse shock treatments and lobotomy
F. **Competency hearing:** Legal hearing that is held to determine a person's ability to make responsible decisions about self, dependents, or property

1. Persons declared incompetent have the legal status of a minor—they cannot
   a. Vote
   b. Make contracts or wills
   c. Drive a car
   d. Sue or be sued
   e. Hold a professional license
2. A guardian is appointed by the court for an incompetent person. Declaring a person incompetent can be initiated by the state or the family.

G. **Insanity:** Legal term meaning the accused is not criminally responsible for the unlawful act committed because he or she is mentally ill

H. **Inability to stand trial:** Person accused of committing a crime is not mentally capable of standing trial. He or she
1. Cannot understand the charge against himself or herself
2. Must be sent to the psychiatric unit until legally determined to be competent for trial
3. Once mentally fit, must stand trial and serve any sentence, if convicted

PATIENT IDENTIFICATION

A. The Joint Commission has implemented new patient identification requirements to meet safety goals (https://www.jointcommission.org/-/media/tjc/documents/standards/r3-reports/r3-report-issue-1-20111.pdf)
B. Use at least two patient identifiers. Ask the client to tell you his or her name and date of birth (DOB) whenever taking blood samples, administering medications, or administering blood products.
C. The patient room number may *not* be used as a form of identification.

Surgical Permit

A. Consent to operate (surgical permit) must be obtained before any surgical procedure, however minor it might be.
B. Legally, the surgical permit must be
1. Written
2. Obtained voluntarily
3. Explained to the client (i.e., informed consent must be obtained)
C. Informed consent means the procedure and treatment, or operation, has been fully explained to the client, including
1. Possible complications, risks, and disfigurements
2. Removal of any organs or parts of the body
3. Benefits and expected results
D. Surgery permits must be obtained as follows:
1. They must be witnessed by an authorized person, such as the health care provider or a nurse.
2. They protect the client against unsanctioned surgery, and they protect the health care provider and surgeon, hospital, and hospital staff against possible claims of unauthorized operations.

3. Adults and emancipated minors may sign their own operative permits if they are mentally competent.
4. Permission to operate on a minor child or an incompetent or unconscious adult must be obtained from a legally responsible parent or guardian. The person granting permission to operate on an adult who lacks capacity to understand information about the proposed treatment (e.g., because of advanced Alzheimer disease or unconscious adult) must be identified in a Durable Power of Attorney or an Advance Health Directive.

> **HESI HINT** Often an NGN-NCLEX-PN question asks who should explain and describe a surgical procedure to the client, including both complications and the expected results of the procedure. The answer is the health care provider. Remember that it is the nurse's responsibility to be sure that the operative permit is signed and is in the client's medical record. It is not the nurse's responsibility to explain the procedure to the client. The nurse must document that the client was given the information and agreed to it.

Consent

A. The law does not *require* written consent to perform medical treatment.
1. Treatment can be performed if the client has been fully informed about the procedure.
2. Treatment can be performed if the client voluntarily consents to the procedure.
3. If informed consent cannot be obtained (e.g., client is unconscious) and immediate treatment is required to save life or limb, the emergency laws can be applied. (See the subsequent section, Emergency Care.)
B. Verbal or written consent
1. When verbal consent is obtained, a notation should be made.
   a. It describes in detail how and why verbal consent was obtained.
   b. It is placed in the client's record or chart.
2. Verbal or written consent can be given by
   a. Alert, coherent, or otherwise competent adults
   b. A parent or legal guardian
   c. A person in loco parentis (a person standing in for a parent with a parent's rights, duties, and responsibilities) in cases of minors or incompetent adults (US Department of Human Services)
C. Consent of minors
1. Minors 14 years of age and older must agree to treatment along with their parents or guardians.
2. Emancipated minors can consent to treatment themselves. Be aware that the definition of an emancipated minor may change from state to state.

Emergency Care

A. Good Samaritan Act: Protects health care providers against malpractice claims for care provided in emergency situations (e.g., the nurse gives aid at the scene to an automobile accident victim).

B. A nurse is required to perform in a "reasonable and prudent manner."

> **HESI HINT** Often NGN-NCLEX-PN questions address the Good Samaritan Act, which is the means of protecting a nurse when she or he is performing emergency care

Prescriptions and Health Care Providers

A. A nurse is required to obtain a prescription (order) to carry out medical procedures from a health care provider.

B. Although verbal telephone prescriptions should be avoided, the nurse should follow the agency's policy and procedures. Failure to follow such rules could be considered negligence. The Joint Commission requires that organizations implement a process for taking verbal or telephone orders that includes a read-back of critical values. The employee receiving the prescription should write the verbal order or critical value on the chart or record it in the computer and then read back the order or value to the health care provider.

C. If a nurse questions a health care provider's (e.g., physician, advanced practice RN, physician's assistant, dentist) prescription because he or she believes that it is wrong (e.g., the wrong dosage was prescribed for a medication), the nurse should do the following:
1. Inform the health care provider.
2. Record that the health care provider was informed and record the health care provider's response to such information.
3. Inform the nursing supervisor.
4. Refuse to carry out the prescription.

D. If the nurse believes that a health care provider's prescription was made with poor judgment (e.g., the nurse believes the client does not need as many tranquilizers as the health care provider prescribed), the nurse should:
1. Record that the health care provider was notified and that the prescription was questioned
2. Notify the nursing supervisor
3. Carry out the prescription because nursing judgment cannot be substituted for a health care provider's judgment.

E. If a nurse is asked to perform a task for which he or she has not been prepared educationally (e.g., obtain a urine specimen from a premature infant by needle aspiration of the bladder) or does not have the necessary experience (e.g., a nurse who has never worked in labor and delivery is asked to perform a vaginal examination and determine cervical dilation), the nurse should do the following:
1. Inform the health care provider that he or she does not have the education or experience necessary to carry out the prescription.

2. Refuse to carry out the prescription.

> **HESI HINT** If the nurse carries out a health care provider's prescription for which he or she is not prepared and does not inform the health care provider of his or her lack of preparation, the nurse is solely liable for any damages.

3. If the nurse informs the health care provider of his or her lack of preparation in carrying out a prescription and carries out the prescription anyway, the nurse *and* the health care provider are liable for any damages.

F. The nurse cannot, without a health care provider's prescription, alter the amount of drug given to a client. For example, if a health care provider has prescribed pain medication in a certain amount and the client's pain is not, in the nurse's judgment, severe enough to warrant the dosage prescribed, the nurse cannot reduce the amount without first checking with the health care provider. Remember, nursing judgment cannot be substituted for medical judgment.

Restraints

A. Patients may be restrained only under the following circumstances:
1. In an emergency
2. For a limited time
3. To protect the client from injury or from harm

B. Nursing responsibilities about restraints
1. The nurse must notify the health care provider immediately that the client has been restrained.
2. It is required and imperative that the nurse accurately document the facts and the client's behavior leading to restraint.

C. When restraining a client, the nurse should do the following:
1. Use restraints (physical or chemical) after exhausting all reasonable alternatives.
2. Apply the restraints correctly and in accordance with facility policies and procedures.
3. Check frequently to see that the restraints do not impair circulation or cause pressure sores or other injuries.
4. Allow for nutrition, hydration, and stimulation at frequent intervals.
5. Remove restraints as soon as possible.
6. Document the need for and application, monitoring, and removal of restraints.
7. Never leave a restrained person alone.

> **HESI HINT** Restraints of any kind may constitute false imprisonment. Freedom from unlawful restraint is a basic human right and is protected by law. Use of restraints must fall within guidelines specified by state law and hospital policy.

Health Insurance Portability and Accountability Act of 1996

A. Congress passed the Health Insurance Portability and Accountability Act of 1996 (HIPAA) to create a national patient-record privacy standard.

B. HIPAA privacy rules pertain to health care providers, health plans, and health clearinghouses and their business partners who engage in computer-to-computer transmission of health care claims, payment and remittance, benefit information, and health plan eligibility information, and who disclose personal health information that specifically identifies an individual and is transmitted electronically, in writing, or verbally.

C. Patient privacy rights are of key importance. Patients must provide written approval of the disclosure of any of their health information for almost any purpose. Health care providers must offer specific information to patients that explains how their personal health information will be used. Patients must have access to their medical records, and they can receive copies of them and request that changes be made if they identify inaccuracies.

D. Health care providers who do not comply with HIPAA regulations or make unauthorized disclosures risk civil and criminal liability.

E. For further information, use this link to the Department of Health and Human Services (DHHS) website, Office of Civil Rights, which contains frequently asked questions about HIPAA standards for privacy of individually identifiable health information: http://aspe.hhs.gov/admnsimp/final/pvcguide1.htm.

? REVIEW OF LEGAL ASPECTS OF NURSING

1. What types of procedures should be assigned to licensed practical nurses?
2. Negligence is measured by reasonableness. What question might the nurse ask when determining such reasonableness?
3. List the four elements that are necessary to prove malpractice (professional negligence).
4. Define an *intentional tort* and give one example.
5. Differentiate between voluntary and involuntary admission.
6. List five activities a person who is declared incompetent cannot perform.
7. Name three legal requirements of a surgical permit.
8. Who may give consent for medical treatment?
9. What law protects the nurse who provides care or gives aid in an emergency?
10. What actions should the nurse take if the nurse questions a health care provider's prescription—that is, believes the prescription is wrong?
11. Describe nursing care of the restrained client.
12. Describe six patient rights guaranteed under HIPAA regulations that nurses must be aware of in practice.

See Answer Key at the end of this text for suggested responses.

DISASTER NURSING AND CRISIS INTERVENTION

Disaster Nursing

A. The role of the nurse takes place at all three levels of disaster management:

1. Disaster preparedness
2. Disaster response
3. Disaster recovery

B. To achieve effective disaster management,
1. Organization is the key.
2. All personnel must be trained.
3. All personnel must know their roles.

Levels of Prevention in Disaster Management

A. Primary prevention
1. Participate in the development of a disaster plan.
2. Train rescue workers in triage and basic first aid.
3. Educate personnel about shelter management.
4. Educate the public about the disaster plan and personal preparation for disaster.

B. Secondary prevention
1. Triage
2. Treatment of injuries
3. Treatment of other conditions, including mental health
4. Shelter supervision

C. Tertiary prevention
1. Follow-up care for injuries
2. Follow-up care for psychological problems
3. Recovery assistance
4. Prevention of future disasters and their consequences

Triage

A. A French word meaning "to sort or categorize"
B. Goal: Maximize the number of survivors by sorting the injured according to treatable and untreatable victims
C. Primary criteria used:
1. Potential for survival
2. Availability of resources

Clinical Judgment and Roles in Triage

A. Triage duties using a systematic approach such as the simple triage and rapid treatment (START) method (Fig 2.1).

B. Treatment of injuries
1. Render first aid for injuries.
2. Provide additional treatment as needed in definitive care areas.

C. Treatment of other conditions, including mental health
1. Determine health needs other than injury.
2. Refer for medical treatment as required.
3. Provide treatment for other conditions based on medically approved protocols (Table 2.7)

Shelter Supervision

A. Coordinate activities of shelter workers.
B. Oversee records of victims admitted and discharged from the shelter.
C. Promote effective interpersonal and group interactions among victims in the shelter.
D. Promote independence and involvement of victims housed in the shelter.

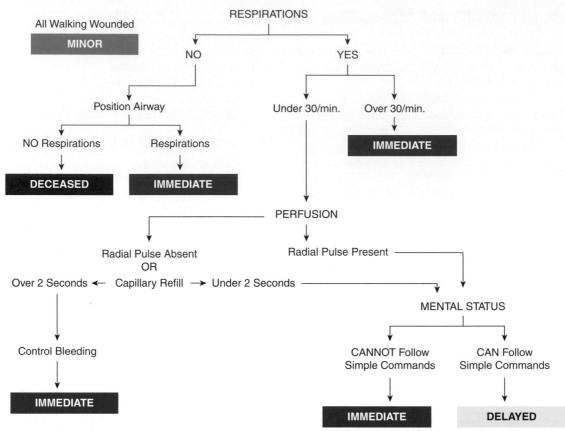

Fig. 2.1 Simple Triage and Rapid Treatment (START) Method for Triage. (From the Critical Illness and Trauma Foundation, Inc.)

TABLE 2.7 **Triage Color Code System**				
	Red	**Yellow**	**Green**	**Black**
Urgency	Most urgent—first priority	Urgent—second priority	Third priority	Dying or dead
Injury type	Life-threatening injuries	Injuries with systemic effects and complications	Minimal injuries with no systemic complications	Catastrophic injuries
May delay treatment?	NO	30–60 min	Several hours	No hope for survival—no treatment

Bioterrorism

A. Learn the symptoms of illnesses that are associated with exposure to likely biologic and chemical agents.

B. Understand that the symptoms could appear days or weeks after exposure.

C. Nurses and other health care providers would be the first responders when victims seek medical evaluation after symptoms manifest. First responders are critical in identifying an outbreak, determining the cause of the outbreak, identifying risk factors, and implementing measures to control and minimize the outbreak.

  1. Biologic agents:
    a. Anthrax
    b. Pneumonic plague
    c. Botulism
    d. Smallpox
    e. Inhalation tularemia
    f. Viral hemorrhagic fever
  2. Chemical agents:
    a. Biotoxin agents: ricin
    b. Nerve agents: sarin
  3. Radiation

> **HESI HINT** In a disaster the nurse must consider both the individual and the community.

Clinical Nursing Judgment

A. Community-disaster risk assessment

B. Measures to mitigate disaster effect

C. Exposure symptom identification

Clinical Nursing Judgment and Interventions

A. Participate in development of a disaster plan.
B. Educate the public on the disaster plan and personal preparation for disaster.
C. Train rescue workers in triage and basic first aid.
D. Educate personnel on shelter management.
E. Practice triage.
F. Treat injuries and illness.
G. Treat other conditions, including mental health.
H. Supervise shelters.
I. Arrange for follow-up care for injuries.
J. Arrange for follow-up care for psychological problems.
K. Assist in recovery.
L. Work to prevent future disasters and their consequences.

Ebola

A. The risk of contracting Ebola in the United States is very low, even when working with West African communities in the United States.
B. Ebola is spread by direct contact with blood or body fluids of a person who is ill with Ebola, has died from Ebola, has had contact with objects such as needles that have been contaminated with the virus.
   1. It is also possible that Ebola virus can be transmitted through the semen of men who have survived infection.
C. The Centers for Disease Control and Prevention (CDC) implemented entry screening at five U.S. airports for travelers arriving from Guinea, Liberia, and Sierra Leone, as well as other African countries. The CDC strongly recommends that travelers from these countries be actively monitored for symptoms by state or local health departments for 21 days after returning from any of these countries.
D. People of West African descent are not at more risk than other Americans if they have not recently traveled to the region. Neither ethnic nor racial backgrounds have anything to do with becoming infected with the Ebola virus.
E. Even if travelers were exposed, they are only contagious after they start to have symptoms (e.g., fever, severe headache, muscle pain, diarrhea, vomiting, and unexplained bleeding).
F. Symptoms:
   1. Fever of greater than 38.6°C or 101.5°F
   2. Severe headache
   3. Muscle pain
   4. Vomiting
   5. Diarrhea
   6. Abdominal pain
   7. Unexplained hemorrhage
G. Diagnosis
   1. CDC recommends testing for all persons with onset of fever within 21 days of having a high-risk exposure. A high-risk exposure includes any of the following:
      a. Percutaneous or mucous membrane exposure or direct skin contact with body fluids of a person with a confirmed or suspected case of Ebola without appropriate personal protective equipment (PPE)
      b. Laboratory processing of body fluids of suspected or confirmed Ebola cases without appropriate PPE or standard biosafety precautions
      c. Participation in funeral rites or other direct exposure to human remains in the geographic area where the outbreak is occurring without appropriate PPE
H. Clinical Judgement interventions
   1. Obtain a thorough history, including recent travel from areas where the virus is present.
   2. Monitor vital signs.
   3. Place the client in strict isolation for 21 days using special precautions identified by the CDC and state.
   4. Notify the CDC.
I. Health care provider protection
   1. Health care providers should wear gloves, gown (fluid resistant or impermeable), shoe covers, eye protection (goggles or face shield), and a facemask.
   2. Additional PPE might be required in certain situations (e.g., copious amounts of blood, other body fluids, vomit, or feces present in the environment), including but not limited to double gloving, disposable shoe covers, and leg coverings.
   3. Avoid aerosol-generating procedures. If performing these procedures, PPE should include respiratory protection (N95 filtering face piece respirator or higher), and the procedure should be performed in an airborne isolation room.
   4. Diligent environmental cleaning, disinfection, and safe handling of potentially contaminated materials is paramount because blood, sweat, emesis, feces, and other body secretions represent potentially infectious materials.

COVID-19

A. COVID-19 information
   1. CDC Guidelines: insert most recent website by CDC here
B. Agent
   1. COVID-19 and multiple variants
C. Transmission
   1. Close personal contact
   2. Droplet infection
   3. Heating and ventilation ductwork spread
D. Incubation Period
   1. Use website: CDC
E. Signs and Symptoms
   1. Fever
   2. Nasal and sinus congestion
   3. Cough
   4. Stomach upset and nausea/vomiting
   5. Chills
F. Treatment
   1. Primary and secondary prevention with vaccination
   2. Tertiary prevention depends on symptoms and patient age
   3. For most children and adults with symptomatic SARS-CoV-2, the virus that causes COVID-19, infection, isolation, and precautions can be discontinued 10 days after symptom onset and after resolution of fever for at least 24 hours and improvement of other symptoms.

4. For people who are severely ill (i.e., those requiring hospitalization, intensive care, or ventilation support) or severely immunocompromised, extending the duration of isolation and precautions up to 10 days after symptom onset and after resolution of fever and improvement of other symptoms may be warranted.

5. For people who are infected but asymptomatic (never develop symptoms), isolation and precautions can be discontinued 10 days after the first positive test.

G. Miscellaneous:

Patients who have recovered from COVID-19 can continue to have detectable SARS-CoV-2 RNA in upper respiratory specimens for up to 3 months after illness onset. However, replication-competent virus has not been reliably recovered and infectiousness is unlikely.

? REVIEW OF DISASTER NURSING

1. List the three levels of disaster management.
2. List examples of the three levels of prevention in disaster management.
3. Define *triage*.
4. Identify three bioterrorism agents.

See Answer Key at the end of this text for suggested responses.

NEXT-GENERATION NCLEX EXAMINATION-STYLE QUESTION

| Health History | Nurses' Notes | Vital Signs | Lab Results |

You are working in the emergency room and Mrs. Lenard is screaming as she runs into the emergency room. You notice that she is holding a young child and she states that her 2-year-old son swallowed something while playing. As you calm Mrs. Lenard down you note that the child has extreme redness on his back and several bruises on his arms. You note that his breathing is normal for his age. You ask Mrs. Lenard about the bruising and redness, and she replies that his skin is always like that. As you assess the child you note that his respirations remain normal, he has stopped crying, however, as you begin to leave the room the child begins to cry and scream. When Mrs. Lenard tries to hold him to calm him down, he screams even louder. You assist Mrs. Lenard by holding the child while you wait for the doctor.

Orders

Chest x-ray, physical exam, implement pediatric safety measures, vital signs q.30 minute, contact social work to assess for child abuse/ may have to separate mom and child.

Instructions

Complete the diagram by selecting from the choices below to specify which potential condition the client is most likely experiencing, 2 actions to take, and 2 parameters the nurse would monitor to assess the client's progress.

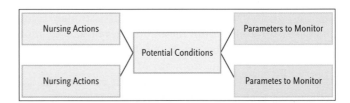

Nursing Actions	Potential Conditions	Parameters to Monitor
Take a temperature	Eczema-related inflammation	Fall precautions
Obtain MRI for suspected head injury	Suspect child abuse	Monitor oximeter
Report suspicion of child abuse to RN and social worker	Lesions due to falls	Observe interaction between mom and child (report to RN as needed)
Provide toys for the child	Cardiac distress	Restrain child for safety
Complete an assessment of the childs friends		Check I & O

REFERENCES AND BIBLIOGRAPHY

Caputi, L. (2020). *Think like a nurse: A handbook* (2nd ed.). LLC: Windy City Publishers. pp.77-79. ISBN:9781941478905; 1941478905; eText ISBN: 9781941478912; 1941478913.

Hersey, P. (2006). *Situational leadership R model*. Escondido, CA: The Center for Leadership Studies, Inc. http://www.situational.com.

Morriss, A., Ely, R. J., & Frei, F. (2014, Fall). Stop holding yourself back. *Harvard Business Review OnPoint*. http://www.necf.org/whitepapers/HBR_Managing_Yourself.pdf

Roussel, L. T., Thomas, P. L., & Harris, J. L. (2020). *Management and leaderhip for nurse administrators* (8th ed.). Burlington, MA: Jones & Bartlett.

The Joint Commission. (2021). Retrieved from https://www.jointcommission.org/media/tjc/documents/standards/r3-reports/r3-report-issue-1-20111.pdf

U. S. Department of Human Services. (2021). *Standards for privacy for individual identifiable health information*. Retrieved from: https://aspe.hhs.gov/standards-privacy-individually-identifiable-health-information.

Yoder-Wise, P. (2019). *Leading and managing in nursing* (7th ed.). St. Louis, MO: Elsevier.

Advanced Clinical Concepts

RESPIRATORY FAILURE

Acute respiratory distress syndrome (ARDS) is also known as acute lung injury (ALI), and noncardiac pulmonary edema.

Acute Respiratory Distress Syndrome

1. ARDS is a serious lung condition that causes hypoxemia in individuals who are usually ill due to another disease or a major injury. In ARDS, fluid builds up inside the alveoli causing inflammation and the breakdown of surfactant. These changes prevent the lungs from filling properly with air and moving enough oxygen into the bloodstream and throughout the body. The lung tissue may have decreased pulmonary compliance.

2. ARDS causes an exchange of oxygen (O_2) for carbon dioxide (CO_2) in the lungs that is inadequate for O_2 consumption and CO_2 production within the body's cells. The increased permeability of the alveolar membrane leads to fluid build-up in the alveoli and interferes with the exchange of CO_2 and O_2 at the capillary beds. Besides pulmonary infection or aspiration, extra-pulmonary sources include sepsis, trauma, massive transfusion, drowning, drug overdose, fat embolism, inhalation of toxic fumes, and pancreatitis. These extra-thoracic illnesses and/or injuries trigger an inflammatory cascade culminating in pulmonary injury (Fig. 3.1).

3. The first symptom of ARDS is usually dyspnea. Other signs and symptoms of ARDS are hypoxemia, tachypnea, and abnormal breath sounds.

4. The diagnosis of ARDS is made based on the following criteria: acute onset, bilateral lung infiltrates on chest radiograph of a non-cardiac origin, and a PaO/FiO ratio of less than 300 mmHg.

5. The causes of ARDS can be direct or indirect. Direct injuries include pneumonia, aspiration of stomach contents, near drowning, lung bruising from trauma (e.g., auto accident), and smoke inhalation. Indirect injuries may be associated with other underlying diseases such as: inflammation of pancreas, medication reactions/overdose, sepsis, and blood transfusions. Regardless of the cause, the overall signs and symptoms of ARDS are the same and often can be life threatening.

A. Signs and symptoms for ARDS may include: (American Lung Association)
   1. Shortness of breath
   2. Tachypnea
   3. Tachycardia
   4. Coughing that produces sputum
   5. Cyanosis
   6. Fatigue
   7. Fever
   8. Crackles and wheezes
   9. Chest pain, especially when trying to breathe deeply
   10. Hypotension
   11. Confusion
   12. Dense pulmonary infiltrates on radiography

B. Risk factors for ARDS
   1. History of smoking
   2. Alcohol abuse
   3. Recent chemotherapy
   4. O_2 use for previous lung conditions
   5. Recent high-risk surgery
   6. Obesity/ Lifestyle habits
   7. Environmental
   8. COVID-19

C. Complications of ARDS
   1. Acid-base imbalance in ARDS: respiratory and metabolic (Tables 3.1–3.3)
   2. Atelectasis: a complete or partial collapse of the lung. It may occur as a result of hospitalization.
   3. Complications of treatment in a hospital: May include a hypercoagulable state, muscle atrophy, infections, stress ulcers, and depression or other mood disorders. Confusion, memory, and judgment impairment also can result from the long-term use of sedative medicines.
   4. Multisystem organ failure: a condition in which two or more of major organs of the body begin to fail due to severe inflammation, infection, or injury.
   5. Pulmonary hypertension (PH): a condition may occur when the blood vessel narrows as a result of damage from inflammation or mechanical ventilation. ARDS may also cause pulmonary embolism (PE).

HESI HINT The initial presentation of ARDS is often subtle. At the time of initial injury, for several hours to 1–2 days afterward, the client may not experience respiratory symptoms or may exhibit only dyspnea, tachypnea, cough, and restlessness. Chest auscultation may be within normal parameters or reveal fine, scattered crackles. The mortality rate in this population is 40% (Atsumi, Y. et al., 2021). Your assessment knowledge will be tested, and you will be asked questions about how to prioritize care for these clients on the examination (Table 3.4).

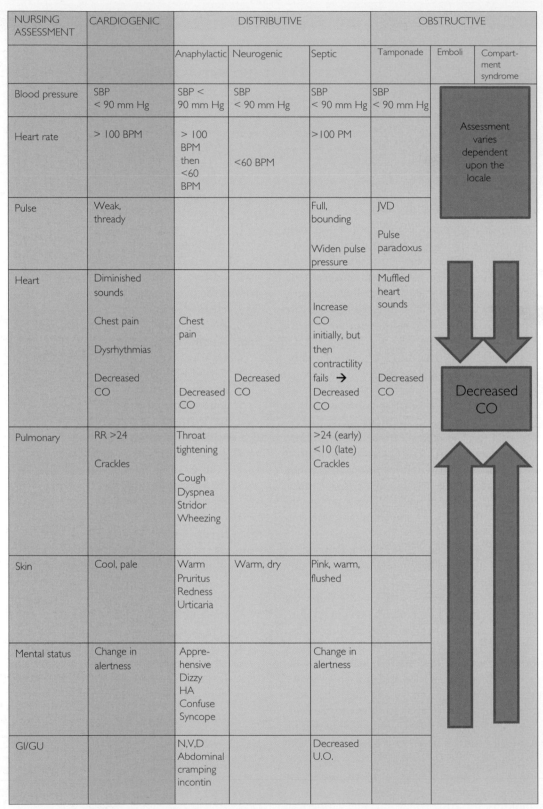

NURSING ASSESSMENT	CARDIOGENIC	DISTRIBUTIVE			OBSTRUCTIVE		
		Anaphylactic	Neurogenic	Septic	Tamponade	Emboli	Compartment syndrome
Blood pressure	SBP < 90 mm Hg	SBP < 90 mm Hg	SBP < 90 mm Hg	SBP < 90 mm Hg	SBP < 90 mm Hg	Assessment varies dependent upon the locale	
Heart rate	> 100 BPM	> 100 BPM then < 60 BPM	< 60 BPM	>100 PM			
Pulse	Weak, thready			Full, bounding Widen pulse pressure	JVD Pulse paradoxus		
Heart	Diminished sounds Chest pain Dysrhythmias Decreased CO	Chest pain Decreased CO	Decreased CO	Increase CO initially, but then contractility fails → Decreased CO	Muffled heart sounds Decreased CO	Decreased CO	
Pulmonary	RR >24 Crackles	Throat tightening Cough Dyspnea Stridor Wheezing		>24 (early) <10 (late) Crackles			
Skin	Cool, pale	Warm Pruritus Redness Urticaria	Warm, dry	Pink, warm, flushed			
Mental status	Change in alertness	Appre-hensive Dizzy HA Confuse Syncope		Change in alertness		Decreased CO	
GI/GU		N,V,D Abdominal cramping incontin		Decreased U.O.			

Fig. 3.1 Clinical Manifestations of Disrupted Acid-base Balance. (From Giddens, J. F. [2017]. *Concepts for nursing practice* [2nd ed.]. St. Louis: Mosby.)

TABLE 3.1 Arterial Blood Gas Values

Blood Gases	Normal Values	Significant Differences
pH	7.35–7.45 (<age 60) 7.31–7.42 (age 60–90) 7.26–7.43 (>age 90)	*Elevations may* indicate metabolic or respiratory alkalosis. *Decreased* levels may indicate metabolic or respiratory acidosis.
Po_2	80–100 mm Hg	Values for older adults may be lower. *Elevations* may indicate excessive O_2 administration. *Decreased* levels may be indicative of asthma, anemia, respiratory distress syndrome, cancer of the lungs, or other causes of hypoxia.
$Paco_2$	35–45 mm Hg	*Elevated* levels may indicate pneumonia, asthma, COPD, anesthesia effects, or use of opioids (respiratory acidosis). *Decreased* levels may indicate hyperventilation/respiratory alkalosis.
HCO_3	21–28 mEq/L	*Elevated levels* may indicate respiratory acidosis as compensation for primary metabolic alkalosis. *Decreased* levels may indicate respiratory alkalosis as compensation for primary metabolic acidosis.
Spo_2 Saturation	95%–100%	Values for older adults may be slightly lower. *Decreased* levels may indicate impaired ability of hemoglobin to release O_2 to tissues.

From Ignatavicius, D. D., & Workman, M. L. (2016). *Medical-surgical nursing: Patient-centered collaborative care* (7th ed., p. 557). St. Louis: Saunders.

TABLE 3.2 Compensation With Blood Gas Values

pH →	$Paco_2$ →	HCO_3 →	Compensation
Normal	*Abnormal*	*Abnormal*	FULLY
Abnormal	*Abnormal*	*Abnormal*	PARTIAL
Abnormal	**Normal**	*Abnormal*	UNCOMPENSATED
Abnormal	*Abnormal*	**Normal**	UNCOMPENSATED

Clinical Assessment

A. Monitor, in conjunction with a registered nurse (RN), the patient on a ventilator.

B. Provide care for either an oral airway or tracheostomy suction.

C. Monitor breath sounds for pneumothorax (diminished or absent breath sounds), especially when positive-end expiratory pressure (PEEP) is delivered via mechanical ventilated the intubated patient.

D. Monitor respiratory effort-rate, depth, and use of accessory muscles.

E. Provide emotional support to decrease anxiety and allow ventilator to "work" the lungs.

F. Monitor hemodynamic status via vital signs and cardiac monitor.

G. Monitor arterial blood gases (ABGs).

H. Monitor vital organ status: central nervous system (CNS), level of consciousness, renal system output, and myocardium (apical pulse and blood pressure [BP]).

I. Monitor metabolic status through routine laboratory work (see Table 3.1).

J. Sedate as per prescription to decrease anxiety and decrease O_2 use.

Respiratory Failure in Children

Pediatric respiratory failure develops when the rate of gas exchange between the atmosphere and the blood is unable to match the body's metabolic demands. Acute respiratory failure remains an important cause of morbidity and mortality in children. Cardiac arrests in children frequently result from respiratory failure.

A. Causes of respiratory failure in children
   1. Congenital heart disease
   2. Respiratory distress syndrome
   3. Infection, sepsis
   4. Neuromuscular diseases
   5. Trauma and burns
   6. Aspiration
   7. Fluid overload and dehydration
   8. Anesthesia and narcotic overdose
   9. Structural anomalies resulting in obstruction of the airway

B. Risk factors for respiratory failure in children
   1. Choking
   2. Cardiac arrest

C. Complications of respiratory failure in children
   1. Death

D. Signs and symptoms of respiratory failure in children are not always evident and are difficult to recognize.
   1. Children may be lethargic, irritable, anxious, or unable to concentrate. Children with respiratory distress commonly sit up and lean forward to improve leverage for the accessory muscles and to allow for easy diaphragmatic movement. Children with epiglottitis sit upright with their neck extended and head forward while drooling and breathing through their mouth.

The respiratory rate and quality can provide diagnostic information, as exemplified by the following:

Bradypnea: Most often observed in central control abnormalities

Tachypnea: Fast and shallow breathing is most efficient in intrathoracic airway obstruction; it decreases dynamic compliance of the lung.

HESI HINT A child in severe respiratory distress should receive 100% oxygen until diagnostic test results, keep in mind the percentage of oxygen the child is receiving.

Clinical Assessment

A. Stridor (an inspiratory sound)
B. Wheezing (an expiratory sound)
C. Crackles
D. Decreased breath sounds (e.g., alveolar consolidation, pleural effusion)
E. Paradoxical movement of the chest wall
F. Accessory muscle use and nasal flaring (Hammer, 2013)

HESI HINT The NGN-NCLEX-PN asks many questions about clinical assessment and related pathophysiology.
Example: The nurse is assessing an infant who grunts during expiration. Which is the likely cause of this finding?
Infants and young children grunt during expiration as respiratory distress begins. Grunting is how the body attempts to create a form of "PEEP" (positive end-expiratory pressure) to help keep the alveoli open.

HESI HINT The NGN-NCLEX-PN tests your ability to assess the child's condition and then subsequently apply and implement actions to address acute life-threatening situations. For example, you need to know acute **respiratory failure** describes any impairment in oxygenation or ventilation in which the arterial oxygen tension falls below 60 mm Hg (acute hypoxemia), the carbon dioxide tension rises above 50 mm Hg (acute hypercarbia, hypercapnia), and the pH drops below 7.35, or both (Hammer, 2013).

? REVIEW OF RESPIRATORY FAILURE

The NGN-NCLEX-PN is NOT based on memorization. PN Nursing school graduates are expected to assess the elements of a given situation and subsequently develop a plan of action that meets the client's needs.

NGN-NCLEX-PN questions are designed for nursing school graduates to demonstrate their ability to apply critical thinking skills to meet the needs based on the contents of the questions.

1. What Po_2 value indicates respiratory failure in adults?
2. What blood value indicates hypercapnia?
3. Identify the condition that exists when the Po_2 is less than 60 mm Hg (acute hypoxemia), the carbon dioxide tension rises above 50 mm Hg (acute hypercarbia, hypercapnia), and the pH drops below 7.35, or both.
4. List three symptoms of respiratory failure in adults.
5. List four common causes of respiratory failure in children.
6. What percentage of O_2 should a child in severe respiratory distress receive?

See Answer Key at the end of this text for suggested responses.

SHOCK

Shock is defined as a state of cellular and tissue hypoxia due to either reduced oxygen delivery, increased oxygen consumption, inadequate oxygen utilization, or a combination of these processes. The state of shock will generally present as hypotensive but may also present as hypertensive or normotensive.

A. Types of shock:
B. Distributive—Distributive shock is characterized by severe peripheral vasodilatation (vasodilatory shock). Molecules that mediate vasodilatation vary such as:
1. Septic shock—Sepsis, defined as a dysregulated host response to infection resulting in life-threatening organ dysfunction, is the most common cause of distributive shock. Septic shock is a subset of sepsis associated with

TABLE 3.3 Clinical Manifestations of Disrupted Acid-Base Balance

Types of Problem	TOO MUCH ACID		TOO LITTLE ACID	
	Too Much Carbonic Acid (Respiratory Acidosis)	Too Much Metabolic Acid (Metabolic Acidosis)	Too Little Carbonic Acid (Respiratory Alkalosis)	Too Little Metabolic Acid (Metabolic Alkalosis)
Common clinical findings	Headache Decreased LOC Hypoventilation (cause of problem) Cardiac dysrhythmias If severe: hypotension	Decreased level of consciousness (LOC) Hyperventilation (compensatory mechanism) Abdominal pain Nausea and vomiting Cardiac dysrhythmias	Excitation and belligerence, light-headedness, unusual behaviors; followed by decreased LOC if severe Perioral and digital paresthesias, carpopedal spasm, tetany Diaphoresis Hyperventilation (cause of problem) Cardiac dysrhythmias	Excitation followed by decreased LOC if severe Perioral and digital paresthesias, carpopedal spasm Hypoventilation (compensatory mechanism) Signs of volume depletion and hypokalemia if present
Blood gas findings	Blood gases; pH decreased (or low normal if fully compensated); $Paco_2$ increased; HCO_3^- increased from compensation	Blood gases; pH decreased (or low normal if fully compensated); $Paco_2$ decreased from compensation; HCO_3^- decreased	Blood gases; pH increased; $Paco_2$ decreased; HCO_3^- decreased if compensation	Blood gases; pH increased; $Paco_2$ increased from compensation; HCO_3^- increased

From Giddens, J. F. (2017). *Concepts for nursing practice* (with Pageburst Digital Book Access on VST) (2nd ed., p. 81). VitalBook file. St. Louis: Mosby.

TABLE 3.4 Clinical Judgment Measures: Acute Respiratory Distress Syndrome

Monitor in conjunction with a Registered Nurse

Clinical Judgment Measure	Assessment Characteristics
Recognize Cues	Monitor Lung sounds: Dyspnea, hyperpnea, crackles (or rales), wheezing, or decreased breath sounds
	Assess for intercostal retractions or substernal retractions
	Note any cyanosis, pallor, mottled skin
	Determine if patient is hypoxic: partial pressure of $O_2(Po_2)$ <50 mm Hg with fraction of inspired O_2 (Fio_2) >60%
	1. Increasing diminished breath sounds
	2. Diffuse pulmonary infiltrates seen on chest radiograph as "white-out" appearance
	3. Verbalization of anxiety, restlessness, confusion, and agitation
Analyze Cues	Determine if lung sounds are emergent.
	Notify intensivist/physician.
	Potential to improve oxygenation with mechanical ventilation
	Treat the underlying cause or injury.
Prioritize Cues	Determine if problem is emergent.
	Determine impact of problem on patient's overall health status.
Solutions	Prevent complications of clients on mechanical ventilation.
	Elevate head of bed (HOB) to at least 30 degrees.
	Assist with daily awakening ("sedation vacation").
	Implement a comprehensive oral hygiene program.
	Monitor hemodynamically with essential vital signs and a cardiac monitor.
	Peaked T waves (early sign) as seen in hyperkalemia; as potassium levels become higher, there are and increased PR intervals.
	Metabolic status through routine laboratory work.
	1. Monitor arterial blood gases (ABGs) routinely.
	2. Then monitor fluid and electrolyte balance.
	a. Monitor needs to determine whether the client is in a respiratory or metabolic state.
	b. The goal is to get the ABG pH level as close to normal as possible.
Actions	Suction oral cavity.
	Give antibiotics as ordered.
	Deep venous thrombosis prophylaxis as ordered.
	Stress ulcer prophylaxis
	Observe for barotrauma.
	Monitor blood chemistry and fluid levels.
	Nursing judgment measures for acute respiratory distress syndrome (ARDS)
	Intensivist for managing the patient on the ventilator and other ICU-related issues like pneumonia prevention, deep vein thrombosis (DVT) prophylaxis, and gastric stress prevention.
	Position the client for maximal lung expansion, proning may be best option if ordered.
	Monitor the client for signs of hypoxemia and O_2 toxicity.
	Monitor vital organ status: central nervous system (CNS) level of consciousness, renal system (urinary output), and myocardium (apical pulse and blood pressure [BP]).
	Dietitian and nutritionist for nutritional support
	Respiratory therapist to manage the ventilator settings
	Pharmacist to manage the medications, which include antibiotics, anticoagulants, diuretics, among others
	Pulmonologist to manage the lung diseases
	Social worker to assess the patient's financial situation, transfer for rehab, and ensure there is an adequate follow-up
	Chaplain for spiritual care
Evaluate Outcomes	The chief treatment strategy is supportive care, along with adequate nutrition.
	Patients are mechanically ventilated, guarded against fluid overload with diuretics, and given nutritional support until evidence of improvement is observed.
	The mode in which a patient is ventilated affects lung recovery. Evidence suggests that some ventilatory strategies can exacerbate alveolar damage and perpetuate lung injury in the context of ARDS. Care is placed in preventing volutrauma (exposure to large tidal volumes), barotrauma (exposure to high plateau pressures), and atelectrauma (exposure to atelectasis).

mortality in the 40% to 50% range that can be identified by the use of vasopressor therapy and the presence of elevated lactate levels (>2 mmol/L) despite adequate fluid resuscitation.

2. Neurogenic shock—Hypotension and overt shock are common in patients with severe traumatic brain injury and spinal cord injury. Interruption of autonomic pathways, that causes decreased vascular resistance and altered vagal tone which is responsible for distributive shock in patients.

3. Anaphylactic shock—Shock from anaphylaxis is most commonly encountered in patients with severe, immunoglobulin-E (Ig-E) mediated allergic reactions to insect stings, food, and drugs.

C. *Cardiogenic*—Cardiogenic shock is due to intracardiac causes of cardiac pump failure that result in reduced cardiac output (CO). Causes of cardiac pump failure are diverse, but can be divided into the following three categories Cardiomyopathic, Arrhythmic, and Mechanical.

D. *Hypovolemic*—Hypovolemic shock is due to reduced intravascular volume (i.e., reduced preload), which reduces CO. There are four stages of hypovolemic shock (Table 3.5). Hypovolemic shock can be divided into two categories: hemorrhagic and nonhemorrhagic.

1. Hemorrhagic—Reduced intravascular volume from blood loss including blunt or penetrating trauma followed by hemorrhage.

2. Nonhemorrhagic—Reduced intravascular volume from fluid loss other than blood can cause shock. Volume depletion from loss of sodium and water can occur from a number of anatomic sites.

E. *Obstructive*—Obstructive shock is mostly due to extracardiac causes of cardiac pump failure and often associated with poor right ventricular output. The causes of obstructive shock can be divided into the following two categories:

1. Pulmonary vascular—Most cases of obstructive shock are due to right ventricular failure from hemodynamically significant PE or severe PH. Patients with severe stenosis or with acute obstruction of the pulmonary or tricuspid valve may also fall into this category.

2. Mechanical—Patients in this category present clinically as hypovolemic shock because their primary physiologic disturbance is decreased preload, rather than pump failure. Mechanical causes of obstructive shock include the following:
   a. Tension pneumothorax
   b. Pericardial tamponade
   c. Constrictive pericarditis)

TABLE 3.5	Stages of Hypovolemic Shock	
Stage	**Signs and Symptoms**	**Clinical Description**
Stage I 1. Initial stage 2. Blood loss of <10% 3. Compensatory mechanisms triggered	• Apprehension and restlessness (first signs of shock) • Increased heart rate • Cool, pale skin • Fatigue	• Arteriolar constriction • Increased production of antidiuretic hormone • Arterial pressure is maintained • Cardiac output usually normal (for healthy individuals) • Selective reduction in blood flow to skin and muscle beds
Stage II • Compensatory stage • Blood volume reduced by 15%–25% • Decompensation begins	• Flattened neck veins and delayed venous filling time • Increased pulse and respirations • Pallor, diaphoresis, and cool skin • Decreased urinary output • Sunken, soft eyeballs • Confusion	• Marked reduction in cardiac output • Arterial pressure decline (despite compensatory arteriolar vasoconstriction) • Massive adrenergic compensatory response resulting in tachycardia, tachypnea, cutaneous vasoconstriction, and oliguria • Decreased cerebral perfusion
Stage III • Progressive stage	• Edema • Increased blood viscosity • Excessively low blood pressure • Dysrhythmia, ischemia, and myocardial infarction • Weak, thready, or absent peripheral pulses	• Rapid circulatory deterioration • Decreased cardiac output • Decreased tissue perfusion • Reduced blood volume
Stage IV • Irreversible stage	• Profound hypotension, unresponsive to vasopressor drugs • Severe hypoxemia, unresponsive to O_2 administration • Anuria, renal shutdown • Heart rate slows, blood pressure falls, with consequent cardiac and respiratory arrest	• Cell destruction so severe that death is inevitable • Multiple organ system failure • It is the nurse's responsibility to recognize the signs and symptoms of shock early in the course of the disease process to prevent the devastating clinical course that the progression of shock can take.

d. Restrictive cardiomyopathy

e. Abdominal compartment syndrome (ACS)

F. Causes of shock

1. Blood loss
2. Trauma
3. Allergic reaction
4. Heatstroke
5. Poisoning
6. Severe burns
7. Severe infection
8. Poisoning

G. Risk factors for shock

1. Very young and very old clients
2. Post—myocardial infarction (MI) or with severe dysrhythmia
3. Adrenocortical dysfunction
4. History of recent hemorrhage or blood loss
5. Burns
6. Massive or overwhelming infection (Ismail & Elbaih, 2017).

> **HESI HINT** If cardiogenic shock exists with the presence of pulmonary edema (i.e., from cardiac pump failure) position the client in high Fowler's with the legs facing downward to reduce venous return to the left ventricle.

H. Complications of shock

1. Refer to Box 3.1

I. Signs and symptoms of shock

1. Weak pulse
2. Rapid shallow breathing
3. Cold and clammy skin
4. Pale skin
5. Rapid heart rate
6. Oliguria/anuria
7. Confusion

J. Clinical assessment of shock: vital signs; tachycardia (pulse more than 100 bpm); tachypnea (respirations more than 24/min); BP decreased (systolic, 80 mm Hg);narrow pulse pressure.

BOX 3.1 Complications of Shock

Early	Severe
Tachycardia	Organ dysfunction
Hypotension	Renal failure
Weakened peripheral pulses	Pleural effusion
Restlessness, agitation, confusion	Respiratory distress
Pale cool, clammy skin	Renal failure
Decreased urine output (M30 mL/h)	Death

Data from Giddens, J. F. (2017). *Concepts for nursing practice* (with Pageburst Digital Book Access on VST) (2nd ed., p. 233,). VitalBook file. St. Louis: Mosby; Harkreader, H. (2007). *Fundamentals of nursing: Caring and clinical judgment* (3rd ed., p. 959). VitalBook file. Philadelphia: Saunders.

Medical Management of Shock

A. **Correct tissue perfusion and restore CO**, cause of shock dictates the type of treatment.

B. Oxygenation and ventilation

1. Optimize O_2 delivery and reduce demand on heart.
2. Increase arterial O_2 saturation with supplemental oxygenation and mechanical ventilation.
3. Space activities that decrease O_2 consumption.

C. Fluid resuscitation

1. Based on laboratory data, lactic acid infusion of volume-expanding fluids is the treatment for hypovolemic shock and anaphylactic shock.
2. Whole blood, plasma, plasma substitutes (colloid fluids) may be used.
3. Isotonic (IV) solutions, such as Ringer's lactate solution and normal saline, may also be used.
4. If shock is cardiogenic in nature, infusion of volume-expanding fluids may be contraindicated and may result in pulmonary edema.

D. Drug therapy

1. Restoration of cardiac function should take priority. Drug selection is based on the effect of the shock on preload, afterload, or contractility.
   a. Drugs that increase preload (e.g., blood products, crystalloids) or decrease preload (e.g., opioids such as morphine, nitrates, diuretics)
   b. Drugs that increase afterload (e.g., vasopressors, dopamine) or decrease afterload (e.g., Vasodilators/Nitrates such as nitroprusside, angiotensin-converting enzyme inhibitor [ACE-I], angiotensin II receptor blocker [ARB])
   c. Drugs that decrease contractility (e.g., beta blockers, calcium channel blockers) or increase contractility (e.g., antiarrhythmic inhibits sodium-potassium adenosine diphosphate (ATPase) such as digoxin, beta 1 stimulator/mild chronotropic arrhythmogenic and vasodilative effects such as dobutamine, cAMP phosphodiesterase inhibitors such as milrinone). Milrinone is a phosphodiesterase 3 inhibitor that increases cardiac inotropy, lusitropy, and peripheral vasodilatation. In contrast, dobutamine is a synthetic catecholamine that acts as a β1 and β2-receptor antagonist and improves BP by increasing cardiac output.

E. Monitoring

1. Central venous monitoring system may be inserted for monitoring shock
2. Serial measurements of cardiopulmonary function (using electrocardiogram [ECG], pulse oximetry, end-tidal CO_2 monitoring, ABGs, and hemodynamic monitoring urinary output, clinical assessment [i.e., mental status] with close monitoring systems)
3. Stabilization and treating the underlying cause of the condition.

F. Clinical nursing judgment measures for shock

1. If cardiogenic shock exists in the presence of pulmonary edema (i.e., from pump failure), position client to reduce venous return (high Fowler position with

legs down) to decrease further venous return to the left ventricle.

2. Sedate as per doctor orders to decrease anxiety and decrease O_2 and the nurse use by being be educated on pump dynamics before being responsible for monitoring a patient with an intra-aortic balloon pump (IABP) is a type of therapeutic device. It helps your heart pump more blood. You may need it if your heart is unable to pump enough blood for your body.).

3. The nurse is also responsible for assessing for potential complications of this device such as limb ischemia, compartment syndrome, aorta dissection, plaque or emboli dislodgement, migration of the catheter, insertion site bleeding, rupture of the balloon, signs and symptoms of infection, and skin breakdown because the client has limited movement.

4. Monitor BP, pulse, respirations, and arrhythmias based on ICU protocols.

5. Monitor arterial pressure by understanding the concepts related to arterial pressure.

6. Assess urine output every hour to maintain at least 30 mL/h (approximately 0.5 mL/kg/h for 70-kg patient) and notify the health care provider if urine output drops below 30 mL/h (reflects decreased renal perfusion and may result in acute renal failure).

7. Monitor IV fluids as prescribed by provider to improve preload: blood, colloids, or electrolyte solutions until designated central venous pressure (CVP) is reached.

8. Remember client's bed position is dependent on cause of shock.

9. Maintain warmth; increase heat in room and use warm blankets (not too hot).

10. Keep side rails up, due to mental confusion and high fall risk.

11. Assist in obtaining blood for laboratory work as prescribed: complete blood count (CBC), electrolytes, blood urea nitrogen (BUN), creatinine (renal damage), lactate (sepsis), and blood gases (oxygenation and ventilation).
    a. Monitor hemodynamic status every 5 to 15 minutes/ or as ordered.
    b. Observe IV site carefully for extravasation and tissue damage.
    c. Assure medications administered are for target mean arterial pressure (MAP) is **the average arterial pressure throughout one cardiac cycle, systole, and diastole.**
    d. Glucose levels should be sustained based on orders and based on the shock.

12. Ensure the pulse oximetry probe is placed appropriately to assure the probe is reading correctly and not cause necrosis due to decreased tissue perfusion.

G. Provide family support
   1. Involve the family in care and facilitate a patient care support person, social worker, or spiritual support.

2. Keep family updated.
3. Collaborate with the health care provider before notifying family of medical interventions.

DISSEMINATED INTRAVASCULAR COAGAULATION

Description: Disseminated intravascular coagulation (DIC) is a life-threatening syndrome characterized by disseminated and often uncontrolled activation of coagulation. This syndrome is associated with a high risk of macro- and microvascular thrombosis and progressive consumption coagulopathy, which leads to an increased bleeding risk. Several pathological conditions may trigger DIC including but not limited to sepsis, cancer, trauma, and obstetric calamity ranking among the most frequent triggering factors (Papageorgiou et al., 2018). DIC is a coagulation disorder characterized by paradoxical thrombosis and hemorrhage that results from abnormally initiated and accelerated clotting. DIC destroys the clotting factors, platelets, and red blood cells (RBCs).

A. DIC is a complication or an effect of the progression of other illnesses and is always secondary to an underlying disorder and is associated with a number of clinical conditions, generally involving activation of systemic inflammation, such as sepsis and severe infection (including COVID-19), trauma (neurotrauma), organ destruction, malignancy, severe transfusion reactions.

B. DIC is most commonly observed in severe sepsis and septic shock. Indeed, the development and severity of DIC correlate with mortality in severe sepsis; bacteremia, both gram-positive and gram-negative organisms, is most commonly associated with DIC; other organisms (e.g., viruses, fungi, and parasites) may also cause DIC.

C. The first phase involves abnormal clotting in the microcirculation, which uses up clotting factors and results in the inability to form clots, so hemorrhage occurs.

D. The diagnosis is based on laboratory findings.
   1. Prothrombin time (PT): prolonged
   2. Partial thromboplastin time (PTT): prolonged
   3. Fibrinogen: decreased
   4. Platelet count: decreased
   5. Fibrin degradation (split) products (FSP or FDP): increased

Clinical Assessment

A. Petechiae, purpura, hematomas
B. Respiratory distress, tachypnea, dyspnea
C. Oozing from IV sites, drains, gums, and wounds
D. Gastrointestinal and genitourinary bleeding
E. Hemoptysis
F. Mental status change
G. Hypotension, tachycardia
H. Pain
I. ABGs and saturation

Clinical Nursing Judgment Measures

A. Treatment should primarily focus on addressing the underlying disorder.

B. Monitor for bleeding.

C. Monitor vital signs.

D. Monitor PT/international normalized ratio (INR).

E. Protect from injury and bleeding.
1. Provide gentle oral care with mouth swabs.
2. Minimize needle sticks; use smallest gauge needle possible.
3. Turn frequently to eliminate pressure points.
4. Minimize number of BP measurements taken by cuff.
5. Use gentle suction to prevent trauma to mucosa.
6. Apply pressure to any oozing site(s).

F. Provide emotional support to decrease anxiety.

> ### ❓ REVIEW OF SHOCK AND DISSEMINATED INTRAVASCULAR COAGULATION
>
> 1. Define *shock*.
> 2. What is the most common cause of shock?
> 3. What causes septic shock?
> 4. What is the goal of treatment for hypovolemic shock?
> 5. What intervention is used to restore cardiac output when hypovolemic shock exists?
> 6. It is important to differentiate between hypovolemic and cardiogenic shock. How might the nurse determine the existence of cardiogenic shock?
> 7. If a client is in cardiogenic shock, what might result from administration of volume-expanding fluids, and what intervention can the nurse expect to perform in the event of such an occurrence?
> 8. List five assessment findings that occur in most shock victims.
> 9. What is the established minimum renal output per hour?
> 10. List four measurable criteria that are the major expected outcomes of a shock crisis.
> 11. What is the effect on PT<PTT platelets and FSPs (FDPs)?
> 12. What medication is used in the treatment of DIC?
> 13. Name four nursing judgment measures to prevent injury in clients with DIC.

See Answer Key at the end of this text for suggested responses.

RESUSCITATION

Cardiopulmonary Arrest

Occurs when the heart malfunctions and stops beating unexpectedly. Cardiac arrest is an "ELECTRICAL" problem.

MI occurs when blood flow to the heart is blocked. A heart attack is a "CIRCULATION" problem.

A. MI is the irreversible death/necrosis of heart muscle secondary to ischemia. Approximately 1.5 million cases of MI occur annually in the United States.

B. Patients with typical MI may have the following symptoms in the days or even weeks preceding the event (although typical STEMI may occur suddenly, without warning):
1. Fatigue
2. Chest discomfort
3. Malaise

C. Typical chest pain in acute MI has the following characteristics:
1. Intense and unremitting for 30 to 60 minutes

2. Substernal, and often radiates up to the neck, shoulder, and jaw, and down the left arm
3. Usually described as a substernal pressure sensation that also may be characterized as squeezing, aching, burning, or even sharp.
4. In some patients, the symptom is epigastric, with a feeling of indigestion or of fullness and gas.
5. Chest pain in a client with known coronary heart disease that is unrelieved by rest or nitroglycerin

D. Prehospital care
1. For patients with chest pain, prehospital care includes the following:
2. Intravenous access, supplemental oxygen if SaO_2 is less than 90%, pulse oximetry
3. Immediate administration of nonenteric-coated chewable aspirin
4. Nitroglycerin for active chest pain, given sublingually or by spray
5. Telemetry and prehospital ECG. The ECG is the most important tool in the initial evaluation and triage of patients in whom an ACS, such as MI, is suspected. It is confirmatory of the diagnosis in approximately 80% of cases. The information in this section is in accordance with the 2020 ESC Guidelines for the Management of Acute Coronary Syndromes (Collet, Thiele, Barbato E, et al., 2021)

> **HESI HINT** NGN-NCLEX-PN questions on cardiopulmonary resuscitation (CPR) often use critical thinking skills to determine prioritization of actions.

E. Chest pain in MI:
1. Typical chest pain in acute MI has the following characteristics:
2. Intense and unremitting for 30 to 60 minutes
3. Substernal, and often radiates up to the neck, shoulder, and jaw, and down the left arm
4. Usually described as a substernal pressure sensation that also may be characterized as squeezing, aching, burning, or even sharp
5. In some patients, the symptom is epigastric, with a feeling of indigestion or of fullness and gas

> **HESI HINT** The nurse must stay current with the American Heart Association (AHA) guidelines for basic life support (BLS) by being certified every 2 years, as required. See the AHA website for current CPR Guidelines and to locate a CPR class.

Clinical Assessment (In-Hospital Care)

A. Diagnostic ABGs

B. Note signs and symptoms:
1. Chest pain/discomfort either at rest or with simple activity
2. Described as crushing, intense pressure, constricting, oppressive or heavy.

3. Tends to increase in intensity over a few minutes.
4. May be substernal or more diffuse.
5. May radiate to shoulders and arms, or to the neck, jaw, or back.
6. Atypical symptoms occur with women and clients diagnosed with diabetes. For example, women experience unexpected shortness of breath, cold sweats, sudden fatigue, nausea, and lightheadedness.
7. Change in previously stable anginal pain—an increase in frequency or severity or rest angina occurring for the first time.
8. Chest pain in a client with known coronary heart disease that is unrelieved by rest and/or nitroglycerin.

Major components of BLS consist of immediate recognition of cardiac arrest and activation of the emergency response system, CPR with emphasis on chest compression, and rapid defibrillation if indicated.

> **HESI HINT** Initiate CPR with BLS guidelines immediately; then move on to advanced cardiac life support (ACLS) guidelines (Merchant, et al., 2020).

Clinical Judgment Interventions

A. Teach patient when to contact the emergency medical system.
B. Determine responsiveness of the patient.
   1. If no response, call a "code" or cardiac arrest, to initiate the response of the cardiac arrest team. Obtain automated external defibrillator or emergency crash cart with defibrillator.
   2. Position patient on cardiac board or put bed in CPR position. If pulse is not identified within 10 seconds, begin chest compressions.
   3. Initiate chest compressions—30 compressions with both hands over the lower half of the sternum at a rate of 100 compressions per minute with a depth of 2 inches (5 cm).
   4. After 20 compressions ventilate by mask or bag over 1 second per breath for 2 breaths.
C. When team leader arrives, team is directed as to what to do.
   1. Without interrupting CPR, apply cardiac portable monitor for a "quick look" paddles or automated external defibrillator (AED) to determine whether defibrillation is necessary or whether asystole has occurred.
   2. Follow hospital policies and procedures to convert client to normal sinus rhythm.
   3. Resume CPR, beginning with compressions, immediately after defibrillations.
   4. O$_2$ is necessary for survival; all other injuries are secondary—except for removal of any source of imminent danger, such as a fire.

Pediatric Resuscitation
Overview of Pediatric Resuscitation

See cardiopulmonary arrest earlier.

For newborn resuscitation, see Maternity Nursing in Chapter 5: Pediatric Nursing

Rapid recognition of cardiac arrest, immediate initiation of high-quality chest compressions, and delivery of effective ventilations are critical to improve outcomes from cardiac arrest.

Lay rescuers should not delay starting CPR in a child with no "signs of life."

Healthcare providers may consider assessing the presence of a pulse as long as the initiation of CPR is not delayed more than 10 seconds.

Palpation for the presence or absence of a pulse is not reliable as the sole determinant of cardiac arrest and the need for chest compressions.

In infants and children, asphyxia cardiac arrest is more common than cardiac arrest from a primary cardiac event; therefore, effective ventilation is important during resuscitation of children.

When CPR is initiated, the sequence is compressions-airway-breathing.

High-quality CPR generates blood flow to vital organs and increases the likelihood of return of spontaneous circulation (ROSC).

The 5 main components of high-quality CPR:
1. adequate chest compression depth,
2. optimal chest compression rate,
3. minimizing interruptions in CPR (i.e., maximizing chest compression fraction or the proportion of time that chest compressions are provided for cardiac arrest)
4. allowing full chest recoil between compressions,
5. avoiding excessive ventilation.

Compressions of inadequate depth and rate, incomplete chest recoil, and high ventilation rates are common during pediatric resuscitation.

For infants, single rescuers (whether lay rescuers or healthcare providers) should compress the sternum with 2 fingers or 2 thumbs placed just below the intermammary line.

For infants, the 2-thumb–encircling hands technique is recommended when CPR is provided by 2 rescuers (Fig. 3.2).

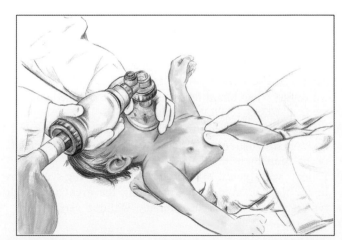

Fig. 3.2 2-Thumb–Encircling Hands Compressions. (From Topjian, A. A., Raymond, T. T., Atkins, D., Chan, M., Duff, J. P., Joyner Jr, B. L., et al. [2021]. Part 4: Pediatric Basic and Advanced Life Support 2020 American Heart Association Guidelines for Cardiopulmonary Resuscitation and Emergency Medical Care. *Pediatrics, 147*[Suppl 1], e2020038505D.)

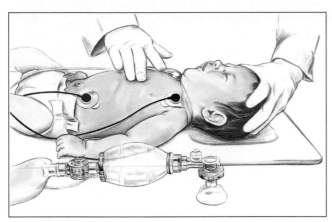

Fig. 3.3 2-Finger Compressions. (From Topjian, A. A., Raymond, T. T., Atkins, D., Chan, M., Duff, J. P., Joyner Jr, B. L., et al. [2021]. Part 4: Pediatric Basic and Advanced Life Support 2020 American Heart Association Guidelines for Cardiopulmonary Resuscitation and Emergency Medical Care. *Pediatrics, 147*[Suppl 1], e2020038505D.)

If the rescuer cannot physically encircle the victim's chest, compress the chest with 2 fingers.

For children, it may be reasonable to use either a 1- or 2-hand technique to perform chest compressions (Fig. 3.3) (Topjian et al., 2021).

The American Heart Association algorithms for CPR (adult and pediatric) and MI can be downloaded at: https://cpr.heart.org/en/resuscitation-science/cpr-and-ecc-guidelines/algorithms.

For infants, if the rescuer is unable to achieve guideline recommended depths (at least one third the anterior-posterior diameter of the chest), it may be reasonable to use the heel of 1 hand (Figs. 3.4–3.6).

> **HESI HINT** In the Pediatric cardiac arrest algorithm know the reversible causes:
> The reversible causes of cardiac arrest include four "H's": **hypoxia**. **hypovolemia**. **hyperkalemia, hypokalemia, other electrolyte disturbances,** and four **"Ts"**: **tension pneumothorax, cardiac tamponade, drug toxicity and therapeutics, thromboembolism and other outflow obstructions**.

> **HESI HINT**
> - For infants and children provide chest compressions that depress the chest at least 1/3 of the anterior posterior diameter of the chest; use chest compression rate of ~100–120/min for infants and children.
> - Single rescuers compression to ventilation rate 30:2; two rescuers 15:2

Management of Foreign Body Airway Obstruction
Adults and Children

Foreign-body airway obstruction. Foreign-body airway obstruction (FBAO), or choking, is an alarming and dramatic emergency.

To confirm a complete FBAO, ask the victim "Are you choking?" If the victim cannot speak or can only make weak, high-pitched sounds, perform abdominal thrust until the object is expelled or the victim becomes unresponsive.
A. Stand behind the victim
B. Make a fist with one hand
C. Place your fist on the victim's abdomen, slightly above the navel and well below the breastbone
D. Grasp your fist with your other hand
E. Deliver quick upward thrusts into the victim's abdomen, Heimlich maneuver
F. Deliver thrusts until the object is expelled or the victim becomes unresponsive. If a choking adult becomes unresponsive while you are doing abdominal thrust, you should ease the victim to the floor and send someone to activate your emergency response system.
G. When a choking victim becomes unresponsive, you begin the steps of CPR, starting with compressions.
H. The only difference is that each time you open the airway, look for the obstructing object before giving each breath.
I. Remove the object if you see it
J. Chest thrust should be used in obese or pregnant patients.

Infants and Children

A. FBAO develops when an object becomes lodged in the airway and blocks the movement of air into and out of the lungs.
B. If the blockage is severe or complete, the victim will be unable to breathe and oxygenate blood supplying the brain, heart, and other vital organs with adequate oxygen to function normally.
C. If the blockage is not relieved, the victim will become unresponsive and can die.
D. Signs of severe or complete FBAO in infants and children include sudden onset of respiratory distress associated with weak or silent cough/cry, inability to speak, stridor, or increasing respiratory difficulty.
E. These signs and symptoms of airway obstruction may also be caused by infections and croup.
F. Typically with FBAO these signs and symptoms will develop suddenly with no other signs of illness or infection.
G. If you suspect a severe (victim not passing air or ineffective cough/cry) or complete FBAO, follow these steps:
H. For a Responsive Infant
I. Pick the infant up from a supine (lying face up) position by lifting the legs with one hand and sliding the other hand all the way to the infant's head. Once this is done, "sandwich" the infant by placing the opposite arm and hand on the infant's stomach and face... grasping the infant's facial cheeks.
J. Supporting the infant—place them face down on your thigh, and make sure the head is lower than the body.
K. Deliver 5 back slaps with the heel of your free hand between the shoulder blades. "Sandwich" the infant between your

Pediatric Basic Life Support Algorithm for Healthcare Providers–Single Rescuer

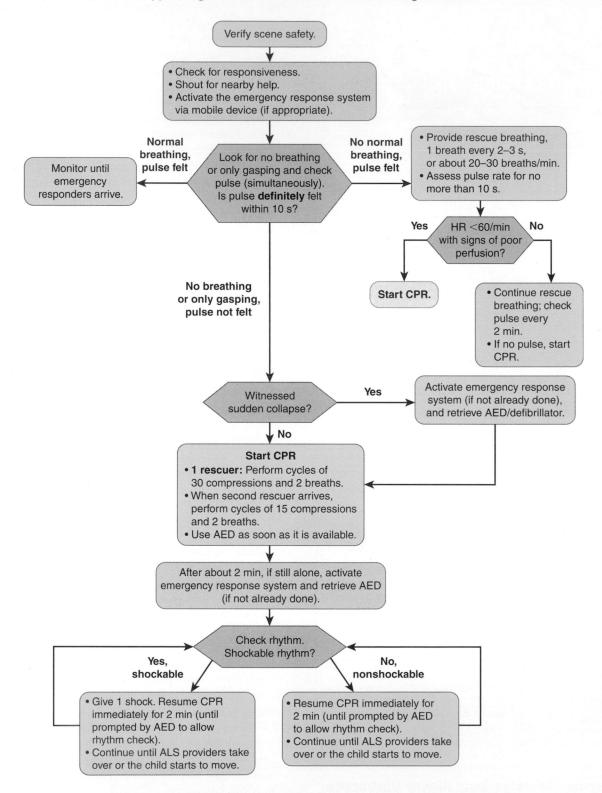

Fig. 3.4 Pediatric Basic Life Support Algorithm for Healthcare Providers—Single Rescuer. *AED,* Automated external defibrillator; *ALS,* advanced life support; *CPR,* cardiopulmonary resuscitation; *HR,* heart rate. (From Topjian, A. A., Raymond, T. T., Atkins, D., Chan, M., Duff, J. P., Joyner Jr, B. L., et al. [2021]. Part 4: Pediatric Basic and Advanced Life Support 2020 American Heart Association Guidelines for Cardiopulmonary Resuscitation and Emergency Medical Care. *Pediatrics, 147*[Suppl 1], e2020038505D.)

Pediatric Basic Life Support Algorithm for Healthcare Providers—2 or More Rescuers

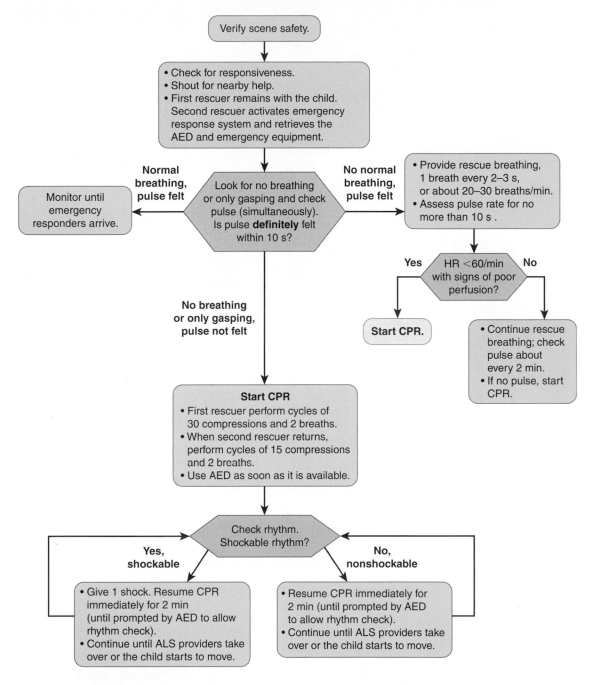

Verify scene safety.

- Check for responsiveness.
- Shout for nearby help.
- First rescuer remains with the child. Second rescuer activates emergency response system and retrieves the AED and emergency equipment.

Normal breathing, pulse felt

Look for no breathing or only gasping and check pulse (simultaneously). Is pulse **definitely** felt within 10 s?

Monitor until emergency responders arrive.

No normal breathing, pulse felt

- Provide rescue breathing, 1 breath every 2–3 s, or about 20–30 breaths/min.
- Assess pulse rate for no more than 10 s .

Yes   HR <60/min with signs of poor perfusion?   **No**

Start CPR.

- Continue rescue breathing; check pulse about every 2 min.
- If no pulse, start CPR.

No breathing or only gasping, pulse not felt

Start CPR
- First rescuer perform cycles of 30 compressions and 2 breaths.
- When second rescuer returns, perform cycles of 15 compressions and 2 breaths.
- Use AED as soon as it is available.

Check rhythm. Shockable rhythm?

Yes, shockable

No, nonshockable

- Give 1 shock. Resume CPR immediately for 2 min (until prompted by AED to allow rhythm check).
- Continue until ALS providers take over or the child starts to move.

- Resume CPR immediately for 2 min (until prompted by AED to allow rhythm check).
- Continue until ALS providers take over or the child starts to move.

©2020 American Heart Association

Fig. 3.5 Pediatric Basic Life Support Algorithm for Healthcare Providers—2 or More Rescuers. *AED,* Automated external defibrillator; *ALS,* advanced life support; *CPR,* cardiopulmonary resuscitation; *HR,* heart rate. (From Topjian, A. A., Raymond, T. T., Atkins, D., Chan, M., Duff, J. P., Joyner Jr, B. L., et al. [2021]. Part 4: Pediatric Basic and Advanced Life Support 2020 American Heart Association Guidelines for Cardiopulmonary Resuscitation and Emergency Medical Care. *Pediatrics, 147*[Suppl 1], e2020038505D.)

arms once again and turn the infant over so that the infant is lying on their back along your arm which should be placed on your thigh for support.

L. Deliver 5-chest thrusts in the same location used for CPR compressions. Alternate 5 back slaps and 5 chest thrusts until the object is expelled or the infant becomes unresponsive.

M. If unresponsive begin the steps of CPR—in this sequence—every time before you administer a breath—check the airway for foreign objects.

N. For a Responsive Child the steps for FBAO in a child are exactly the same as you would use with an adult FBAO victim.

Pediatric Cardiac Arrest Algorithm

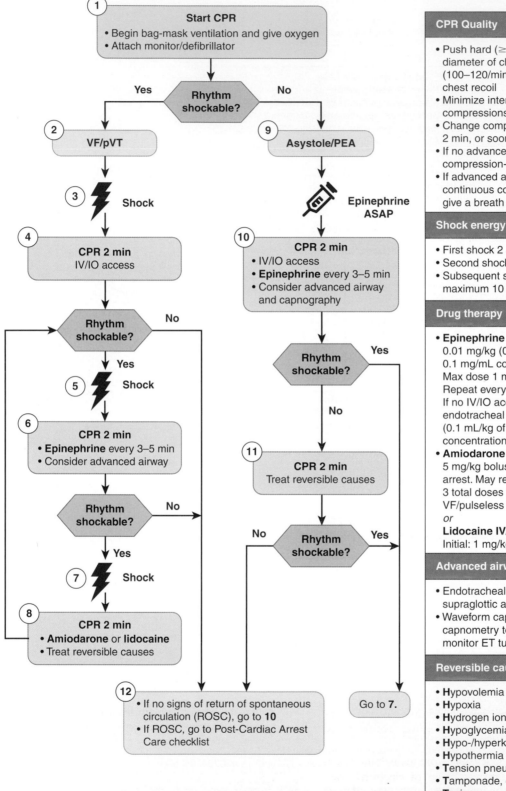

CPR Quality

- Push hard (≥$\frac{1}{3}$ of anteroposterior diameter of chest) and fast (100–120/min) and allow complete chest recoil
- Minimize interruptions in compressions
- Change compressor every 2 min, or sooner if fatigued
- If no advanced airway, 15:2 compression-ventilation ratio
- If advanced airway, provide continuous compressions and give a breath every 2–3 s

Shock energy for defibrillation

- First shock 2 J/kg
- Second shock 4 J/kg
- Subsequent shocks ≥4 J/kg, maximum 10 J/kg or adult dose

Drug therapy

- **Epinephrine IV/IO dose:** 0.01 mg/kg (0.1 mL/kg of the 0.1 mg/mL concentration). Max dose 1 mg. Repeat every 3–5 min. If no IV/IO access, may give endotracheal dose: 0.1 mg/kg (0.1 mL/kg of the 1 mg/mL concentration).
- **Amiodarone IV/IO dose:** 5 mg/kg bolus during cardiac arrest. May repeat up to 3 total doses for refractory VF/pulseless VT

  or

  Lidocaine IV/IO dose: Initial: 1 mg/kg loading dose

Advanced airway

- Endotracheal intubation or supraglottic advanced airway
- Waveform capnography or capnometry to confirm and monitor ET tube placement

Reversible causes

- **H**ypovolemia
- **H**ypoxia
- **H**ydrogen ion (acidosis)
- **H**ypoglycemia
- **H**ypo-/hyperkalemia
- **H**ypothermia
- **T**ension pneumothorax
- **T**amponade, cardiac
- **T**oxins
- **T**hrombosis, pulmonary
- **T**hrombosis, coronary

©2020 American Heart Association

Fig. 3.6 Pediatric Cardiac Arrest Algorithm. *ASAP,* As soon as possible; *CPR,* cardiopulmonary resuscitation; *ET,* endotracheal; *HR,* heart rate; *IO,* intraosseous; *IV,* intravenous; *PEA,* pulseless electrical activity; *VF/pVT,* ventricular fibrillation/pulseless ventricular tachycardia. (From Topjian, A. A., Raymond, T. T., Atkins, D., Chan, M., Duff, J. P., Joyner Jr, B. L., et al. [2021]. Part 4: Pediatric Basic and Advanced Life Support 2020 American Heart Association Guidelines for Cardiopulmonary Resuscitation and Emergency Medical Care. *Pediatrics, 147*[Suppl 1], e2020038505D.)

O. Please review previous information
See Figs. 3.4–3.6.

FLUID AND ELECTROLYTE BALANCE

Electrolytes play a vital role in maintaining homeostasis within the body.

- Electrolytes help to regulate myocardial and neurological functions, fluid balance, oxygen delivery, acid–base balance, and much more.
- The most serious electrolyte disturbances involve abnormalities in the levels of sodium, potassium, and/or calcium.
- Kidneys work to keep the electrolyte concentrations in the blood constant despite changes in the body.
- Homeostasis: The ability of a system or living organism to adjust its internal environment to maintain a stable equilibrium, such as the ability of warm-blooded animals to maintain a constant temperature.
- Electrolyte: Any of the various ions (such as sodium or chloride) that regulate the electric charge on cells and the flow of water across their membranes.
- Sodium: A chemical element with symbol Na (from Latin: natrium) and atomic number 11. It is a soft, silvery white, highly reactive metal and is a member of the alkali metals.

Importance of Electrolyte Balance

Electrolytes maintain voltages across their cell membranes, especially those of the nerve, heart, and muscle and carry electrical impulses across nerve impulses, muscle contractions, and to other cells.

Electrolyte imbalances can develop from dehydration and over hydration. The most common cause of electrolyte disturbances is renal failure. The most serious electrolyte disturbances involve abnormalities in the levels of sodium, potassium, and/or calcium.

Other electrolyte imbalances are less common, and often occur in conjunction with major electrolyte changes. Chronic laxative abuse or severe diarrhea or vomiting (gastroenteritis) can lead to electrolyte disturbances combined with dehydration. People suffering from bulimia or anorexia nervosa are especially at high risk for an electrolyte imbalance.

Kidneys work to keep the electrolyte concentrations in blood constant despite changes in your body. For example, during heavy exercise electrolytes are lost through sweating, particularly sodium and potassium, and sweating can increase the need for electrolyte (salt) replacement. It is necessary to replace these electrolytes to keep their concentrations in the body fluids constant.

Dehydration

There are three types of dehydration:

1. Hypotonic or hyponatremic (primarily a loss of electrolytes, sodium in particular).
2. Hypertonic or hypernatremic (primarily a loss of water).
3. Isotonic or isonatremic (an equal loss of water and electrolytes).
4. Hypotonic or hyponatremic (primarily a loss of electrolytes, sodium in particular).
5. Hypertonic or hypernatremic (primarily a loss of water).
6. Isotonic or isonatremic (an equal loss of water and electrolytes).

Solutions used for intravenous rehydration must be isotonic or hypotonic.

Fig. 3.7 illustrates the mechanism for the transportation of water and electrolytes across the epithelial cells in the secretory glands.

For review, see Table 3.6.

> **HESI HINT** The most common type of dehydration is isotonic (isonatremic) dehydration, which effectively equates with hypovolemia; but the distinction of isotonic from hypotonic or hypertonic dehydration may be important when treating people with dehydration.
>
> Physiologically, dehydration is both loss of water and solutes (mainly sodium) and are usually lost in roughly equal quantities as to how they exist in blood plasma.

> **HESI HINT**
> 1. Hypotonic or hyponatremic (primarily a loss of electrolytes, sodium in particular).
> 2. Hypertonic or hypernatremic (primarily a loss of water).
> 3. Isotonic or isonatremic (an equal loss of water and electrolytes).
> 4. Hypotonic or hyponatremic (primarily a loss of electrolytes, sodium in particular).
> 5. Hypertonic or hypernatremic (primarily a loss of water).
> 6. Isotonic or isonatremic (an equal loss of water and electrolytes

Fluid Volume Deficit: Dehydration

- *Fluid volume deficit* (FVD) or hypovolemia (may be acute or chronic); fluid output exceeds the fluid intake; the body

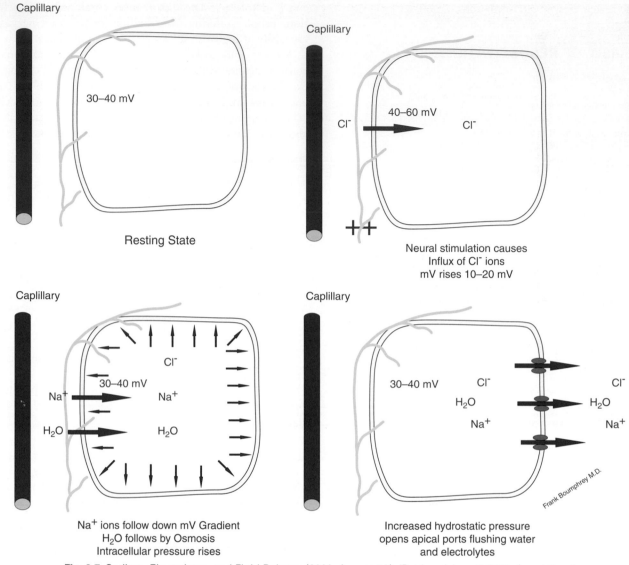

Fig. 3.7 Sodium, Electrolytes, and Fluid Balance (2020, August 13). (Retrieved June 7, 2021, from https://med.libretexts.org/@go/page/8178.)

loses both water and electrolytes from the ECF in similar proportions.

- Common sources of fluid loss are the gastrointestinal tract, polyuria, and increased perspiration.
- Risk factors for FVD: vomiting, diarrhea, GI suctioning, sweating, decreased intake, nausea, inability to gain access to fluids, adrenal insufficiency, osmotic diuresis, hemorrhage, coma, third-space fluid shifts, burns, ascites, and liver dysfunction
- Appropriate management is vital to prevent potentially life-threatening hypovolemic shock.
- Elderly patients are more likely to develop fluid imbalances.
- The goals of management are to treat the underlying disorder and return the extracellular fluid compartment to normal, to restore fluid volume, and to correct any electrolyte imbalances.

Causes of Fluid Volume Deficit

- Abnormal losses through the skin, GI tract, or kidneys.
- Decrease in intake of fluid (e.g., inability to intake fluid due to oral trauma)
- Bleeding
- Movement of fluid into third space.
- Diarrhea
- Diuresis
- Abnormal drainage
- Inadequate fluid intake
- Increased metabolic rate (e.g., fever, infection)

Organ Function

A. Kidneys
   1. Main function of the kidneys is to filter blood and adjust the amount and composition of fluids in the body. The

TABLE 3.6 Fluid Volume

Variable	Deficit	Excess
Description	• Occurs when the body loses water and electrolytes isotonically—(i.e., in the same proportion as exists in the normal body fluid) • Serum electrolyte levels remain normal • Dehydration: state in which the body loses water and serum sodium levels increase	• Occurs when the body retains water and electrolytes isotonically • Water intoxication: state in which the body retains water and serum sodium levels decrease
Causes	• Vomiting • Diarrhea • Gastrointestinal suctioning • Sweating • Inadequate fluid intake • Massive edema, as in initial stage of major burns • Ascites • Older adults forgetting to drink	• Heart failure (HF) • Renal failure • Cirrhosis, liver failure • Excessive ingestion of table salt • Overhydration with sodium-containing fluid • Poorly controlled intravenous (IV) therapy, especially in young and old clients
Symptoms	• Weight loss (1 L of fluid weight loss or gain is approximately equal to 2.2 pounds or 1 kg) • Decreased skin turgor • Oliguria (concentrated urine) • Dry and sticky mucous membranes • Postural hypotension or weak, rapid pulse	• Peripheral edema • Increased bounding pulse • Elevated BP • Distended neck and hand veins • Dyspnea; moist crackles heard when lungs auscultated • Attention loss, confusion, aphasia • Altered level of consciousness
Laboratory findings	• Elevated blood urea nitrogen (BUN) and creatinine • Increased serum osmolarity • Elevated hemoglobin and hematocrit	• Decreased BUN • Decreased hemoglobin and hematocrit • Decreased serum osmolality • Decreased urine osmolality and specific gravity
Treatment and nursing care	• Strict I&O • Replacement of fluids isotonically, preferably orally • *Water is a hypotonic fluid.* • If intravenous hydration is needed, isotonic fluids are used.	• Diuretics • Fluid restriction • Strict I&O • Sodium-restricted diet • Weighed daily • Serum K^+ monitored

total blood volume is determined by a client's gender, height, and weight. The average healthy adult has approximately 5.2 to 6 L of circulating blood in the body.

2. As a result of this filtration process, the kidney selectively maintains and excretes body fluids, producing approximately 1 to 2 L of urine (30 mL/h).
3. Regulates sodium and potassium levels and maintains the pH level by excreting or maintaining hydrogen ions and bicarbonate
4. Excretes metabolic wastes and toxic substances.
5. The kidneys are also responsible for manufacturing the hormone erythropoietin (EPO) (Fig. 3.8).

B. Lungs
   1. Regulate CO_2 concentration as a result of O_2 and CO_2 gas exchange at the alveolar capillary beds, thus influencing the acid-base balance.
   2. Water loss via lung is affected by the external temperature and humidity.

At 35°C and humidity at 75% respectively, the loss of water via the lung during inspiration and expiration is ∼7 mL/h. When the parameters change for example and this can increase or decrease the lung excretion to minus 10°C and 25% lung excretion of H_2O increases up to 20 mL/h (Zieliński & Przybylski, 2012).

C. Heart
   1. Pumps blood with sufficient force to perfuse the kidneys, allowing the kidneys to work effectively.
   2. Potassium, sodium, and calcium electrolyte levels are crucial in maintaining adequate electrical conductivity to help with efficient myocardial pumping action.

D. Adrenal glands
   1. Secretes aldosterone when the body's BP becomes low, resulting in sodium retention (leading to water retention), thereby increasing BP and potassium excretion to maintain homeostasis.

E. Parathyroid glands
   1. Regulates calcium and phosphorus balance levels in blood by increasing or decreasing the manufacture of parathyroid hormone, which influences transference of calcium and phosphorous from the bones.

F. Pituitary gland
   1. Secretes antidiuretic hormone (ADH), which causes the body to retain water by signaling the kidneys to increase the water absorption when filtering the blood.

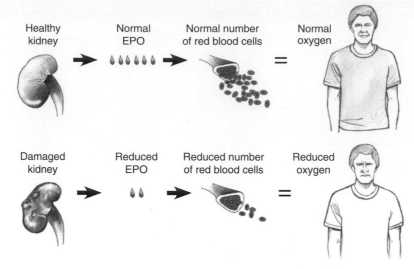

Fig. 3.8 Top: Kidney → normal EPO → normal number RBCs → normal O_2. **Bottom**: Damaged kidney → reduced EPO → fewer RBCs → reduced O_2. *EPO,* Erythropoietin. (From Brugnara, C., & Eckardt, K. U. [2011]. *Hematologic aspects of kidney disease.* In Taal MW [Ed.], *Brenner and Rector's: The kidney* [9th ed., pp. 2081–2120]. St. Louis: Saunders. National Kidney and Urologic Diseases Information Clearinghouse from National Institute of Diabetes and Digestive and Kidney Diseases.)

Electrolyte Imbalance
Clinical Assessment and Clinical Judgment Measures
See (Table 3.7).

HESI HINT Potassium imbalances are potentially life threatening and must be corrected immediately. A low magnesium level often accompanies a low potassium level, especially with the use of diuretics. Magnesium must be corrected to normalize potassium.

INTRAVENOUS THERAPY

Overview: Although the PN may not administer IV solutions and medications, it is important for the PN to apply the following information to assist the RN and other health care providers to monitor the client receiving IV therapy. IV solutions are used to supply electrolytes, nutrients, and water.

Administration of Intravenous Therapy
A. The purpose and duration of the IV therapy is determined by the underlying condition/situation. This also determines the type of equipment, such as vascular access device, including IV tubing and the size of the catheter.
B. Types of vascular devices for IV administration
  1. Peripheral
  2. Central
C. Gloves *must* be worn during venipunctures and when discontinuing an IV line.
D. Assess the IV and insertion site frequently (minimum of every 2 hours) for the prescribed rate of infusion and for patency.
E. Intermittent IV therapy may be given through a saline lock; flushing per facility policy.
F. IV tubing and dressing should be changed according to facility policy.
G. When the IV catheter is discontinued, apply pressure to the site for 1 to 3 minutes for peripheral lines and 5 to 10 minutes for central lines after the catheter is removed (central lines are only removed by provider orders and nurses must be educated on removal to prevent air embolism), and inspect the tip of the catheter to ensure it is intact; then document. It is not appropriate for a PN to remove a central line.

Complications Associated With Intravenous Administration
Infections such as septicemia
1. Aseptic and antiseptic technique should be used when starting an IV and caring for the IV site.
2. Inspect all fluids and containers before use to ensure that they have not been opened, contaminated, or expired.
3. Change administration sets per agency policy or at least every 96 hours.
4. Primary IV solution bags should not hang for more than 24 hours.
5. Do not irrigate blocked cannulas.
  A PE occurs when a substance or clot is propelled by venous circulation to the right side of the heart and subsequently into the pulmonary artery.
1. Special blood tubing with a clot filter is used when infusing blood or blood products.

TABLE 3.7 Electrolyte Imbalances

Abnormalities and Common Causes	Signs and Symptoms	Treatment
Hyponatremia (↓Na) • Diuretics • GI fluid loss • Hypotonic tube feeding • D$_5$W or hypotonic IV fluids • Diaphoresis	• Craving for salt • Anorexia, nausea, and vomiting • Weakness • Lethargy • Confusion • Muscle cramps, twitching • Seizures • Na <135 mEq/L	• Restrict fluids (safer) • If IV saline solutions prescribed, the solution should be administered very slowly; use isotonic saline if fluid restriction is not effective
Hypernatremia (↑Na) • Water deprivation • Hypertonic tube feeding • Diabetes insipidus • Heatstroke • Hyperventilation • Watery diarrhea • Renal failure • Cushing syndrome	• Thirst • Hyperpyrexia • Sticky mucous membranes • Dry mouth • Hallucinations • Lethargy • Irritability • Seizures • Na >145 mEq/L	• Restrict sodium in the diet • Beware of "hidden" sodium in foods and medications • Increase water intake
Hypokalemia (↓K) • Diuretics • Diarrhea • Vomiting • Gastric suction • Steroid administration • Hyperaldosteronism • Amphotericin B • Bulimia • Cushing syndrome	• Fatigue • Anorexia • Nausea, vomiting • Muscle weakness • Decreased GI motility • Dysrhythmias • Paresthesia • Flat T waves on ECG • K$^+$ <3.5 mEq/L	• Potassium supplements can be given both orally or IV • Oral forms of potassium are unpleasant tasting and are irritating to the GI tract (do not give on empty stomach; dilute) • Potassium IV should *never* be given as a bolus • Assess renal status—that is, urinary • Encourage foods high in potassium, such as bananas, oranges, cantaloupe, avocadoes, spinach, potatoes
Hyperkalemia (↑K) • Hemolyzed serum sample produces pseudohyperkalemia • Oliguria • Acidosis • Renal failure • Addison disease • Multiple blood transfusions	• Muscle weakness • Bradycardia • Dysrhythmias • Flaccid paralysis • Intestinal colic • Tall T waves on ECG • K$^+$ >5 mEq/L	• Do not give parenteral potassium • 50% glucose with regular insulin can be given to reduce the potassium level • Kayexalate can also be used to reduce serum potassium • Monitor ECG • Calcium gluconate is given to protect the heart • IV loop diuretics may be prescribed • Renal dialysis may be required
Hypocalcemia (↓Ca) • Renal failure • Hypoparathyroidism • Malabsorption • Pancreatitis • Alkalosis	• Diarrhea • Numbness • Tingling of extremities • Convulsions • Positive Trousseau sign • Chvostek sign • Calcium (Ca) <8.5 mEq/L • At risk for tetany	• Administer calcium supplements orally 30 min before meals • IV calcium should be given slowly and can cause tissue necrosis • Increase calcium intake, such as dairy products, greens

Continued

TABLE 3.7 Electrolyte Imbalances—cont'd

Abnormalities and Common Causes	Signs and Symptoms	Treatment
Hypercalcemia (↑Ca)		
• Hyperparathyroidism	• Muscle weakness	• Eliminate parenteral calcium
• Malignant bone disease	• Constipation	• Administer agents to reduce calcium such as calcitonin
• Prolonged immobilization	• Anorexia	• Avoid calcium-based antacids
• Excess calcium supplementation	• Nausea, vomiting	• Loop diuretics may be used
• Diuretic phase of acute renal failure	• Polyuria	• Renal dialysis may be required
	• Polydipsia	
	• Neurosis	
	• Dysrhythmias	
	• Ca >10.5 mEq/L	
Hypomagnesemia (↓Mg)		
• Alcoholism	• Anorexia, distention	• Magnesium sulfate IV should be given
• Malabsorption	• Neuromuscular irritability	• Encourage foods high in magnesium, such as meats, nuts, legumes, fish, and vegetables
• Diabetic ketoacidosis	• Depression	
• Prolonged gastric suction	• Disorientation	
• Diuretics	• Mg <1.5 mEq/L	
Hypermagnesemia (↑Mg)		
• Renal failure	1. Flushing	• Avoid magnesium-based antacids and laxatives
• Adrenal insufficiency	2. Hypotension	• Restrict dietary intake of foods high in magnesium
• Excess replacement	3. Drowsiness, lethargy	
	4. Hypoactive reflexes	
	5. Depressed respirations	
	6. Bradycardia	
	7. Mg >2.5 mEq/L	
Hypophosphatemia (↓pH)		
• Refeeding after starvation	• Paresthesias	• Correct underlying cause
• Alcohol withdrawal	• Muscle weakness	• Administer oral replacement of phosphates with vitamin D
• Diabetic ketoacidosis	• Muscle pain	
• Respiratory alkalosis	• Mental changes	
	• Cardiomyopathy	
	• Respiratory failure	
	• pH <2 mEq/L	
Hyperphosphatemia (↑pH)		
• Renal failure	• Short term: tetany symptoms	• Administer aluminum hydroxide with meals to bind phosphorus
• Excess intake of phosphorus	• Long term: phosphorus precipitation in nonosseous sites	• Dialysis may be required if renal failure is underlying cause
	• pH >4.5 mEq/L	

ECG, Electrocardiogram; *GI*, gastrointestinal; *IV*, intravenous.

2. Lower extremity veins should be avoided for cannulation.
3. Do not irrigate plugged cannulas.
4. If a blood clot has occurred, subsequent IVs should not be started below the site of occurrence.

> **HESI HINT** An air embolism can be fatal if the pulmonary capillaries are blocked. Watch for empty IV fluid containers and ensure all central lines are capped and locked if not in use.

Circulatory overload is especially hazardous for patients with impaired renal or cardiac functioning.
1. The infusion rate should be maintained at the prescribed rate.

2. Observe for signs of circulatory overload: weight gain; edema; pulmonary edema, which is characterized by dyspnea, cough, sweating and frothy pinkish sputum; decreased SAO$_2$; puffy eyelids and ascites. REPORT findings of circulatory overload to the RN and decrease the IV fluid rate as directed.

Phlebitis can occur because of mechanical, chemical, and/or septic causes.
1. Cannulation sites should not be placed over a joint.
2. Cannulas should be well anchored to prevent motion, thereby reducing the risk of entry of microorganisms into the puncture wound.

3. The cannula size should be smaller than the vein.
4. Use aseptic and antiseptic technique.

Remove the cannula within 96 hours or immediately if one of the following occurs: erythema, induration, tenderness when palpating the vein, or leaking at the insertion site.

> **HESI HINT** If an IV catheter is suspected as the causative factor of sepsis, the catheter should be removed and blood cultures drawn and sent to the laboratory.

> **HESI HINT** Flushing a saline lock: Attach NS prefilled Luer **lock** syringe by twisting the syringe to the positive pressure cap. Inject 3–5 mL of solution using turbulent stop-start technique. **Flush** until visibly clear. Do not bottom out syringe (leave 0.2–0.5 mL in the syringe).

> **HESI HINT** Laws for licensed PN (LPN) in many states limit IV and blood product administration. The PN needs to be aware of the Scope of Practice in his or her state and the agency's policies. In some states, additional IV classes may be required for the PN to start IVs.

Acid-Base Balance

Description: An acid-base balance must be maintained in the body because alterations can result in alkalosis or acidosis.

A. Maintaining the acid-base balance is imperative and involves three systems:
   1. Chemical buffer system
   2. Kidneys
   3. Lungs
B. Acid-base balance is determined by the hydrogen ion concentration in body fluids.
   1. Normal range is 7.35 to 7.45 expressed as the pH (Fig. 3.9).
   2. A pH level below 7.35 indicates acidosis.
   3. A pH level above 7.45 indicates alkalosis.
   4. Measurement is made by examining ABGs (see Fig. 3.1 and Table 3.8).

Chemical Buffer System

Chemical buffers act quickly to prevent major changes in body fluid pH by removing or releasing hydrogen ions. The buffer systems in the human body are extremely efficient, and different systems work at different rates taking seconds for the chemical buffers in the blood to make adjustments to pH.

The respiratory tract can adjust the blood pH upward in minutes by exhaling CO_2 from the body.

The renal system can also adjust blood pH through the excretion of hydrogen ions (H^+) and the conservation of bicarbonate, but this process takes hours to days to have an effect.

The buffer systems functioning in blood plasma include plasma proteins, phosphate, and bicarbonate and carbonic acid buffers.

The kidneys help control acid-base balance by excreting hydrogen ions and generating bicarbonate that helps maintain

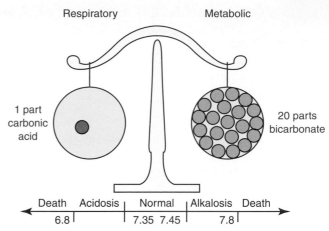

Fig. 3.9 Relationship of Sodium Bicarbonate to Carbonic Acid. (From Potter, P. A., & Perry, A. G. [2009]. *Fundamentals of nursing* [7th ed.]. St. Louis: Mosby.)

TABLE 3.8 Arterial Blood Gas Comparisons

Acid-Base Conditions	pH	Pco$_2$ (mm Hg)	HCO$_3$ (mEq/L)
Normal	7.35–7.45	35–45	21–28
Respiratory acidosis	↓	↑	Normal
Respiratory alkalosis	↑	↓	Normal
Metabolic acidosis	↓	Normal	↓
Metabolic alkalosis	↑	Normal	↑

blood plasma pH within a normal range. Protein buffer systems work predominantly inside cells.

A. The main chemical buffer is the bicarbonate—carbonic acid (HCO_3–H_2CO_3) system.
B. The bicarbonate-carbonic acid buffer works in a fashion similar to phosphate buffers. The bicarbonate is regulated in the blood by sodium, as are the phosphate ions. When sodium bicarbonate ($NaHCO_3$) comes into contact with a strong acid, such as HCl, carbonic acid (H_2CO_3), which is a weak acid, and NaCl are formed. When carbonic acid comes into contact with a strong base, such as NaOH, bicarbonate and water are formed.

$$NaHCO_3 + HCl \rightarrow H_2CO_3 + NaCl$$

(sodium bicarbonate) + (strong acid) → (weak acid) + (salt)

$$H_2CO_3 + NaOH \rightarrow HCO_3^- + H_2O$$

(weak acid) + (strong base) → (bicarbonate) + (water)

   1. With 20 times more bicarbonate than carbonic acid, this capture system is most efficient at buffering changes that would make the blood more acidic. This is useful because most of the body's metabolic wastes, such as lactic acid and ketones, are acids. Carbonic acid levels in the blood are controlled by the expiration of CO_2 through the lungs.

2. Excess CO_2 in the body alters the ratio and creates an imbalance. Other chemical buffers involve:
   a. Phosphate
   b. Protein
   c. Hemoglobin
   d. Plasma

Lungs

A. Control CO_2 content through respirations (carbonic acid content).
B. Control, to a small extent, water balance ($CO_2 + H_2O = H_2CO_3$).
C. Release excess CO_2 by increasing respiratory rate.
D. Retain CO_2 by decreasing respiratory rate.

Kidneys

A. Regulate bicarbonate levels by retaining and reabsorbing bicarbonate as needed.
B. Provide a very slow compensatory mechanism (can require hours or days).
C. Cannot help with compensation when metabolic acidosis is created by renal failure.

Determining Acid-Base Disorders

A. In uncompensated acid-base disturbances:
B. Arrows are used to indicate whether the pH, Pco_2, or HCO_3 is high ($\uparrow$), low ($\downarrow$), or within normal limits (WNL) ($\leftarrow \rightarrow$).
C. When pH is high ($\uparrow$), alkalosis is present.
D. In respiratory disorders, the HCO_3 is normal, and the arrows for pH and Pco_2 point in opposite directions. The tables should demonstrate the arrows
E. In metabolic disorders, the Pco_2 is normal, and the arrows for pH and HCO_3 point in the same direction or are equal (see Table 3.8) Please add arrows
F. The body will begin to compensate in acid-base disorders to bring the pH back within the normal range of 7.35 to 7.45 (see Table 3.8).
G. Example: For a client with a pH of 7.29 ($\downarrow$), a Pco_2 of 50 ($\uparrow$), and an HCO_3 of 28 ($\leftarrow \rightarrow$):
   1. Determine the pH: acidosis.

2. Determine the Pco_2: respiratory.
3. Determine HCO_3: not metabolic.
4. Respiratory acidosis is the disorder (see Table 3.8)
5. Determine state of compensation: The client's ABG reflects an uncompensated state $\rightarrow$ indicating more interventions need to be implemented (Biga et al., 2020).

> **HESI HINT** The acronym "ROME" can help you remember: respiratory, opposite, metabolic, equal.

? REVIEW OF FLUID AND ELECTROLYTE BALANCE

1. List four common causes of fluid volume deficit.
2. List four common causes of fluid volume overload.
3. Identify two examples of isotonic IV fluids.
4. List three systems that maintain acid-base balance.
5. Cite the normal ABGs for the following:
   A. pH
   B. Pco_2
   C. HCO_3

See Answer Key at the end of this text for suggested responses.

ELECTROCARDIOGRAM

Description: The visual representation of the electrical activity of the heart reflected by changes in the electrical potential at the skin surface, which is a record of the heart's electrical events that precede them. The visual representation of an ECG can be recorded as a tracing on a strip of graph paper or seen on an oscilloscope (Fig. 3.10).
A. The following conditions can interfere with normal heart functioning:
   1. Disturbances of rate or rhythm
   2. Disorders of conductivity
   3. Enlarged heart chambers
   4. Presence of MI
   5. Fluid and electrolyte imbalances

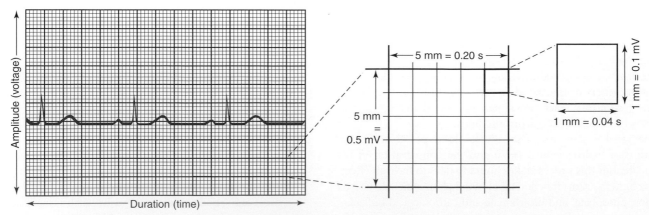

Fig. 3.10 Composition of Electrocardiogram Paper. (Electrocardiograph waveforms are measured in amplitude (voltage) and duration (time). From Ignatavicius, D. D., & Workman, M. L. [2016]. *Medical-surgical nursing: client-centered collaborative care* [8th ed.]. St. Louis: Saunders.)

B. Each ECG should include identifying information:
1. Patient's name and identification number
2. Location, time, and date of recording
3. Age, gender, and current cardiac and noncardiac medications
4. Height, weight, and BP
5. Clinical diagnosis and current clinical status
6. Any unusual position of the client during the recording
7. If present, thoracic deformities, respiratory distress, and muscle tremor

---

HESI HINT Blood flow through the heart

Superior/inferior VENA CAVA (unoxygenated) → Right ATRIUM → (Tricuspid Valve) → Right

VENTRICLE → (Pulmonic Valve) Pulmonary Artery → LUNGS (gas exchanged at alveoli—oxygenated) → Left ATRIUM → (Mitral Valve) → Left VENTRICLE → (Aortic Valve) → Aorta

Review the three structures that control the one-way flow of blood through the heart:

Atrioventricular valves
Tricuspid (right side)
Mitral (left side)
Semilunar valves
Pulmonic (in pulmonary artery)
Aortic (in aorta)
Chordae tendineae
Papillary muscles

From Patton, K. T., Bell, F., Thompson, T., & Williamson, P. (2010). From Anatomy and physiology (11th ed.). St. Louis: Mosby. *Anatomy and physiology* (11th ed.). St. Louis: Mosby.

C. The standard ECG is the 12-lead ECG.
D. Bedside monitoring through telemetry is more commonly seen in the clinical setting.
1. Telemetry uses three or five leads transmitted to an oscilloscope.
2. Graphic information is printed either on request or at any time the set parameters are transcended.
E. A portable continuous monitor (Holter monitor) can be placed on the client to provide a magnetic tape recording. While wearing a Holter monitor, the client is instructed to keep a diary concerning:
1. Activity

2. Medications
3. Chest pains
F. The ECG graph paper consists of small and large squares (see Fig. 3.10).
1. The small squares represent 0.04 second each; five of these small squares combine to form one large square.
2. Each large square represents 0.20 second (0.04 second × 5). Five large squares represent 1 second. Calculation of heart rate uses the 6-second rule (Box 3.2):
   a. Easiest means of calculating the heart rate.
   b. This cannot be used when the heart rate is irregular.
   c. Thirty large squares equal one 6-second time interval.
   d. Count the number of regular rate (RR) intervals in the 30 large squares and multiply by 10 to determine the heart rate for 1 minute (the R is the high peak on the strip; (see Fig. 3.10 and Box 3.2).
G. Composition of the ECG: normal **ECG** contains waves, intervals, segments, and one complex, as defined below. Wave: A positive or negative deflection from baseline that indicates a specific electrical event. The waves on an **ECG** include the P wave, Q wave, R wave, S wave, T wave, and U wave.
1. P wave: atrial systole
   a. Represents depolarization of the atrial muscle
   b. Should be rounded and without peaking or notching
2. QRS complex: ventricular systole
   a. Represents depolarization of the ventricular muscle
   b. Normally follows the P wave
   c. Is measured from the beginning of the QRS to the end of the QRS (normal <0.12 second)
   d. T wave: ventricular diastole
      1) Represents repolarization of the ventricular muscle
      2) Follows the QRS complex
      3) Usually is slightly rounded, without peaking or notching

---

HESI HINT The T wave represents repolarization of the ventricle, so this is a critical time in the heartbeat. This action represents a resting and regrouping stage so that the next heartbeat can occur. If defibrillation occurs during this phase, the heart can be thrust into a life-threatening dysrhythmia.

BOX 3.2   Methods for Estimating Heart Rate Using an Electrocardiogram Tracing

1. Measure the interval between consecutive QRS complexes, determine the number of small squares, and divide 1500 by that number. This method is used only when the heart rhythm is regular.
2. Measure the interval between consecutive QRS (Q wave, R wave and S wave) complexes, determine the number of large squares, and divide 300 by that number. This method is used only when the heart rhythm is regular.
3. Determine the number of RR intervals within 6 s and multiply by 10. The ECG paper is conveniently marked at the top with slashes that represent 3-s intervals. This method can be used when the rhythm is irregular. If the rhythm is extremely irregular, an interval of 30–60 s should be used.

4. Count the number of big blocks between the same points in any two successive QRS complexes (usually R wave to R wave) and divide by 300 because there are 300 big blocks in 1 min. It is easiest to use a QRS that falls on a dark line. If little blocks are left over when counting big blocks, count each little block as 0.2, add this to the number of big blocks, and then divide by 300.
5. The memory method relies on memorization of the following sequence: 300, 150, 100, 75, 60, 50, 43, 37, 33, 30. Find a QRS complex that falls on the dark line representing 0.2 s or a big block, and count backward to the next QRS complex. Each dark line is a memorized number. This is the method most widely used in hospitals for calculating heart rates for regular rhythms.

Adapted from Monahan, F. D., & Phipps, W. J. (2007). *Phipps' medical-surgical nursing: health and illness perspectives* (8th ed.). St. Louis: Mosby; and Ignatavicius, D. D., & Workman, M. L. (2010). *Medical-surgical nursing: Client-centered collaborative care* (6th ed.). St. Louis: Saunders.

3. ST segment
   a. Represents early ventricular repolarization
   b. Is measured from the end of the S wave to the beginning of the T wave
4. PR interval
   a. Represents the time required for the impulse to travel from the atria (sinoatrial node), through the atrioventricular (AV) node, to the Purkinje fibers in the ventricles
   b. Is measured from the beginning of the P wave to the beginning of the QRS complex
   c. Represents AV nodal function (normal 0.12 to 0.20 second)
5. U wave
   a. Is not always present
   b. Is most prominent in the presence of hypokalemia
6. QT interval
   a. Represents the time required to completely depolarize and repolarize the ventricles
   b. Is measured from the beginning of the QRS complex to the end of the T wave
7. RR interval
   a. Reflects the regularity of the heart rhythm
   b. Is measured from one QRS to the next QRS

HESI HINT NGN-NCLEX-RN questions are likely to relate to early recognition of abnormalities and associated clinical actions. Remember to monitor the patient as well as the machine! Feel the pulse! Listen to the heart. Evaluate the blood pressure. If the ECG monitor shows a severe dysrhythmia but the client is sitting up quietly watching television without any sign of distress, assess to determine whether the leads are attached properly.

⚡ REVIEW OF ELECTROCARDIOGRAM

1. Identify the waveforms found in a normal ECG.
2. In an ECG reading, which wave represents depolarization of the atrium?
3. In an ECG reading, what complex represents depolarization of the ventricle?
4. What does the PR interval represent?
5. If the U wave is most prominent, what condition might the nurse suspect?
6. Describe the calculation of the heart rate using an ECG rhythm strip (see Fig. 3.10).
7. What is the most important assessment data for the nurse to obtain in a client with an arrhythmia?
8. What are the possible lethal dysrhythmias?

See Answer Key at the end of this text for suggested responses.

PERIOPERATIVE CARE

Description: The perioperative period includes client care before surgery (preoperative), during surgery (intraoperative), and after surgery (postoperative).
A. The nurse's role is to

1. Educate and advocate
2. Reduce anxiety
3. Promote an uncomplicated perioperative period for the client and family
B. Surgery is performed under aseptic conditions in either a hospital or an alternative hospital setting (ambulatory surgical center or health care provider's office).
C. Patient safety is a serious concern during the perioperative period. Steps should be implemented to ensure safety.
D. Surgical Risk Factors Refer to
1. Age: very young and very old
2. Nutrition: obesity and malnutrition increase surgical risk
3. Fluid and electrolyte status: dehydration and hypovolemia increase surgical risk because of imbalances in calcium, magnesium, potassium, and phosphorus.
4. General health: any infection or pathology increases surgical risk.
   a. Cardiac conditions: angina, coronary artery disease, MIs, valvular problems, hypertension, dysrhythmias, health failure (well-controlled cardiac problems pose little risk).
   b. Blood coagulation disorders can lead to severe bleeding, hemorrhage, and shock or blood clotting disorders.
   c. Upper respiratory tract infections (surgery is usually delayed when the patient has an upper respiratory disorder) and chronic obstructive pulmonary disease (COPD) are exacerbated by general anesthesia and adversely affect pulmonary function. If the client has had a history of asthma, inquire about inhaled or oral corticosteroid and bronchodilators. Inquire about smoking status.
   d. Renal disease, such as a renal insufficiency, impairs fluid and electrolyte regulation. Many drugs are metabolized and excreted by the kidneys, so a decrease in renal function can lead to an altered response to drugs and unpredictable drug elimination.
   e. Endocrine disorders, such as diabetes mellitus, predispose patients to wound infection and delayed healing. History of thyroid dysfunction (either hyper or hypo) can place the client at surgical risk because of alterations in the metabolic rate. Addison disease requires special consideration during surgery. Addisonian crisis or shock can occur if patient abruptly stops taking replacement corticosteroids and stress of surgery may require additional IV corticosteroid therapy.
   f. Liver disease impairs the liver's ability to detoxify medications used during surgery to produce prothrombin or to metabolize nutrients for wound healing. Consider the presence of liver disease if there is a history of jaundice, hepatitis, alcohol abuse, or obesity.
   g. Impairment of the immune system can lead to delayed wound healing and increased risk for postoperative infections. Chronic infections like hepatitis B

or C, AIDS, human immunodeficiency virus (HIV), and tuberculosis (TB) require infection control precautions for the protection of the patient and staff.

E. Current medications: Prescription and over-the-counter drugs. Medications that increase surgical risk include:
1. Anticoagulants (increase blood coagulation time).
2. Tranquilizers (may cause hypotension).
3. Heroin, other recreational drugs, and alcohol abuse (decrease CNS response).
4. Antibiotics (may be incompatible with anesthetics).
5. Diuretics (may precipitate electrolyte imbalance.
6. Steroids (decreased wound healing).
7. Over-the-counter natural supplements.
8. Vitamin E (may increase the risk of bleeding when used with warfarin or other herbal medications such as ginkgo, ginger, and garlic).
9. Nonsteroidal antiinflammatory drugs (NSAIDs) inhibit platelet aggregation.

Preoperative Care

Description: Care provided from the time the client and family make the decision to have surgery until the client is taken to the operative suite

Data to Obtain When Taking a Preoperative Clinical History

A. Age
B. Allergies to medications, foods, and topical antiseptics (iodine, betadine, hibiclens)
C. Current medications: prescriptions, over-the-counter, and herbal preparations
D. History of medical and surgical problems of the patient and immediate family members
E. Previous surgical experiences
F. Previous experience with anesthesia
G. Tobacco, alcohol, and drug abuse
H. Understanding of surgical procedure and risks involved
I. Coping resources
J. Cultural and ethnic factors that may affect surgery

Key Components of Preoperative Teaching Plans

A. Regulations concerning valuables, jewelry, dentures, and hearing aids
B. Food and fluid restrictions such as nothing by mouth (NPO) timing or exceptions per prescription by health care provider.
C. Invasive procedures such as urinary catheters, IVs, nasogastric (NG) tubes, enemas, and vaginal preparations
D. Preoperative medications
E. OR, transportation, skin preparation, postanesthesia
F. Postoperative procedures:
1. Respiratory care, such as ventilator, incentive spirometer, deep breather, splinting
2. Activity, such as range of motion, leg exercises, early ambulation, turning

3. Pain control, such as IM medications, patient-controlled analgesia (PCA)
4. Dietary restrictions
5. ICU or post anesthesia care unit (PACU) orientation (recovery room)

Preoperative Checklist Information

A. Informed consent, surgical consent, signed by the surgeon and the client, and witnessed by the nurse. Consent to treatment must be obtained before administration of any narcotics or other medications affecting the client's cognition. (Follow facility policy for consent validity.)
B. Site is marked by the person performing surgery. Before the incision is initiated, all team members confirm identity, procedure, site of surgery, and consents.
C. History and physical examination (by health care provider) are noted in chart with validity per facility policy.
D. Preop lab or diagnostic tests completed as ordered.
E. Identification band is on client and allergies are noted.
F. Contact lenses, glasses, dentures, partial plates, wigs, jewelry, artificial eyes, prostheses, makeup, and nail polish have been removed per facility policy or as prescribed by health care provider.
G. Client has voided or been catheterized.
H. Client is in hospital gown.
I. Vital signs: BP, temperature, pulse, and respirations have been taken.
J. Premedications, including antibiotics, have been given; types and times have been noted.
K. Skin preparation has been performed (if prescribed by health care provider or physician): Based on facility policy
L. Vital signs completed
M. Signature of nurse certifies completion of list.

HESI HINT Marking the operative site is required for procedures involving right/left distinctions, multiple structures (fingers, toes), and levels (spinal procedures). Site marking should be done with the involvement of the client.

Intraoperative Care

Description: From the time the client is received in the operative suite until admission to the PACU, an OR nurse is in charge of care. "If the circulating nurse is not an RN, the licensed PN or surgical technician must have immediate access to the RN at all times."

A. Maintain quiet during induction.
B. Maintain safety:
1. Conduct client identification: right client, right procedure, right anatomic site.
2. Ensure that sponge, needle, and instrument counts are accurate. Counts are to be done and verified and

documented by two personnel before, during, before closing incision(s), and end of the surgery.

3. Position client during procedure to prevent injury.
4. Strictly adhere to asepsis during all intraoperative procedures.
5. Ensure adequate functioning suction setups are in place.
6. Take responsibility for correct labeling, handling, and deposition of any and all specimens.

C. Monitor physical status.
1. If excessive blood loss occurs, calculate effect on client.
2. Report changes in pulse, temperature, respirations, and BP to surgeon, in conjunction with anesthesiologist/certified registered nurse anesthetist (CRNA).
3. Positioning the patient is a critical part of every procedure and usually follows administration of the anesthetic.

D. Provide psychological support:
1. Provide emotional support to client and family immediately before, during, and after surgery.
2. Arrange with physician to provide information to the family if surgery is prolonged or complications or unexpected findings occur.
3. Communicate emotional state of client to other health care team members.

Postoperative Care

Description: From admission to discharge or until client has recovered

A. Initially, the patient may go PACU.
B. On arrival, the client is assessed for vital signs (BP, pulse, respirations, temperature), level of consciousness, skin color and condition, dressing location and condition, IV fluids, drainage tubes, position, and O_2 saturation levels.
C. When client has been stabilized, and it has been prescribed by the health care provider, the client is then discharged or transferred to the general clinical unit or the ICU.
D. Immediate postoperative clinical care should include:
1. Monitoring for signs of shock and hemorrhage: hypotension, narrow pulse pressure, rapid weak pulse, cold moist skin, increased capillary filling time, and decreased urine output (Table 3.9)
2. Positioning client on side (if not contraindicated) to prevent aspiration and to allow client to cough out airway; side rails should be up at all times
3. Providing warmth with heated blanket
4. Managing nausea and vomiting with antiemetic drugs and NG suctioning
5. Managing pain with analgesics

TABLE 3.9 Common Postoperative Complications

Postoperative Complication	Occurrence	Interventions for Preventions
• Urinary retention	• 8—12 h postoperatively	• Monitor hydration status and encourage oral intake if allowed • Monitor for first void after surgery • Offer bedpan or assist to commode • Catheterize as needed per prescription
• Pulmonary problems • Atelectasis • Pneumonia • Embolus	• 1—2 days postoperatively	• Assist client to turn, cough, deep breathe every 2 h • Keep client hydrated • Early ambulation • Early incentive spirometer (per hospital protocol)
• Wound-healing problems	• 5—6 days postoperatively	• Splint incision when client coughs • Monitor for signs of infection, malnutrition, dehydration • High-protein diet • Maintain dressing per prescription • Keep wound clean and dry
• Urinary tract infections	• 5—8 days postoperatively	• Oral fluid intake • Emptying of bladder every 4—6 h • Monitor intake and output • Avoid catheterizations if possible
• Thrombophlebitis	• 6—14 days postoperatively	• Leg exercises every 2 h while in bed • Early ambulation • Apply antiembolic (TED) stockings or sequential hose as prescribed; remove TEDs every 8 hours and reapply • Apply alternating compression devices • Avoid pressure that may obstruct venous flow; do not raise knee gatch on bed, do not place pillows beneath knees, avoid crossing legs at knees • Low-dose heparin may be used prophylactically
• Decreased gastrointestinal peristalsis • Constipation • Paralytic ileus	• 2—4 days postoperatively	• Nasogastric tubing to decompress gastrointestinal tract • Client to limit use of narcotic analgesics that decrease peristalsis • Encourage early ambulation • Encourage oral fluid intake if allowed

6. Checking with anesthesiologist about intraoperative medications before administering pain medications.
7. Determining intraoperative irrigations and instillations with drains to help evaluate amount of drainage on dressing and in drainage collection devices
8. Assess bladder for urinary retention if the client does not have a catheter.
9. Most PACU settings use a scoring system to determine whether the client meets the criteria to be discharged from the PACU.
10. Handoff report should be in an SBAR[a] format:

HESI HINT Wound dehiscence is separation of the wound edges; it is more likely to occur with vertical incisions. Wound dehiscence usually occurs after the early postoperative period, when the client's own granulation tissue is "taking over" the wound, after absorption of the sutures has begun. Evisceration of the wound is protrusion of intestinal contents (in an abdominal wound) and is more likely in clients who are older, diabetic, obese, or malnourished, and who have prolonged paralytic ileus.

HESI HINT NGN-NCLEX-PN items may focus on the nurse's role in terms of the entire perioperative process.

Example: A 43-year-old mother of two teenage daughters enters the hospital to have her gallbladder removed in a same-day surgery using an endoscope instead of an incision. What clinical needs will dominate each phase of her short hospital stay?

Preoperative phase: education about postoperative care, including NPO, assistance with meeting family needs

Operative phase: assessment, management of the operative suite

Postanesthesia phase: pain management, postanesthesia precautions

Postoperative phase: prevention of complications, assessment for pain management, and teaching about dietary restrictions and activity levels.

HESI HINT NGN-NCLEX-PN items may focus on delivery of safe effective care.

Time Out and Hand-Off (SBAR) communication are best practices implemented to prevent serious medical error during the perioperative period. **Time Out** occurs before making the incision, and the entire surgical team pauses as the surgical site listed on the consent is read aloud. The entire team confirms that this information is correct. The **Hand-Off** (SBAR) communication is the transfer of relevant patient information during the perioperative period, which is standardized and must include an opportunity to ask and to respond to questions.

---

[a]The SBAR (**Situation-Background-Assessment-Recommendation**) technique provides a framework for communication between members of the health care team about a patient's condition. S = Situation (a concise statement of the problem) B = Background (pertinent and brief information related to the situation) A = Assessment (analysis and considerations of options—what you found/think) R = Recommendation (action requested/recommendation)

❓ REVIEW OF PERIOPERATIVE CARE

1. List five variables that increase surgical risk.
2. Why is a patient with liver disease at increased risk for operative complications?
3. Preoperative teaching should include demonstration and explanation of expected postoperative client activities. What activities should be included?
4. What items should the nurse assist the patient in removing before surgery?
5. How is the patient positioned in the immediate postoperative period, and why?
6. List three nursing judgment measures that prevent postoperative wound dehiscence and evisceration.
7. Identify three nursing judgment measures that prevent postoperative urinary tract infections.
8. Identify nursing judgment measures that prevent postoperative paralytic ileus.
9. List four nursing judgment measures that prevent postoperative thrombophlebitis.
10. During the intraoperative period, what activities should the OR nurse perform to ensure safety during surgery?
11. How is handoff given?

See Answer Key at the end of this text for suggested responses.

HIV INFECTION

Description: Infection with HIV. The infection is a retrovirus which is blood-borne and attracted to CD4+T cells. Exposure to this blood pathogen is generally acquired through contact of infected blood or blood products, unprotected sex with an infected individual, or fetal exposure from an infected mother through placental transmission or exposure of maternal bodily fluids during birth. In the United States, according to the Centers for Disease Control (CDC), an estimated 1.2 million people in the United States had HIV at the end of 2018, the most recent year for which this information is available. Of those people, about 14%, or 1 in 7, did not know they had HIV. HIV is a virus that attacks the body's immune system. If HIV is not treated, it can lead to AIDS (acquired immunodeficiency syndrome) (Box 3.3).

There is currently no effective cure. Once people get HIV, they have it for life and with proper medical care, HIV can be controlled. People with HIV who get effective HIV treatment can live long, healthy lives and protect their partners. By taking HIV medicine (called antiretroviral therapy or ART), people with HIV can live longer and prevent transmitting HIV to their sexual partners. In addition, there are effective methods to prevent getting HIV through sex or drug use, including preexposure prophylaxis (PrEP) and post-exposure prophylaxis (PEP).

A. HIV is caused by a retrovirus, which destroys CD4 cells (also called T cells or helper cells), which are critical to the immune system. CD4 cells are responsible for keeping people healthy and protecting them from common diseases and infections.

B. The virus enters the cell and begins to replicate. CD4+ T cells are known to be the central facilitators for both

---

BOX 3.3　Stages of Human Immunodeficiency Virus

When people with HIV don't get treatment, they typically progress through three stages. But HIV medicine can slow or prevent progression of the disease. With the advancements in treatment, progression to Stage 3 is less common today than in the early days of HIV.

Stage 1: Acute HIV Infection

- People have a large amount of HIV in their blood. They are very contagious.
- Some people have flu-like symptoms. This is the body's natural response to infection.
- But some people may not feel sick right away or at all.
- If you have flu-like symptoms and think you may have been exposed to HIV, seek medical care and ask for a test to diagnose acute infection.
- Only antigen/antibody tests or nucleic acid tests (NATs) can diagnose acute infection.

Stage 2: Chronic HIV Infection

- This stage is also called asymptomatic HIV infection or clinical latency.
- HIV is still active but reproduces at very low levels.

- People may not have any symptoms or get sick during this phase.
- Without taking HIV medicine, this period may last a decade or longer, but some may progress faster.
- People can transmit HIV in this phase.
- At the end of this phase, the amount of HIV in the blood (called *viral load*) goes up and the CD4 cell count goes down. The person may have symptoms as the virus levels increase in the body, and the person moves into Stage 3.
- People who take HIV medicine as prescribed may never move into Stage 3.

Stage 3: Acquired Immunodeficiency Syndrome (AIDS)

- The most severe phase of HIV infection.
- People with AIDS have such badly damaged immune systems that they get an increasing number of severe illnesses, called opportunistic infections.
- People receive an AIDS diagnosis when their CD4 cell count drops below 200 cells/mm, or if they develop certain opportunistic infections.
- People with AIDS can have a high viral load and be very infectious.
- Without treatment, people with AIDS typically survive about three years.

From Centers for Disease Control and Prevention. About HIV. Available at: https://www.cdc.gov/hiv/basics/whatishiv.html.

---

cellular and humoral immune responses against exogenous antigens and are kept constant in the human body by homeostatic mechanisms. HIV binds to the CD4 molecule on the surface of helper T cells and replicates within them. This results in destruction of CD4+ T cells and leads to a steady decline in the population of T cells. In normal healthy adults the CD4 count ranges from 500 to 1200 cells/mm^3, depending on the laboratory (Diao et al., 2020).

C. Individuals experiencing an acute infection that includes fever, lymphadenopathy, and sore throat which are also symptoms of acute HIV and referral for testing is suggested.

Complications

HIV infection weakens your immune system, making you much more likely to develop many infections and certain types of cancers.

Infections Common to Human Immunodeficiency Virus/Acquired Immunodeficiency Syndrome

A. *Pneumocystis pneumonia (PCP)*. This fungal infection can cause severe illness. Although it is declined significantly with current treatments for HIV/AIDS, in the United States. PCP is still the most common cause of pneumonia in people infected with HIV (Table 3.11).

B. Candidiasis (thrush). Candidiasis is a common HIV-related infection. It causes inflammation and a thick, white coating on your mouth, tongue, esophagus, or vagina.

C. TB. In resource-limited nations, TB is the most common opportunistic infection associated with HIV. It is a leading cause of death among people with AIDS.

D. Cytomegalovirus (CMV). This common herpes virus is transmitted in body fluids such as saliva, blood, urine, semen, and breast milk. A healthy immune system

inactivates the virus, and it remains dormant in your body. If your immune system weakens, the virus resurfaces—causing damage to your eyes, digestive tract, lungs, or other organs.

E. Cryptococcal meningitis. Meningitis is an inflammation of the membranes and fluid surrounding your brain and spinal cord (meninges). Cryptococcal meningitis is a common CNS infection associated with HIV, caused by a fungus found in soil.

F. Toxoplasmosis. This potentially deadly infection is caused by Toxoplasma gondii, a parasite spread primarily by cats. Infected cats pass the parasites in their stools, which may then spread to other animals and humans. Toxoplasmosis can cause heart disease, and seizures occur when it spreads to the brain.

Cancers Common to Human Immunodeficiency Virus/Acquired Immunodeficiency Syndrome

A. Lymphoma. This cancer starts in the white blood cells. The most common early sign is painless swelling of the lymph nodes in your neck, armpit, or groin.

B. Kaposi sarcoma. A tumor of the blood vessel walls, Kaposi sarcoma usually appears as pink, red, or purple lesions on the skin and mouth. In people with darker skin, the lesions may look dark brown or black. Kaposi sarcoma can also affect the internal organs, including the digestive tract and lungs (Table 3.10).

Other Complications

A. Wasting syndrome. Untreated HIV/AIDS can cause significant weight loss, often accompanied by diarrhea, chronic weakness, and fever.

TABLE 3.10 Opportunistic Infections

Pneumocystis carinii Pneumonia	Kaposi Sarcoma	Cryptosporidiosis	Candidiasis of OralCavity and Esophagus
• Fever • Dry cough • Dyspnea at rest • Chills	• Purple-blue lesions on skin, often arms and legs • Invasion of gastrointestinal tract, lymphatic system, lungs, and brain	• Severe, watery diarrhea (may be 30–40 stools per day) • Abdominal cramps • Nausea • Electrolyte imbalance • Malaise	• Thick, white exudate in the mouth • Unusual taste to food • Retrosternal burning • Oral ulcers
Cryptococcal Meningitis	**Cytomegalovirus (CMV) Retinitis**	**CMV Colitis**	**Disseminated CMV**
• Headache • Changes in level of consciousness • Nausea, vomiting • Stiff neck • Blurred vision	• Most common CMV infection in persons with AIDS • Impaired vision in one or both eyes • Can lead to blindness	• Diarrhea • Malabsorption of nutrients • Weight loss	• Malaise • Fever • Pancytopenia • Weight loss • Positive cultures from blood, urine, or throat
Perirectal Mucocutaneous Herpes Simplex Viral Infections	**Lymphomas of Central Nervous System**	**Tuberculosis (TB)**	**HIV Encephalopathy**
• Severe pain • Bleeding, rectal discharge • Ulceration in the rectal area	• Change in mental status • Apathy • Psychomotor slowing • Seizures	• Pulmonary and extrapulmonary • Lymphatic and hematogenous TB are common; negative skin testing does not rule out TB • TB skin test is positive if induration of 5 mm or more if client is immunosuppressed	• Memory loss and impaired concentration • Apathy • Depression • Psychomotor slowing (most prominent symptom) • Incontinence • CT scan findings: diffuse atrophy and ventricular enlargement

CT, Computed tomography.

B. Neurological complications. HIV can cause neurological symptoms such as confusion, forgetfulness, depression, anxiety, and difficulty walking. HIV-associated neurocognitive disorders (HAND) can range from mild symptoms of behavioral changes and reduced mental functioning to severe dementia causing weakness and inability to function.

C. Kidney disease. HIV-associated nephropathy (HIVAN) is an inflammation of the tiny filters in your kidneys that remove excess fluid and wastes from your blood and pass them to your urine. It most often affects black or Hispanic people.

D. Liver disease. Liver disease is also a major complication, especially in people who also have hepatitis B or hepatitis C.

E. No HIV test can detect HIV immediately after infection. If there has been an exposure to HIV in the last 72 hours, discuss PEP.

F. The time between when a person gets HIV and when a test can accurately detect it is called the **window period**. The window period varies from person to person and also depends on the type of HIV test.

G. Initial symptoms may occur 2 to 4 weeks post first exposure to HIV, after which the person becomes asymptomatic. Persons infected with HIV can transmit the virus to others any time after infection has occurred, whether they are symptomatic or asymptomatic.

H. Nucleic Acid Test (NAT)—A NAT can usually tell you if you have HIV infection 10 to 33 days after exposure.

I. Antigen/Antibody Test—An antigen/antibody test performed by a laboratory on blood from a vein can usually detect HIV infection 18 to 45 days after exposure. Antigen/antibody tests done with blood from a finger prick take longer to detect HIV (18 to 90 days after an exposure). CDC tracks HIV diagnoses among racial and ethnic groups such as: American Indian/Alaska Native, Asian, Black/African American, Hispanic/Latino, Native Hawaiian and other Pacific Islander, White, and multiracial people. The CDC site that is most helpful is: https://www.cdc.gov/hiv/statistics/overview/index.html.

Clinical Assessment of Adult Human Immunodeficiency Virus Infection

Initially, an individual commonly experiences an acute infection that includes fever, lymphadenopathy, and sore throat, which are also symptoms of acute HIV. Health care providers can refer clients and recommend access to laboratory-based follow-up or immediate testing with point-of-care tests performed on finger-stick whole blood or oral secretions or immediate HIV repeat testing with an additional HIV point-of-care test. The following symptoms may occur:

- Extreme fatigue
- Loss of appetite and unexplained weight loss of greater than 10 lbs in 2 months.
- Swollen glands, sore throat, headache, and malaise
- Muscle weakness and joint pain
- Unexplained fever for more than a week.
- Night sweats.
- Unexplained chronic diarrhea
- Dry cough: may represent PCP
- White spots in the mouth and throat; may represent candidiasis.
- Painful blisters may represent shingles
- Painless, purple-blue lesions on the skin.
- Confusion, disorientation
- In women, recurrent vaginal infections that are resistant to treatment.
- Opportunistic infections.

When people with HIV don't get treatment, they typically progress through three stages (Table 3.11). But HIV medicine can slow or prevent progression of the disease. With the advancements in treatment, progression to Stage 3 is less common today than in the early days of HIV. **Untreated, HIV** typically turns into **AIDS** in about 8 to 10 years. When **AIDS** occurs, your immune system has been severely damaged. You'll be more likely to develop opportunistic infections or opportunistic cancers—diseases that wouldn't usually cause illness in a person with a healthy immune system.

Risk groups for acquiring HIV include the following:
1. Have sex with many partners (men or women).
2. Have unsafe sex with an infected person.
3. Share needles to take drugs or steroids.
4. Have unprotected sex for drugs or money.
5. *Have another* sexually transmitted infection (STI).

There are several treatment options available to help patients prevent the spread of HIV. Depending on the stage of HIV, often patients may be prescribed a variety of options (Box 3.4).

Clinical Assessment

A. Obtain prescription for and review laboratory testing. CDC recommends that everyone between the ages of 13 and 64 get tested for HIV at least once. People at higher risk should get tested more often.
   1. All pregnant women should be tested to begin treatment as early as possible to reduce the risk of transmitting HIV to the child.
   2. Refer to the CDC for current testing guidelines: https://www.cdc.gov/hiv/guidelines/testing.html.
   3. HIV treatment should be initiated as quickly as possible after diagnosis.

> **HESI HINT** An individual exposed to HIV may remain asymptomatic for many years dependent on various factors and if he or she is actively under a medical regimen of ART. The stages of HIV infection are presented in Table 3.11.
>
> Patients are only admitted to the hospital for treatment until their HIV status has progressed to an "AIDS" diagnosis because their nursing care is much more demanding (see Box 3.3).

When people with HIV don't get treatment, they typically progress through three stages. But HIV medicine can slow or prevent progression of the disease. With the advancements in treatment, progression to Stage 3 is less common today than in the early days of HIV (see Box 3.3).

TABLE 3.11   Stages of Human Immunodeficiency Virus Infection

Stage	Clinical Symptoms
Stage 1: Acute HIV Infection	1. People have a large amount of HIV in their blood. They are very contagious. 2. Some people have flu-like symptoms. This is the body's natural response to infection. 3. But some people may not feel sick right away or at all. 4. If you have flu-like symptoms and think you may have been exposed to HIV, seek medical care and ask for a test to diagnose acute infection. 5. Only antigen/antibody tests or nucleic acid tests (NATs) can diagnose acute infection.
Stage 2: Chronic HIV Infection	1. This stage is also called asymptomatic HIV infection or clinical latency. 2. HIV is still active but reproduces at very low levels. 3. People may not have any symptoms or get sick during this phase. 4. Without taking HIV medicine, this period may last a decade or longer, but some may progress faster. 5. People can transmit HIV in this phase. 6. At the end of this phase, the amount of HIV in the blood (called viral load) goes up and the CD4 cell count goes down. The person may have symptoms as the virus levels increase in the body, and the person moves into Stage 3. 7. People who take HIV medicine as prescribed may never move into Stage 3.
Stage 3: Acquired Immunodeficiency Syndrome (AIDS)	1. The most severe phase of HIV infection. 2. People with AIDS have such badly damaged immune systems that they get an increasing number of severe illnesses, called opportunistic infections. 3. People receive an AIDS diagnosis when their CD4 cell count drops below 200 cells/mm, or if they develop certain opportunistic infections. 4. People with AIDS can have a high viral load and be very infectious. 5. Without treatment, people with AIDS typically survive about three years.

HIV Testing. Linkage to Care. The Time Is Now

Diagnosing HIV quickly and linking people to treatment immediately are crucial to achieving further reduction in new HIV infections. Usually, it is the primary care providers (PCPs are the first to detect and assist in the prevention and spread of HIV (Box 3.4). The Centers for Disease Control and prevention recommend that PCPs do the following:

- Perform HIV screening when indicated
- Adequately screen patients who are at risk for HIV
- Assist patients who test positive with HIV treatment, care, and prevention.

> **HESI HINT** HIV clients with tuberculosis require respiratory isolation. Tuberculosis can be transmitted in virtually any setting. Clinicians should be aware that transmission has been documented in health care settings where health care workers (HCWs) and patients come in contact with persons with infectious TB who:
> - Have unsuspected TB disease,
> - Have not received adequate or appropriate treatment, or
> - Have not been separated from others.

From https://www.cdc.gov/tb/education/corecurr/pdf/chapter7.pdf; Center for Disease Control (CDC). (n.d.). Tuberculosis infection control (Chapter 7). Retrieved October 12, 2021, from https://www.cdc.gov/tb/education/corecurr/pdf/chapter7.pdf.

BOX 3.4 Prevention Options for Human Immunodeficiency Virus Infection

Use treatment as prevention (TasP). If you're living with HIV, taking HIV medication can keep your partner from becoming infected with the virus. If you make sure your viral load stays undetectable—a blood test doesn't show any virus—you won't transmit the virus to anyone else. Using TasP means taking your medication exactly as prescribed and getting regular checkups.

Use post-exposure prophylaxis (PEP). *Use post-exposure prophylaxis (PEP) if you've been exposed to HIV.* If you think you've been exposed through sex, needles, or in the workplace, contact your doctor or go to the emergency department. Taking PEP as soon as possible within the first 72 hours can greatly reduce your risk of becoming infected with HIV. You will need to take medication for 28 days.

Use a new condom every time you have sex. Use a new condom every time you have anal or vaginal sex. Women can use a female condom. If using a lubricant, make sure it's water-based. Oil-based lubricants can weaken condoms and cause them to break. During oral sex use a nonlubricated, cut-open condom or a dental dam—a piece of medical-grade latex.

Consider preexposure prophylaxis (PrEP). The combination drugs emtricitabine plus tenofovir (Truvada) and emtricitabine plus tenofovir alafenamide (Descovy) can reduce the risk of sexually transmitted HIV infection in people at very high risk. PrEP can reduce your risk of getting HIV from sex by more than 90% and from injection drug use by more than 70%, according to the Centers for Disease Control and Prevention. Descovy hasn't been studied in people who have receptive vaginal sex.

Clinical Assessment and Interventions for Human Immunodeficiency Virus Patients With Tuberculosis

A. Assess respiratory functioning frequently.
B. Avoid known sources of infection.
C. Use strict asepsis for all invasive procedures.
D. Obtain vital signs frequently.
E. Plan activities to allow for rest periods.
F. Elevate head of bed (HOB).
G. Refer client to nutritionist.
H. Offer small, frequent feedings.
I. Weigh daily.
J. Encourage client to avoid fatty foods.
K. Monitor for skin breakdown and offer good skin care.
L. Use safety precautions for clients with neurologic symptoms or loss of vision.
M. Orient client who is confused.

> **HESI HINT**
> **Standard Precautions**
> - Wash hands, even if gloves have been worn to give care.
> - Wear examination gloves for touching blood or body fluids or any nonintact body surface.
> - Wear gowns during any procedure that might generate splashes (e.g., changing clients with diarrhea).
> - Use masks and eye protection during activity that might disperse droplets (e.g., suctioning).

N. Provide emotional, cultural, and spiritual support for the grieving client who is losing all relationships and skills.
O. Provide emotional support for significant others: family, family of choice, partners, and friends.
P. Administer IV fluids for hydration, as prescribed.
Q. Administer total parenteral nutrition (TPN) as prescribed.
R. Administer agents that treat specific opportunistic infections and medications for HIV (Table 3.12). Educate the client about the need to maintain compliance with medication regimen even if the client does not feel ill.
S. Assist with pain management; administer prescribed narcotics or analgesics.
T. Collaborate with RN to develop and implement client/family teaching about ways to avoid infection.
See Table 3.13.

> **HESI HINT** The CDC does not recommend excluding pregnant health care workers from caring for patients with known CMV infection. Health care workers should be careful with all patients they encounter. Spread of CMV requires direct contact with virus-containing secretions. Hand washing and using gloves are excellent ways to prevent infection.

TABLE 3.12 Human Immunodeficiency Virus Drugs

Drugs	Indications	Adverse Reactions	Nursing Implications
• NRT (NucleoTide) Inhibitors • Tenofovir	HIV infection classifications used in various combinations to reduce viral load and slow development of resistance	• Headache • Renal insufficiency • Fever, rash, N/V, abdominal cramps	• Monitor for lactic acidosis
• Non-NRT Inhibitors • Efavirenz • Delavirdine • Nevirapine • Etravirine		• CNS changes • Nausea • Rash • Triglycerides • Hepatotoxicity	• Many drug–drug interactions • Monitor liver function tests • Reduces contraceptive effects
• Protease Inhibitors • Indinavir • Amprenavir • Saquinavir • Ritonavir • Nelfinavir • Lopinavir + ritonavir • Fosamprenavir (Lexiva) • Atazanavir		• Depression • Ketoacidosis • Seizures • Angioedema • Stevens-Johnson syndrome	• Many drug–drug interactions • High-fat, high-protein foods reduce absorption • Give most of these with food • Reduces contraceptive effects
• Combination Products • Lamivudine + zidovudine • ○Zidovudine + lamivudine + abacavir • Emtricitabine + tenofovir • Tenofovir + emtricitabine + efavirenz		• Monitor for side effects associated with the individual drugs	• Note implications of the individual drugs in the combination product
• CCR5 Inhibitors • Maraviroc		• Hepatotoxicity • Cough, fever, rash, hypotension • Increased risk of infection	• Use cautiously in clients with underlying liver, renal, and cardiac disease
• Fusion Inhibitors • Enfuvirtide		• Infection risk and lipodystrophy if injection site is not rotated	• Monitor skin reactions at injection site
• Antiprotozoals • Atovaquone • Trimethoprim/sulfamethoxazole • Pentamidine isethionate	Atovaquone used for PCP in those unable to tolerate trimethoprim/sulfamethoxazole prophylaxis Prophylaxis for PCP Treatment of PCP	1. CNS disturbances 2. Agranulocytosis 3. Phlebitis if IV 4. Renal calculi with Bactrim 5. Leukopenia 6. ECG abnormalities	• Enhances effects of oral hypoglycemics • Increases thrombocytopenia risk if given with thiazide diuretics • Check for allergy to sulfonamide • IV or aerosol; not oral • Use careful precautions against potential spread of TB
• Antivirals • Acyclovir sodium • Valacyclovir • Famciclovir • Ganciclovir • Valganciclovir	Herpes simplex CMV retinitis	• Granulocytopenia • Thrombocytopenia	• Give with or without food • Many incompatibilities: IV, PO, topical • Monitor liver function tests
• Antifungals • Amphotericin B • Caspofungin • Fluconazole • Flucytosine • Anidulafungin • Posaconazole • Itraconazole • Micafungin • Voriconazole	IV: Cryptococcal meningitis PO: Oral candidiasis	• Nephrotoxicity • Hypotension • Hypokalemia • Febrile reaction • Muscle cramps • Circulatory problems	• Many drug–drug interactions • Vesicant: monitor IV site closely; premedicate with antipyretic; give slowly • Swish as long as possible before swallowing PO form

Note: Client should have regular blood counts to track CD4 levels and viral load.
CMV, Cytomegalovirus; *CNS,* central nervous system; *ECG,* electrocardiogram; *IV,* intravenous; *N/V, nausea and vomiting*; *PCP, Pneumocystis carinii* pneumonia; *PO,* by mouth.

TABLE 3.13 HIV Drugs

Drug Class	Generic Name (Other Names and Acronyms)	Brand Name
Nucleoside Reverse Transcriptase Inhibitors (NRTI) are antiviral drugs used against HIV block reverse transcriptase, an enzyme HIV needs to make copies of itself.	abacavir (abacavir sulfate, ABC)	Ziagen
	emtricitabine (FTC)	Emtriva
	lamivudine (3TC)	Epivir
	tenofovir disoproxil fumarate (tenofovir DF, TDF)	Viread
	zidovudine (azidothymidine, AZT, ZDV)	Retrovir
Nonnucleoside reverse transcriptase inhibitors (NNRTIs) are small molecule drugs that bind directly to the active site of HIV-1 reverse transcriptase bind to and later alter reverse transcriptase, an enzyme HIV needs to make copies of itself.	doravirine (DOR)	Pifeltro
	efavirenz (EFV)	Sustiva
	etravirine (ETR)	Intelence
	nevirapine (extended-release nevirapine, NVP)	Viramune / Viramune XR (extended release)
	rilpivirine (rilpivirine hydrochloride, RPV)	Edurant
Protease inhibitors (PIs) are medications that work with antiretroviral drugs to treat HIV. block HIV protease, an enzyme HIV needs to make copies of itself.	atazanavir (atazanavir sulfate, ATV)	Reyataz
	darunavir (darunavir ethanolate, DRV)	Prezista
	fosamprenavir (fosamprenavir calcium, FOS-APV, FPV)	Lexiva
	ritonavir* (RTV)	Norvir
	*Although ritonavir is a PI, it is generally used as a pharmacokinetic enhancer as recommended in the Guidelines for the Use of Antiretroviral Agents in Adults and Adolescents Living with HIV and the Guidelines for the Use of Antiretroviral Agents in Pediatric HIV Infection.	
	saquinavir (saquinavir mesylate, SQV)	Invirase
	tipranavir (TPV)	Aptivus
Fusion inhibitors block HIV from entering the CD4 T lymphocyte (CD4 cells) of the immune system.	enfuvirtide (T-20)	Fuzeon
CCR5 antagonists block CCR5 coreceptors on the surface of certain immune cells that HIV needs to enter the cells.	maraviroc (MVC)	Selzentry
Integrase inhibitors block HIV integrase, an enzyme HIV needs to make copies of itself.	cabotegravir (cabotegravir sodium, CAB)	Vocabria
	dolutegravir (dolutegravir sodium, DTG)	Tivicay
	raltegravir (raltegravir potassium, RAL)	Isentress / Isentress HD
Attachment inhibitors bind to the gp120 protein on the outer surface of HIV, preventing HIV from entering CD4 cells.	fostemsavir (fostemsavir tromethamine, FTR)	Rukobia
Post-attachment inhibitors block CD4 receptors on the surface of certain immune cells that HIV needs to enter the cells.	ibalizumab-uiyk (Hu5A8, IBA, Ibalizumab, TMB-355, TNX-355)	Trogarzo

Continued

TABLE 3.13   HIV Drugs—cont'd

Drug Class	Generic Name (Other Names and Acronyms)	Brand Name
Pharmacokinetic enhancers are used in HIV treatment to increase the effectiveness of an HIV medicine included in an HIV treatment regimen. Combination HIV medicines contain two or more HIV medicines from one or more drug classes.	cobicistat (COBI, c)	Tybost
	abacavir and lamivudine (abacavir sulfate/lamivudine, ABC/3TC)	Epzicom
	abacavir, dolutegravir, and lamivudine (abacavir sulfate/dolutegravir sodium/lamivudine, ABC/DTG/3TC)	Triumeq
	abacavir, lamivudine, and zidovudine (abacavir sulfate/lamivudine/zidovudine, ABC/3TC/ZDV)	Trizivir
	atazanavir and cobicistat (atazanavir sulfate/cobicistat, ATV/COBI)	Evotaz
	bictegravir, emtricitabine, and tenofovir alafenamide (bictegravir sodium/emtricitabine/tenofovir alafenamide fumarate, BIC/FTC/TAF)	Biktarvy
	cabotegravir and rilpivirine (CAB and RPV, CAB plus RPV, Cabenuva kit, cabotegravir extended-release injectable suspension and rilpivirine extended-release injectable suspension)	Cabenuva
	darunavir and cobicistat (darunavir ethanolate/cobicistat, DRV/COBI)	Prezcobix
	darunavir, cobicistat, emtricitabine, and tenofovir alafenamide (darunavir ethanolate/cobicistat/emtricitabine/tenofovir AF, darunavir ethanolate/cobicistat/emtricitabine/tenofovir alafenamide, darunavir/cobicistat/emtricitabine/tenofovir AF, darunavir/cobicistat/emtricitabine/tenofovir alafenamide fumarate, DRV/COBI/FTC/TAF)	Symtuza
	dolutegravir and lamivudine (dolutegravir sodium/lamivudine, DTG/3TC)	Dovato
	dolutegravir and rilpivirine (dolutegravir sodium/rilpivirine hydrochloride, DTG/RPV)	Juluca
	doravirine, lamivudine, and tenofovir disoproxil fumarate (doravirine/lamivudine/TDF, doravirine/lamivudine/tenofovir DF, DOR/3TC/TDF)	Delstrigo
	efavirenz, emtricitabine, and tenofovir disoproxil fumarate (efavirenz/emtricitabine/tenofovir DF, EFV/FTC/TDF)	Atripla
	efavirenz, lamivudine, and tenofovir disoproxil fumarate (EFV/3TC/TDF)	Symfi
	efavirenz, lamivudine, and tenofovir disoproxil fumarate (EFV/3TC/TDF)	Symfi Lo
	elvitegravir, cobicistat, emtricitabine, and tenofovir alafenamide (elvitegravir/cobicistat/emtricitabine/tenofovir alafenamide fumarate, EVG/COBI/FTC/TAF)	Genvoya
	elvitegravir, cobicistat, emtricitabine, and tenofovir disoproxil fumarate (QUAD, EVG/COBI/FTC/TDF)	Stribild
	emtricitabine, rilpivirine, and tenofovir alafenamide (emtricitabine/rilpivirine/tenofovir AF, emtricitabine/rilpivirine/tenofovir alafenamide fumarate, emtricitabine/rilpivirine hydrochloride/tenofovir AF, emtricitabine/rilpivirine hydrochloride/tenofovir alafenamide, emtricitabine/rilpivirine hydrochloride/tenofovir alafenamide fumarate, FTC/RPV/TAF)	Odefsey
	emtricitabine, rilpivirine, and tenofovir disoproxil fumarate (emtricitabine/rilpivirine hydrochloride/tenofovir disoproxil fumarate, emtricitabine/rilpivirine/tenofovir, FTC/RPV/TDF)	Complera
	emtricitabine and tenofovir alafenamide (emtricitabine/tenofovir AF, emtricitabine/tenofovir alafenamide fumarate, FTC/TAF)	Descovy
	emtricitabine and tenofovir disoproxil fumarate (emtricitabine/tenofovir DF, FTC/TDF)	Truvada
	lamivudine and tenofovir disoproxil fumarate (Temixys, 3TC/TDF)	Cimduo
	lamivudine and zidovudine (3TC/ZDV)	Combivir
	lopinavir and ritonavir (ritonavir-boosted lopinavir, LPV/r, LPV/RTV)	Kaletra

PEDIATRIC HUMAN IMMUNODEFICIENCY VIRUS INFECTION

Description: Infection with HIV in infants and children

A. Sources of infection in pediatric clients

B. The risk of mother-to-child transmission of HIV during pregnancy, delivery, and breastfeeding is as high as 25% to 30% in the absence of treatment. With the implementation of HIV testing, counseling, antiretroviral medication, delivery by cesarean section prior to onset of labor, and discouraging breastfeeding, vertical transmission has decreased to less than 2% in the United States.

C. For infants acquiring HIV before or around delivery, disease progression occurs rapidly in the first few months of life and often leads to death. Over 80% of HIV-infected infants who are well at 6 weeks progress to become eligible to start ART before 6 months of age. *Early determination of HIV exposure and definitive diagnosis is thus critical.*

D. All infants and children should have their *HIV exposure status* established at their first contact with the health system, ideally before 6 weeks of age. To facilitate this, all Maternal, Neonatal and Child service delivery points in health facilities should offer HIV serological testing to mothers and their infants and children. In most cases the HIV status is established by: asking about maternal HIV testing in pregnancy, labor, or postpartum period; checking the child's and/or mother's health card; offering a rapid antibody test to all infants and/or mothers whose HIV status is unknown, especially where the national HIV prevalence is greater than 2% in the United States (Nesheim et al., 2019).

E. The exact mechanism of mother-to-child transmission of HIV remains unknown. Transmission may occur during intrauterine life, delivery, or breastfeeding. The greatest risk factor for vertical transmission is thought to be advanced maternal disease, such as AIDS, likely because of a high maternal HIV viral load. Unfortunately, it has been reported that 30% of pregnant women are not tested for HIV during pregnancy, and another 15% to 20% receive no or minimal prenatal care, thereby allowing for potential newborn transmission (Peterson & Ramus, 2020; Rahangdale & Cohan, 2008).

F. Viral testing (e.g., PCR) should be conducted at 4 to 6 weeks of age for infants known to be HIV-exposed, or at the earliest possible opportunity for those seen after 4 to 6 weeks of age.

G. Urgent HIV antibody testing should be carried out for any infant or child presenting with signs, symptoms, or medical conditions that indicate HIV.

H. Infants with detectable HIV antibodies should go on for a viral test.

I. Every child should be evaluated for HIV exposures (Rivera & Frye, 2020).

Clinical Judgment

A. Risk groups
  1. Infants born to mothers who are HIV-positive
  2. Hemophiliacs
  3. Infants and children who have received blood transfusions

B. Clinical Symptoms
  1. Failure to thrive
  2. Lymphadenopathy
  3. Organomegaly
  4. Neuropathy
  5. Cardiomyopathy
  6. Chronic recurrent infections such as thrush
  7. Unexplained fevers

> **HESI HINT**
> - Because of the persistence of the maternal HIV antibody, infants younger than 18 months require virologic assays that directly detect HIV in order to diagnose HIV infection.
> - Preferred virologic assays include HIV bDNA polymerase chain reaction (PCR) and HIV RNA assays. The HIV PCR DNA qualitative test is usually less expensive.
> - Further virologic testing in infants with known perinatal HIV exposure is recommended at 2 weeks, 4 weeks, and 4 months.
> - An antibody test to document seroreversion to HIV antibody—negative status in uninfected infants is no longer recommended (Rivera & Frye, 2020).

> **HESI HINT** The focus of NGN-NCLEX-RN questions are likely to be assessment of early signs of the disease and management of complications associated with HIV.

Clinical Interventions

A. Avoid exposure to persons with infections

B. Administer *no* live virus vaccines.

C. Teach the family to
  1. Use gloves when diapering the child.
  2. Clean any soiled surfaces (wearing gloves)
  3. Identify signs of opportunistic infections.

D. Monitor growth parameters.

E. Support use of social services.

F. Support child's attending school as much as child is able.

G. Assist in community and school education programs.

> **? REVIEW OF HUMAN IMMUNODEFICIENCY VIRUS INFECTION**
>
> 1. Identify the ways HIV is transmitted.
> 2. Vertical transmission (from mother to fetus) occurs how often if the mother is not treated during pregnancy? Change answer <2% in US
> 3. Describe standard precautions.
> 4. What does the CD4 T-cell count describe?
> 5. Why does the CD4 T-cell count drop in HIV infections?
> 6. Describe the ways a pediatric client might acquire HIV infection.

See Answer Key at the end of this text for suggested responses.

PAIN

Pain: In light of research documenting the dramatic rise of opioid addiction and opioid-related deaths, delegates at the 2016 American Medical Association (AMA) meeting voted to stop treating pain as the fifth vital sign because they believe it is likely that the initiative, along with other factors, has exacerbated the opioid crisis (Anson, 2016)

A. Description: An individual's subjective experience of physical discomfort from illness or injury. Consider multidimensional pain questionnaire used to measure patients' response to post-operative pain therapy is the Overall Benefit of Analgesic Score (OBAS) comprises simple seven questions to assess pain intensity, adverse effects, and patients' satisfaction with analgesia. (OBAS) comprises simple seven questions to assess pain intensity, adverse effects, and patients' satisfaction with analgesia. Client's pain often goes unrecognized and untreated.
1. Health care professionals are increasingly better educated about identifying, assessing, and managing pain.

B. An individual's response to pain is influenced by several factors:
1. Anxiety: Reduction of anxiety can help to control pain.
2. Past experience with pain: The more pain experienced in childhood, the greater the perception of pain in adulthood.
3. Culture and religion: Cultural and religious practices learned from one's family play an important role in determining how a person experiences and expresses pain.
4. Gender affects the expression of pain.
5. Communication, whether it is a language barrier and/or a client who is unable to speak
6. Altered level of consciousness

C. Pain is classified as either acute or chronic.
1. Acute pain
   a. Is temporary (30 days in relationship to injury; no longer than 6 months)
   b. Occurs after an injury to the body
   c. Includes postoperative pain, labor pain, and renal calculus pain
2. Chronic pain (usually lasting beyond 6 months after initial injury)
   a. Nonmalignant (e.g., low back pain, rheumatoid arthritis)
   b. Intermittent (e.g., migraine headaches)
   c. Malignant, associated with neoplastic diseases

Theory of Pain

A. Gate control theory: Pain impulses travel from the periphery to the gray matter in the dorsal horn of the spinal cord along small nerve fibers.

A "gating" mechanism called the *substantia gelatinosa,* a collection of cells in the gray area (dorsal horns) of the spinal cord. Found at all levels of the cord, it receives direct input from the dorsal (sensory) nerve roots, especially those fibers from pain and thermoreceptors, which will either open to or close off the transmission of pain impulses to the brain.

1. Stimulation of large, fast-conducting sensory fibers opposes the input from small pain fibers, thus blocking pain transmission.
2. Modalities used: Stimulation of large fibers by massage, heat, cold, acupuncture, transcutaneous electrical nerve stimulation (TENS)

B. Endorphin/enkephalin theory
1. Endorphins: naturally occurring compounds that have morphinelike qualities; they modulate pain by preventing the conduction of pain impulses in the CNS.
2. Enkephalins: specific neurotransmitters that bind with opiate receptors in the dorsal horn of the spinal cord; they modulate pain by closing the gate and stopping the pain impulse.
3. Modalities used: stimulation of endogenous opiate release through acupuncture, placebos, TENS

Clinical Assessment for Pain

A. Location: Pain may be localized, radiating, or referred.
B. Intensity: Ask client to rate pain before and after an intervention such as medication (use scale such as 0 to 10, with 0 being no pain).
C. Comfort: Often clients can describe what relieves pain better than they can describe the pain itself.
D. Quality: Pain may be sharp, dull, aching, sore, etc.
E. Chronology: Ask client when pain started, what time of day it occurs, how often it appears, how long it lasts, whether it is constant or intermittent, whether the intensity changes.
F. Subjective experience: Determine what decreases or aggravates pain, what other symptoms are associated with pain, what interventions provide relief, what limitations the pain inflicts.

HESI HINT The alphabet mnemonic "PQRST" is an easy tool to use when assessing and documenting a client's experience of pain.

P Provocative and Palliative or Aggravating Factors	What provokes the painful sensation? What makes it worse or better?
Q Quality	Type of sensation → dull, aching, sharp, stabbing, burning
R Region or Location, Radiation	Where is the pain located and does it radiate anywhere?
S Severity	Ask the client to rate pain on a scale.
T Timing	How long has it been hurting? How often does it occur? When did it occur?
U Understanding	Ask the client what he or she thinks may be the cause or the problem causing the pain.

From Ignatavicius, D. D., Workman, L., & Rebar, C. (2018). *Medical-surgical nursing: Concepts for interprofessional collaborative care* (9th ed.). St. Louis: Saunders.

Clinical Judgment Measures for Pain Management

A. Pharmacologic interventions (Table 3.14)
  1. Non-narcotics, NSAIDs
  2. Act by means of a peripheral mechanism at level of damaged tissue by inhibiting prostaglandin and other chemical mediator syntheses involved in pain
  3. Show antipyretic activity through action on the hypothalamic heat-regulating center to reduce fever
  4. Examples: salicylate—aspirin nonsalicylates, acetaminophen ibuprofen
B. Narcotic mixed agonists/antagonists
  1. Bind to both a receptor that produces pain relief, which is the agonist portion, and to another receptor that does not produce a physiologic effect, which is the antagonist portion. Patients are less likely to have respiratory depression.
  2. May cause withdrawal symptoms if administered after client has been receiving narcotics.
  3. Produce side effects, including drowsiness, occasionally nausea and psychomimetic effects, such as hallucinations and euphoria.
  4. Examples: butorphanol nalbuphine

C. Narcotics
  1. Act as opioids, binding with specific opiate receptors throughout the CNS to reduce pain perception.
  2. Cause such side effects as nausea and vomiting, constipation, respiratory depression, and CNS depression.
  3. Examples: hydromorphone morphine sulfate (Table 3.15)

> **HESI HINT** For narcotic-induced respiratory depression, naloxone may be administered as prescribed by the health care provider.

D. Adjuvants to analgesics
  1. Are given in combination with an analgesic to potentiate or enhance the analgesic's effectiveness
  2. Are helpful in controlling discomfort associated with pain, such as nausea, anxiety, and depression (e.g., promethazine)

> **HESI HINT**
> - Use noninvasive methods for pain management when possible:
> - Relaxation exercises

TABLE 3.14 Routes of Administration for Analgesics

Route	Administration
Oral	• Preferred method of administration • Drug levels usually peak at 1–2 h
Intramuscular	• Acceptable method of managing acute, short-term pain • Onset 30 min, peak effect 1–3 h, duration of action 4 h
Rectal	• Useful with clients who are nauseated and unable to take analgesics by mouth • Useful for home care and with elderly clients as an alternative to oral and intravenous (IV) administration; reduced effectiveness with constipation
IV bolus (IV push)[a]	• Provides the most rapid onset (5 min), but with the shortest duration (1 h) • Useful with acute pain, such as a client in labor
Patient-controlled analgesia (PCA)[a]	• Ideal method of pain control in that the client is able to prevent pain by administering to himself/herself smaller doses of the narcotic (usually morphine) as soon as the first sign of discomfort arises • Usually administered IV • A predetermined dose and a set lockout interval (5–20 min) are prescribed by physician, and pump is calibrated to deliver the specified dose for bolus, basal, and whenever client presses the button. • Pump can deliver a bolus amount as a loading dose, a basal rate, intermittent doses, or a combination of any of the above • Lockout mechanism prevents overdosage • Pump can record number of times the client uses the pump and the cumulative dose delivered • Danger of respiratory depression • Teach family members at bedside to not push PCA if client is sleeping
Continuous subcutaneous narcotic infusion	• Useful with clients who cannot take anything by mouth and who require prolonged administration of parenteral narcotics • Provides a constant level of analgesia by continuous infusion of a narcotic • Site should be inspected every 8 h and changed at least every 7 days • Risk for respiratory depression
Continuous epidural analgesia (management of this route of administration is not within the scope of the PN)	• Catheter threaded into epidural space with continuous infusion of fentanyl citrate, morphine, or other narcotic analgesics • Risk of respiratory depression
Transdermal patches	• Applied to skin (self-adhesive or with overlay to secure patch) • Also used to deliver hormonal therapy, nitroglycerin, and nicotine • Sites for application and frequency of application are specific to each medication • Document removal of old patch as well as site and application date/time of new patch

[a]Depending on the state where you practice, administration of intravenous medications and blood products may not be within the practical nurse (PN's) Scope of Practice. Monitoring the client's response to the medication and blood product should be done by the PN.

TABLE 3.15   Onset of Commonly Administered Narcotics[a]

Medication	Mode	Onset	Comments
Codeine	Oral	30—45 min	• Do *not* administer discolored injection solutions
	IM or SQ	10—30 min	• May also be prescribed as an antitussive or antidiarrheal
Hydromorphone	Oral	30 min	• Fast-acting, potent narcotic
	IM	15 min	• More likely to cause appetite loss than other narcotics
	IV	10—15 min	
Morphine sulfate	Oral	60—90 min	• Drug of choice in relieving pain associated with myocardial infarction
	IM	10—30 min	• May cause transient decrease in blood pressure
	IV	10 min	• Drug of choice for use with chronic cancer pain
Fentanyl citrate	IM	7—15 min	• Synthetic narcotic, morphine sulfate-like
	IV	Within 5 min	• Acts more quickly; shorter duration
	Intradermal	Within 12 h	
	Intrabuccal	5—15 min	
	Intrathecal	Immediate	

IM, Intramuscular; *IV,* intravenous; *SQ,* subcutaneously.
[a]Although IV medication administration may not be within the PN's Scope of Practice, the IV mode is included for readers' information.

- Distraction
- Imagery
- Biofeedback
- Interpersonal skills
- Physical care: altering positions, touch, hot and cold applications

Clinical Assessment of Pain Relief Techniques

A. Pain (Table 3.16)

B. Response to pharmacologic intervention: Tolerance to pharmacologic interventions may occur—that is, the client physiologically requires increasingly larger doses to provide the same effect.

   1. The first sign of tolerance is a decreased duration of a drug's effectiveness.

   2. The need for increased doses can be the result of increased pain rather than tolerance (e.g., clients with advanced cancer) (see Table 3.16).

HESI HINT Narcotic analgesics are preferred for pain relief because they bind to the various opiate receptor sites in the CNS. Morphine is often the preferred narcotic (*remember*, it causes respiratory depression).

Another agonist is methadone. Narcotic antagonists block the attachment of narcotics such as naloxone to the receptors. Once naloxone has been given, additional narcotics cannot be given until the naloxone effects have passed.

❓ REVIEW OF PAIN

1. What modalities are associated with the gate control pain theory?
2. How does past experience with pain influence current pain experience?
3. What modalities are thought to increase the production of endogenous opiates?
4. What six factors should the nurse include when assessing the pain experience?
5. What mechanism is involved in the reduction of pain through the administration of NSAIDs?
6. If narcotic agonist/antagonist drugs are administered to a client already taking narcotic drugs, what may be the result?
7. List four side effects of narcotic medications.
8. What is the antidote for narcotic-induced respiratory depression?
9. What is the first sign of tolerance to pain analgesics?
10. Which route of administration for pain medications has the quickest onset and the shortest duration?
11. List the six modalities that are considered noninvasive, nonpharmacologic pain relief measures.

See Answer Key at the end of this text for suggested responses.

DEATH AND GRIEF

Description: Death completes the life cycle. Grief is the process an individual goes through to deal with loss. How each person deals with these situations depends on the individual. An individual's past experience and coping skills and what other stresses he or she may have going on in his or her life can largely affect how the person responds and reacts to these situations.

Clinical Assessment

Types of Death

There are five modes of **death** (natural, accident, suicide, homicide, and undetermined)

TABLE 3.16 Pain Relief Techniques

Noninvasive: Cutaneous stimulation that is useful alone or in combination with other pain-management techniques

- Heat and cold applications decrease pain and muscle spasm.
- Transcutaneous electrical nerve stimulation provides continuous mild electrical current to the skin via electrodes.
- Massage provides a simple, inexpensive, and effective method of pain relief.
- Distraction diverts client's attention from the pain; useful during short periods of pain or during painful procedures such as intravenous venipunctures.
- Relaxation can be used as a distraction and to facilitate sedation or sleep; rarely decreases pain sensation.
- Biofeedback techniques: control of autonomic responses (tachycardia, muscle tension) to pain through electrical feedback.
- Positioning, guided imagery meditation.

Invasive: Any procedure used to relieve pain that invades the body

- Nerve blocks: injection of anesthetic into or near a nerve to decrease pain pathways—for example, "deadening" area for dental work, regional anesthesia used in obstetrics.
- Neurosurgical procedures: surgical or chemical (alcohol) interruption of nerve pathways; commonly used in clients with cancer who have severe pain.
- Acupuncture: insertion of needles at various points into the body to relieve pain.

A. Stages of preparing for an expected death may not be sequential. An individual may fluctuate between the stages. An individual may not experience every stage.
  1. Denial
     a. Coping style used to protect self/ego
     b. Noncompliance, refusal to seek treatment, ignoring of symptoms
     c. Changing the subject when speaking about illness
     d. Stating, "Not me, it must be a mistake."
  2. Anger
     a. Often directing it at family or health care team members
     b. Stating, "Why me? It's not fair."
  3. Bargaining
     a. Making a deal with God to prolong life
     b. Usually not sharing this with anyone, keeping it a very private experience
  4. Depression
     a. Results from the losses experienced because of health status and hospitalization
     b. Anticipating the loss of life
  5. Acceptance
     a. Accepting of the inevitable
     b. Beginning to separate emotionally

Clinical Assessment of Death and Grief

A. Shock, disbelief, rejection, or denial
  1. Anger and crying
  2. Conflicting emotions
  3. Anger toward the deceased
  4. Guilt
  5. Preoccupation with loss
B. Resolution
  1. Process taking up to 1 year or more
  2. Renewed interest in activities
C. Complicated grief
  1. Unresolved grief
     a. Determine level of dysfunction

  2. Physical symptoms similar to those of the deceased
  3. Clinical depression
  4. Social isolation
  5. Failure to acknowledge loss

Clinical Judgment Measures

A. Encourage client to express anger in a supportive, nonthreatening environment.
B. Discourage rumination.
C. Assist client in giving up idealized perception of deceased; point out misrepresentations.
D. Encourage interaction with others.
E. Assist client with identification of support systems.
F. Consult spiritual leader as indicated by client need and preference.
G. Assist client toward a comfortable, peaceful death.

HESI HINT Do not take away the coping style used in a crisis state. Denial is a very useful and needed tool for some at the initial stage. Support, do not challenge, unless it hinders or blocks treatment, endangering the patient.

? REVIEW OF DEATH AND GRIEF

1. Identify the five stages of grief associated with dying.
2. A client has been told of a positive breast biopsy report. She asks no questions and leaves the health care provider's office. She is overheard telling her husband, "The doctor didn't find a thing." What coping style is operating at this stage of grief?
3. Your client, an incest survivor, is speaking of her deceased father, the perpetrator. "He was a wonderful man, so good and kind. Everyone thought so." What would be the most useful intervention at this time?
4. Your client feels responsible for his sister's death because he took her to the hospital where she died. "If I hadn't taken her there, they couldn't have killed her." It has been 1 month since her death. Is this response indicative of a normal or a complicated grief reaction?

5. Mrs. Green lost her husband 3 years ago. She has not disturbed any of his belongings and continues to set a place at the table for him nightly. Is this response indicative of a normal or a complicated grief reaction?

See Answer Key at the end of this text for suggested responses.

For further review, go to http://evolve.elsevier.com/HESI/RN for HESI's online study examinations.

NEXT-GENERATION NCLEX® EXAMINATION-STYLE QUESTIONS

| Health History | Nurses' Notes | Vital Signs | Lab Results |

Mrs. James, 35-year-old female, has been brought to the emergency room for chest pain. She was out jogging with her friend and became short of breath and had difficulty breathing. The EMTs had her on 2 L of O2, heart monitor (telemetry) and had started an IV. The PN enters the room to do vital signs, helps her undress and while she was getting undressed she became pale, fainted, and fell forward into the arms of the PN. The PN called for help from the other healthcare providers so that she could be immediately assessed. When the ER physician arrived at her bedside he ordered: nitroglycerin 2.5 mg. sublingual × 3 per day, 2 mg. morphine IV, lab work, chest x-ray, and a 12 lead EKG. Mrs. James became alert and stated that she was in extreme pain and that her chest felt like a brick was sitting on it.

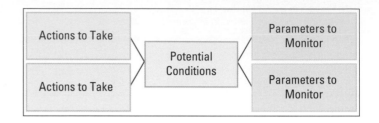

Orders

2L O_2, IV, 12-lead EKG, chest X-ray, CBC, SMA-12, nitroglycerin 2.5 mg. 3 × per day, morphine 2 mg IV for pain as needed (not to exceed 8 mg within 1 hour), safety parameters, vital signs q.15 min.

Instructions

Complete the diagram by selecting from the choices below to specify what condition the client is most likely experiencing; 2 actions the nurse should take to address that condition and 2 parameters the nurse should monitor to assess the clients progress.

Actions to Take	Potential Conditions	Parameters to Monitor
Start the IV and monitor amount of fluids	Anxiety	Heart rate and cuff blood pressure
Obtain CT scan	Pulmonary embolism	Monitor for internal bleeding
Assess level of chest pain and report to RN	Myocardial infarction (MI)	Assess the skin for any bruises or petechiae
Monitor ECG and contact RN if immediate change occurs	Gastrointestinal discomfort or GERD	Chest discomfort/pain
Do bedside sonogram		Monitor antibiotic use

REFERENCES AND BIBLIOGRAPHY

2021 ESC guidelines for the management of acute coronary syndromes in patients presenting without persistent ST-segment elevation: The Task force for the management of acute coronary syndromes in patients presenting without persistent ST-segment elevation of the European Society of Cardiology (ESC). *European Heart Journal*, August 29. [Epub ahead of print].

Ackley, B. J., Ladwig, G. B., Msn, R. N., Makic, M. B. F., Martinez-Kratz, M., & Zanotti, M. (2019). *Nursing diagnosis handbook E-book: An evidence-based guide to planning care.* St. Louis: Mosby.

American Heart Association. (n.d.). *Study Guide 2017 BLS for healthcare providers CPR emphasis as of February 2016 for Healthcare Providers.* Retrieved October 12, 2021, from https://www.hinman.org/Clinicians/Handouts/2017/Th113-Th114-Fr141-Fr142.pdf.

Anson, P. (2016). *AMA drops the pain as the fifth vital sign.* Retrieved December 6, 2021 from: https://www.painnewsnetwork.org/stories/2016/6/16/ama-drops-pain-as-vital-sign.

Atsumi, Y., Morikawa, Y., & Hataya, H. (2021, July). Accuracy of shorter respiratory rate measurement times in the pediatric population. *Pediatrics, 63*(7), 764–769. https://doi.org/10.1111/ped.14513. Epub 2021 Apr 25. PMID: 33070406.

Biga, L., Dawson, S., Harwell, A., Hopkins, R., Kaufmann, J., LeMaster, M., et al. (n.d.). 26.4 acid-base balance. *Anatomy Physiology.* Retrieved October 12, 2021, from: https://open.oregonstate.education/aandp/chapter/26-4-acid-base-balance/.

Centers for Disease Control and Prevention. (2021, March 15). *Benefits of routine screening.* Centers for Disease Control and Prevention. Retrieved October 12, 2021, from https://www.cdc.gov/hiv/clinicians/screening/benefits.html.

Centers for Disease Control and Prevention. (2021, October 1). *Basic statistics*. Centers for Disease Control and Prevention. Retrieved October 12, 2021, from https://www.cdc.gov/hiv/basics/statistics.html.

Centers for Disease Control and Prevention. (2021, June 24). *Statistics overview*. Centers for Disease Control and Prevention. Retrieved October 12, 2021, from https://www.cdc.gov/hiv/statistics/overview/index.html.

Collet, J. P., Thiele, H., & Barbato, E. (2021, April 7). 2020 ESC guidelines for the management of acute coronary syndromes in patients presenting without persistent ST-segment elevation. ESC Scientific Document Group. *European Heart Journal, 42*(14), 1289−1367. https://doi.org/10.1093/eurheartj/ehaa575. PMID: 32860058.

Diao, B., Wang, C., Tan, Y., Chen, X., Liu, Y., Ning, L., et al. (2020). Reduction and functional exhaustion of T cells in patients with Coronavirus disease 2019 (COVID-19). *Frontiers in Immunology, 11*, 827. https://doi.org/10.3389/fimmu.2020.00827.

Gloria, M.,, Paulina, J., & Krista. (2021). *Deficient fluid volume (dehydration) nursing care plan*. Nurseslabs. Retrieved October 12, 2021, from https://nurseslabs.com/deficient-fluid-volume/.

Hammer, J. (2013). Acute respiratory failure in children. *Paediatric Respiratory Reviews, 14*(2), 64−69.

Ignatavicius, D. D., Workman, L., & Rebar, C. (2018). *Medical-surgical nursing: Concepts for interprofessional collaborative care* (9th ed.). St. Louis: Saunders.

Ignatavicius, D. D., Workman, L., Rebar, C., & Heimgartner, N. M. (2021). *Medical-surgical nursing: Concepts for interprofessional collaborative care* (10th ed.). St. Louis: Saunders.

Ismail, M., & Elbaih, A. (2017). Pathophysiology and management of different types of shock. *Narayana Medical Journal, 6*, 14−39. https://doi.org/10.5455/nmj./00000120.

Medicine Library. (2020, August 13). *25.3A sodium, electrolytes, and fluid balance*. From https://med.libretexts.org/@go/page/8178.

Merchant, R. M., Topjian, A. A., Panchal, A. R., Cheng, A., Aziz, K., Berg, K. M., et al., Adult Basic and Advanced Life Support, Pediatric Basic and Advanced Life Support, Neonatal Life Support, Resuscitation Education Science, and Systems of Care Writing Groups. (2020). Part 1: Executive summary: 2020 American heart association guidelines for cardiopulmonary resuscitation and emergency cardiovascular care. *Circulation, 142*(16_Suppl. 2), S337−S357. https://doi.org/10.1161/CIR.0000000000000918.

Mount Sinai Health System. (n.d.). *T-cell count*. Retrieved October 12, 2021, from https://www.mountsinai.org/health-library/tests/t-cell-count.

Nesheim, S. R., FitzHarris, L. F., Mahle Gray, K., & Lampe, M. A. (2019). Epidemiology of perinatal HIV transmission in the United States in the Era of its elimination. *The Pediatric Infectious Disease Journal, 38*(6), 611−616. https://doi.org/10.1097/INF.0000000000002290.

Patton, K. T., Bell, F., Thompson, T., & Williamson, P. (2010). *From anatomy and physiology* (11th ed.). St. Louis: Mosby. Anatomy and physiology (11th ed.). St. Louis: Mosby.

Papageorgiou, C., Jourdi, G., Adjambri, E., Walborn, A., Patel, P., Fareed, J., et al. (2018). Disseminated intravascular coagulation: An update on pathogenesis, diagnosis, and therapeutic strategies. *Clinical and Applied Thrombosis, 24*(Suppl. 9), 8S−28S. https://doi.org/10.1177/1076029618806424.

Peterson, A., & Ramus, R. (2020). *HIV in pregnancy*. Retrieved December 6, 2021 from https://emedicine.medscape.com/article/1385488-overview#a2.

Rahangdale, L., & Cohan, D. (2008). Rapid human immunodeficiency virus testing on labor and delivery. *Obstetrics & Gynecology, 112*(1), 159−163.

Rivera, D., & Frye, R. (2020). *Pediatric HIV infection: Practice essentials*. Retrieved December 6, 2021 from https://www.ncbi.nlm.nih.gov/books/NBK304129/.

U.S. Department of Health and Human Services. (n.d.). *FDA-approved HIV medicines*. National Institutes of Health. Retrieved October 12, 2021, from https://hivinfo.nih.gov/understanding-hiv/fact-sheets/fda-approved-hiv-medicines.

Vo, P., & Kharasch, V. S. (2014). Respiratory failure. *Pediatrics in Review, 35*(11), 476−486.

Zieliński, J., & Przybylski, J. (2012). How much water is lost during breathing? *Pneumonologia i Alergologia Polska, 80*(4), 339−342. Polish. PMID: 22714078.

Medical-Surgical Nursing

CARING AND NURSING

Four common goals of nursing are to promote wellness, prevent illness, facilitate coping, and restore health. To achieve these objectives, the practical nurse (PN) takes on the role of caregiver, teacher, collaborator, and advocate. Both caring and knowledge are needed to care for clients effectively and safely. Caring represents the art of nursing. Knowledge represents the science in nursing. Historically caring has been a basic tenet of nursing.

> **HESI HINT** NCLEX will focus on cultural diversity and the inclusion of both spiritual and complementary and alternative medicine (CAM) associated with individuals' family and cultural practices.

It is important for modern PNs to recognize that the client is not static but is made up of diverse parts that require the PN to encompass both the art and science of nursing. Providing care encompasses observation and interaction, as well as developing caring and trusting relationships. In order to elicit information from a client, it is important for the PN to use active listening as well as other therapeutic communication techniques that help the client consider possible solutions when a problem occurs. Establishing a good nurse-client relationship through therapeutic communication is necessary to gain the client's trust so that obtaining information, providing teaching, and other communications are well received. Through active listening, the PN may learn how the client and family have been managing care via conventional treatment, alternative treatments, and herbal medications or what some clients describe as folk remedies.

> **HESI HINT** Care for the client is planned jointly by all members of the health care team. In order to enhance the care of the client, the PN collaborates with the registered nurse (RN) and other members of the health care team, including the client and the family, to provide continuity of care. The PN provides information to the team members regarding the client's use of CAM, folk remedies, or other treatment options garnered via therapeutic communication.

CULTURAL DIVERSITY

PNs frequently provide care for clients of different cultural backgrounds. PNs need to be cognizant of their own cultural biases because everyone has biases and, if the nurse is not alert, those biases are discerned by clients. How PNs communicate with clients may be influenced by bias and may create a barrier between the client and PN. Therefore, PNs must learn to accept that differences exist and to set aside those cultural differences when interacting with clients and their families. The use of nontraditional and herbal treatments should be implemented if the client and health care provider (HCP) include these requests in the treatment plan.

> **HESI HINT** Culture influences how clients seek medical attention or treat themselves. Obtain a cultural and spiritual assessment and include cultural and spiritual preferences in the plan of care when appropriate and feasible. PNs are expected to provide care for all clients. It is important to note that clients are culturally diverse, regardless of their ethnicity, race, or socioeconomic status and to note that in every culture, subgroups may form. Since the 2000 census, there has been a notable change in the cultural, ethnic, and racial alignment of the United States.

> **HESI HINT** Reasons why clients use herbal medications:
> - Cultural influence
> - Perception that supplements are safer and "healthier" than conventional drugs
> - Sense of control over one's care
> - Emotional comfort from taking action
> - Limited access to professional care
> - Lack of health insurance
> - Convenience
> - Media hype and aggressive marketing
> - Recommendation from family and friends

The Institute of Medicine (IOM) was actively involved in studying "innovative" treatments such as acupuncture, yoga, and therapeutic use of animals. Acupuncture and massage have also been successfully implemented to decrease pain or the need for pain medication (Stussman et al., 2020). In the treatment for posttraumatic stress disorder, for example, the use of eye movement desensitization reprocessing emphasizes the focus on mental images and muscle tension, creating positive images and thoughts while following particular eye movements that create different scenarios for the reality of the traumatic event.

Furthermore, conventional medicine treats premenstrual syndrome with selective serotonin reuptake inhibitors (SSRIs) such as fluoxetine, paroxetine, sertraline, and citalopram or a tricyclic antidepressant related to SSRI such as clomipramine (Boyles & Baxter, 2021). However, in some CAM circles it is said that "A simpler but almost as effective method can be a large block of chocolate! Chocolate has been found to increase serotonin and has been dubbed the Prozac of plants" by *Forbes* magazine (Farrar & Farrar, 2020). However, ongoing research supported by National Institutes of Health remains inconclusive.

Acupressure and herbal medicines are among the traditional medical practices used by Asian clients to reestablish the balance between yin and yang. In some Asian countries, healers use a process of "coining," in which a coin is heated and vigorously rubbed on the body to draw illness out of the body. The resulting welts can mistakenly be attributed to child abuse if this practice is not understood. Traditional healers, such as Buddhist monks, acupuncturists, and herbalists, also may be consulted when someone is ill (Arnold & Boggs, 2019; Stussman et al., 2020).

A Japanese technique used to promote healing, reduce stress, and induce relaxation is called reiki. The process for administering reiki is by "laying on hands" and is based on the idea that an unseen "life force energy" flows through us and is what causes us to be alive. It is believed that when a person's "life force energy" is low, the person is more apt to become ill or feel stress. When the life force energy is high, an individual is believed to be more prone to being happy and healthy.

Smell connects to the part of the brain that controls the autonomic nervous system. Aromatherapy is the introduction of essential oils, such as sweet orange to grapefruit scents, which are effective in managing the odor of dressing changes in some hospice settings. It is believed that essential oils stimulate the release of neurotransmitters in the brain. Specific types of essential oils may induce pain reduction, induce sedation, or stimulate clients to a sense of well-being (Clark, 2021). Many clients also use herbal medications that they used in their country of origin or that they learned about from family traditions. To maintain client safety, nurses need to be aware of those herbal medications, their mechanisms of action, side effects, and food or drug interactions. (See Fig. 4.1 and Table 4.1; Farrar & Farrar, 2020.)

SPIRITUAL ASSESSMENT

During times of illness, religious or spiritual practices may be a source of comfort for the client. While obtaining a spiritual assessment, the PN can discover information about the client's preference for a personal clergy member or the hospital chaplain. A spiritual assessment tool may assist the nurse to integrate a spiritual assessment into the client's plan of care. FICA is an acronym for Faith and Belief: Importance, Community, and address in Care (Puchalsk, 2022).

Sometimes a simple question can be used to obtain a spiritual history. Ask the client, "Do you have any spiritual needs or concern's related to your health?"

> **HESI HINT** Cultural and Spiritual Assessment (questions to ask clients to assess spiritual or cultural aspects that may affect their health care):
> 1. What do you think caused this illness?
> 2. What problems has the illness created for you?
> 3. What traditional remedies or rituals might be used in your culture to treat this illness?
> 4. Is there anything we (the nursing staff) should know about your religious practices or your spiritual needs?
> 5. Is there a spiritual or religious leader (priest, rabbi, pastor, imam) with whom you would like to meet? Would you like to talk with the chaplain?

RESPIRATORY SYSTEM

Pneumonia

Description: Pneumonia is an inflammation of the lower respiratory tract.

A. Pneumonia is commonly caused by infectious agents.
B. Organisms that cause pneumonia reach the lungs by three methods: aspiration, inhalation, or hematogenous spread.
C. Pneumonia is generally classified according to causative agents: bacterial, viral, fungal (rare), chemical.
D. Pneumonia may be community-acquired or health care-associated pneumonia (hospital/agency acquired).
E. High-risk groups include individuals who are:
   1. Debilitated with accumulated lung secretions
   2. Cigarette smokers
   3. Immobile
   4. Immunosuppressed
   5. Experiencing a depressed gag reflex and/or cough
   6. Sedated (including suspected oral/intravenous [IV] drug abuse/use)
   7. Impaired by neuromuscular disorders
   8. Nasogastric (NG)/orogastric tracheal intubation (endotracheal tube and tracheostomy)
   9. Hospitalized client or recent resident of a long-term care facility.

Nursing Assessment

A. Tachypnea: shallow respirations, often with use of accessory muscles
B. Grunting, crackles, dullness on percussion over consolidated areas
C. Abrupt onset of fever with shaking and chills (not reliable with older adults)

Essential Oil	Disorder Treated
True lavender	Anxiety
True lavender	Breast tenderness
Juniper	Fluid retention
Juniper	Breast tenderness
Clary sage	Low-back pain
Geranium	Mood swings
Geranium	Nervous tension

Fig. 4.1 Examples of Essential Oils. (Clark, C. [2021]. Aromatherapy: Essential oils and nursing: Explore this option for enhancing well-being. *American Nurse Journal, 16*[8].)

TABLE 4.1	Nursing Considerations for Commonly Ingested Herbs		
Herb	**Uses**	**Nursing Implications**	**Herbal Interactions**
Echinacea Other names: Ephedra, ma huang, ephedrine	Nonspecific immunostimulant to treat cold symptoms, urinary tract infections, and difficult-to-heal superficial wounds. Used as a bronchodilator for asthma, nasal decongestant, and central nervous system stimulant.	May interfere with immunosuppressive therapy (multiple sclerosis, lupus erythematosus, or AIDS). Not recommended for concurrent use with immunosuppressants (cyclosporine). May impair hepatic metabolism of certain anesthesia medications. Contraindicated in clients with cardiac conditions, hypertension, diabetes, and thyroid disease.	Enhances toxic effects of: monoamine oxidase inhibitors (MAOIs) such as isocarboxazid, phenelzine. Concurrent therapy with methyldopa and reserpine is not recommended because it inhibits activity of those agents.
Garlic	Research shows effectiveness in reducing serum cholesterol and triglycerides. May modestly lower hypertension. Has properties of antiplatelet activity similar to aspirin.	Monitor clients for signs of bleeding. Taste and odor often result in halitosis.	Since garlic reduces platelet aggregation it has the potential to increase bleeding. Use with extreme caution with clients receiving platelet inhibitors (for example, aspirin) (warfarin) or herbal medicines (such as ginkgo, ginger, feverfew, ginseng)
Ginkgo biloba	Used to increase cerebral blood flow in older adults, to enhance alertness and brain function. Alleviates tension. Useful for erectile dysfunction. Improves peripheral blood flow for clients diagnosed with diabetes mellitus.	Potential for increased bleeding; monitor clients for signs of bleeding Therapy must be continued for at least 6 months to assess optimal responses.	Reduces platelet aggregation; therefore, use caution for clients receiving platelet inhibitors (aspirin, clopidogrel), anticoagulants (warfarin), and herbal medicines (ginger, garlic, feverfew, and ginseng).
Ginseng	Useful for diabetes. Promotes overall well-being.	Monitor for signs of bleeding. Potential for hypoglycemia for clients taking insulin or oral diabetic agents.	Use with caution in clients receiving platelet inhibitors (aspirin), anticoagulants, and herbal medicines (e.g., garlic, feverfew, ginger, ginkgo). May raise insulin levels; may induce hypoglycemia.
St. John's wort	Antidepressant Antiviral properties Anti-inflammatory	May stimulate manic behavior Serious effects when mixed with MAOIs	Should not be used with other psychoactive medications, MAOIs, or serotonin reuptake inhibitors (SSRIs).

Buckle, J. (2015). *Clinical aromatherapy: Essential oils in practice* (3rd ed.). St. Louis: Elsevier.

D. Productive cough with pleuritic pain
1. Secretions may be pink, rusty, purulent, green, yellow, or white
2. Sputum may range from scant to large amounts
E. Rapid, bounding pulse
F. In the older adults, symptoms include:
1. Confusion
2. Lethargy/malaise
3. Anorexia
4. Rapid respiratory rate (tachypnea)
5. Rapid heart rate (tachycardia)
6. Pain and dullness noted with percussion over the affected lung area
7. Bronchial breath sounds; crackles
8. Chest x-ray indication of infiltrates with consolidation or pleural effusion
9. Elevated white blood cell (WBC) count
10. Arterial blood gases (ABGs) indicate hypoxemia (decreased PaO_2; decreased $PaCO_2$; decreased pH)
11. A drop in oxygen saturation when using a pulse oximetry (should be >90%, ideally >95%)
12. Positive sputum; Gram stain and culture

HESI HINT Fever can cause dehydration from excessive fluid loss in diaphoresis. Increased temperature also increases metabolism and oxygen demand.

HESI HINT: HIGH RISK FOR PNEUMONIA Any person who has an altered level of consciousness, has depressed or absent gag and cough reflexes, or is susceptible to aspirating oropharyngeal secretions (including alcoholics, anesthetized individuals, those with brain injury, those in a state of drug overdose, stroke victims, those with asplenia, and those who are immunocompromised) is at high risk.

Nursing Plans and Interventions

A. Examine and report sputum for volume (amount), color, consistency, clarity, and odor.
B. Assist client to cough productively by:
1. Deep breathing every 2 hours (may use incentive spirometer).

2. Using humidity to loosen secretions (may be oxygenated).
3. Suctioning the airway, if necessary.
4. Chest physiotherapy as prescribed.
C. Provide fluids up to 3 L/day unless contraindicated (helps liquefy lung secretions).
D. Auscultate lung sounds before and after coughing.
E. Monitor rate, depth, and pattern of respirations regularly (normal adult rate is 16 to 20 breaths/min). Assess for accessory muscle use.
F. Monitor ABGs (normal range: P_{O_2} >80 mm Hg; P_{CO_2} <45 mm Hg).
G. Monitor O_2 saturation with pulse oximetry (ideally >95%).
H. Report skin color.
1. Assess nail color, mucous membrane color for appropriate ethnic population.
2. Cyanosis is a late sign of decreased oxygenation

I. Monitor mental status, restlessness, and irritability.
J. Administer humidified O_2 as prescribed.
K. Monitor temperature regularly.
L. Provide adequate rest periods throughout the day, including uninterrupted sleep.
M. Administer antibiotics as prescribed (Table 4.2).
N. Collaborate with RN to develop a client/family teaching plan about risk factors and include preventive measures.
O. Encourage at-risk groups to obtain required pneumonia and annual flu vaccine immunizations.
P. Promote rest and conserve energy.

HESI HINT Bronchial breath sounds are heard over areas of density or consolidation. Sound waves are easily transmitted over consolidated tissue.

TABLE 4.2 Anti-infectives

Drugs	Indications	Adverse Reactions	Nursing Implications
Penicillins • Procaine penicillin G (Wycillin) • Benzathine penicillin (Bicillin L-A) • Penicillin V (Pen-Vee K)	• Anti-infectives • Used primarily for Gram-positive infections	• Allergic reactions • Anaphylaxis • Phlebitis at IV site • Diarrhea • GI distress • Superinfection • False-positive for glucose using Clinitest	• Use with caution in clients allergic to cephalosporins • Monitor for allergic reactions • Observe all clients for at least 30 min after parenteral administration • Oral penicillin G should be taken on an empty stomach • Probenecid decreases renal excretion, thereby resulting in an increased blood level of the drug • Alters contraceptive effectiveness
Semisynthetic • Oxacillin sodium • Nafcillin sodium • Cloxacillin sodium • Dicloxacillin sodium	• Anti-infectives • Used primarily for Gram-positive infections	• Allergic reactions • Anaphylaxis • Superinfection • *See Penicillins*	• Cannot be used in clients allergic to penicillin • Caution in clients allergic to cephalosporins • Monitor for superinfection (sore mouth, vaginal discharge, diarrhea, cough) • *See Penicillins*
Antipseudomonal Penicillins and Combinations • Ampicillin • Ticarcillin + clavulanate (Timentin) • Piperacillin + tazobactam (Zosyn) • Ampicillin + sulbactam (Unasyn)	• Anti-infectives • Broad spectrums	• Similar to penicillin • Ampicillin rash	• Contraindicated in clients allergic to penicillin • *See Penicillins*
Tetracyclines • Tetracycline HCL • Doxycycline hyclate (Vibramycin) • Minocycline (Minocin)	• Anti-infectives	• Hypersensitivity reactions • Photosensitivity	• Decreases the effectiveness of oral contraceptives • Avoid concurrent use of antacids, milk products • Inspect IV site frequently • Monitor for superinfections • Avoid exposure to sunlight during use • Avoid use in pregnant clients and children under 8 years; can cause yellow-brown discoloration of teeth and growth retardation

Continued

Aminoglycosides
- Gentamicin sulfate
- Tobramycin sulfate (Nebcin)
- Amikacin sulfate
- Miscellaneous agents
- Vancomycin hydrochloride
- Metronidazole (Flagyl)

- Anti-infectives
- Used with Gram-negative bacteria

- Neuromuscular blockade
- Nephrotoxicity
- Ototoxicity

- Monitor renal function, BUN, creatinine, and I&O
- Monitor for ototoxicity; headache, dizziness, hearing loss, tinnitus
- Monitor for superinfection
- Monitor vancomycin serum drug concentrations
- Red-neck syndrome

Cephalosporins
- First generation:
  - Cefazolin (Kefzol)
  - Cephalexin (Keflex)
- Second generation:
  - Cefaclor (Ceclor)
  - Cefamandole (Mandol)
  - Cefuroxime (Ceftin-PO, Zinacef-IV)
  - Cefoxitin (Mefoxin)
  - Cefotetan (Cefotan)
  - Cefprozil (Cefzil)
- Third generation:
  - Cefotaxime (Claforan)
  - Ceftriaxone (Rocephin)
  - Ceftazidime (Fortaz)
  - Cefdinir (Omnicef)
  - Cefixime (Suprax)
  - Cefpodoxime (Vantin)
  - Ceftibuten (Cedax)
- Fourth generation
  - Cefepime (Maxipime)

- Anti-infectives

- Allergic reactions
- Thrombophlebitis
- GI distress
- Superinfection

- Use with caution in clients allergic to penicillin and cephalosporins
- *See Penicillins*

Carbapenems
- Imipenem (Primaxin)
- Meropenem (Merrem IV)
- Ertapenem (Invanz)

- Used for the treatment of infections known or suspected to be caused by multidrug-resistant (MDR) bacteria
- Their use is primarily in people who are hospitalized

- Serious allergic reactions can occur in people treated with carbapenems
- Seizures are a dose-limiting toxicity for both imipenem and meropenem
- *Clostridium difficile* —related diarrhea

- Monitor for allergic reactions, seizures, and diarrhea
- Caution with penicillin and cephalosporin allergy

Monobactam
- Aztreonam (Azactam)

- *Pseudomonas aeruginosa* + many otherwise resistant organisms
- Most effective against Gram-negatives

- Phlebitis
- Pseudomembranous colitis
- CNS changes
- EEG changes
- Headache/diplopia
- Hypotension

- Monitor renal and hepatic function, especially in older adults
- Carefully monitor for diarrhea
- Assess motor sensory function and cardiac rhythm

Macrolides
- Clarithromycin (Biaxin)
- Azithromycin (Zithromax)
- Erythromycin

- Biaxin (oral): URI, including Strep; as adjunct treatment for *Helicobacter pylori*
- Zithromax (IV): Gram-negative and Gram-positive organisms

- Pseudomembranous colitis
- Phlebitis—a vesicant
- Superinfections
- Dizziness
- Dyspnea

- Give Biaxin XL with food
- Space MAOIs 14 days before start and after end of Biaxin
- Report diarrhea, abdominal cramping—all macrolides
- Monitor liver, renal laboratory results
- Oral Zithromax—give on empty stomach

Continued

TABLE 4.2 Anti-infectives—cont'd

Drugs	Indications	Adverse Reactions	Nursing Implications
Fluoroquinolones • Ciprofloxacin (Cipro) • Levofloxacin (Levaqin) • Moxifloxacin (Avelox)	• All three of the most difficult to treat respiratory infections, UTIs, skin, bone, and joint infections • Has been used as conjunctive treatment for TB and AIDS	• Superinfections • CNS disturbances • Arroyos and cataracts possible with Cipro • Cipro—a vesicant	• Prompt onset • Crosses placenta and found in breast milk • Can lower seizure threshold • Monitor liver, renal, and blood counts • Safety for children not known • Many drug—drug interactions
Lincosamides • Clindamycin HCl (Cleocin HCl)	• *Pneumocystis carinii* pneumonia (PCP) in AIDS • Soft tissue infections caused by streptococci, staphylococci, and anaerobes • Severe infections resistant to penicillins and cephalosporins • Used in penicillin or erythromycin-sensitive clients	• Agranulocytosis • Pseudomembranous colitis • Superinfections	• Highly toxic drug; use only when absolutely necessary • Periodic liver, renal, and blood counts • Report diarrhea immediately
Streptogramin • Quinupristin/dalfopristin (Synercid)	• Life-threatening vancomycin-resistant enterococcus (VRE)	• Arthralgia, myalgia • Severe vesicant • Pseudomembranous colitis • Nausea/vomiting, diarrhea • Rash, pruritus	• Incompatible with any saline solutions or heparin • Functionally related to both macrolides and lincosamides • Monitor total bilirubin • Many drug—drug interactions
Oxazolidinone Linezolid (Ziox)	Life-threatening VRE and methicillin- resistant *Staphylococcus aureus* (MRSA)	GI disturbances Headache Pancytopenia Pseudomembranous colitis Superinfections	Monitor renal and liver labs, + blood count May exacerbate hypertension, especially if foods ingested with tyramine Report diarrhea immediately

BUN, Blood urea nitrogen; *CNS,* central nervous system; *EEG,* Electroencephalogram; *GI,* gastrointestinal; *I&O,* intake and output; *IV,* intravenous; *MAOIs,* monoamine oxidase inhibitors; *TB,* tuberculosis; *URI,* upper respiratory infection; *UTIs,* urinary tract infections.

HESI HINT Hydration enables liquefaction of mucus trapped in the bronchioles and alveoli, facilitating expectoration, and is essential for clients experiencing fever. It is important because 300—400 mL of fluid is lost daily by the lungs through evaporation.

HESI HINT Irritability and restlessness are early signs of cerebral hypoxia; the client's brain is not getting enough oxygen.

HESI HINT: Pneumonia Preventatives
• **Older adults:** Flu shots; pneumonia immunizations; avoiding sources of infection and indoor pollutants (dust, smoke, and aerosols); no smoking
• **Immunosuppressed and debilitated persons:** Flu shots, pneumonia immunizations, infection avoidance, sensible nutrition, adequate fluid intake, balance of rest and activity

• **Comatose and immobile persons:** Elevate the head of the bed at least 30 degrees to feed and for 1 h after feeding; position on the side to prevent aspiration; frequently turn client
• **Ventilated clients:** Elevate the head of the bed 30—45 degrees to prevent aspiration and ventilator-associated pneumonia

Chronic Airflow Limitation

Description: Chronic airflow limitation (CAL) includes chronic bronchitis, pulmonary emphysema, and asthma (Table 4.3).

A. Emphysema and bronchitis, termed *chronic obstructive pulmonary disease* (COPD), are characterized by bronchospasm and dyspnea. The damage to the lung is not reversible and increases in severity over time.

B. Asthma, unlike COPD, is an intermittent disease with reversible airflow obstruction.

TABLE 4.3   Chronic Airflow Limitation

Chronic Bronchitis	Emphysema	Asthma
• Cough with sputum production on a daily basis for a minimum of 3 months/year • Chronic hypoxemia, cor pulmonale • Increase in mucus, cilia production • Increase in bronchial wall thickness (obstructs air flow) • Reduced responsiveness of respiratory center to hypoxemic stimuli	• Reduced gas exchange surface area • Increased air trapping (increased A-P diameter) • Decreased capillary network • Increased work, increased O_2 consumption	• Narrowing or closure of the airway due to a variety of stimulants
Precipitating Factors • Higher incidence in smokers	• Cigarette smoking • Environment and/or occupational exposure • Genetic	• Mucosal edema • V/Q abnormalities • Increased work of breathing • Beta-blockers • Respiratory infection • Allergic reaction • Emotional stress • Exercise • Environmental or occupational exposure • Reflux esophagitis
Assessment • Generalized cyanosis "Blue Bloaters" • Right-sided heart failure • Distended neck veins • Crackles • Expiratory wheezes	• "Pink Puffers" • Barrel chest • Pursed-lip breathers • Distant, quiet breath sounds • Wheezes • Pulmonary blebs on radiograph	• Dyspnea, wheezing, chest tightness • Monitor precipitating factors • Medication history
Nursing Plans and Interventions • Lowest Fio_2 possible to prevent CO_2 retention • Monitor for s/s of fluid overload • Maintain PaO_2 between 55 and 60 • Baseline arterial blood gases (ABGs) • Teach pursed-lip breathing and diaphragmatic breathing • Teach tripod position	• Lowest Fio_2 possible to prevent CO_2 retention • Monitor for s/s of fluid overload • Maintain PaO_2 between 55 and 60 • Baseline ABGs • Teach pursed-lip breathing and diaphragmatic breathing • Teach tripod position	• Administer bronchodilators • Administer fluids and humidification • Reinforce teaching (causes, medication regimen) • ABGs • Ventilatory patterns

C. Alveoli beyond the chronic obstruction are overinflated, causing chronic hypoxemia, hypoxia, and hypercapnia (in emphysema).

HESI HINT Respiratory compensation happens through the lungs, most often to correct acid–base imbalances.

Nursing Assessment

A. Changes in breathing pattern (e.g., an increase in rate with a decrease in depth)

B. Barrel chest as a result of long-term hyperinflation of the lungs

C. Generalized cyanosis of lips, mucous membranes, face, and nail beds ("blue bloater")

D. Cough (dry or productive)

E. Higher CO_2 than average

F. Low O_2, as determined by pulse oximetry (<90% to 92%)

G. Decreased breath sounds (noting location in the lung fields; e.g., right upper quadrant)

H. Coarse crackles in lung fields, which tend to disappear after coughing; wheezing

I. Dyspnea, orthopnea

J. Poor nutrition, weight loss

K. Activity intolerance

L. Anxiety concerning breathing, manifested by:
1. Anger
2. Fear of being alone
3. Fear of not being able to "catch breath"

HESI HINT Productive cough and comfort can be facilitated by semi-Fowler or high Fowler positions, which lessen pressure on the diaphragm from abdominal organs. Managing gastric distention becomes a priority in these clients because it elevates the diaphragm and inhibits full lung expansion.

HESI HINT Normal ABG Values

Blood Gas	Adult	Child
PH	7.35–7.45	7.36–7.44
P_{CO_2}	35–45 mm Hg	Same as adult
P_{O_2}	80–100 mm Hg	Same as adult
HCO_3	22–26 mEq/L	Same as adult

HESI HINT A **barrel chest** is indicative of emphysema and is caused by using overinflated muscles to breathe, which causes the person to work harder to breathe, but the amount of O_2 taken in is inadequate to oxygenate the tissues (there may be a pink tinge to the skin).

Insufficient oxygenation occurs with chronic bronchitis and leads to generalized cyanosis and often right-sided heart failure (HF; cor pulmonale). The client may appear cyanotic (blue-tinged skin).

HESI HINT: Health Promotion

Eating consumes energy needed for breathing. Offer mechanical soft diets that do not require as much chewing and digestion. Consider frequent small meals and providing fluids between meals instead of during meals. Assist with feeding if needed.

Prevent secondary infections—avoid crowds, contact with persons who have infectious diseases, and respiratory irritants (tobacco smoke).

Reinforce client teaching to report any change in characteristics of sputum.

Encourage client to hydrate well and to obtain immunizations needed (flu and pneumonia).

HESI HINT Cells of the body depend on oxygen to carry out their functions. Inadequate arterial oxygenation is manifested by cyanosis and slow capillary refill (>3 s). A chronic sign is clubbing of the fingernails, and a late sign is clubbing of the fingers.

Nursing Plans and Interventions

A. Collaborate with RN to develop and implement a client teaching plan about sitting upright and bending slightly forward to promote breathing.
1. In bed—sitting with arms resting on or over the bed table (tripod position)
2. In chair—leaning forward with elbows resting on knees (tripod position; Fig. 4.2)

B. Reinforce the client teaching plan regarding diaphragmatic and pursed-lip breathing.

C. Collaborate with RN to develop and implement a client teaching plan about prolonged expiratory phase to clear trapped air.

D. Administer O_2 at 1 to 2 L per nasal cannula (Table 4.4).

HESI HINT Caution must be taken in administering O_2 to a client with COPD. The stimulus to breathe is hypoxia (hypoxic drive), not the usual hypercapnia, the stimulus to breathe for healthy persons. Therefore, if too much oxygen is given, the client may stop breathing.

A. Pace activities to conserve energy.

B. Maintain adequate dietary intake, but do not overfeed.
1. Small, frequent meals
2. Favorite foods
3. Dietary supplements (protein-rich shakes, vitamins)

C. Provide an adequate fluid intake (3 L/day) unless contraindicated.

D. Collaborate with the RN to develop and implement a client/family teaching plan about relaxation techniques.

E. Reinforce the teaching plan regarding prevention of secondary infections.

F. Collaborate with RN to develop and implement a client/family teaching plan about medication regimen (Table 4.5).

G. Collaborate with RN to develop and implement a client/family teaching plan about proper technique for inhalers.

H. Smoking cessation is imperative.

I. Encourage health promotion activities.

HESI HINT When asked to prioritize nursing actions, use the ABC rule.
• A: Airway first
• B: Breathing
• C: Circulation
In cardiopulmonary resuscitation (CPR) circumstances, follow the CAB guidelines.
• C: Circulation first
• A: Then airway
• B: Then breathing

HESI HINT *Look and listen!* If breath sounds are clear, but the client is cyanotic and lethargic, adequate oxygenation is not occurring.

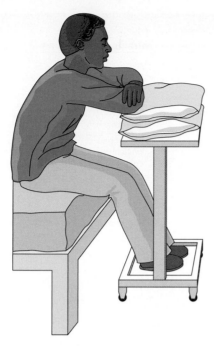

Sitting on the edge of a bed with the arms folded and placed on two or three pillows positioned over a nightstand.

A

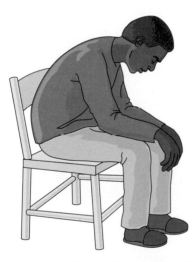

Sitting in a chair with the feet spread shoulder-width apart and leaning forward with the elbows on the knees. Arms and hands are relaxed.

B

Fig. 4.2 Forward-leaning Position. (A) The client sits on the edge of the bed with arms folded on a pillow placed on the elevated bedside table. (B) Client in three-point position. The client sits in a chair with the feet approximately 1 foot apart and leans forward with elbows on knees. (Ignatavicius, D. D., Workman, L., & Rebar, C. [2016]. *Medical-surgical nursing: Concepts for interprofessional collaborative care* [9th ed.]. St. Louis: Elsevier.)

HESI HINT The key to respiratory status is to auscultate breath sounds as well as visualize the client. Breath sounds are better "described," not named (e.g., sounds should be described as "crackles," "wheeze," "high-pitched whistling sound," rather than "rales," "rhonchi," etc., which may not mean the same thing to each clinical professional).

TABLE 4.4 Nursing Skills: Respiratory Client

Suctioning (Tracheal)
- Suction when adventitious breath sounds are heard, when secretions are present at endotracheal tube, or when gurgling sounds are noted.
- Use aseptic/sterile technique throughout the procedure.
- Wear mask and goggles.
- May liquefy secretions with 3 mL saline instilled before suctioning.
- Advance catheter until resistance is felt.
- Apply suction only when withdrawing catheter (gently rotate catheter when withdrawing).
- Never suction more than 10–15 s, and only pass the catheter three or fewer times.
- Oxygenate with 100% O_2 for 1–2 min before and after suctioning to prevent hypoxia.

Maintain Ventilator Setting
- Verify that alarms are on.
- Maintain settings and check often to ensure they are specifically set as prescribed by health care provider.
- Verify functioning of ventilator at least every 4 h.

Oxygen Administration
- Nasal cannula: low oxygen flow for low oxygen concentrations (good for chronic obstructive pulmonary disease).
- Simple face mask: low flow but effectively delivers high oxygen concentrations; cannot deliver less than 40% O_2.
- Nonrebreather mask: low flow but delivers high oxygen concentrations (60%–90%).
- Partial rebreather mask: low flow oxygen reservoir bag attached; can deliver high oxygen concentrations.
- Venturi mask: high-flow system; can deliver exact oxygen concentration.

Pulse Oximetry
- Easy measurement of oxygen saturation.
- Should be greater than 90%, ideally greater than 95%.
- Noninvasive, fastens to finger, toe, or earlobe.

Tracheostomy Care
- Aseptic technique (remove inner cannula only).
- Clean disposable inner cannula with hydrogen peroxide—rinse with sterile saline.
- 4 × 4 gauze dressing is butterfly folded.

Respiratory Isolation Technique
- Mask required for anyone entering room.
- Private room required.
- Client must wear mask if leaving room.

Proper Use of an Inhaler
- Have client exhale completely.
- Only grip (in mouth) if client has a spacer, otherwise keep mouth open to bring in volume of air with misted medication. While inhaling slowly, push down firmly on the inhaler to release the medication.
- Use bronchodilator inhaler before steroid inhaler and rinse mouthpiece after every use.

TABLE 4.5   Bronchodilators/Corticosteroids

Drugs	Indications	Adverse Reactions	Nursing Implications
Adrenergics/Sympathomimetics			
• Epinephrine • Isoproterenol HCL (Isuprel) • Albuterol (Proventil) • Isoetharine (Bronkometer) • Terbutaline (Brethine) • Salmeterol (Serevent) • Metaproterenol (inhaled) (Alupent) • Levalbuterol (Xopenex)	• Bronchodilator	• Anxiety • Increased heart rate • Nausea, vomiting • Urinary retention	• Check heart rate • Monitor for urinary retention, especially in men older than 40 years • Reinforce teaching in proper use of inhaler • Use bronchodilator inhaler before steroid inhaler • May cause sleep disturbance
Methylxanthines			
• Aminophylline (IV) • Theophylline (oral)	• Bronchodilator	• GI distress • Sleeplessness • Cardiac dysrhythmias • Hyperactivity	• Administer oral forms with food • Avoid foods containing caffeine • Can also be administered intravenously • Check heart rate • Reinforce teaching in proper use of inhaler • Monitor therapeutic range 10–20 mg/mL • Crosses placenta
Corticosteroids			
• Prednisone (oral) • Methylprednisolone (Solu-Medrol) (IV) • Beclomethasone dipropionate (inhaled) (Vanceril) • Budesonide (inhaled) (Pulmicort) • Fluticasone (inhaled) (Flovent) • Triamcinolone (inhaled) (Azmacort) • Flunisolide (inhaled) (AeroBid) • Mometasone (inhaled) (Asmanex)	• Anti-inflammatory	• Cardiac dysrhythmias that occur with long-term steroid use	• Reinforce teaching in proper use of inhaler
Anticholinergics			
• Ipratropium (Atrovent) • Tiotropium (Spiriva)	• Bronchodilator • Control of rhinorrhea	• Dry mouth • Blurred vision • Cough	• Do not exceed 12 doses in 24 h (Ipratropium)
Combination Products			
• Fluticasone + albuterol (Advair) • Ipratropium + albuterol (Combivent) • Budesonide + formoterol (Symbicort)	• See individual drugs	• See individual drugs	• See individual drugs
Phosphodiesterase 4 Inhibitors			
• Roflumilast (Daliresp)	• Reduced lung inflammation in severe COPD	• Insomnia • Weight loss • Depression	• Many drug–drug interactions

GI, Gastrointestinal; *COPD,* chronic obstructive pulmonary disease.

HESI HINT Watch for NCLEX-PN questions that deal with oxygen delivery. In adults, O_2 must bubble through some type of water solution so it can be humidified if given at greater than 4 L/min or delivered directly to the trachea. If given at 1–4 L/min or by mask or nasal prongs, the oropharynx and nasal pharynx provide adequate humidification.

Cancer of the Larynx

Description: Neoplasm occurring in the larynx, most commonly squamous cell in origin.

A. The combined effects of prolonged use of alcohol and/or tobacco are directly related to development.

B. Other contributing factors include the following:
1. Vocal straining
2. Chronic laryngitis
3. Family predisposition
4. Industrial exposure to carcinogens
5. Nutritional deficiencies; riboflavin

C. Men are affected eight times more often than women.

D. Diagnosis usually occurs between ages 55 and 70.

E. Earliest sign is hoarseness or a change in vocal quality that lasts greater than 2 weeks.

Medical management includes radiation therapy, often with adjuvant chemotherapy or surgical removal of the larynx (laryngectomy).

Nursing Assessment

A. Hoarseness for greater than 2 weeks (early)
B. Color changes in mouth or tongue
C. Later changes include dysphagia, dyspnea, cough, hemoptysis, weight loss, neck pain radiating to the ear, enlarged cervical nodes, and halitosis.

> **HESI HINT** With cancer of the larynx, the tongue and mouth often appear white, gray, dark brown, or black, and also patchy.

A. Direct laryngoscopy
B. X-ray films of head, neck, and chest
C. Computed tomography (CT) scan of the neck and biopsy
D. Magnetic resonance imaging (MRI)

Nursing Plans and Interventions

A. Collaborate with the RN to develop and implement a client/family perioperative teaching plan.
  1. Allow client/family to observe and handle tracheostomy tubes and suctioning equipment.
  2. Explain how and why suctioning will take place after surgery.
  3. Plan for acceptable communication method after surgery. Consider literacy level.
  4. Coordinate referral to speech pathologist.
  5. Discuss the planned rehabilitation program.
B. Provide postoperative care.
  1. Simplify communications.
  2. Use planned alternate communication method.
  3. Keep the call bell/light within reach at all times.
  4. Ask client yes/no questions whenever possible.
  5. Invite a family member to remain at bedside to provide support.
C. Promote respiratory functioning.
  1. Monitor respiratory rate and characteristics every 1 to 2 hours.
  2. Keep bed in semi-Fowler position at all times.
  3. Keep laryngeal airway humidified at all times.
  4. Auscultate lung sounds every 2 to 4 hours.
  5. Provide tracheostomy care every 2 to 4 hours and as needed (PRN).
    a. Suction excess secretions from oral cavity and tracheostomy PRN.
    b. Immediately after surgery, secretions may increase.

> **HESI HINT** Tracheostomy care involves cleaning the inner cannula, suctioning, and applying a clean dressing. Suctioning is performed as needed but it is not required every time tracheostomy care is provided.

D. Administer tube feedings as prescribed.
E. Encourage ambulation as early as possible.
F. Coordinate referral for speech rehabilitation with artificial larynx and/or to learn esophageal speech.
G. Humidification of environment.

> **HESI HINT** Air entering the lungs is humidified along the nasobronchial tree. This natural humidifying pathway is gone for the client who has had a laryngectomy. If the air is not humidified before entering the lungs, secretions tend to thicken and become crusty.

> **HESI HINT** A laryngectomy tube has a larger lumen and is shorter than the tracheostomy tube. Observe the client for any signs of bleeding or occlusion, which are the greatest immediate postoperative risks (first 24 h).

> **HESI HINT** Fear of choking is very real for laryngectomy clients. They cannot cough as before because the glottis is gone. Teach the "glottal stop" technique to remove secretions (take a deep breath, momentarily occlude the tracheostomy tube, cough, and simultaneously remove the finger from the tube).

Pulmonary Tuberculosis

Description: Pulmonary tuberculosis (TB) is a communicable lung disease caused by an infection with the *Mycobacterium tuberculosis* bacteria.

A. Airborne transmission.
B. After initial exposure, the bacteria encapsulate (form tuberculoma).
C. Bacteria remain dormant until a later time when clinical symptoms appear.

Nursing Assessment

A. Often asymptomatic.
B. Symptoms include:
  1. Fever with night sweats
  2. Anorexia, weight loss
  3. Malaise, fatigue
  4. Cough, hemoptysis
  5. Dyspnea, pleuritic chest pain with inspiration
  6. Cavitation or calcification as evidenced on chest x-ray film

7. Sputum culture is positive for *M. tuberculosis*
8. Repeated upper respiratory infections (URIs)

HESI HINT: TB Skin Test
Some HCPs may use serum blood testing using interferon-gamma release assay to detect TB. However, other HCPs may use TB skin tests. A positive TB skin test in a healthy client is exhibited by an induration ≤10 mm in diameter 48 h after the skin test. Anyone who has received a bacillus Calmette-Guerin vaccine will have a positive skin test and must be evaluated with an initial chest radiograph. A health history with a signs and symptoms form may be filled out annually until signs and symptoms arise; then another chest x-ray is required. Chest x-rays are required on new employment; an employer may require an x-ray every 5 years.

Nursing Plans and Interventions

A. Collaborate with the RN to develop and implement a client/family teaching plan.
   1. Cough into tissues and immediately dispose of them into special bags.
   2. Take all prescribed medications daily for 9 to 12 months.
   3. Conduct hand hygiene using proper technique.
   4. Report symptoms of deteriorating condition, especially hemorrhage.
B. Collect sputum cultures as needed; client may return to work after three negative cultures.
C. Place client in respiratory isolation while hospitalized. All personnel should wear a particulate respirator mask to filter the small tuberculosis organism.
D. Administer anti-TB medications as prescribed (Table 4.6).
E. Coordinate referral for client and high-risk persons to local or state health department for testing and prophylactic treatment.
F. Promote adequate nutrition.

Lung Cancer

Description: Neoplasm occurring in the lung.
A. Lung cancer is the leading cause of cancer-related deaths in men and women in the United States.
B. Cigarette smoking is responsible for 80% to 90% of all lung cancers.
C. Exposure to occupational hazards such as asbestos and radioactive dust poses significant risk.
D. Lung cancer tends to appear years after exposure; it is most commonly seen in persons in the fifth or sixth decade of life.

Nursing Assessment

A. Dry, hacking cough early, with cough turning productive as disease progresses
B. Hoarseness
C. Dyspnea
D. Hemoptysis; rust-colored or purulent sputum
   1. Pain in the chest area

2. Diminished breath sounds, occasional wheezing
3. Abnormal chest x-ray
4. Positive sputum for cytology

Nursing Plans and Interventions

A. Nursing interventions are similar to those implemented for the client with COPD.
B. Place client in semi-Fowler position.
C. Collaborate with RN to develop and implement a client/family teaching plan for pursed-lip breathing to improve gas exchange.
D. Collaborate with RN to develop and implement a client/family teaching plan for relaxation techniques; client often becomes anxious about breathing difficulty.
E. Administer oxygen, as indicated by pulse oximetry or ABGs.
F. Take measures to allay anxiety.
   1. Keep client/family informed of impending tests and procedures.
   2. Give client as much control as possible over personal care.
   3. Encourage client/family to verbalize concerns.
G. Decrease pain to manageable level by administering analgesics PRN (within safety range for respiratory difficulty).
H. Surgery
   1. Thoracotomy for clients who have a resectable tumor. Unfortunately, detection is often so late that the tumor is no longer localized and not amenable to resection.
   2. Pneumonectomy—removal of entire lung
      a. Position on back or operative side to facilitate expansion of remaining lung.
      b. Chest tubes may be clamped.
      c. Never turn to inoperative side.
   3. Lobectomy and segmental resection
      a. Position on back.
      b. Check to ensure tubing is not kinked or obstructed.
      c. Chest tubes usually inserted (Fig. 4.3).

HESI HINT Some tumors are so large that they fill entire lobes of the lung. When removed, large spaces are left. Chest tubes are not usually used with these clients because it is helpful if the mediastinal cavity, where the lung used to be, fills up with fluid. This fluid helps prevent a shift of the remaining chest organs to fill the empty space.

I. Chest tubes
   1. Keep all tubing coiled loosely below chest level, with connections tight and taped.
   2. Keep water seal and suction control chamber at the appropriate water levels.
   3. Monitor the fluid drainage, and mark the time of measurement and the fluid level.
   4. Observe for air bubbling in the water seal chamber and fluctuations (tidaling).
   5. Monitor the client's clinical status.

TABLE 4.6 Drug Therapy for Tuberculosis

Drug	Mechanisms of Action	Side Effects	Comments
First-Line Drugs			
• Isoniazid (INH)	• Interferes with DNA metabolism of tubercle bacillus	• Peripheral neuritis, hepatotoxicity, hypersensitivity (skin rash, arthralgia, fever), optic neuritis, vitamin B_6, neuritis	• Metabolism primarily by liver and excretion by kidneys, pyridoxine (vitamin B_6) administration during high-dose therapy as prophylactic measure • Use as single prophylactic agent for active TB in individuals whose PPD (purified protein) converts to positive • Ability to cross blood–brain barrier
• Rifampin (Rifadin)	• Has broad-spectrum effects • Inhibits RNA polymerase of tubercle bacillus	• Hepatitis, febrile reaction, GI disturbance, peripheral neuropathy, hypersensitivity	• Most common use with isoniazid • Low incidence of side effects • Suppression of effect of birth control pills • Possible orange urine
• Ethambutol (Myambutol)	• Inhibits RNA synthesis and is bacteriostatic for the tubercle bacillus	• Skin rash, GI disturbance, malaise, peripheral neuritis, optic neuritis	• Side effects uncommon and reversible with discontinuation of drug • Most common use as substitute drug when toxicity occurs with isoniazid or rifampin
• Streptomycin	• Inhibits protein synthesis and is bactericidal	• Ototoxicity (eighth cranial nerve), nephrotoxicity, hypersensitivity	• Cautious use in older adults, those with renal disease, and pregnant women • Must be given parenterally
• Pyrazinamide	• Bactericidal effect (exact mechanism is unknown)	• Fever, skin rash, hyperuricemia, jaundice (rare)	• High rate of effectiveness when used with streptomycin or capreomycin
• Rifapentine (Priftin)	• Inhibits DNA-dependent RNA polymerase	• Red discoloration of body fluids and tissues	• Many drug interactions • Always use in conjunction with at least one other antituberculosis drug
Second-Line Drugs			
• Ethionamide (Trecator)	• Inhibits protein synthesis	• GI disturbance, hepatotoxicity, hypersensitivity	• Valuable for treatment of resistant organisms; contraindicated in pregnancy
• Capreomycin (Capastat)	• Inhibits protein synthesis and is bactericidal	• Ototoxicity, nephrotoxicity	• Cautious use in older adults
• Kanamycin (Kantrex) and amikacin	• Interferes with protein synthesis	• Ototoxicity, nephrotoxicity	• Use in selected cases for treatment of resistant strains
• Para-aminosalicylic acid (PAS)	• Interferes with metabolism of tubercle bacillus	• GI disturbance (frequent), hypersensitivity, hepatotoxicity	• Interferes with absorption of rifampin; infrequent use
• Streptomycin • Levofloxacin (Levaquin) and moxifloxacin (Avelox)	• Inhibits protein synthesis and is bactericidal • Inhibits DNA gyrase	• Ototoxicity (eighth cranial nerve), nephrotoxicity, hypersensitivity • Increased risk of tendinitis	• Cautious use in older adults, those with renal disease, and pregnant women; must be given parenterally • Many drug–drug interactions
• Cycloserine (Seromycin)	• Inhibits cell-wall synthesis	• Personality changes, psychosis, rash	• Contraindicated in individuals with a history of psychosis; use in treatment of resistant strains

GI, Gastrointestinal; *TB,* tuberculosis.

6. Check the position of the chest drainage system.
7. Encourage the client to breathe deeply periodically.
8. Do not empty collection container. Replace unit when full.
9. Do not strip or milk chest tubes.
10. Chest tubes are not clamped routinely. If the drainage system breaks, place the distal end of the chest tubing connection in a sterile water container at a 2-cm level as an emergency water seal.
11. Maintain dry occlusive dressing.

HESI HINT: Chest Tubes
- If the chest tube becomes disconnected, do not clamp! Immediately place the end of the tube in a container of sterile saline or water until a new drainage system can be connected.
- If the chest tube is accidentally removed from the client, the nurse should cover with a dry sterile dressing. If a chest tube becomes disconnected, immediately reestablish the water-seal system and attach a new drainage system as soon as possible.
- Notify the HCP immediately.

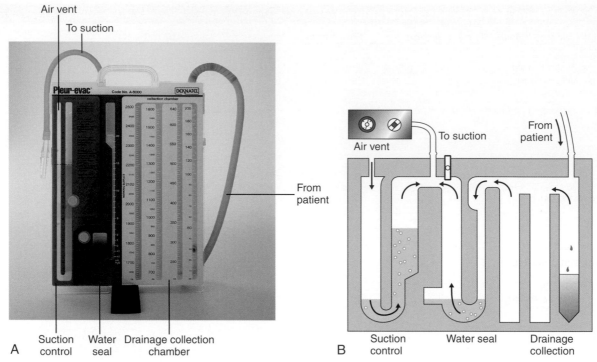

Fig. 4.3 Chest Tubes. Chest tubes are used to remove or drain blood or air from the intrapleural space, to expand the lung after surgery, or to restore subatmospheric pressure to the thoracic cavity. Many brands of commercial chest drainage systems are available; all are based on the traditional three-bottle water seal system. (A) Commonly used disposable chest drainage system. (B) Diagram of chambers of water-seal chest drainage. (Ignatavicius, D. D., Workman, L., & Rebar, C. [2020]. *Medical-surgical nursing: Concepts for inter-professional collaborative care* [10th ed.]. St. Louis: Elsevier.)

HESI HINT: NCLEX-PN Content on Chest Tubes
Fluctuations (tidaling) in the fluid will occur if there is no external suction. These fluctuating movements are a good indicator that the system is intact and should move upward with each inspiration and downward with each expiration (continuous bubbling indicates an air leak when the chest tube is hooked to suction). If fluctuations cease, check for kinked tubing, accumulation of fluid in the tubing, occlusions, or change in the client's position because expanding lung tissue may be occluding the tube opening. Remember, when external suction is applied, the fluctuations cease. Most hospitals *do not milk* chest tubes as a means of clearing or preventing clots. It is too easy to remove chest tubes. Mediastinal tubes may have orders to be stripped because of location, compared with larger thoracic cavity tubes.

HESI HINT Various pathophysiologic conditions can be related to the nursing diagnosis "ineffective breathing patterns."
- Inability of air sacs to fill and empty properly (emphysema, cystic fibrosis)
- Obstruction of the air passages (carcinoma, asthma, chronic bronchitis)
- Accumulation of fluid in the air sacs (pneumonia)
- Respiratory muscle fatigue (COPD, pneumonia, degenerative diseases such as multiple sclerosis [MS], myasthenia gravis [MG])

J. Chemotherapy
1. Nursing care for immunosuppression (see Oncology).
2. Administer antiemetics before administration of chemotherapy as prescribed.
3. Only RNs are certified to administer chemotherapy.
K. Radiation therapy
1. Provide skin care according to HCP's request.
2. Reinforce instructions to the client to not wash off the lines drawn by the radiologist.
3. Reinforce instructions to the client to wear soft, cotton garments only.
4. Avoid the use of powders or creams to radiation site unless specified by radiologist.

💡 REVIEW OF RESPIRATORY SYSTEM

1. List four common symptoms of pneumonia the nurse might note on physical examination.
2. State four nursing interventions for assisting the client to cough productively.
3. What symptoms of pneumonia might the nurse expect to see in an older client?
4. What should the O_2 flow rate be for the client with COPD?
5. How does the nurse prevent hypoxia during suctioning?
6. During mechanical ventilation, what are three major nursing interventions?
7. When examining a client with emphysema, what physical findings is the nurse likely to see?
8. What is the most common risk factor associated with lung cancer?
9. Describe the preoperative nursing care for a client undergoing a laryngectomy.
10. List five nursing interventions to implement after chest tube insertion.

11. What immediate action should the nurse take when a chest tube becomes disconnected from a bottle or suction apparatus? What should the nurse do if a chest tube is accidentally removed from the client?
12. What instructions should be given to a client after radiation therapy?
13. What precautions are required for clients with TB when placed on respiratory isolation?
14. List four components of teaching for the client with TB.
See Answer Key at the end of this text for suggested responses.

RENAL SYSTEM

Acute Kidney Injury

Description: Acute kidney injury (AKI) is the abrupt deterioration of the renal system; may be a reversible syndrome.

HESI HINT Normally, kidneys excrete approximately 1 mL of urine per kg of body weight per hour, which is about 1–2 L/24 h for adults.

A. AKI occurs when metabolites accumulate in the body and urinary output changes.
B. There are three major types of AKI (Table 4.7).
C. There are three phases of AKI:
   1. Oliguric phase
   2. Diuretic phase
   3. Recovery phase

Nursing Assessment

A. History of taking nephrotoxic drugs (salicylates, antibiotics, nonsteroidal anti-inflammatory drugs [NSAIDs], angiotensin-converting enzyme [ACE] inhibitors, angiotensin receptor blocker)
B. Alterations in urinary output
C. Edema, weight gain (ask if waistbands have suddenly become too tight)
D. Change in mental status
E. Hematuria
F. Dry mucous membranes
G. Drowsiness, headache, muscle twitching, seizures

HESI HINT Electrolytes are profoundly affected by kidney problems (a favorite NCLEX-PN topic). There must be a balance between the extracellular fluid and intracellular fluid to maintain homeostasis. A change in the number of ions or in the amount of fluid will cause a shift in one direction or the other. Sodium and chloride are the primary extracellular ions. Potassium and phosphate are the primary intracellular ions.

H. Diagnostic findings in the oliguric phase:
   1. Increased blood urea nitrogen (BUN) and creatinine
   2. Increased potassium (hyperkalemia)

TABLE 4.7 Acute Kidney Injury

Types	Description	Etiologic Factors
• Prerenal	• Interference with renal perfusion	• Hemorrhage • Hypovolemia • Decreased cardiac output • Decreased renal perfusion
• Intrarenal	• Damage to renal parenchyma	• Prolonged prerenal state • Nephrotoxins • Intratubular obstruction • Infections (glomerulonephritis) • Renal injury • Vascular lesions • Acute pyelonephritis
• Postrenal	• Obstruction in the urinary tract anywhere from the tubules to the urethral meatus	• Calculi • Prostatic hypertrophy • Tumors

   3. Decreased sodium (hyponatremia)
   4. Decreased pH (acidosis)
   5. Fluid overloaded (hypervolemic)
   6. High urine specific gravity greater than 1.020 g/mL
I. Diagnostic findings in the diuretic phase:
   1. Decreased fluid volume (hypovolemia)
   2. Decreased potassium (hypokalemia)
   3. Further decrease in sodium (hyponatremia)
   4. Low urine specific gravity less than 1.020 g/mL
J. Diagnostic laboratory work returns to normal range in recovery phase.

HESI HINT In some cases, a person with AKI may not experience the oliguric phase but may progress directly to the diuretic phase, during which the urine output may be as much as 10 L/day.

Nursing Plans and Interventions

A. Monitor intake and output (I&O) accurately; give only enough fluids in oliguric phase to replace losses—usually 400 to 500 mL/24 hours.
B. Document and report any change in the fluid volume status.
C. Monitor laboratory values for both serum and urine to assess electrolyte status, especially hyperkalemia indicated by serum potassium levels greater than 7 mEq/L and electrocardiogram (ECG) changes.
D. Identify changes in the level of consciousness.
E. Weigh daily—in oliguric phase, gain up to 1 lb/day.
F. Prevent cross infection.

G. Sodium polystyrene (Kayexalate) may be prescribed if K$^+$ too high.

H. Provide low-protein, moderate-fat, and high-carbohydrate diet.

HESI HINT Body weight is a good indicator of fluid retention and renal status. Obtain accurate weights on all clients with kidney failure, done on the same scale at the same time every day.

1 kg of weight = 1 L of water

HESI HINT: Fluid Volume Alterations

Excess fluid symptoms:
- Dyspnea
- Tachycardia
- Jugular vein distention (JVD)
- Peripheral edema
- Pulmonary edema

Deficient fluid symptoms:
- Decreased urine output
- Reduction in body weight
- Decreased skin turgor
- Dry mucous membranes
- Hypotension
- Tachycardia

HESI HINT Watch for signs of hyperkalemia: dizziness, weakness, cardiac irregularities, muscle cramps, diarrhea, and nausea.

HESI HINT Potassium has a critical safe range (3.5–5.0 mEq/L) because it affects the heart, and any imbalance must be corrected by medications or dietary modification. Limit high-potassium foods (e.g., bananas, avocados, spinach, and fish) and salt substitutes, which are high in potassium.

HESI HINT Clients with kidney injury retain sodium. With water retention, the sodium becomes diluted, and serum levels may appear near normal. With excessive water retention, the sodium levels appear decreased (dilution). Limit fluid and sodium intake in clients with AKI.

I. Monitor cardiac rate and rhythm (acute cardiac dysrhythmias are usually related to hyperkalemia).

J. Monitor drug levels and interactions.

HESI HINT During the oliguric phase, minimize protein breakdown and prevent rise in BUN by limiting protein intake. When BUN and creatinine levels return to normal, AKI is determined to be resolved.

Chronic Kidney Disease/End-Stage Renal Disease

Description: Chronic kidney disease/end-stage renal disease (ESRD) is progressive, irreversible damage to the nephrons and glomeruli, resulting in uremia.

A. Causes of chronic kidney disease are multitudinous.

B. As renal function diminishes, dialysis becomes necessary.

C. Transplantation is an alternative to dialysis for some clients.

Nursing Assessment

A. History of high medication usage

B. Family history of kidney disease

C. Increased blood pressure (BP) and/or chronic hypertension

D. Peripheral edema, pulmonary edema

E. Neurologic impairment (weakness, drowsiness)

F. Decreasing urinary function
1. Hematuria
2. Proteinuria
3. Cloudy urine
4. Oliguria (100 to 400 mL/day)
5. Anuria (<100 mL/day)

G. Jaundice

H. Gastrointestinal (GI) upsets

I. Metallic taste in mouth

J. Ammonia breath

K. Pain, discomfort

L. Peripheral neuropathy

M. Dialysis (Table 4.8)

N. Previous kidney transplant

O. Laboratory information
1. Azotemia (accumulation of nitrogenous waste products [urea nitrogen, creatinine] in the blood)
2. Increased creatinine and BUN
3. Decreased calcium
4. Elevated phosphorus and magnesium
5. Anemia

HESI HINT Accumulation of waste products from protein metabolism is the primary cause of uremia. Protein must be restricted in clients with ESRD. However, if protein intake is inadequate, a negative nitrogen balance occurs, causing muscle wasting. The glomerular filtration rate is most often used as an indicator of the level of protein consumption.

HESI HINT: Dialysis Covered by Medicare
- All persons in the United States are eligible for Medicare as of their first day of dialysis under special ESRD funding.
- Medicare card will indicate ESRD.
- Transplantation is covered by Medicare procedure; coverage terminates 6 months postoperative if dialysis is no longer required.

TABLE 4.8 Renal Dialysis

Type of Dialysis	Description	Nursing Implications
• Hemodialysis	• Requires venous access (arteriovenous shunt, fistula, or graft) • Treatment is 3–8 h in length, three times a week • Correction of fluid and electrolyte imbalance is rapid • Potential blood loss • Does not result in protein loss	• Heparinization is required • Requires expensive equipment • Inconvenient for home use • Rapid shifts of fluid and electrolytes can lead to disequilibrium syndrome (an unpleasant sensation and potentially dangerous situation) • Potential for hepatitis B and C • Do NOT take blood pressure or perform venipunctures on the arm with the arteriovenous (AV) shunt, fistula, or graft • Monitor the access site for thrill and bruit
• Continuous arteriovenous hemofiltration	• Requires vascular access: usually femoral or subclavian catheters • Slow process • Correction of fluid and electrolyte imbalance is slow • Does not cause blood loss • Does not result in protein loss	• Requires heparinization of filter tubing • Filters are costly • Equipment is simple to use • Limited to special care units, NOT for home use • Filter may rupture, causing blood loss

• Peritoneal	• Surgical placement of abdominal catheter is required (Tenckhoff, Gore-Tex, column-disk)
	• Slow process
	• Correction of fluid and electrolyte imbalance is slow
	• Does not cause blood loss
	• Protein is lost in dialysate
		• Heparinization is NOT required
		• Fairly expensive
		• Simple to perform
		• Easy to use at home
		• Dialysate is similar to intravenous fluid and is prescribed for the individual client's electrolyte needs
		• Potential complications:
		  • Bowel or bladder perforation
		  • Exit site and tunnel infection
		  • Peritonitis

Nursing Plans and Interventions

A. Monitor serum electrolyte levels.
B. Weigh daily.
C. Maintain strict I&O.
D. Check for JVD and other signs of fluid overload: periorbital edema, edema in lower legs, sacral area, etc.
E. Monitor edema, pulmonary edema (listen to breath sounds for crackles).
F. Provide low-protein, low-sodium, low-potassium, and low-phosphate diet.

G. Administer phosphate binders with food because client is unable to excrete phosphates (no magnesium-based antacids). Timing is important.
H. Encourage protein intake of high biologic value (eggs, milk, and meat) because the client is on a low-protein diet.
I. Alternate periods of rest with periods of activity.
J. Encourage strict adherence to medication regimen; teach client to obtain HCP's permission before taking any over-the-counter medications.
K. Observe for complications.
　1. Anemia, administer antianemic drug (Table 4.9)
　2. Renal osteodystrophy (abnormal calcium metabolism causes bone pathology)
　3. Severe, resistant hypertension
　4. Infection
　5. Metabolic acidosis
　6. Bleeding because of anticoagulants used during dialysis

HESI HINT Protein intake is restricted until blood chemistry shows the ability to handle protein catabolites—urea and creatinine. Ensure high-calorie intake so protein is spared for its own work; give hard candy, jellybeans, flavored carbohydrate powders.

TABLE 4.9 Antianemic: Biologic Response Modifier

Drug	Indications	Adverse Reactions	Nursing Interventions
• Erythropoietin (Epogen)	• Anemia resulting from decreased production of erythropoietin in end-stage renal disease • Stimulates RBC production, increases Hgb, reticulocyte count, and Hct	• Use with caution in older clients because of increased risk of thrombosis	• Monitor Hct weekly; report levels over 30%—33% or increases of more than 4 points in less than 2 weeks • Explain that pelvic and limb pain should dissipate after 12 h • Do not shake vial; shaking may inactivate the glycoprotein • Discard unused contents—does not contain preservatives

Hct, Hematocrit; *Hgb,* hemoglobin; *RBC,* red blood cell.

TABLE 4.10   Postoperative Care: Kidney Surgery

Assessment	Nursing Interventions	Rationale
• Respiratory status	• Auscultate lung sounds to detect "wet" sounds indicating infection • Demonstrate method of splinting incision for comfort when coughing and deep breathing	• Flank incision causes pain with BOTH inspiration and expiration; therefore, client avoids deep breathing and coughing, which can lead to respiratory difficulties, including pneumonia
• Circulatory status	• Check vital signs to detect early signs of bleeding, shock • Monitor skin color and temperature (pallor and cold skin are signs of shock) • Monitor urinary output (will decrease with circulatory collapse) • Monitor surgical site for frank bleeding	• The kidney is very vascular • Bleeding is a constant threat • Circulatory collapse will occur with hemorrhage and can occur very quickly
• Pain relief status	• Administer narcotic analgesics as needed to relieve pain	• Relief of pain will improve the client's cooperation with deep breathing exercises • Relief of pain will improve client's cooperation with early ambulation
• Urinary status	• Check urinary output and drainage from ALL tubes inserted during the surgery • Maintain accurate intake and output	• Mechanical drainage of bladder will be implemented after surgery

L. Living-related or cadaver kidney transplant (Table 4.10).
   1. Monitor for rejection.
   2. Monitor for infection.
   3. Reinforce client teaching about meticulously maintaining immunosuppressive drug therapy.

Urinary Tract Infections

Description: Infection or inflammation at any site in the urinary tract. (Kidney = pyelonephritis, urethra = urethritis, bladder = cystitis, prostate = prostatitis.)
A. Normally, the entire urinary tract is sterile.
B. The most common infectious agent is *Escherichia coli*.
C. Persons at highest risk for acquiring urinary tract infection (UTI):
   1. Clients diagnosed with diabetes
   2. Pregnant women
   3. Men with prostatic hypertrophy
   4. Immunosuppressed persons
   5. Catheterized clients
   6. Anyone with urinary retention, either short term or long term
   7. Older women (bladder prolapse)
   8. Sexually active women, who are more vulnerable to UTIs and kidney stones
D. Diagnosis
   1. Clean-catch midstream urine collection for culture to identify specific causative organism (before administering anti-infective medications)
   2. IV pyelogram to determine kidney functioning
   3. Cystogram to determine bladder functioning
   4. Cystoscopy to determine bladder or urethral abnormalities

Nursing Assessment

A. Signs of infection including malaise, fever, and chills
B. Urinary frequency, urgency, or dysuria

C. Hematuria
D. Pain at the costovertebral angle
E. Elevated serum WBC (>10,000)
F. Urinalysis with red blood cells (RBCs) and WBCs
G. Characteristics of urine: cloudy, dark, and foul smelling
H. Bladder spasms
I. Nausea and vomiting

Nursing Plans and Interventions

A. Administer prescribed antibiotics specific to infectious agent.
B. Instruct client in the appropriate medication regimen.
C. Encourage fluid intake of 3000 mL fluid per day.
D. Maintain I&O.
E. Administer mild analgesics (acetaminophen or aspirin).
F. Encourage voiding every 2 to 3 hours to prevent residual urine from stagnating in bladder.
G. Avoid caffeine, alcohol, citrus juices, chocolate, and highly spicy foods/beverages.

> **HESI HINT** The key to resolving UTIs with most antibiotics is to keep the blood level of the antibiotic constant. It is important to tell the client to take the antibiotics around the clock and not to skip doses so a consistent blood level can be maintained for optimal efficacy.

H. Collaborate with RN and implement a teaching plan.
   1. Take entire prescription as directed.
   2. Encourage oral fluid intake to 3000 mL/day (water, juices). Should not consume citrus juices.
   3. Shower rather than bathe as a preventive measure. If bathing is necessary, never take a bubble or oil bath.
   4. Women/girls should cleanse from front to back after toileting.

5. Avoid urinary tract irritants: alcohol, sodas, citrus juices, spices.
6. Women should void immediately after intercourse.
7. Void every 2 to 3 hours during the day.
8. Wear cotton undergarments and loose clothing to help decrease perineal moisture.
9. Practice good handwashing technique.
10. Obtain follow-up care.

Urinary Tract Obstruction

Description: Partial or complete blockage of the urine flow at any point in the urinary system.
A. Urinary tract obstruction is usually caused by:
   1. Foreign body (calculus)
   2. Tumor
   3. Stricture
   4. Functional (e.g., neurogenic bladder)
B. When urinary tract obstruction occurs, urine is retained above the point of obstruction.
   1. Hydrostatic pressure builds, causing dilation of the organs above the obstruction.
   2. If hydrostatic pressure continues to build, then hydronephrosis develops, which can lead to kidney failure.

Nursing Assessment

A. Pain, usually quite severe, acute
   1. May experience renal colic
   2. Radiating down the thigh and to the genitalia
B. Symptoms of obstruction
   1. Fever, chills
   2. Nausea, vomiting, diarrhea
   3. Abdominal distention

> **HESI HINT** Location of the pain can help determine location of the stone.
> Flank pain usually means the stone is in the kidney or upper ureter. If it radiates to the abdomen or scrotum, the stone is likely to be in the ureter or bladder.
> Excruciating, spastic-type pain is called colic.
> During kidney stone attacks, it is preferable to administer pain medications at regularly scheduled intervals rather than PRN to prevent spasms and optimize comfort.

C. Change in voiding pattern.
   1. Dysuria, hematuria
   2. Urgency, frequency, hesitancy, nocturia, dribbling
   3. Difficulty in starting a stream
   4. Incontinence
D. Those with the following conditions are at risk for developing calculi:
   1. Strictures
   2. Prostatic hypertrophy
   3. Neoplasms

4. Congenital malformations
5. History of calculi
6. Family history of calculi

Nursing Plans and Interventions

A. Administer narcotic analgesics or NSAIDs as prescribed.
B. Apply moist heat to the painful area unless prescribed otherwise.
C. Encourage high oral fluid intake to help dislodge the stone.
D. Monitor IV antibiotics if infection is present.
E. Strain all urine.
F. Send any stones found from straining to the laboratory for analysis.
G. Accurately document I&O.
H. Endourologic procedures:
   1. Cystoscopy
   2. Cystolitholapaxy
   3. Ureteroscopy
   4. Percutaneous nephrolithotomy
I. Lithotripsy
   1. Electrohydraulic lithotripsy
   2. Laser
   3. Extracorporeal shock wave
J. Surgical therapy
   1. Nephrolithotomy
   2. Ureterolithotomy
   3. Cystectomy

> **HESI HINT: Percutaneous Nephrostomy**
> A needle/catheter is inserted through the skin into the calyx of the kidney. The stone may be dissolved by percutaneous irrigation with the liquid that will dissolve the stone, or ultrasonic sound waves (lithotripsy) can be directed through the needle/catheter to break up the stone, which can be then eliminated through the urinary tract.

K. Collaborate with the RN and implement a teaching plan to include the following:
   1. Encourage follow-up care because stones tend to recur.
   2. Maintain a high fluid intake of 3 to 4 L/day.
   3. Follow prescribed diet (based on composition of stone).
   4. Avoid long periods of supine position.

Benign Prostatic Hyperplasia

(Sometimes called *hypertrophy of the prostate.*)
Description: Benign prostatic hyperplasia is enlargement or hypertrophy of the prostate.
A. Tends to occur in men aged greater than 40 years.
B. Intervention is required when symptoms of obstruction occur.
C. The most common treatment is transurethral resection of the prostate gland (TURP). The prostate is removed by endoscopy (no surgical incision is made), allowing for a shorter hospital stay.

Nursing Assessment

A. Increased urgency and frequency with a decrease in the amount of each voiding

B. Nocturia

C. Hesitancy (need to stop and start several times while voiding)

D. Terminal dribbling

E. Changes in size and force of urinary stream

F. Acute urinary retention

G. Bladder distention and pain

H. Dribbling

I. Hematuria

J. UTIs

Nursing Plans and Interventions

A. Assist with preoperative teaching to include information concerning pain from bladder spasms that occur postoperatively.

B. Postoperatively maintain patent urinary drainage system to decrease the spasms.

C. Provide pain relief as prescribed: analgesics, narcotics, and antispasmodics.

> **HESI HINT** Bladder spasms frequently occur after TURP. Inform the client that the presence of the oversized balloon on the catheter (30 –45 mL inflate) will cause a continuous feeling of needing to void. The client should not try to void around the catheter because that can precipitate bladder spasms. Medications to reduce or prevent spasms should be given.

D. Minimize catheter manipulation by taping catheter to the abdomen or leg or by using a leg strap.

E. Maintain gentle traction on urinary catheter.

F. Check the urinary drainage system for clots.

G. Irrigate bladder as prescribed (may be continuous or intermittent). If continuous, keep indwelling urinary bag emptied to avoid retrograde pressure.

> **HESI HINT** Instillation of the hypertonic or hypotonic solution into a body cavity will cause a shift in the cellular fluid. Use only sterile saline for bladder irrigation after TURP because the irrigation must be isotonic to prevent fluid and electrolyte imbalance.

H. Observe the color and content of urinary output.

1. Normal drainage after prostate surgery is reddish pink clearing to light pink within 24 hours after surgery.

2. Monitor for bright red bleeding with large clots and increased viscosity (suspect hemorrhage).

I. Monitor vital signs frequently for indication of circulatory collapse (indicated by increased pulse with decreased BP).

J. Monitor hemoglobin (Hgb) and hematocrit (Hct) for pattern of decreasing values that indicates bleeding.

K. After catheter is removed:

1. Monitor amount and number of times the client voids.

2. Have the client use urine cups to provide a specimen with each voiding.

3. Observe for hematuria after each voiding (urine should progress to clear yellow color by the fourth day).

4. Inform client that burning on urination and urinary frequency are usually experienced in the first postoperative week.

5. Generally the client is not impotent after surgery, but sterility may occur.

6. Reinforce instructions for client to immediately report any frank bleeding to HCP.

7. Monitor for signs of urethral stricture: straining, dysuria, weak urinary stream.

8. Administer antispasmodics as prescribed.

> **HESI HINT** Inform the client before discharge that some bleeding is expected after TURP. Large amounts of blood or frank, bright bleeding should be reported. However, it is normal for the client to pass small amounts of blood during the healing process, as well as small clots. He should rest quietly and continue drinking large amounts of fluid.

L. Encourage the client to increase fluid intake to 3000 mL/day.

M. Prepare client for discharge with instructions to:

1. Continue to drink 12 to 14 glasses of water per day.

2. Avoid constipation, straining.

3. Avoid strenuous activity, lifting, intercourse, or engaging in sports during the first 3 to 4 weeks after surgery.

4. Schedule a follow-up appointment.

? REVIEW OF RENAL SYSTEM

1. Differentiate between AKI and chronic kidney failure.

2. During the oliguric phase of AKI, protein should be severely restricted. What is the rationale for this restriction?

3. Identify two nursing interventions for the client on hemodialysis.

4. What is the highest-priority nursing diagnosis for clients in any type of kidney failure?

5. A client with kidney failure asks why he is being given antacids. What should the nurse reply?

6. List four essential elements of a teaching plan for clients with frequent UTIs.

7. What are the most important nursing interventions for clients with possible renal calculi?

8. What discharge instructions should be given to a client who has had urinary calculi?

9. After TURP, hematuria should subside by what postoperative day?

10. After the urinary catheter is removed in the TURP client, what are three priority nursing actions to be taken?

11. After kidney surgery, what are the primary assessments the nurse should make?

See Answer Key at the end of this text for suggested responses.

CARDIOVASCULAR SYSTEM

> **HESI HINT** What is the relationship of the kidneys with the cardiovascular system?
> - The kidneys filter about a liter of blood per minute.
> - If cardiac output (CO) is decreased, the amount of blood going through the kidneys is decreased; urinary output is decreased. Therefore, a decreased urinary output may be a sign of cardiac problems.
> - When the kidneys produce and excrete 0.5 mL of urine per kg of body weight or average 30 mL/h output, the blood supply is considered to be minimally adequate to perfuse the vital organs.

Angina

Description: Angina is chest discomfort or pain occurring when myocardial oxygen demands exceed supply. This temporary deficiency of blood flow is called ischemia. Common causes include:

A. Atherosclerotic heart disease, hypertension, coronary artery spasm, hypertrophic cardiomyopathy
B. Any activity that increases the heart's oxygen demand: physical exertion, cold temperatures

Nursing Assessment

A. Pain
1. Mild to severe intensity, described as heavy, squeezing, pressing, burning, choking, aching, and feeling of apprehension
2. Substernal, radiating to left arm and/or shoulder, jaw, or right shoulder
3. Transient or prolonged, with gradual or sudden onset; typically short duration
4. Often precipitated by exercise, exposure to cold, a heavy meal, mental tension, sexual intercourse
5. Relieved by rest and/or nitroglycerin
B. Dyspnea, tachycardia, palpitations
C. Nausea, vomiting
D. Fatigue
E. Diaphoresis, pallor, weakness
F. Syncope
G. Dysrhythmias
H. Diagnostic information
1. ECG: generally at client baseline unless taken during anginal attack, when ST depression and T-wave inversion may occur.
2. Exercise stress test shows ST segment depression and hypotension.
3. Stress echocardiogram: looks for changes in wall motion (indicated in women).
4. Coronary angiogram: detects coronary artery spasms.
5. Cardiac catheterization: detects arterial blockage.
I. Risk factors
1. Nonmodifiable
   a. Heredity

b. Gender: risk greater for male than female until menopause, then equal risk
c. Ethnic background: African Americans have greater risk
d. Age (increasing risk with increasing age)
2. Modifiable
a. Hyperlipidemia
b. Those with serum cholesterol greater than 300 mg/dL have four times greater risk of developing coronary artery disease (CAD) than those with levels less than 200 mg/dL (desirable level).
c. Low-density lipoprotein (LDL) "bad" cholesterol. A molecule of LDL is approximately 50% cholesterol by weight (<100 mg/dL optimal, <130 mg/dL desirable).
d. High-density lipoprotein (HDL) "good cholesterol." HDL is inversely related to the risk of developing CAD (>60 mg/dL is desirable). In fact, HDL may serve to remove cholesterol from tissues.
e. Hypertension, cigarette smoking, obesity, physical inactivity, metabolic syndrome, stress, elevated homocysteine level, substance abuse

Nursing Plans and Interventions

A. Monitor medications and instruct client in proper administration.
B. Determine factors precipitating pain and assist client/family in adjusting lifestyle to decrease these factors.
C. Collaborate with RN to develop and implement client/family teaching plan about risk factors and identify client's own risk factors.
D. During an attack:
1. Provide immediate rest, take vital signs, and record an ECG.
2. Administer no more than three sublingual nitroglycerin tablets, 5 minutes apart (Table 4.11).
3. Seek emergency treatment if no relief has occurred after taking nitroglycerin.
E. Physical activity
1. Avoid isometric activity.
2. Implement an exercise program.
3. Sexual activity may be resumed after exercise is tolerated, usually when able to climb two flights of stairs without exertion. Nitroglycerin can be taken prophylactically before intercourse.
F. Provide nutritional information concerning modifying fats (saturated) and sodium. Antilipemic medications may be prescribed to lower cholesterol levels (Table 4.12).
G. Medical interventions include:
1. Percutaneous coronary intervention: a balloon catheter is repeatedly inflated to split or fracture plaque and the arterial wall is stretched, enlarging the diameter of the vessel.
2. Arthrectomy: a catheter with a collection chamber is used to remove plaque from a coronary artery by shaving, cutting, or grinding.

TABLE 4.11   Antianginals

Drugs	Indications/Actions	Adverse Reactions	Nursing Implications
Nitrates			
• Nitroglycerin (NTG) for acute attacks (sub lingual—one tablet for acute attacks of angina every 5 min not to exceed three tablets) • Isosorbide dinitrate (Isordil) for anginal prophylaxis • Isosorbide mononitrate (Imdur)	• Acute attack • Anginal prophylaxis • Reduces vascular resistance	• Headache • Flushing • Dizziness • Weakness • Hypotension • Nausea	• Monitor relief • Have client rest • Monitor vital signs • Store in original container • Replace NTG tablets every 3–5 months
Beta-Blockers			
• Propranolol HCL (Inderal) • Atenolol (Tenormin) • Nadolol (Corgard)	• Anginal prophylaxis • Reduce oxygen demand	• Fatigue • Lethargy • Hallucinations • Impotence • Bradycardia • Hypotension • HF • Wheezing	• Monitor apical heart rate • Watch for a decreased BP • Do not stop abruptly • Clients with HF, bronchitis, asthma, COPD, renal or hepatic insufficiency have an increased likelihood of incurring adverse reactions
Calcium Channel Blockers			
• Verapamil (Calan) • Nifedipine HCL (Procardia) • Diltiazem HCL (Cardizem, Norvasc)	• Anginal prophylaxis • Inhibits influx of calcium ions	• Dizziness • Hypotension • Fatigue • Headache • Syncope • Peripheral edema • Hypokalemia • Dysrhythmia • HF	• Clients with HF and older adults have an increased likelihood of incurring adverse reactions • Watch for a decreased BP • Monitor serum potassium • Swallow pills whole • Store at room temperature • Do not stop abruptly • Take 1 h before meals or 2 h after meals
Other			
• Ranolazine (Ranexa)	• Anginal prophylaxis • Inhibits influx of sodium ions	• Dysrhythmia • Constipation	• Many drug-drug interactions • Contraindication in all levels of hepatic cirrhosis

BP, Blood pressure; *COPD*, chronic obstructive pulmonary disease; *HF*, heart failure.

3. Coronary artery bypass graft (CABG).
4. Transcardial laser revascularization.
5. Coronary artery drug-eluting stents.

Myocardial Infarction

Description: Myocardial infarction (MI) is the disruption or deficiency of coronary artery blood supply resulting in necrosis (death) of myocardial tissue.
A. Causes of MI
   1. Thrombus or clotting
   2. Shock or hemorrhage

Nursing Assessment

A. Sudden onset of pain in the lower sternal region (substernal)
   1. Severity increases until it becomes nearly unbearable.

   2. Heavy and viselike pain often radiates to the shoulders and down the arms and/or to the neck, jaw, and back. Common locations for pain are substernal, retrosternal, or epigastric areas.
   3. MI pain differs from angina pain in its sudden onset.
   4. Pain is not relieved by rest.
   5. Pain may occur during rest.
   6. Pain is not relieved by nitroglycerin.
   7. Pain may persist for hours or days.
   8. Client may not have pain (silent MI), especially those with diabetic neuropathy.
B. Rapid, irregular, and thready pulse
C. Decreased level of consciousness, indicating decreased cerebral perfusion
D. Left heart shift sometimes occurs post-MI
E. Cardiac dysrhythmias occur in about 90% of clients with MI

TABLE 4.12 Antilipemics

Drugs	Indications	Adverse Reactions	Nursing Implications
Bile Sequestrants • Colestipol HCL (Colestid) • Colesevelam (Welchol) • Cholestyramine (Questran)	• Treat type IIA hyperlipidemia (hypercholesterolemia) when dietary changes fail	• Abdominal pain, nausea and vomiting, distention, flatulence, belching, constipation • Reduced absorption of lipid-soluble vitamins: A, D, E, and K • Alters absorption of other oral medications	• Reinforce teaching plan to mix powder forms with liquid or fruits high in moisture content such as applesauce to prevent accidental inhalation or esophageal distress • Monitor prothrombin times • Report visual changes and rickets • Administer other oral medications 1 h before or 6 h after giving bile sequestrants
HMG-CoA Reductase Inhibitors (Statins) • Atorvastatin (Lipitor) • Fluvastatin (Lescol) • Pravastatin (Pravachol) • Simvastatin (Zocor) • Lovastatin (Mevacor) • Pitavastatin (Livalo) • Rosuvastatin (Crestor)	• Diagnosis of cardiac disease • Extremely high LDL • Middle-aged with diagnosis of type 2 diabetes • High risk of cardiac disease	• Side effects similar to bile sequestrants • May elevate liver enzymes • Hepatitis and/or pancreatitis • Rhabdomyolysis	• Obtain liver enzymes baseline and monitor every 6 months • Monitor creatine phosphokinase (CPK) levels • Review specific drug/food interactions; avoid grapefruit juice • Timing with or without food varies with drug • Reinforce teaching with client to report any muscle tenderness • Monitor dose limits when interacting medications prescribed
Fibric Acid Derivatives • Gemfibrozil (Lopid) • Fenofibrate (Tricor) • Fenofibric acid (Trilipix) • Clofibrate (Claripex)	• Used with diet changes to lower both elevated cholesterol and triglycerides	• Abdominal/epigastric pain, diarrhea—most common • Flatulence, nausea and vomiting • Heartburn • Dyspepsia • Gallstones • TriCor: weakness, fatigue, H/A • Myopathy	• Obtain baseline labs: liver function, complete blood count (CBC), and electrolytes and monitor every 3–6 months • Administer: • Lopid: 30 min before breakfast and dinner • TriCor: with meals
Water-Soluble Vitamins • Niacin (Niaspan) • Nicotinic acid (Nicobid)	• Large doses decrease lipoprotein and triglyceride synthesis and increase HDL	• Flushing of face/neck • Pruritus • H/A • Orthostatic hypotension • Extended-release form: hepatotoxicity • Hyperglycemia • Hyperuricemia • Upper GI distress	• Give with milk or food to avoid GI irritation • Client to change positions slowly • Reinforce teaching with clients taking extended-release form to report darkened urine, light-colored stools, anorexia, yellowing of eyes or skin, severe stomach pain

GI, Gastrointestinal; *LDL,* low-density lipoprotein.

F. Cardiogenic shock or fluid retention

G. Narrowed pulse pressure—for example, 90/80

H. Bowel sounds absent or high-pitched, indicating possibility of mesenteric artery thrombosis, which acts as an intestinal obstruction (see Gastrointestinal System).

I. HF indicated by wet lung sounds.

J. ECG changes; occur as early as 2 hours post-MI or as late as 72 hours post-MI (Table 4.13).

K. Nausea, vomiting, gastric discomfort, indigestion

L. Anxiety, restlessness, feeling of impending doom or death

M. Cool, pale, diaphoretic skin

N. Dizziness, fatigue, syncope

O. Women more commonly experience dyspnea, unusual fatigue, and sleep disturbances.

HESI HINT: Signs of Cardiogenic Shock
- Hypotension
- Urine output of less than 30 mL/h
- Tachycardia
- Cool, moist skin
- Decreased level of consciousness

TABLE 4.13 Post-Myocardial Infarction Cardiac Enzyme Elevations

Enzyme/Marker	Onset	Peak (h)	Return to Normal
CK-MB (recognized indicator of MI by most clinicians)	4–8 h	12–24	48–72 h
Myoglobin	1–4 h (elevate before CK-MB)	12	24 h
Cardiac troponins	As early as 1 h post injury	10–24	5–14 days

Nursing Plans and Interventions

A. Administer and/or monitor medications as prescribed.
  1. For pain and to increase O_2 perfusion, IV morphine sulfate (acts as a peripheral vasodilator and decreases venous return) is the drug of choice.
  2. Other medications often prescribed include (see Table 4.11):
     a. Nitrates (nitroglycerin)
     b. ACE inhibitors
     c. Beta blockers
     d. Calcium channel blockers (when beta blockers are contraindicated)
     e. Aspirin
     f. Antiplatelet aggregates
B. Obtain vital signs, including ECG rhythm strip, regularly per agency policy.
C. Administer oxygen at 2 to 5 L per nasal cannula.
D. Obtain cardiac enzymes as prescribed.
E. Provide a quiet, restful environment.
F. Auscultate breath sounds for rales (indicating pulmonary edema).
G. Monitor the patency of the IV line for administration of emergency medications.
H. Monitor fluid balance.
I. Keep in semi-Fowler position to assist with breathing.
J. Patient is ambulatory shortly after the procedure.
K. Encourage client to gradually resume activity.
L. Encourage verbalization of fears.
M. Provide information about the disease process and cardiac rehabilitation.
N. Medical interventions (see Angina).
  1. Thrombolytic agents, within 1 to 4 hours of the start of an MI (used in intensive care unit [ICU] only)
  2. Intraaortic balloon pump to improve myocardial perfusion (ICU only)
  3. Surgical reperfusion with CABG

Hypertension

Description: Hypertension is persistent BP levels greater than 140/90.
A. Essential (primary) hypertension has no known cause (idiopathic).

B. Secondary hypertension develops in response to an identifiable mechanism or another disease.

> **HESI HINT** BP is created by the difference in the pressure of the blood as it leaves the heart and the resistance it meets flowing out to the tissues. Therefore, any factor that alters CO or peripheral vascular resistance will alter BP (prehypertension BP is 120–139/80–89). Diet and exercise, smoking cessation, weight control, and stress management can control many factors that influence the resistance blood meets as it flows from the heart.

Nursing Assessment

A. BP greater than 140/90 or diastolic BP greater than or equal to 90 on three separate occasions
  1. Obtain BP with client lying, sitting, and standing.
  2. Compare readings taken lying, sitting, and standing. A difference of more than 10 mm Hg of either systolic or diastolic indicates postural hypotension. Take in both arms.
B. Genetic risk factors (nonmodifiable)
  1. Positive family history for hypertension
  2. Sex (men have greater risk of being hypertensive at an earlier age than women)
  3. Age (increasing risk with increasing age)
  4. Ethnicity (African Americans at greater risk than whites)
C. Lifestyle and habits that increase risk of becoming hypertensive (modifiable)
  1. Use of alcohol, tobacco, and caffeine
  2. Sedentary lifestyle, obesity
  3. Socioeconomic level (incidence is greater in lower socioeconomic groups)
  4. Nutrition history of high salt and fat intake
  5. Use of oral contraceptives or estrogens
  6. Diabetes mellitus (DM)
  7. Stress

> **HESI HINT** Remember the risk factors for hypertension: heredity, race, age, alcohol abuse, increased salt intake, obesity, and use of oral contraceptives.

D. Associated physical problems
  1. Kidney failure
  2. Impaired kidney function
  3. Respiratory problems (especially COPD)
  4. Cardiac problems (especially valvular disorders)
  5. Dyslipidemia
  6. Diabetes
E. Pharmacologic history
  1. Steroids (increase BP)
  2. Estrogens (increase BP, for example, birth control pills, NSAIDs, and cocaine)
     a. Gather data related to headache, edema, nocturia, nosebleeds, and vision changes (may be asymptomatic).

b. Assist the client to identify the level and source of stress (job-related, economic, or family).

c. Recognize personality type—determine whether client exhibits "Type A" behavior.

Nursing Plans and Interventions

A. Collaborate with RN and implement a teaching plan to include:

1. Information about disease process
   a. Risk factors
   b. Causes
   c. Long-term complications
   d. Lifestyle modifications
   e. Relationship between treatment and prevention of complications
2. Information about treatment plan
   a. How to take own BP

b. Reasons for each medication (Tables 4.14 and 4.15)

c. How and when to take each medication

d. Necessity of consistency with medication regimen

e. Need for ongoing assessment while taking antihypertensives

> **HESI HINT** The number one cause of cerebral vascular accident (CVA) with hypertensive clients is noncompliance with medication regimen. Hypertension is often symptomless, and antihypertensive medications are expensive and have side effects. Studies have shown that the more clients know about their antihypertensive medications, the more likely they are to take them; teaching and reinforcement are important.

3. Monitor serum electrolytes every 90 to 120 days for duration of treatment.

TABLE 4.14 Diuretics

Drugs	Indications	Adverse Reactions	Nursing Implications

Thiazides
• Chlorthalidone (Hygroton)
• Hydrochlorothiazide (Esidrix, Microzide)
• Indapamide (Lozol)
• Metolazone (Zaroxolyn)
	• To decrease fluid volume
	• Inexpensive
	• Effective
	• Useful in severe hypertension
	• Effective orally
	• Enhances other antihypertensives
		• Hypokalemia symptoms include:
		  • Dry mouth
		  • Thirst
		  • Weakness
		  • Drowsiness
		  • Lethargy
		  • Muscle aches
		  • Tachycardia
		  • Hyperuricemia
		  • Glucose intolerance
		  • Hypercholesterolemia
		  • Sexual dysfunction
			• Observe for postural hypotension, can be potentiated by:
			  • Alcohol
			  • Barbiturates
			  • Narcotics
			• Caution with:
			  • Renal failure
			  • Gout
			  • Client taking lithium
			  • Hypokalemia increases risk of digitalis toxicity
			  • Administer potassium supplements

Loop • Furosemide (Lasix) • Furosemide (Demadex) • Bumetanide (Bumex)	• Rapid action • Potent for use when thiazides fail • Cause volume depletion	• Hypokalemia • Hyperuricemia • Glucose intolerance • Hypercholesterolemia • Hypertriglyceridemia • Sexual dysfunction • Weakness	• Volume depletion and electrolyte depletion are rapid • All nursing implications cited for Thiazides
Potassium-Sparing • Spironolactone (Aldactone) • Amiloride (Midamor) • Triamterene (Dyrenium) • Eplerenone (Inspra)	• Volume depletion without significant potassium loss	• Hyperkalemia • Gynecomastia • Sexual dysfunction	• Watch for hyperkalemia or renal failure in those treated with ACE inhibitors or NSAIDs • Watch for increase in serum lithium levels • Give after meals to decrease GI distress
Combination Thiazide and Potassium-Sparing • HCTZ and triamterene (Maxide) • Hydrochlorothiazide (HCTZ) + amiloride (Moduretic) • HCTZ + spironolactone (Aldactazide)	• Decreases fluid volume while minimizing K+ loss	• Side effects of individual drug offset or minimized by its partner	• Caution client previously on a loop or thiazide alone not to overdo K+ foods now because of K+ sparing component in new drug • Follow scheduling dosage to avoid sleep disruption

ACE, Angiotensin-converting enzyme; *GI*, gastrointestinal; *NSAIDs*, nonsteroidal anti-inflammatory drugs.

TABLE 4.15 Antihypertensives

Drugs	Indications	Adverse Reactions	Nursing Implications
Alpha-Adrenergic Blockers • Prazosin HCL (Minipress) • Terazosin (Hytrin) • Phentolamine mesylate (Regitine) • Doxazosin (Cardura)	• Used as peripheral vasodilator that acts directly on the blood vessels • Used in extreme hypertension of pheochromocytoma	• Orthostatic hypotension • Weakness • Palpitations	• Use cautiously in older clients • Occasional vomiting and diarrhea • Warn clients of possible: • Drowsiness • Lack of energy • Weakness
Combined Alpha Beta-Blockers • Labetalol (Normodyne) • Carvedilol (Coreg)	• Produces decrease in BP without reflex tachycardia or bradycardia	• HF • Ventricular dysrhythmias • Blood dyscrasias • Bronchospasm • Orthostatic hypotension	• Contraindicated with: • HF • Heart block • COPD
Beta-Blockers • Metoprolol tartrate (Lopressor) • Nadolol (Corgard) • Propranolol HCL (Inderal) • Timolol maleate (Blocadren) • Atenolol (Tenormin) • Bisoprolol (Zebeta) • Metoprolol (Lopressor, Toprol)	• Blocks the sympathetic nervous system, especially to the heart • Produces a slower heart rate • Lowers BP • Reduces O_2 consumption during myocardial contraction	• Bradycardia • Fatigue • Insomnia • Bizarre dreams • Sexual dysfunction • Hypertriglyceridemia • Decreased HDL • Depression	• Check apical or radial pulse daily • Monitor for GI distress • Do not discontinue abruptly • Watch for shortness of breath; give cautiously with bronchospasm • Do not vary how taken (with or without food) • Do not vary time taken • May mask symptoms of hypoglycemia or may prolong a hypoglycemic reaction
Central-Acting Inhibitors • Clonidine (Catapres) • Guanabenz acetate (Wytensin) • Guanfacine (Tenex) • Methyldopa (Aldomet)	• Decrease BP by stimulating central alpha receptors resulting in decreased sympathetic outflow from the brain	• Drowsiness • Dry mouth • Fatigue • Sexual dysfunction	• Watch for rebound hypertension if abruptly discontinued • Caution to make position changes slowly, avoid standing still, or taking hot baths and showers
Vasodilators • Hydralazine HCL (Apresoline) • Minoxidil (Loniten)	• Decrease BP by decreasing peripheral resistance	• Headache • Tachycardia • Fluid retention (HF, pulmonary edema) • Postural hypotension	• Monitor BP, pulse routinely • Observe for peripheral edema • Monitor I&O • Weigh daily
Angiotensin II Receptor Antagonists • Losartan (Cozaar) • Valsartan (Diovan) • Irbesartan (Avapro) • Azilsartan (Edarbi) • Candesartan (Atacand) • Eprosartan (Teveten) • Olmesartan (Benicar) • Telmisartan (Micardis)	• Blocks the vasoconstrictor and aldosterone producing effects of angiotensin II at various sites (vascular smooth muscle and adrenal glands)	• Hypotension • Fatigue • Hepatitis • Renal failure • Hyperkalemia (rare)	• Monitor liver enzymes, electrolytes • Monitor for angioedema in those with history of it when on ACE inhibitors previously
Angiotensin-Converting Enzyme (ACE) Inhibitors • Captopril (Capoten) • Enalapril maleate (Vasotec) • Lisinopril (Zestril) • Ramipril (Altace) • Benazepril (Lotensin) • Quinapril (Accupril) • Fosinopril (Monopril) • Moexipril (Univasc) • Trandolapril (Mavik)	• Decreases BP by suppressing renin—angiotensin-aldosterone system and inhibiting conversion of angiotensin I to angiotensin II • Useful with diabetics	• Proteinuria • Neutropenia • Skin rash • Cough	• Watch for acute renal failure (reversible) • Routine renal function tests • Remain in bed 3 h after first dose

Continued

Calcium Channel Blockers			
• Diltiazem (Cardizem) • Nifedipine (Procardia, Adalat) • Verapamil HCL (Calan, Isoptin) • Nisoldipine (Sular) • Felodipine (Plendil) • Nicardipine (Cardene) • Amlodipine (Norvasc)	• Inhibits calcium ion influx during cardiac depolarization • Decreases SA/AV node conduction	• Headache • Hypotension • Dizziness • Edema • Nausea • Constipation • Tachycardia • HF • Dry cough	• Check BP and pulse routinely • Limit caffeine consumption • Take medications before meals • Avoid grapefruit juice with these drugs as it will increase serum levels, causing hypotension • High-fat meals elevate serum levels

BP, Blood pressure; *COPD*, chronic obstructive pulmonary disease; *GI*, Gastrointestinal; *HDL*, high-density lipoprotein; *HF*, heart failure.

4. Monitor renal functioning (BUN and creatinine) every 90 to 120 days for duration of treatment.
5. Monitor BP and pulse rate, usually weekly.
B. Encourage client to implement nonpharmacologic measures to assist with BP control.
   1. Stress reduction
   2. Weight loss
   3. Tobacco cessation
   4. Exercise
   5. Diabetes control (normalize blood glucose levels)
C. Determine medication side effects experienced by client.
   1. Impotence
   2. Insomnia
D. Provide nutritional guidance, including a sample meal plan and how to eat at restaurants (low-salt, low-fat/low-cholesterol diet).

Peripheral Vascular Disease

Description: Peripheral vascular disease (PVD) involves circulatory problems that can be due to either arterial or venous pathology.

Nursing Assessment

The signs, symptoms, and treatment of PVD can be opposite, depending on the source of the pathology. Therefore, careful assessment is very important.
A. Predisposing factors
   1. Arterial
      a. Arteriosclerosis: 95% of all cases are caused by atherosclerosis
      b. Advanced age
   2. Venous
      a. History of deep vein thrombosis (DVT)
      b. Valvular incompetence
B. Associated diseases
   1. Arterial
      a. Raynaud disease (nonatherosclerotic, triggered by extreme heat or cold, spasms of the arteries)
      b. Buerger disease (occlusive inflammatory disease, strongly associated with smoking)
      c. Diabetes
      d. Acute occlusion (emboli/thrombi)
   2. Venous
      a. Varicose veins
      b. Thrombophlebitis
      c. Venous stasis ulcers
C. Skin
   1. Arterial
      a. Smooth
      b. Shiny
      c. Loss of hair
      d. Thick nails
      e. Dry, thin skin
   2. Venous—brown pigment around ankles
D. Color
   1. Arterial
      a. Pallor on elevation
      b. Rubor when dependent
   2. Venous—cyanotic when dependent
E. Temperature
   1. Arterial—cool
   2. Venous—warm
F. Pulses
   1. Arterial—decreased or absent
   2. Venous—normal
G. Pain
   1. Arterial
      a. Sharp
      b. Increase with walking and elevation
      c. Intermittent claudication: CLASSIC presenting symptom, occurs in skeletal muscles during exercise; relieved by rest
      d. Rest pain: occurs when the extremities are horizontal; may be relieved by dependent position; often appears when collateral circulation fails to develop
   2. Venous
      a. Persistent, aching, full feeling, dull sensation
      b. Pain relieved when horizontal (elevate extremities and use elastic stockings)
      c. Nocturnal cramps
H. Ulcers
   1. Arterial
      a. Client may describe as very painful
      b. Occur on lateral lower leg, toes, and heel
      c. Demarcated edges

d. Small, but deep
e. Circular in shape
f. Necrotic
g. Not edematous
2. Venous
   a. Described by client as dull ache or heaviness
   b. Occur on medial leg, ankle
   c. Uneven edges
   d. Superficial, but large
   e. Marked edema
   f. Highly exudative

Nursing Plans and Interventions

A. Noninvasive treatment
  1. Arterial
    a. Elimination of smoking
    b. Topical antibiotic
    c. Bed rest/immobilization
    d. Fibrinolytic agents: if clots are the problem—not used for Raynaud or Buerger disease (see Table 4.14)
  2. Venous
    a. Systemic antibiotics
    b. Compression dressing (snug)

c. Limb elevation
d. For thrombosis (Table 4.16)
B. Surgery
  1. Arterial
    a. Embolectomy: removal of clot
    b. Endarterectomy: removal of clot and stripping of plaque
    c. Arterial bypass: Teflon/Dacron graft or autograft
    d. Percutaneous transluminal angioplasty: compression of plaque
    e. Amputation: removal of extremity
  2. Venous
    a. Vein ligation
    b. Thrombectomy
    c. Debridement
C. Monitor extremities at designated intervals.
  1. Color
  2. Temperature
  3. Sensation and pulse quality in extremities
D. Schedule activities within client's tolerance level.
E. Encourage rest at the first sign of pain.
F. Encourage keeping extremities elevated (if venous) when sitting, and change position often.
G. Encourage client to avoid crossing legs and to wear nonrestrictive clothing.

TABLE 4.16 Anticoagulants

Drug	Indications	Adverse Reactions	Nursing Implications
• Heparin sodium (Hepalean, Heplock)	• Administered parenterally (subcutaneous or IV) as an antagonist to thrombin and to prevent the conversion of fibrinogen to fibrin	• Hemorrhage • Agranulocytosis • Leukopenia • Hepatitis	• Monitor PTT, Hgb, Hct, platelets • Obtain stools for occult blood • Avoid IM injection • Notify anyone performing diagnostic testing of medication • *Antagonist:* protamine sulfate
• Warfarin sodium (Coumadin)	• Blocks the formation of prothrombin from vitamin K	• Hemorrhage • Agranulocytosis • Leukopenia • Hepatitis	• See heparin • Given orally • Monitor PT • Avoid sudden change in intake of foods high in vitamin K • Antagonist: vitamin K
• Antiplatelet Agent • Ticlopidine (Ticlid) • Dipyridamole (Persantine) • Clopidogrel (Plavix) • Prasugrel (Effient) • Ticagrelor (Brilinta)	• Short-term use after cardiac interventions • Reduce risk of thrombolytic stroke for those intolerant to aspirin • Prevention of thrombolytic disorders	• Neutropenia • Thrombocytopenia • Agranulocytosis • Leukopenia • Hemorrhage • GI irritation, bleeding • Pancytopenia	• Give pc with food to decrease gastric irritation (Ticlid) • Advise not to take antacids within 2 h of taking ticlopidine • Monitor CBC every 2 weeks for 3 months, and thereafter if signs of infection develop • Monitor for signs of bleeding • Give 1 h ac (Persantine); (Plavix) no regard for meals
• Low molecular weight heparin enoxaparin (Lovenox) • Tinzaparin (Innohep) • Dalteparin (Fragmin)	• Prevention of thrombolytic formation (deep vein)	• Hemorrhage • GI irritation, bleeding • Thrombocytopenia	• Monitor for signs of bleeding • Given subcutaneously • Monitor CBC • Use soft toothbrush; avoid cuts
• Factor Xa inhibitor • Fondaparinux	• Prevention of thrombolytic formation (deep vein)	• Hemorrhage • GI irritation, bleeding	• Monitor for signs of bleeding • Give subcutaneously • Monitor CBC • Use soft toothbrush; avoid cuts

GI, Gastrointestinal; *Hct,* hematocrit; *Hgb,* hemoglobin; *IM,* intramuscular; *IV,* intravenous; *PT,* prothrombin time; *PTT,* partial thromboplastin time.

H. Encourage client to keep the extremities warm by wearing extra clothing such as socks and slippers. Do not use external heat sources such as electric heating pads.
I. Collaborate with RN to develop and implement a client/family teaching plan about methods to prevent further injury.
   1. Change position frequently.
   2. Wear nonrestrictive clothing.
   3. Avoid crossing legs or keeping legs in a dependent position.
   4. Wear shoes when ambulating.
   5. Obtain proper foot and nail care.

> **HESI HINT** Decreased blood flow results in diminished sensation in the lower extremities. Any heat source can cause severe burns before the client actually realizes the damage is being done.

J. Discourage cigarette smoking (causes vasoconstriction and spasm of arteries).
K. Provide preoperative and postoperative care if surgery is required.
   1. Preoperative: maintain affected extremity at a level position, if venous, or at a slightly dependent position, if arterial (15 degrees); at room temperature; and protected from trauma.
   2. Postoperative: assess surgical site frequently for hemorrhage.
   3. Monitor peripheral pulses.
   4. Anticoagulants may be continued after surgery to prevent thrombosis of affected artery and to diminish development of thrombi at the initiating site.

Abdominal Aortic Aneurysm

Description: An abdominal aortic aneurysm (AAA) is dilation of the abdominal aorta caused by an alteration in the integrity of its wall.
A. The most common cause of AAA is atherosclerosis.
B. Without treatment, rupture and death will occur.
C. AAA is often asymptomatic.
D. The most common symptom is abdominal pain or low back pain with the complaint that the client can feel "heart beating."
E. Those taking antihypertensive drugs are at risk of developing AAA.

> **HESI HINT** A client is admitted with severe chest pain and states that he feels a terrible, tearing sensation in his chest. He is diagnosed with a dissecting aortic aneurysm. What assessment should the nurse obtain in the initial assessment?
> • Vital signs every 1 h
> • Neurologic vital signs
> • Respiratory status
> • Urinary output
> • Peripheral pulses

Nursing Assessment

A. Bruit (swooshing sound heard over a constricted artery when auscultated) heard over abdominal aorta, pulsation in the upper abdomen
B. Abdominal or lower back pain
C. Abdominal x-ray study will confirm diagnosis if aneurysm is calcified (aortogram, angiogram, and abdominal ultrasound).
D. Symptoms of rupture: hypovolemic or cardiogenic shock with sudden, severe abdominal pain

Nursing Plans and Interventions

A. Palpate and report findings of all peripheral pulses and vital signs regularly.
   1. Radial
   2. Femoral
   3. Popliteal
   4. Posterior tibial
   5. Dorsalis pedis
B. Observe for signs of occlusion after graft.
   1. Change in pulses
   2. Severe pain
   3. Cool to cold extremities below graft
   4. White or blue extremities
C. Observe renal functioning for signs of kidney damage (artery clamped during surgery may result in kidney damage).
   1. Output of less than 30 mL/h
   2. Amber-colored urine
   3. Elevated BUN and creatinine (early signs of kidney failure)
D. Observe for postoperative ileus.
   1. Maintain NG tube for up to 1 to 2 days postoperative (may help prevent ileus).
   2. Check bowel sounds every shift.

> **HESI HINT** Thrombophlebitis is inflammation of the venous walls with formation of a clot. It is also known as venous thrombosis, phlebothrombosis, or DVT.

Thrombophlebitis
Nursing Assessment

A. Calf or groin pain
B. Functional impairment of extremity
C. Edema and warmth in extremity
D. Asymmetry
   1. Inspect legs from groin to feet.
   2. Measure the diameter of calf.
E. Tender areas noted on the affected extremity with very gentle palpation
F. Occlusion noted with diagnostic testing
   1. Venogram
   2. Doppler ultrasound
   3. Fibrinogen scanning

G. Risk factors
1. Prolonged strict bed rest
2. General surgery
3. Leg trauma
4. Previous venous insufficiency
5. Obesity
6. Oral contraceptives
7. Pregnancy
8. Malignancy

> **HESI HINT** Heparin prevents conversion of fibrinogen to fibrin and prothrombin to thrombin, thereby inhibiting clot formation. Because the clotting mechanism is prolonged, do not cause tissue trauma, which may lead to bleeding when heparin is given subcutaneously. Do not massage area or aspirate; give in the abdomen between the pelvic bones; 2 inches from umbilicus; rotate sites.

Nursing Plans and Interventions

A. Administer anticoagulant therapy as prescribed (see Table 4.16).

> **HESI HINT: Anticoagulants**
> **Heparin**
> - Antagonist: protamine sulfate
> - Laboratory: partial thromboplastin time (PTT) or activated PTT determines efficacy, international normalized ratio (INR)
> - Keep 1.5—2.5 times normal control
>
> **Warfarin**
> - Antagonist: vitamin K
> - Laboratory: prothrombin time (PT) determines efficacy
> - Keep 1.5—2.5 times normal control
> - INR
>   - Desirable therapeutic level usually 2—3 (reflects how long it takes a blood sample to clot)

1. Observe for side effects, especially bleeding.
2. Collaborate with the RN to develop and implement a client teaching plan regarding the side effects of medications included in treatment regimen.
3. Monitor laboratory data to determine the efficacy of medications included in treatment regimen.
4. Include information on all laboratory requests that client is receiving anticoagulants.
5. PTT determines efficacy of heparin.
6. PT or INR determines efficacy of warfarin (Coumadin).
7. Maintain pressure on venipuncture sites to minimize hematoma formation.
8. Notify HCP of any unusual bleeding.
   a. Abnormal vaginal bleeding
   b. Nose bleeds
   c. Melena
   d. Hematuria
   e. Bleeding gums
   f. Hemoptysis
9. Advise client to use soft toothbrush and floss with waxed floss.
10. Encourage client to wear medical alert bracelet.
11. Encourage client to avoid alcoholic beverages.
12. Advise client to avoid safety razor if taking warfarin (Coumadin).
13. Tell client to avoid acetylsalicylic acid.
B. Use antiembolic stockings. Elevate extremity and/or use shock blocks for foot of bed.
C. Bed rest; strict, if prescribed, means no bathroom privileges! Prevent straining.
D. Monitor for decreasing symptomatology: pain and edema.
E. Monitor for pulmonary embolus (chest pain, shortness of breath).
F. Reinforce client teaching that there is increased risk for DVT formation in the future.
G. Dietary precautions if taking warfarin.

Dysrhythmias

Description: Dysrhythmias are a disturbance in the heart rate and/or heart rhythm.
A. Dysrhythmias are caused by a disturbance in the electrical conduction of the heart, *not* by abnormal heart structure.
B. Client is often asymptomatic until CO is altered.
C. Common causes of dysrhythmias:
1. Drugs—for example, digoxin, quinidine, caffeine, nicotine, alcohol
2. Acid—base and electrolyte imbalances (potassium, calcium, and magnesium)
3. Marked thermal changes
4. Disease and trauma
5. Stress

Nursing Assessment

A. Change in the pulse rate and/or rhythm
1. Tachycardia: fast rates (>100 beats/min)
2. Bradycardia: slow rates (<60 beats/min)
3. Irregular rhythm
4. Pulselessness
B. ECG changes
C. Complaints of:
1. Palpitations
2. Syncope
3. Pain
4. Dyspnea
D. Diaphoresis
E. Hypotension
F. Electrolyte imbalances

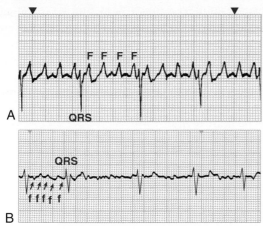

Fig. 4.4 (A) Atrial fibrillation. Note the chaotic fibrillatory (f) waves between the QRS complexes. Note: Recorded from lead V1. (B) Atrial flutter with a 4:1 conduction (four flutter [F] waves to each QRS complex). (A, From Urden, L., Stacy, K., & Lough, M. [2020]. *Priorities in critical care nursing* [6th ed.]. St. Louis: Elsevier/Mosby; B, From Sole, M., Klein, D., & Moseley, M. [2020]. *Introduction to critical care nursing* [7th ed.]. St. Louis: Elsevier/Saunders.)

Selected Dysrhythmias

A. Atrial fibrillation (Fig. 4.4B): Chaotic activity in the atrioventricular node
   1. No true P waves visible
   2. Irregular ventricular rhythm
   3. Assessment and treatment
   4. Anticoagulant therapy is needed due to risk for CVA and/or pulmonary embolism.
   5. Administer antidysrhythmic drugs.

HESI HINT Blood pools in the atria because of the decrease in CO due to ineffective atrial contractions (loss of atrial kick). An embolized clot may develop and move to the brain, causing a stroke.

---

   a. Cardioversion may be used to treat atrial dysrhythmias.
B. Atrial flutter (see Fig. 4.4A)
   1. Saw-toothed wave form
   2. Fluttering in chest
   3. Ventricular rhythm usually remains regular
   4. Assessment and treatment
      a. May use cardioversion to treat either atrial dysrhythmia
      b. Administer antidysrhythmic drugs
      c. Radiofrequency catheter ablation
C. Ventricular tachycardia
   1. Wide bizarre QRS
   2. Assessment and treatment
      a. Assess whether the client has a pulse; if the client has no pulse, start CPR immediately.

   b. Prepare for synchronized cardioversion (if client is stable with pulse and BP; defibrillation as soon as possible is the usual treatment).
   c. Administer antidysrhythmic drugs.
D. Ventricular fibrillation
   1. Cardiac emergency.
   2. No CO (there is no pulse or BP).
   3. Assessment and treatment
      a. Start CPR.
      b. Defibrillate as quickly as possible.
      c. Administer antidysrhythmic drugs.

Nursing Plans and Interventions

A. Determine medications client is currently taking.
B. Determine serum drug levels, especially digitalis.
C. Determine serum electrolyte levels, especially K^+ and Mg^{++}.
D. Obtain ECG reading on admission and monitor continuously via Holter monitor, event monitor, or loop recorder.

HESI HINT A Holter monitor offers continuous observation of the client's heart rate. To make assessment of the rhythm strips most meaningful, teach the client to keep a record of:
• Medication times and doses
• Chest pain episodes—type and duration
• Valsalva maneuver (straining at stool, sneezing, coughing)
• Sexual activity

E. Approach client in a calm, reassuring manner.
F. Monitor client's activity and observe for any symptoms occurring during activity.
G. Ensure proper administration of medications, and monitor for side effects (Table 4.17).
H. Be prepared for emergency measures such as cardioversion or defibrillation.

HESI HINT Cardioversion is the delivery of synchronized electrical shock to the myocardium.

I. Be prepared for pacemaker insertion.
   1. Temporary pacemaker—used temporarily in emergency situations. Pacing wire is threaded into the right ventricle via the superior vena cava, or an epicardial wire is put in place (through the client's chest incision) during cardiac surgery.
   2. Permanent internal pacemaker with pulse generator implanted in the abdomen or shoulder. May be single or dual chambered. Programmable pacemakers can be reprogrammed by placing a magnetic device over the generator.
   3. Collaborate with RN to develop and implement a client/family teaching plan to:

a. Report pulse rate lower than the set rate of the pacemaker.

b. Avoid leaning over an automobile with the engine running.

c. Stand 4 to 5 feet away from high-output generators (electromagnetic sources), such as radar detectors that are operating.

d. When traveling via air, notify security of presence of pacemaker. Handheld screening wand should not be placed directly over the pacemaker.

e. Avoid MRI diagnostic testing.

HESI HINT Synchronous or demand pacemaker fires only when the client's heart rate falls below a rate set on the generator (Fig. 4.5).

J. Assist in the treatment of premature ventricular contractions (PVCs) as prescribed (tend to be precursors of ventricular tachycardia and ventricular fibrillation; Fig. 4.6).

1. Occur more often than once in 10 beats.

2. Occur in groups of two and/or three (three PVCs in a row equals ventricular tachycardia).

3. Occur near the T wave (R on T phenomenon).

4. Take on multiple configurations (this is an ominous sign that indicates more than one irritable area in the ventricle).

Heart Failure

Description: HF is the inability of the heart to pump enough blood to meet the tissue's oxygen demands. Primary underlying conditions causing HF include:

A. Ischemic heart disease

B. MI

C. Cardiomyopathy

D. Valvular heart disease

E. Hypertension

Nursing Assessment

A. Observe for symptoms associated with left- or right-sided HF.

   1. Left-sided HF—pulmonary edema (left ventricular failure):

      a. Description: results in pulmonary congestion due to the inability of the left ventricle to pump blood to the periphery.

      b. Symptoms: dyspnea, orthopnea, crackles ("wet" lung sounds), cough, fatigue, tachycardia, anxiety; restlessness, confusion, and paroxysmal nocturnal dyspnea.

TABLE 4.17 Antidysrhythmics

Drugs	Indications	Adverse Reactions	Nursing Implications
Class I (A, B, C) • Quinidine • Disopyramide phosphate (Norpace) • Procainamide (Pronestyl) • Moricizine (Ethmozine) • Lidocaine HCL (Xylocaine) • Mexiletine (Mexitil) • Tocainide HCL (Tonocard) • Phenytoin sodium (Dilantin) • Propafenone (Rythmol) • Flecainide acetate (Tambocor)	• Premature beats • Atrial flutter, fibrillation • Contraindicated in heart block • Ventricular dysrhythmias • Unlabeled use: Digitalis-induced dysrhythmias • Ventricular dysrhythmias	• Diarrhea • Hypotension • ECG changes • Cinchonism • Interacts with many common drugs • Hypotension • CNS effects • Seizures • GI distress • Bradycardia • Dizziness • Slurred speech • Ventricular dysrhythmias	• Instruct client to monitor pulse rate and rhythm • Monitor ECG • Monitor for tinnitus and visual disturbances • Lidocaine administered by IV bolus and infusion • Monitor for confusion, drowsiness, slurred speech, seizures with lidocaine • Administer oral drugs with food • May cause digoxin toxicity
Class II • Propranolol HCL(Inderal) • Adenosine (Adenocard) • Metoprolol (Lopressor) • Atenolol (Tenormin)	• Supraventricular and ventricular tachydysrhythmias	• Hypotension • Bradycardia • Bronchospasm • Facial flushing	• Monitor vital signs • Contraindicated in asthma, COPD
Class III (Intropics) • Amiodarone HCL (Cordarone) • Milrinone (Primacor) • Inamrinone (Inocor) • Sotalol (Betapace) • Dofetilide (Tykosin) • Dronedarone (Multaq) • Ibutilide (Corvert) IV	• Ventricular dysrhythmias	• Dysrhythmias • Hypertension or hypotension • Muscle weakness, tremors • Photophobia	• Amiodarone is now one of the first-choice drugs • Monitor vital signs, ECG • Instruct client taking amiodarone to wear sunglasses and sunscreens when outside

Continued

Class IV
- Verapamil HCL (Isoptin, Calan)
- Diltiazem (Cardizem)

- Supraventricular dysrhythmias

- Hypotension
- Bradycardia
- Constipation

- Monitor BP and pulse
- Instruct client to change positions slowly

Miscellaneous Agents
- Atropine sulfate (Atropisol)

- Bradycardia

- Chest pain
- Urinary retention
- Dry mouth

- Monitor heart rate and rhythm
- Report chest pain
- Watch for urinary retention
- Avoid use in glaucoma

- Digoxin (Lanoxin)
- Digitoxin (Crystodigin)

- Supraventricular dysrhythmias
- Atrial fibrillation

- Bradycardia
- Dysrhythmias
- Anorexia, nausea, vomiting, diarrhea, visual disturbances

- Monitor pulse rate and rhythm
- Instruct client to report signs of toxicity
- Hypokalemia increases the risk of toxicity
- Causes hypercalcemia

- Epinephrine (Adrenaline)

- Cardiac arrest

- Tachycardia
- Hypertension

- Impaired renal function can cause toxicity—monitor BUN and creatinine
- Monitor pulse return in asystole
- Monitor vital signs

Additional Drugs that Promote Cardiovascular Perfusion in the Failing Heart
Vasopressors
- Norepinephrine (Levophed)

- Dilates coronary arteries and causes peripheral vasoconstriction for emergency hypotensive states not caused by blood loss, vascular thrombosis, or anesthesia using cyclopropane or halothane

- Can cause SEVERE tissue necrosis, sloughing, and gangrene if infiltrates (blanching along vein pathway = preliminary sign of extravasation)

- Rapidly inactivated by various body enzymes; need to ensure IV patency
- Use cautiously in previously hypertensive clients
- Check BP every 2—5 min
- Encourage the use of large veins to avoid complications of prolonged vasoconstriction
- Pressor effects potentiated by many drugs; check drug-drug interactions
- Have phentolamine (Regitine) diluted per protocol for local injection if infiltrates

Cardiotonic/Vasodilator (Human B-Type Natriuretic Peptide: HBNP)
- Nesiritide (Natrecor)

- Treatment of acutely decompensated HF in clients who have dyspnea at rest or with minimal activity
- Reduces pulmonary capillary wedge pressure and reduces dyspnea

- Hypotension is primary side effect and can be dose limiting
- Dysrhythmias
- H/A, dizziness, insomnia, tremors, paresthesias
- Abdominal pain, nausea, and vomiting

- Many drug—drug interactions
- Monitor BP and telemetry
- As diuresis occurs, monitor electrolytes, especially K^+
- Watch for overresponse to treatment in older adults

Group IIa—IIIb Inhibitor (Platelet Antiaggregate)
- Eptifibatide (Integrilin)
- Tirofiban (Aggrastat)
- Abciximab (Reopro)

- Acute coronary syndrome (unstable angina or non-Q waver MI)
- Used in combination with heparin, aspirin, and in selected situations, Ticlid and Plavix

- Bleeding, most frequent
- Hypotension
- Thrombocytopenia
- Acute toxicity: decreased muscle tone, dyspnea, loss of righting reflex (unable to maintain balance)

- Check drug-drug interactions before giving other meds
- Obtain baseline PT/aPTT, Hemoglobin & Hematocrit (H&H), platelet count, and monitor
- Dose adjusted by weight for older adults
- Same client teaching as with heparin: review activities to avoid
- Watch for bleeding
- Quickly reversible, so emergency procedures may still be performed shortly after discontinuing infusion

aPTT, Activated partial thromboplastin time; *BP*, blood pressure; *BUN*, blood urea nitrogen; *CNS*, central nervous system; *COPD*, chronic obstructive pulmonary disease; *ECG*, electrocardiogram; *GI*, gastrointestinal; *IV*, intravenous; *MI*, myocardial infarction; *PT*, prothrombin time.

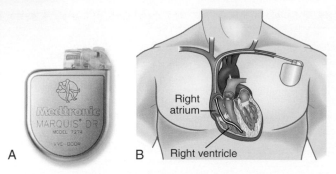

A

B

Right
atrium

Right ventricle

Fig. 4.5 (A) The implantable cardioverter-defibrillator (ICD) pulse generator from Medtronic, Inc. (B) The ICD is placed in a subcutaneous pocket over the pectoral muscle. A single-lead system is placed transvenously from the pulse generator to the endocardium. The single lead detects dysrhythmias and delivers an electric shock to the heart muscle. (From Lewis, S., Dirksen, S., Heitkemper, M., & Bucher, L. [2019]. *Medical-surgical nursing: Assessment and management of clinical problems* [11th ed.]. St. Louis: Mosby.)

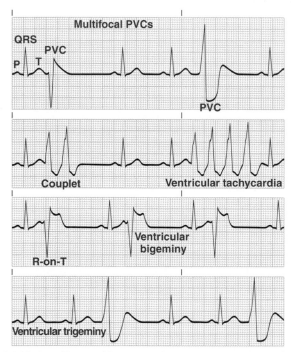

Fig. 4.6 Various Forms of Premature Ventricular Contractions (PVCs). (Note: Recorded from lead II. Sole, M., Klein, D., & Moseley, M. [2020]. *Introduction to critical care nursing* [7th ed.]. St. Louis: Elsevier/Saunders.)

2. Right-sided HF—peripheral edema (right ventricular failure):
   a. Description: results in peripheral congestion due to the inability of the right ventricle to pump blood out to the lungs. Often results from left-sided failure or pulmonary disease.
   b. Symptoms: peripheral edema, weight gain, distended neck veins, anorexia, nausea, nocturia, weakness, hepatomegaly, and ascites.

B. Enlargement of ventricles as indicated by chest x-ray.

> **HESI HINT** Restricting sodium reduces salt and water retention, thereby reducing vascular volume and preload.

Nursing Plans and Interventions

A. Monitor vital signs at least every 4 hours for changes.
B. Monitor apical heart rate with vital signs to detect dysrhythmias or abnormal heart sounds such as S3 or S4.
C. Assess for hypoxia.
   1. Restlessness
   2. Tachycardia
   3. Angina
D. Auscultate lungs for indication of pulmonary edema (wet sounds/crackles).
E. Administer oxygen as needed.
F. Elevate head of the bed to assist with breathing.
G. Observe for signs of edema.
   1. Weigh daily.
   2. Monitor I&O.
   3. Measure abdominal girth; observe ankles and fingers.
H. Limit sodium intake.
I. Elevate lower extremities while sitting.
J. Obtain apical heart rate before administration of digitalis; withhold medication and call HCP if the rate is less than 60 beats/min (Table 4.18).
K. Administer diuretics in the morning if possible (see Table 4.14).
L. Provide periods of rest after periods of activity.

Inflammatory and Infectious Heart Disease

Description: Inflammatory and infectious process involving the endocardium and pericardium.

A. Endocarditis is an inflammatory disease involving the inner surface of the heart, including the valves. Organisms travel through the blood to the heart where vegetations adhere to the valve surface or endocardium. These vegetations can break off and become emboli.
B. Causes of endocarditis
   1. Rheumatic heart disease
   2. Congenital heart disease
   3. IV drug abuse
   4. Cardiac surgery
   5. Immunosuppression
   6. Dental procedures
   7. Invasive procedures
C. Pericarditis is an inflammation of the outer lining of the heart.
   1. Causes of pericarditis
      a. Post-MI, trauma, neoplasm, connective tissue disease, after heart surgery, idiopathic
      b. Infections, such as pleurisy, bacteremia, *Streptococcus pneumonia*, or *Haemophilus influenza*

TABLE 4.18 Digitalis Preparations

Drugs	Indications	Adverse Reactions	Nursing Implications
• Digitoxin (Crystodigin, Purodigin) • Digoxin (Lanoxin, Lanoxicaps)	• Heart failure • Increases the contractility of cardiac muscle • Slow heart rate and conduction	• Severe: AV block • Headache • Dysrhythmias • Nausea • Vomiting • Blurred vision • Yellow-green halos • Hypotension • Fatigue	• Monitor serum electrolytes; hypokalemia increases risk of digoxin toxicity • Monitor serum digitalis levels if any side effects are present • Check apical pulse before administration; call health care provider if rate is below 60 beats/min • Teach client to take radial pulse before administration and call health care provider if below 60 beats/min in adults • Therapeutic range: 0.5–2 ng/mL
• Digoxin-immune • FAB (Digibind)	• Antidote for digitalis toxicity • Binds with digitoxin or digoxin to prevent binding at their site of action	• Decreased cardiac output • Atrial tachydysrhythmias • Use with caution in children and older adults	• Use with 0.22-micron filter • Place client on continuous cardiac monitor • Have resuscitation equipment at bedside before giving first dose

Nursing Assessment

A. Endocarditis
1. Fever
2. Chills, malaise, night sweats, fatigue
3. New onset murmurs
4. Symptoms of HF
5. Atrial embolization (CVA or pulmonary embolism)

B. Pericarditis
1. Pain: sudden, sharp, severe
   a. Substernal, radiating to the back or arm
   b. Aggravated by coughing, inhalation, deep breathing
   c. Relieved by leaning forward
2. Pericardial friction rub heard best at left lower sternal border
3. Fever

HESI HINT: Pericarditis
The presence of a friction rub is an indication of pericarditis (inflammation of the lining of the heart). ST segment elevation and T wave inversion are also signs of pericarditis.

Nursing Plans and Interventions

A. Endocarditis
1. Monitor hemodynamic status (vital signs, level of consciousness, urinary output).
2. IV antibiotics are usually prescribed for 4 to 6 weeks. Clients may be instructed in IV therapy for home health care. The American Heart Association no longer recommends the administration of antibiotics before dental or genitourinary procedures, except for clients who are at the highest risk of adverse outcomes from infective (bacterial) endocarditis. See www.americanheart.org/.
3. Collaborate with RN to develop and implement a client/family teaching plan about anticoagulant therapy if prescribed.

4. Encourage client to maintain good hygiene.
5. Reinforce client instructions to inform dentist or other HCPs of history.

B. Pericarditis
1. Provide rest and maintain position of comfort.
2. Administer analgesics and anti-inflammatory drugs.

Valvular Heart Disease

Description: Heart valves are unable to fully open (stenosis) or fully close (insufficiency or regurgitation).

A. Valve dysfunction most commonly occurs on the left side of the heart, with the mitral valve most frequently involved, followed by the aortic valve.

HESI HINT With mitral valve stenosis, blood is regurgitated back into the left atrium from the left ventricle. In the early period, there may be no symptoms, but as the disease progresses, the client will exhibit excessive fatigue, dyspnea on exertion, orthopnea, dry cough, hemoptysis, or pulmonary edema. There will be a rumbling apical diastolic murmur, and atrial fibrillation is common.

B. Common causes of valvular disease
1. Rheumatic fever
2. Congenital heart diseases
3. Syphilis
4. Endocarditis
5. Hypertension

C. Prevention of rheumatic heart disease would reduce the incidence of valvular heart disease.

Nursing Assessment

A. Fatigue; dyspnea, orthopnea; hemoptysis and pulmonary edema; murmurs; irregular cardiac rhythm; and angina
B. Pericardial effusion with possible tamponade requires pericardiocentesis.

Nursing Plans and Interventions

A. See Heart Failure.

B. Monitor client for changes in the ECG pattern.

C. Collaborate with RN to develop and implement a teaching plan to help client/family determine the necessity for prophylactic antibiotic therapy before any invasive procedure (e.g., dental procedures).

D. Prepare the client for surgical repair or replacement of heart valves.

E. Reinforce instruction for client who will be receiving a mechanical valve replacement on the need for lifelong anticoagulant therapy to prevent thrombus formation. Tissue (biologic) valves and autografts do not require lifelong anticoagulant therapy.

⚡ REVIEW OF CARDIOVASCULAR SYSTEM

1. How do clients experiencing angina describe that pain?
2. Develop a teaching plan for the client taking nitroglycerin.
3. List the parameters of BP for diagnosing hypertension.
4. Differentiate between essential and secondary hypertension.
5. Develop a teaching plan for the client taking antihypertensive medications.
6. Describe intermittent claudication.
7. Describe the nurse's discharge instructions to a client with venous PVD.
8. What is often the underlying cause of AAA?
9. What laboratory values should be monitored daily for the client with thrombophlebitis who is undergoing anticoagulant therapy?
10. When do PVCs present a grave danger?
11. Differentiate between the symptoms of left-sided and right-sided HF.
12. List three symptoms of digitalis toxicity.
13. What condition increases the likelihood of digitalis toxicity occurring?
14. What lifestyle changes can the client who is at risk for hypertension initiate to reduce the likelihood of becoming hypertensive?
15. What immediate actions should the nurse implement when a client is having an MI?
16. What symptoms should the nurse expect to find in the client with hypokalemia?
17. Bradycardia is defined as a heart rate less than _____ beats/min. Tachycardia is defined as a heart rate greater than _____ beats/min.
18. What precautions should clients with valve disease who have the highest risk for adverse outcomes from infective (bacterial) endocarditis take before invasive procedures or dental work?

See Answer Key at the end of this text for suggested responses.

GASTROINTESTINAL SYSTEM

Hiatal Hernia and Gastroesophageal Reflux Disease

A. Hiatal hernia is herniation of the stomach and other abdominal viscera through an enlarged esophageal opening in the diaphragm.
   1. Sliding hernia is the most common type, accounting for 75% to 90% of adult hiatal hernias.

B. Gastroesophageal reflux disease (GERD) is the result of an incompetent lower esophageal sphincter that allows regurgitation of acidic gastric contents into the esophagus.
   1. Multiple factors determine whether GERD is present.
      a. Efficiency of antireflux mechanism
      b. Volume of gastric contents
      c. Potency of refluxed material
      d. Efficiency of esophageal clearance
      e. Resistance of the esophageal tissue to injury and the ability to repair tissue

C. The client must have several episodes of reflux for GERD to be present.

Nursing Assessment

A. Heartburn after eating
B. Dyspepsia
C. Feeling of fullness and discomfort after eating
D. Regurgitation (hot, bitter, or sour liquid coming into the throat/mouth)
E. GERD-related chest pain described as burning, squeezing or radiating to the back, neck, jaw or arms
F. Positive diagnosis determined by history and fluoroscopy or endoscopy

Nursing Plans and Interventions

A. Determine an eating pattern that alleviates symptoms.
   1. Encourage small, frequent low-fat meals.
   2. Encourage the client to eliminate foods or habits that are determined to aggravate symptoms (these foods are client-specific—for example, avoid alcohol, smoking, and caffeinated beverages).
   3. Encourage the client to sit up while eating and remain in upright position for at least 2 to 3 hours after eating.
   4. Encourage the client to stop eating 3 hours before bedtime.
   5. Elevate the head of the bed on 6- to 8-inch blocks.
   6. Assist with teaching about frequently prescribed medications (H_2 antagonists, antacids, and proton pump inhibitors [PPIs]).
   7. Encourage weight reduction, if appropriate.

> **HESI HINT** A Fowler or semi-Fowler position is beneficial in reducing the amount of regurgitation and preventing the encroachment of the stomach tissue upward through the opening in the diaphragm.

B. Assist with the teaching plan for client/family that should include the following:
   1. Differentiate between the symptoms of hiatal hernia and MI.

2. Be alert to the possibility of aspiration.

3. Head-of-bed elevation increased by using 6-inch blocks.

4. Encourage weight loss if the client is overweight.

Peptic Ulcer Disease

Peptic ulcer disease (PUD) is ulceration that penetrates the mucosal wall of any portion of the GI tract in contact with hydrogen chloride.

A. Gastric ulcers tend to occur in the lesser curvature of the stomach. Pain intensifies with food consumption.

B. Duodenal ulcers occur in the duodenum, often near the pylorus. Eating relieves pain.

C. Esophageal ulcers occur in the esophagus.

D. The etiology of some PUD is unknown. A significant number of gastric ulcers are caused by an organism, *Helicobacter pylori*, and can be successfully treated with drug therapy. Risk factors for development of peptic ulcers include:

1. Drugs (NSAIDs, corticosteroids)

2. Alcohol

3. Cigarette smoking

4. Acute medical crisis or trauma

5. Familial tendency

6. Blood type O

E. Symptoms common to all types of ulcers include the following:

1. Epigastric pain radiating to the back (not associated with the type of food eaten) and relieved by antacids

2. Belching

3. Bloating

F. Gastric ulcer signs/symptoms

1. Burning/gaseous pain aggravated by food

2. Location in antrum, body and fundus of stomach

3. Pain 1 to 2 hours after meals

G. Duodenal ulcer signs/symptoms

1. Occur 2 to 5 hours after a meal

2. Pain described as burning or cramp-like

3. Located in midepigastric region

Nursing Assessment

A. Determine how food intake affects pain

B. History of antacid, histamine antagonist, or PPI use

C. Hematemesis

D. Melena (black, tarry stools)

E. Presence and/or location of peptic ulcers as determined by:

1. Barium swallow

2. Upper GI endoscopy

3. Gastric analysis indicating increased levels of stomach acid

F. Potential complications: hemorrhage, perforation (always demands surgery), obstruction, and cancer

Nursing Plans and Interventions

A. Determine symptom onset and how symptoms are relieved.

B. Monitor color, quantity, consistency of stools and emesis, and test for occult blood.

C. Administer medications as prescribed, usually 1 to 2 hours after meals and at bedtime (Table 4.19).

> **HESI HINT** Gastric emptying can be delayed by withholding fluids with meals, by eating in a recumbent or semi-recumbent position, or by lying down after meals.

D. Administer mucosal healing agents at least 1 hour before meals, as prescribed (see Table 4.19).

E. Encourage small, frequent meals with no bedtime snack. Avoid beverages containing caffeine or alcohol. Avoid "irritating" foods.

F. Prepare for surgery if uncontrolled bleeding, obstruction, or perforation occurs.

1. Partial gastrectomy

2. Vagotomy

3. Pyloroplasty

G. Anticipate dumping syndrome.

1. Secondary to rapid entry of hypertonic food into jejunum (pulls water out of bloodstream).

2. Occurs 5 to 30 minutes after eating.

3. Characterized by vertigo, syncope, sweating, pallor, tachycardia, or hypotension.

4. Provide small, frequent meals: high-protein, high-fat, low-carbohydrate diet.

5. Avoid liquids with meals, and encourage client to lie down after eating.

6. This syndrome can also be observed in clients on hypertonic tube feeding.

H. Reinforce the teaching plan related to the importance of avoiding medications that increase the risk for developing peptic ulcers.

1. Salicylates

2. NSAIDs such as ibuprofen

3. Corticosteroids in high doses

4. Anticoagulants

I. Emphasize to the client the importance of informing all health care personnel of ulcer history.

J. Assist the client to recognize signs and symptoms of GI bleeding.

1. Dark, tarry stools; coffee-ground emesis; bright red, rectal bleeding; fatigue; and pallor

2. Severe abdominal pain should be reported immediately (could indicate perforation)

K. Emphasize the importance of smoking cessation and stress management.

> **HESI HINT** Stress can cause or exacerbate ulcers. Reinforce teaching about stress reduction methods and encourage those with a family history of ulcers to obtain medical surveillance for ulcer formation.

TABLE 4.19 Antiulcer Drugs

Drugs	Indications	Adverse Reactions	Nursing Implications
Antacids			
• Aluminum hydroxide/ magnesium hydroxide (Maalox, Mylanta, Riopan, Gelusil II)	• Treatment of peptic ulcers • Work by neutralizing or reducing acidity of stomach contents • Differences in absorption rate	• Constipation • Diarrhea • Drug interactions	• Need to take several times a day • Administer after meals • Review client's history of renal diseases when client is taking magnesium products; electrolyte readjustment occurs and can result in renal insufficiency and calcinosis
Histamine₂ Antagonists			
• Ranitidine HCL (Zantac) • Cimetidine (Tagamet) • Famotidine (Pepcid) • Nizatidine (Axid)	• Treatment of peptic ulcers • Prophylactic treatment for clients at risk for developing ulcers (those on steroids, or highly stressed)	• Multiple drug interactions	• Cigarette smoking interferes with drug action • Expensive
Mucosal Healing Agents			

• Sucralfate (Carafate)	• Treatment of peptic ulcers	• Constipation
		• Drug interaction with:
		  • Tetracycline
		  • Phenytoin sodium
		  • Digoxin
		  • Cimetidine
			• Medication to be taken at least 1 h before meals or other medications
			• Antacids interfere with absorption

Proton Pump Inhibitors			

• Lansoprazole (Prevacid) (PO only)
• Pantoprazole (Protonix) (available oral and IV)
• Esomeprazole (Nexium) (oral only)
• Omeprazole (Prilosec)
• Rabeprazole (Aciphex)
• Dexlansoprazole (Kapidex)
	• Treatment of erosive esophagitis associated with gastroesophageal reflux disease	• Constipation
		• Heartburn
		• Anxiety
		• Diarrhea
		• Abdominal pain, hepatocellular damage, pancreatitis, gastroenteritis
		• Tinnitus, vertigo, confusion, H/A
		• Blurred vision, hypokinesia
		• Chest pain, dyspnea
			• Taken before meals
			• Do not crush or chew
			• Pantoprazole IV:
			  • Resume oral therapy as soon as feasible
			  • Long-lasting effects of drug may inhibit absorption of other drugs
			  • Not removed by hemodialysis
			  • Monitor for indications of adverse reactions

HESI HINT: CLINICAL MANIFESTATIONS OF GI BLEEDING
- Pallor: conjunctival, mucous membranes, and nail beds
- Dark, tarry stools
- Bright red or coffee-ground emesis
- Abdominal mass or bruit
- Decreased BP, rapid pulse, cool extremities (shock)

Inflammatory Bowel Diseases

Inflammatory bowel diseases consist of Crohn disease and ulcerative colitis.

Crohn Disease (Regional Enteritis)

Description: Crohn disease (regional enteritis) is subacute, chronic inflammation extending throughout the entire intestinal mucosa (most frequently found in terminal ileum).

Nursing Assessment

A. Abdominal pain (unrelieved by defecation)
B. Diarrhea and weight loss, with client becoming emaciated because of malabsorption
C. Constant fluid loss
D. Perforation of the intestine may occur because of severe inflammation and constitutes a medical emergency.

HESI HINT The GI tract usually accounts for only 100–200 mL fluid loss per day, although it filters up to 8 L/day. Large fluid losses can occur if vomiting and/or diarrhea occurs.

Ulcerative Colitis

Description: Ulcerative colitis is a disease that affects the superficial mucosa of the colon, causing the bowel to eventually narrow, shorten, and thicken due to muscular hypertrophy. It occurs in the large bowel and rectum.

Nursing Assessment

A. Diarrhea
B. Abdominal pain (unrelieved by defecation), right lower quadrant
C. Intermittent tenesmus (anal contractions) and rectal bleeding
D. Liquid stools containing blood, mucous, and pus (may pass 10 to 20 liquid stools per day)
E. Weakness and fatigue
F. Anemia
G. Stress

Nursing Plans and Interventions

A. Determine bowel elimination pattern and control diarrhea with diet and medication as indicated.
B. Provide a nutritious, well-balanced, low-residue, low-fat, high-protein, high-calorie diet. *No dairy products.*
C. Administer vitamin and iron supplements.
D. Encourage the client to avoid foods that are known to cause diarrhea, such as milk products and spicy food.
E. Encourage the client to avoid smoking, caffeinated beverages, pepper, and alcohol.
F. Provide complete bowel rest with IV total parenteral nutrition if necessary.
G. Administer medications as prescribed, often corticosteroids, antidiarrheals, sulfasalazine (Azulfidine), mesalamine (various brands), and infliximab (Remicade) or other biologic treatments, if there is no response to previous medications.
H. Monitor I&O and serum electrolytes.
I. Weigh at least twice a week.
J. Provide emotional support and encourage use of support groups such as local Ileitis and Colitis Foundation.
K. Encourage client to talk with the enterostomal therapists *before* surgery.
L. If ileostomy is performed, collaborate with RN to develop and implement a teaching plan for client/family about stoma care (see Stoma Care).

> **HESI HINT** Opioid drugs tend to depress gastric motility. However, they should be given with care, and those receiving them should be closely monitored because a distended intestinal wall accompanied by decreased muscle tone may lead to intestinal perforation.

Diverticular Diseases

Description: Diverticular diseases manifest in two clinical forms: diverticulosis and diverticulitis.
A. Diverticulosis: bulging pouches in the GI wall (diverticula) push the mucosa lining through the surrounding muscle.
B. Diverticulitis: inflamed diverticula (may cause obstruction, infection, and/or hemorrhage).

> **HESI HINT** Diverticulosis is the presence of pouches in the wall of the intestine. There is usually no discomfort, and the problem goes unnoticed unless seen on radiologic examination (usually prompted by some other condition). Diverticulitis is an inflammation of the diverticula (pouches), which can lead to perforation of the bowel.

Nursing Assessment

A. Left lower quadrant pain; increased flatus; rectal bleeding
B. Signs of intestinal obstruction
   1. Constipation alternating with diarrhea
   2. Abdominal distention
   3. Anorexia
   4. Low-grade fever
C. Barium enema or colonoscopy positive for diverticular disease
D. Obstruction, ileus, or perforation confirmed with abdominal x-ray film. Barium enema not done during acute phase of illness.

Nursing Plans and Interventions

A. Provide a well-balanced, high-fiber diet unless inflammation is present, at which time client is NPO (nothing by mouth) followed by low-residue, bland foods.

> **HESI HINT** A client admitted with complaints of severe lower abdominal pain, cramping, and diarrhea is diagnosed with diverticulitis. What are the nutritional needs of this client throughout recovery?
> - Acute phase—NPO, graduating to liquids.
> - Recovery phase—no fiber or foods that irritate the bowel.
> - Maintenance phase—high-fiber diet, with stool softeners, bulk-forming laxatives to prevent pooling of foods in the pouches where they can become inflamed. Avoid small, poorly digested foods such as popcorn, nuts, seeds, and so on.

B. Include bulk-forming laxatives such as Metamucil in daily regimen.
C. Increase fluid intake to 3 L/day.
D. Monitor I&O and bowel elimination; avoid constipation.
E. Observe for complications.
   1. Obstruction
   2. Peritonitis
   3. Hemorrhage (with ruptured diverticula, a temporary colostomy is performed and maintained for approximately 3 months to allow the bowel to rest)

Intestinal Obstruction

Description: Partial or complete blockage of intestinal flow (fluids, feces, gas) that occurs mostly in the small intestines.

A. Mechanical causes of intestinal obstruction
1. Adhesions (most common cause)
2. Strangulated hernia
3. Volvulus (twisting of the gut)
4. Intussusception (telescoping of the gut within itself)
5. Tumors that develop slowly; usually mass of feces becomes lodged against the tumor
B. Neurogenic causes of intestinal obstruction
1. Paralytic ileus (usually occurs in postoperative clients)
2. Spinal cord lesion
C. Vascular cause: mesenteric artery occlusion (leads to gut infarct)

HESI HINT: BOWEL OBSTRUCTIONS
- **Mechanical:** Caused by disorders outside the bowel (hernia, adhesions); disorders within the bowel (tumors, diverticulitis); or blockage of the lumen in the intestine (intussusception, gallstone).
- **Nonmechanical:** Paralytic ileus, which does not involve any actual physical obstruction but results from inability of the bowel to function.

Nursing Assessment

A. Sudden onset of abdominal pain, tenderness, or guarding.
B. History of abdominal surgeries.
C. History of obstruction.
D. Distention.
E. Increased peristalsis when obstruction first occurs, then peristalsis becomes absent when paralytic ileus occurs. Assessed by listening to bowel sounds.
F. Bowel sounds are high-pitched with early mechanical obstruction and diminished to absent with neurogenic, or late, mechanical obstruction.
G. Nausea or vomiting.

HESI HINT Blood gas analysis will show an alkalotic state if the bowel obstruction is high in the small intestine where gastric acid is secreted. If the obstruction is in the lower bowel where base solutions are secreted, the blood will be acidic.

Nursing Plans and Interventions

A. NPO, IV fluids, and electrolyte therapy
B. I&O, indwelling urinary catheter to maintain strict output
C. NG intubation
1. Attach to low suction (intermittent 80 mm Hg).
2. Document output every 8 hours.
3. Irrigate with normal saline if policy dictates.
4. Cantor, Miller-Abbott, or Harris tubes are passed through the nose and the stomach and advanced into the intestinal tract by the HCP.
   a. Advance tube every 1 to 2 hours.

b. Do not secure to nose until the tube reaches the specified position.
c. Reposition client every 2 hours to assist with advancement of the tube.
d. Connect the tube to suction as prescribed.
e. Irrigate with 20 to 30 mL of normal saline.
f. Label lumen of Miller-Abbott tube. Do *not* put anything with mercury in lumen.
g. Note amount, color, consistency, pH, and any unusual odor of drainage.
5. Document pain; medicate as prescribed.
6. Monitor abdomen regularly for distention, rigidity, and change in the status of bowel sounds.
7. If conservative medical interventions fail, surgery will be required to remove obstruction (see Perioperative Care in Chapter 3: *Advanced Clinical Concepts*).

HESI HINT A client admitted with complaints of constipation, thready stools, and rectal bleeding over the past few months is diagnosed with a rectal mass. What are the nursing interventions for this client?
- NPO
- Nasogastric tube (possibly an intestinal tube such as a Miller-Abbott)
- IV fluids
- Surgical preparation of bowel (if obstruction is complete)
- Teaching (preoperative, nutrition, etc.)

Cancer of the Colon

Description: Tumors occurring in the colon.
A. Cancer of the colon is the fourth most common cancer in the United States.
B. The estimated cure rate for cancer of the colon is 50%.
C. About 45% of cancerous tumors of the colon occur in the rectal or sigmoid area, 25% in the cecum and ascending colon, and 30% in the remainder of the colon.
D. The highest incidence is in persons older than 60 years.
E. A diet of high-fiber, low-fat foods, including cruciferous vegetables, may be a factor in the prevention of colon cancer.

HESI HINT Diet recommended by the American Cancer Society to prevent bowel cancer:
- Eat more cruciferous vegetables (from the cabbage family such as broccoli, cauliflower, Brussels sprouts, cabbage, and kale).
- Increase fiber intake.
- Maintain average body weight.
- Eat less animal fat.

F. Early detection is important.
G. Usual treatment is surgical removal of the tumor with adjuvant radiation or antineoplastic chemotherapy.

H. Diagnosis is made by test for occult blood in the stool, digital examination, flexible fiberoptic sigmoidoscopy with biopsy, colonoscopy, CT scan of the abdomen, MRI, ultrasound, and barium enema.

I. Carcinoembryonic antigen serum level is used to evaluate the effectiveness of treatment.

Nursing Assessment

A. Rectal bleeding

B. Change in bowel habits

C. Sense of incomplete evacuation

D. Abdominal pain, nausea, vomiting

E. Weight loss, cachexia

F. Fatigue

G. Abdominal distention or ascites

H. Family history of cancer, particularly cancer of the colon

I. History of polyps

Nursing Plans and Interventions

A. Treatment
   1. Prepare client for surgery, surgical removal of the tumor and reanastomosis, if possible, followed by chemotherapy/radiation therapy (see Perioperative Care in Chapter 3: *Advanced Clinical Concepts*).
   2. Bowel preparation may include laxatives and gut lavage with polyethylene glycol (GoLYTELY).
   3. If colostomy is performed, collaborate with RN to develop and implement a teaching plan for client/family about stoma care (see Stoma Care).

B. Prevention
   1. Provide high-calorie, high-protein diet.
   2. Promote prevention of constipation with high-fiber diet.
   3. Encourage early detection by screening with Hemoccult (guaiac) tests.

HESI HINT American Cancer Society recommendations for early detection of colon cancer in adults with average risk:
- A digital rectal examination every year starting at age 45.
- A stool blood test every year starting at age 45.
- A colonoscopy or sigmoidoscopy examination every 10 years after the age of 50 in average-risk clients, or more often based on the advice of a physician.
- Individuals in good health and with a life expectancy of greater than 10 years should continue regular colorectal cancer screening through the age of 75.

Stoma Care

A. Assess stoma for color (should be rose pink or brick-red in color).
   1. Normal to have some swelling immediately after surgery.
   2. Oozing from stoma when touched is normal because of its large amount of blood vessels.

B. The more distal the stoma is, the greater the chance for continence.
   1. An ileostomy drains liquid material; peristomal skin is prone to breakdown from enzymes.
   2. As the stoma's location descends the GI tract, the effluence (stoma drainage) becomes more solid or formed.
   3. The greatest chance for continence is with a stoma created from the sigmoid colon on the left side of the abdomen.
   4. Consultation with an enterostomal therapist is essential.

C. Preoperative care
   1. Reinforce a teaching plan related to postoperative expectations of client and family.
   2. Proposed location of the stoma.
   3. Approximate size.
   4. What it will look like; provide a picture if indicated.
   5. Support for the family but emphasize that the client is ultimately responsible for his or her own care.

D. Pouch care
   1. Ostomates will often wear pouches.
   2. The adhesive-backed opening, designed to cover the stoma, should provide about ⅛-inch clearance from the stoma.
   3. Use rubber band or clip to secure the bottom of the pouch and prevent leakage.
   4. Use simple squirt bottle to remove effluence from the sides of the bag. Change pouch system every 3 to 7 days.
   5. Maintain an extra supply of pouches so they never run out.
   6. Change the pouch when bowel is inactive.
   7. Empty pouch when $^{3}/_{1}$ to $^{1}/_{2}$ full.

E. Irrigation
   1. Those with descending colon colostomies can irrigate to provide control over effluence.
   2. Irrigate at approximately the same time daily.
   3. Use warm water (cold or hot water will cause cramping).
   4. Lubricate stoma cone, insert cone gently into stoma and hold tip securely in place.
   5. Allow irrigation solution to flow in steadily for 5 to 10 minutes; if cramping occurs, slow the flow rate. Allow 30 to 45 minutes for solution and feces to be expelled.
   6. Wash around stoma with lukewarm water and a mild soap.
   7. Commercial skin barriers may be purchased for home use.
   8. Odor control
   9. Commercial preparations are available.
   10. Eliminate foods in diet that cause offensive odors.

F. Diet
   1. Ileostomy
      a. Reinforce client instructions to chew food thoroughly.
      b. High-fiber foods can cause severe diarrhea and may need to be eliminated (popcorn, peanuts, unpeeled vegetables).

2. Colostomy: reinforce client instructions to resume the regular diet gradually. Foods that were a problem preoperatively should be tried cautiously.

Cirrhosis

Description: Cirrhosis is damage to the liver tissue, causing enlargement, fibrosis, scarring, and loss of effective hepatic functioning.

A. Etiology of cirrhosis includes the following:
  1. Chronic alcohol ingestion (Laennec cirrhosis)
  2. Viral hepatitis
  3. Exposure to hepatotoxins (including medications)
  4. Infections
  5. Congenital abnormalities
  6. Chronic biliary tree obstruction
  7. Chronic severe right-sided HF
  8. Idiopathic
B. Initially, hepatomegaly occurs; later, the liver becomes hard and nodular. May be detectable on palpation of right upper quadrant.

Nursing Assessment

A. History of alcohol use, prescriptive, and street drug use
B. Work history of exposure to toxic chemicals (pesticides, fumes, etc.)
C. Medication history of long-term use of hepatotoxic drugs
D. Family health history of liver abnormalities
E. Weakness, malaise
F. Anorexia, weight loss
G. Palpable liver (early), abdominal girth increases as liver enlarges
H. Jaundice
I. Fetor hepaticus (fruity or musty breath)

HESI HINT: CLINICAL MANIFESTATIONS OF JAUNDICE
- Yellow skin, sclera, and/or mucous membranes (bilirubin in skin)
- Dark-colored urine (bilirubin in urine)
- Chalky or clay-colored stools (absence of bilirubin in stools)

HESI HINT Fetor hepaticus is a distinctive breath odor of chronic liver disease. It is characterized by a fruity or musty odor that results from the damaged liver's inability to metabolize and detoxify mercaptan, which is produced by the bacterial degradation of methionine, a sulfurous amino acid.

J. Asterixis (hand-flapping tremor that often accompanies metabolic disorders)
K. Mental and behavioral changes
L. Bruising, erythema, or bleeding abnormalities like esophageal and gastric varices

M. Dry skin, spider angiomas
N. Gynecomastia (breast development), testicular atrophy
O. Ascites and peripheral edema
P. Peripheral neuropathy
Q. Hematemesis
R. Palmar erythema (redness in palms of the hands [hepatic encephalopathy])

HESI HINT For treatment of ascites, paracentesis and peritoneovenous shunts (LeVeen and Denver shunts) may be indicated.

HESI HINT Esophageal varices may rupture and cause hemorrhage. Immediate management includes insertion of an esophagogastric balloon tamponade—a Blakemore-Sengstaken or Minnesota tube. Other therapies include vasopressors, vitamin K, coagulation factors, and blood transfusions.

S. Elevated bilirubin, aspartate transaminase (AST), alanine transaminase (ALT), alkaline phosphatase, PT, and ammonia
T. Decreased Hgb, Hct, electrolytes, and albumin

HESI HINT Ammonia is not broken down as usual in the damaged liver; therefore, the serum ammonia level rises, which causes neurologic symptoms, including confusion. Because of possible altered mental state, the nurse should include safety precautions in the client's plan of care.

U. Complications
  1. Ascites, edema
  2. Portal hypertension
  3. Esophageal varices
  4. Encephalopathy
  5. Respiratory distress
  6. Coagulation defects

Nursing Plans and Interventions

A. Eliminate causative agent (alcohol, hepatotoxin).
B. Administer vitamin supplements (A, B complex, C, K) and assist with teaching the client/family the need for continuing these supplements.
C. Administer prescribed medications like vasopressin to control bleeding, beta blockers to reduce portal venous pressure thus reducing risk for bleeding, neomycin to decrease bacterial flora and decrease formation of ammonia, and diuretics to decrease fluids.
D. Monitor mental status frequently (at least every 2 hours); note any subtle changes.

E. Avoid initiating bleeding and observe for bleeding tendencies.
  1. Avoid injections whenever possible.
  2. Provide small-bore needles for IV insertion.
  3. Maintain pressure to venipuncture sites for at least 5 minutes.
  4. Use electric razor.
  5. Provide a soft-bristle toothbrush and encourage careful mouth care.
  6. Check stools and emesis for frank or occult blood.
  7. Prevent straining at stool.
    a. Administer stool softeners as prescribed.
    b. Provide high-fiber diet.
F. Provide special skin care.
  1. Avoid soap, rubbing alcohol, and perfumed products (which are drying to the skin).
  2. Apply moisturizing lotion or baby oil frequently.
  3. Observe skin for any lesions, including scratch marks.
  4. Turn frequently and apply lotion to exposed skin.
G. Monitor fluid and electrolyte status daily.
  1. I&O (accurate output may require indwelling urinary catheter).
  2. Observe for peripheral edema, pulmonary edema.
  3. Measure abdominal girth (determines increase or decrease of ascites).
  4. Weigh daily (determines increase or decrease of edema and ascites).
  5. Restrict fluids to 1500 mL/day (may help to reduce edema and ascites).
  6. Monitor dietary intake carefully, especially protein intake. Restrict protein if client has hepatic coma; otherwise, encourage foods with high biologic protein.
H. Reinforce teaching plan related to dietary restrictions: low sodium, low potassium, low fat, high carbohydrate.
I. If encephalopathy is present, lactulose is used to decrease ammonia levels (Table 4.20).
J. If esophageal varices are present, esophagogastric balloon tamponade (Blakemore tube), sclerotherapy, and/or portal systemic shunts may be used for treatment.

Hepatitis

Description: Hepatitis is widespread inflammation of liver cells, usually caused by a virus (Table 4.21).

Nursing Assessment

A. Known exposure to hepatitis

B. Individuals at risk for contracting hepatitis:
  1. Those having unprotected sex
  2. IV drug users (disease transmitted by dirty needles)
  3. Those who have recently had body piercings or tattoos (disease transmitted by dirty needles)
  4. Those living in crowded conditions
C. Fatigue, malaise, weakness
D. Anorexia, nausea, and vomiting
E. Jaundice, dark urine, clay-colored stools
F. Myalgia (muscle aches), joint pain
G. Dull headaches, irritability, depression
H. Abdominal tenderness in right upper quadrant
I. Fever with hepatitis A
J. Elevation of liver enzymes (ALT, AST, alkaline phosphatase), bilirubin

Nursing Plans and Interventions

A. Observe and report client's response to activity and plan periods of rest after periods of activity.
B. Assist client with care as needed, and encourage client to get help with daily activities at home (caring for children, preparing meals, etc.).
C. Provide high-calorie, high-carbohydrate diet with moderate fats and proteins.
  1. Serve small, frequent meals.
  2. Provide vitamin supplements.
  3. Provide foods the client prefers.
D. Administer medications as prescribed, for example, interferon, antiemetics, nucleoside and neurotide analogs, as needed.

HESI HINT: PROVIDE AN ENVIRONMENT CONDUCIVE TO EATING For clients who are anorexic and/or nauseated:
- Remove strong odors immediately; they can be offensive and increase nausea.
- Encourage client to sit up for meals; this can decrease the propensity to vomit.
- Serve small, frequent meals.

E. Emphasize to the client the importance of adhering to personal hygiene, using individual drinking and eating utensils, toothbrushes, and razors. Prevention of spread to others must also be emphasized.
F. Client should avoid hepatotoxic substances such as alcohol, aspirin, acetaminophen, and sedatives.

TABLE 4.20   Ammonia Detoxicant/Stimulant Laxative

Drug	Indications	Adverse Reactions	Nursing Implications
• Lactulose (Cephulac)	• Encephalopathy Used to decrease ammonia levels and bowel pH	• Diarrhea	• Reinforce client instruction regarding need for medication • Observe for diarrhea • Monitor ammonia levels

TABLE 4.21   Comparison of Three Types of Hepatitis

Characteristics	Hepatitis A	Hepatitis B	Hepatitis C
• Source of infection	• Contaminated food • Contaminated water	• Contaminated blood products • Contaminated needles or surgical instruments	• Contaminated blood products • Contaminated needles; intravenous drug use • Dialysis
• Route of infection	• Oral • Fecal • Parenteral	• Parenteral • Oral • Fecal • Direct contact • Breast milk • Sexual contact	• Parenteral • Sexual contact
• Incubation period	• 2–6 weeks	• 6–20 weeks	• Average: 6–7 weeks
• Onset	• Abrupt	• Insidious	• Insidious
• Seasonal variation	• Autumn • Winter	• All year	• All year
• Age group affected	• Children • Young adults	• Any age	• Any age
• Vaccine	• Yes	• Yes	• No
• Inoculation	• Yes	• Yes	• Yes
• Potential for chronic liver disease	• No	• Yes	• Yes
• Immunity	• Yes	• Yes	• No

HESI HINT Liver tissue is destroyed by hepatitis. Rest and adequate nutrition are necessary for regeneration of liver tissue being destroyed by the disease. Because many drugs are metabolized in the liver, drug therapy must be scrutinized carefully. Caution the client that recovery takes many months and that previously taken medications should not be resumed without the HCP's directions.

Pancreatitis

Description: Pancreatitis is nonbacterial inflammation of the pancreas.

A. Acute pancreatitis occurs when there is digestion of the pancreas by its own enzymes, primarily trypsin.

B. Alcohol ingestion and biliary tract disease are major causes of acute pancreatitis.

C. Chronic pancreatitis is a progressive, destructive disease with permanent dysfunction.

D. Long-term alcohol use is the major factor in chronic pancreatitis.

E. Alcohol consumption should be avoided for both acute and chronic pancreatitis.

Nursing Assessment

A. Acute pancreatitis
   1. Severe midepigastric pain radiating to back, usually related to excessive alcohol ingestion or a fatty meal
   2. Abdominal guarding; rigid, board-like abdomen, and abdominal pain
   3. Decreased or absent bowel sounds
   4. Nausea and vomiting
   5. Elevated temperature, tachycardia, decreased BP
   6. Bluish discoloration of flanks (Grey Turner sign) or periumbilical area (Cullen sign)
   7. Elevated amylase, lipase, and glucose levels, triglycerides, and low serum calcium
   8. Shock because of hemorrhaging into the pancreas

B. Chronic pancreatitis
   1. Continuous burning or gnawing abdominal pain
   2. Recurring attacks of severe upper abdominal and back pain
   3. Ascites
   4. Steatorrhea, diarrhea
   5. Frothy urine and stool
   6. Weight loss
   7. Jaundice, dark urine
   8. Signs and symptoms of DM

Nursing Plans and Interventions

A. Acute pancreatitis
   1. Nothing taken orally.
   2. Maintain NG tube to suction; total parenteral nutrition given.
   3. Administer hydromorphone (Dilaudid) or fentanyl (Sublimaze) PRN.
   4. Administer antacids, histamine-2 receptor-blocking drugs, anticholinergics, and PPIs.
   5. Assist client to assume position of comfort on side with legs drawn up to chest.
   6. Reinforce teaching: avoid alcohol, caffeine, fatty and spicy foods.

7. If severe, blood sugar monitoring and regular insulin coverage may be needed temporarily.
8. Place in semi-Fowler position to decrease pressure on the diaphragm.
9. Encourage client to cough and deep breathe; incentive spirometry.
10. Monitor bowel sounds every 4 hours.

HESI HINT Acute pancreatic pain is located retroperitoneally. Any enlargement of the pancreas causes the peritoneum to stretch tightly. Therefore, sitting up or leaning forward will reduce the pain.

B. Chronic pancreatitis
1. Administer analgesics such as hydromorphone (Dilaudid), fentanyl (Sublimaze), and morphine (narcotic tolerance and dependency may be a problem).
2. Administer pancreatic enzymes such as pancreatin (Creon) or pancrelipase (Viokase) with meals or snacks. i.e. should be mixed with fruit juice or applesauce (mixing with proteins should be avoided).
3. Monitor client's stools for number and consistency to determine effectiveness of enzyme replacement.
4. Reinforce client/family instructions about eating a bland, low-fat diet and avoiding rich foods, alcohol, and caffeine.
5. Monitor for signs and symptoms of diabetes mellitus.
6. Monitor ECG for dysrhythmias related to electrolyte imbalances.

Cholecystitis and Cholelithiasis

Description: Cholecystitis is an acute inflammation of the gallbladder. Cholelithiasis is the formation or presence of stones in the gallbladder.
A. Incidence of these diseases is greater in females who are multiparous and overweight.
B. Treatment for cholecystitis consists of IV hydration, administration of antibiotics, and pain control with morphine.
C. Treatment for cholelithiasis consists of nonsurgical removal of stones.
   1. Dissolution therapy (administration of bile salts, used rarely).
   2. Endoscopic retrograde cholangiopancreatography.
   3. Lithotripsy (not covered by many insurance carriers, thereby limiting its use).
D. Cholecystectomy is performed if stones are not removed nonsurgically and inflammation is *absent*. May be done through laparoscope.

HESI HINT After an endoscopic retrograde cholangiopancreatography, the client may feel sick. The scope is placed in the gallbladder, and the stones are crushed and left to pass on their own. These clients may be prone to pancreatitis.

Nursing Assessment

A. Pain, anorexia, vomiting, and/or flatulence precipitated by ingestion of fried, spicy, or fatty foods
B. Fever, elevated WBC, and other signs of infection (cholecystitis)
C. Abdominal tenderness
D. Jaundice and clay-colored stools (blockage)
E. Elevated liver enzymes, bilirubin, and WBC
F. Biliary colic

Nursing Plans and Interventions

A. Administer analgesics PRN for pain.
B. NPO.
C. Maintain NG tube to suction if indicated.
D. Monitor client's response to IV antibiotics.
E. Monitor I&O.
   1. Monitor electrolyte status regularly.
   2. Collaborate with the RN to develop and implement a teaching plan for client/family about avoiding fried, spicy, or fatty foods and reducing intake of calories if indicated.

HESI HINT Nonsurgical management of the client with cholecystitis includes the following:
- Low-fat diet
- Medications for pain if required
- Decompression of the stomach via nasogastric tube

F. Provide preoperative and postoperative care if surgery is indicated (see Perioperative Care in Chapter 3: *Advanced Clinical Concepts*).
G. Monitor T-tube drainage and safeguard the placement of the T-tube.

❓ REVIEW OF GASTROINTESTINAL SYSTEM

1. List four nursing interventions for the client with a hiatal hernia.
2. List three categories of medications used in the treatment of PUD.
3. List the symptoms of upper and lower GI bleeding.
4. What bowel sound disruptions occur with an intestinal obstruction?
5. List four nursing interventions for postoperative care of the client with a colostomy.
6. List the common clinical manifestations of jaundice.
7. What are the common food intolerances for clients with cholelithiasis?
8. List three classic initial signs of colorectal cancer.
9. In a client with cirrhosis, it is imperative to prevent further bleeding and observe for bleeding tendencies. List six relevant nursing interventions.
10. What is the main side effect of lactulose, which is used to reduce ammonia levels in clients with cirrhosis?
11. List four groups who have a high risk of contracting hepatitis.
12. How should the nurse administer pancreatic enzymes?
See Answer Key at the end of this text for suggested responses.

ENDOCRINE SYSTEM

Hyperthyroidism (Graves Disease, Goiter)

Description: Hyperthyroidism is excessive activity of thyroid gland, resulting in an elevated level of circulating thyroid hormones. Possibly long-term or lifelong treatment.

A. Hyperthyroidism can result from a primary disease state, replacement hormone therapy, or excess thyroid-stimulating hormone (TSH) from anterior pituitary tumor.

B. Graves disease is thought to be an autoimmune process and accounts for most cases.

C. Diagnosis is made by evaluating serum hormone levels.

D. Common treatment for hyperthyroidism; goal is to create a euthyroid state.
1. Thyroid ablation with medication
2. Radioactive iodine therapy
3. Thyroidectomy
4. Adenectomy of portion of anterior pituitary where TSH-producing tumor is located

E. *All* treatments leave the client in a hypothyroid state, requiring hormone replacement

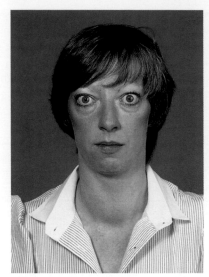

Fig. 4.7 Graves disease. This woman has a diffuse goiter and exophthalmos. (From Stevens, A., Lowe, J., & Scott, I. [2010]. *Core pathology* [3rd ed.]. London: Mosby.)

Nursing Assessment

A. Enlarged thyroid gland

B. Acceleration of body processes
1. Weight loss
2. Increased appetite
3. Diarrhea
4. Heat intolerance
5. Tachycardia, palpitations, increased systolic BP
6. Diaphoresis, wet moist skin
7. Nervousness, insomnia
8. Exophthalmos—abnormal protrusion of the eyes (Fig. 4.7)
9. T_3 elevated above 220 ng/dL
10. T_4 elevated above 12 mcg/dL
11. Radioactive iodine uptake (I_{131}) indicates presence of goiter
12. Thyroid scan indicates presence of goiter

Nursing Plans and Interventions

A. Provide a calm, restful atmosphere.

B. Monitor for signs of thyroid storm (life-threatening, sudden oversecretion of thyroid hormone).

HESI HINT Thyroid storm is a life-threatening event that occurs with uncontrolled hyperthyroidism caused by Graves disease. Symptoms include fever, tachycardia, agitation, anxiety, and hypertension. Primary nursing interventions include maintaining an airway and adequate ventilation.

Propylthiouracil (PTU) or methimazole (Tapazole) are antithyroid drugs used to treat thyroid storm. Propranolol (Inderal) may be given to decrease excessive sympathetic stimulation.

C. Collaborate with RN to develop and implement a teaching plan for client/family about the following:
1. After treatment, resulting hypothyroidism will require daily hormone replacement.
2. Client should wear medical alert bracelet in case of emergency.
3. Signs of hormone replacement overdosage are the signs for hyperthyroidism (see Nursing Assessment under Hyperthyroidism).
4. Signs of hormone replacement underdosage are the signs for hypothyroidism (see Nursing Assessment under Hypothyroidism).

D. Reinforce the teaching plan related to the recommended diet: high-calorie, high-protein, low-caffeine, low-fiber (if diarrhea is present) diet.

E. Perform eye care for exophthalmos.
1. Artificial tears to maintain moisture
2. Sunglasses when in bright light
3. Annual eye examinations

F. Prepare client for treatment of hyperthyroidism.
1. Thyroid ablation
   a. PTU or methimazole (Tapazole) acts by blocking synthesis of T_3 and T_4.
   b. Dosage is calculated based on body weight and given over several months.
   c. Client should take medication exactly as prescribed so the desired effect can be achieved.
   d. The expected effect is to make the client euthyroid; often given to prepare the client for thyroidectomy.
2. Radiation
   a. Iodine$_{131}$ is given to destroy thyroid cells.
   b. Iodine$_{131}$ is very irritating to the GI tract.
   c. Clients often vomit (vomitus is radioactive).

d. Place client on radiation precautions. Use time, distance, and shielding as means of protection against radiation (see Reproductive System in Chapter 5: *Pediatric Nursing*).

HESI HINT: POSTOPERATIVE THYROIDECTOMY Be prepared for the possibility of laryngeal edema. Put a tracheostomy set at bedside along with oxygen and a suction machine; Ca^{++} gluconate easily accessible in the event the parathyroid glands were removed.

3. Thyroidectomy
   a. Monitor respirations.
   b. Check frequently for bleeding.
   c. Support the neck when moving client. (Do not hyperextend.)
   d. Watch for laryngeal edema damage by assessing for hoarseness or inability to speak clearly.
   e. Observe for hypocalcemia if parathyroid glands have been removed.
   f. Keep drainage devices compressed/empty
4. Adenectomy: TSH-secreting pituitary tumors resected using transnasal approach (transsphenoidal hypophysectomy).

HESI HINT Normal serum calcium is 9—10.5 mEq/L. The best indicator of parathyroid problems is a decrease in the client's calcium compared with the preoperative value.

HESI HINT If two or more parathyroid glands have been removed, the chance of tetany increases dramatically:
- Monitor serum calcium levels (9—10.5 mg/dL is normal range).
- Check for tingling of toes and fingers and around the mouth.

Hypothyroidism (Hashimoto Disease, Myxedema)

Description: Hypothyroidism is a hypofunction of the thyroid gland with resulting insufficiency of thyroid hormone.
A. Early symptoms of hypothyroidism are nonspecific but gradually intensify.

B. Treated with hormone replacement.
C. Endemic goiters occur in individuals living in areas where there is deficient iodine. Iodized salt has helped to prevent this problem.

HESI HINT Myxedema coma can be precipitated by acute illness, withdrawal of thyroid medication, anesthesia, use of sedatives, or hypoventilation (with the potential for respiratory acidosis and carbon dioxide narcosis). The airway must be kept patent and ventilator support used as indicated.

Nursing Assessment

A. Fatigue
B. Thin, dry hair; dry skin
C. Thick, brittle nails
D. Constipation
E. Bradycardia, hypotension
F. Goiter
G. Periorbital edema, facial puffiness
H. Cold intolerance
I. Weight gain
J. Dull emotions and mental processes
K. Diagnosed by
   1. Low T_3 (below 70)
   2. Low T_4 (below 5)
   3. T_4 antibody present, indicating that T_4 is being destroyed by the body
   4. Low blood glucose
L. Husky voice
M. Slow speech

Nursing Plans and Interventions

A. Collaborate with RN to develop and implement a teaching plan for client or family about:
   1. Medication regimen: daily dosage of prescribed hormone replacement
   2. Medication effects and side effects (Table 4.22)
   3. Ongoing follow-up with serum hormone levels
   4. Signs and symptoms of myxedema coma (hypotension, hypothermia, hyponatremia, hypoglycemia, hypoventilation, respiratory failure)

TABLE 4.22 Thyroid Preparations			
Drugs	**Indications**	**Adverse Reactions**	**Nursing Implications**
• Levothyroxine (Synthroid) • Liothyronine sodium (Cytomel) • Desiccated thyroid (Armour Thyroid)	• Action is to increase metabolic rates • Synthetic T_4	• Anxiety • Insomnia • Tremors • Tachycardia • Palpitations • Angina • Dysrhythmias	• Check serum hormone levels routinely • Monitor blood pressure and pulse regularly • Weigh daily • Report side effects to health care provider • Avoid foods and products containing iodine • Initiate cautiously in clients with cardiovascular disease

TABLE 4.23 Corticosteroids

Drugs	Indications	Adverse Reactions	Nursing Implications
Steroids • Hydrocortisone • Prednisone • Dexamethasone • Methylprednisolone (Medrol)	• Hormone replacement • Severe rheumatoid arthritis • Autoimmune disorders	• Emotional lability • Impaired wound healing • Skin fragility • Abnormal fat deposition • Hyperglycemia • Hirsutism • Moon face • Osteoporosis • All symptoms of Cushing syndrome if overdosage occurs	• Wean slowly (administer a high dose, then taper off)—careful monitoring required during withdrawal • Monitor serum potassium, glucose (can become diabetic), and sodium • Weigh daily; report weight gain of greater than 5 pounds/week • Administer with antiulcer drugs or food • Use care to prevent injuries • Reinforce the teaching plan related to the symptoms of Cushing syndrome • Monitor blood pressure and pulse closely

B. Assist in the implementation of a bowel elimination plan to prevent constipation.
1. Increase fluid intake to 3 L/day.
2. Encourage high-fiber diet, including fresh fruits and vegetables.
3. Increase activity.
4. Discourage use of enemas and laxatives.
C. Avoid sedation, which can lead to respiratory difficulties.

Addison Disease (Primary Adrenocortical Deficiency)

Description: Addison disease is an autoimmune process often found in conjunction with other endocrine diseases of an autoimmune nature—a primary disorder; hypofunction of the adrenal cortex.
A. Sudden withdrawal from corticosteroids may precipitate symptoms of Addison disease (Table 4.23).
B. Addison disease is characterized by lack of cortisol, aldosterone, and androgens.
C. Definitive diagnosis is made using an adrenocorticotropic hormone (ACTH) stimulation test.
D. If ACTH production failure by anterior pituitary is found, it is considered secondary Addison.

> **HESI HINT** People take steroids for various conditions. Clients should be cautioned against suddenly stopping the medications and be informed that it is necessary to taper off taking steroids.

Nursing Assessment

A. Fatigue, weakness
B. Weight loss, anorexia, nausea, vomiting
C. Postural hypotension
D. Hypoglycemia
E. Hyponatremia
F. Hyperkalemia

G. Hyperpigmentation of mucous membranes and skin (only if primary Addison disease; not seen in secondary Addison disease)
H. Signs of shock when in Addison crisis (see Shock in Chapter 3: *Advanced Clinical Concepts*)
I. Loss of body hair
J. Hypovolemia; signs include: hypotension, tachycardia, and fever

Nursing Plans and Interventions

A. Take vital signs frequently (every 15 minutes if in crisis).
B. Monitor I&O and weigh daily.
C. Instruct client to rise slowly because of the possibility of postural hypotension.
D. During Addison crisis, monitor the client's response to IV glucose with parenteral glucocorticoids. This condition requires large fluid volume replacement.
E. Monitor serum electrolyte levels.
F. Collaborate with RN to develop and implement a teaching plan for client/family about:
1. Need for lifelong hormone replacement
2. Need for close medical supervision
3. Need for medical alert jewelry
4. Signs and symptoms of over- and underdosage of medication
5. High-sodium, low-potassium, and high-carbohydrate diet (complex carbohydrates)
6. Encourage fluid intake of at least 3 L/day.
G. Provide ulcer prophylaxis because of exogenous source of corticosteroid.

> **HESI HINT** Addison crisis is a *medical emergency* brought on by the sudden withdrawal of a steroid or by a stressful event (trauma, severe infection).
> • Vascular collapse: hypotension and tachycardia occur; administer IV fluids until stabilized.
> • Hypoglycemia: administer IV glucose.

- Administer parenteral hydrocortisone: *essential to reversing the crisis.*
- Aldosterone replacement: administer fludrocortisone acetate (Florinef) orally (only available as oral preparation) with simultaneous administration of salt (sodium chloride) if client has a sodium deficit.

Cushing Syndrome

Description: Cushing syndrome is excess adrenal corticoid activity.

A. Etiology is usually chronic administration of corticosteroids.

B. Cushing syndrome can also be caused by adrenal, pituitary, or hypothalamus tumors.

Nursing Assessment

A. Physical symptoms include
  1. Moon face
  2. Truncal obesity
  3. Buffalo hump
  4. Abdominal striae
  5. Muscle atrophy
  6. Thinning of the skin
  7. Hirsutism in female
  8. Hyperpigmentation
  9. Amenorrhea
  10. Edema, poor wound healing, easy bruising
B. Impotence
C. Hypertension
D. Susceptible to multiple infections
E. Osteoporosis
F. Peptic ulcer formation
G. Many false-positives and false-negatives in laboratory testing
H. Laboratory data often include the following findings:
  1. Hyperglycemia
  2. Hypernatremia
  3. Hypokalemia
  4. Decreased eosinophils and lymphocytes
  5. Increased plasma cortisol
  6. Increased urinary 17-hydroxycorticoids

Nursing Plans and Interventions

A. Protect from exposure to infection.
B. WASH HANDS; use good hand hygiene technique.
C. Monitor for signs of infection: fever, oral candidiasis, yeast infections, adventitious lung sounds, skin lesions, elevated WBCs
D. Collaborate with RN to develop and implement a teaching plan for client/family about safety measures.
  1. Position bed close to floor with easy access to call light.
  2. Encourage use of side rails.
  3. Ensure walkways are unobstructed.
  4. Encourage wearing shoes when ambulating.
E. Provide low-sodium diet; encourage foods with vitamin D and calcium.

F. Provide good skin care.
G. Discuss weaning from steroids after surgery. (If weaning occurs too quickly, Addison disease symptoms will occur.)
H. Encourage selection of clothing that minimizes visible aberrations; encourage maintenance of normal physical appearance.
I. Monitor I&O and weigh daily.
J. Provide ulcer prophylaxis.
K. Preoperative and postoperative care for hypophysectomy or adrenalectomy

> **HESI HINT** Instruct clients to take steroids with meals to prevent gastric irritation. They should never skip doses. If they have nausea or vomiting for more than 12–24 h, they should contact the HCP.

Diabetes Mellitus

Description: DM is a metabolic disorder characterized by high levels of glucose resulting from defects in insulin secretion or insulin action or both.

A. DM is characterized by hyperglycemia.
B. DM affects the metabolism of protein, carbohydrate, and fat.
C. Four ways to diagnose DM:
  1. Fasting plasma glucose $\geq$126 mg/dL
  2. Glycosylated Hgb $\leq$6.5%
  3. Random blood glucose $\leq$200 mg/dL in a client with classic symptoms of hyperglycemia
  4. Oral glucose tolerance test greater than 200 (use plasma glucose, not fingersticks, to diagnose diabetes)
D. Diabetes is majorly classified as: (Table 4.24)
  1. Type 1: results from B-cell destruction
  2. Type 2: results from progressive secretory insulin deficit and/or defect in insulin uptake
  3. Other: transplant-related diabetes, cystic fibrosis-related diabetes, iatrogenic-induced diabetes (stress, hospital); steroid-induced diabetes
  4. Gestational diabetes
  5. Prediabetes: blood glucose levels when fasting are 100 to 125 mg/dL or A1c of 5.7% to 6.4%
E. Many clients diagnosed with type 2 DM use insulin but retain some degree of pancreatic function.
F. Obesity is a major risk factor in type 2 DM.

Nursing Assessment

A. Type 1
  1. Description: results from the progressive autoimmune-based destruction of beta cells.
    a. Client can become hyperglycemic and ketosis prone relatively easily.
    b. Precipitating factors for diabetic ketoacidosis (DKA) include infection and inadequate management or undermanagement of glucose.
  2. Clinical characteristics of DKA:
    a. Serum glucose of $\leq$250

TABLE 4.24   Comparison of Type 1 and Type 2 Diabetes Mellitus

Variable	Type 1 DM	Type 2 DM
Prevalence	5% of US population with DM	90%–95% of US population with DM
Pathology	Beta cell destruction leading to absolute insulin deficiency	Basic defect is insulin resistance and usually has relative rather than absolute insulin deficiency
Onset	Sudden	Gradual, insidious
Signs and symptoms	• Polyuria • Polydipsia • Polyphagia • Weight loss	• Polydipsia • Polyuria • Polyphagia • Weight loss • Fatigue • Frequent infections • Blurred vision • Impotence
Age at onset	Any age but mostly younger than 21	Any age but mostly adults
Weight	• Thin • Slender	• Overweight • Obese
Ketosis	Common	Rare
Pathology	• Autoimmune and viral component	• Obesity, cardiovascular disease an equal comorbidity • Genetic predisposition
Lifestyle management	• Medical nutrition therapy: carbohydrate counting • Physical activity	• Medical nutrition therapy: heart-healthy, portion-controlled diet • Physical activity

Pharmacologic management	• Intensive insulin therapy	• Typically a stepwise approach:
		  1. Diet
		  2. Exercise
		  3. Oral agents
		  4. Oral agents and insulin

DM, Diabetes mellitus.

b. Ketonuria in large amounts

c. Arterial pH of less than 7.30 and HCO_3 less than 15 mEq/dL; nausea, vomiting, dehydration, abdominal pain; Kussmaul respirations; acetone odor to breath

3. Treatment

a. Usually with isotonic IV fluids 0.9% NaCl solution 1 L/h until BP stabilized and urine output 30 to 60 mL/h

b. Slow IV infusion by IV pump of regular insulin; too rapid infusion of insulin to lower serum glucose can lead to cerebral edema

c. Careful replacement of potassium based on laboratory data

B. Type 2

1. Description: results from either the inadequate production of insulin by the body or lack of sensitivity to the insulin being produced.

a. Rare development of ketoacidosis

b. With extreme hyperglycemia, hyperosmolar hyperglycemia nonketotic syndrome develops

2. Clinical characteristics

a. Hyperglycemia greater than 600 mg/dL

b. Plasma hyperosmolality

c. Dehydration

d. Changed mental status

e. Absent ketone bodies

3. Treatment

a. Usually with isotonic IV fluid replacement and careful monitoring of potassium and glucose levels

b. IV insulin given until blood glucose stable at 250 mg/dL

Nursing Assessment

A. Integumentary system

1. Skin infections

2. Wounds that do not heal

3. Acanthosis (thickening of the skin)

B. Oral cavity

1. Periodontal disease

2. Candidiasis (raised, white patchy areas on mucous membranes)

C. Eyes

1. Cataracts

2. Retinopathy

D. Cardiopulmonary system

1. Angina

2. Dyspnea

3. Hypertension

E. Periphery

1. Hair loss on extremities, indicating poor perfusion

2. Other signs of poor peripheral circulation:

a. Coolness

b. Skin shininess and thinness

c. Weak or absent peripheral pulses

d. Ulcerations on extremities

d. Pallor

e. Thick nails with ridges

F. Kidneys

1. Edema of face, hands, and feet

2. Symptoms of UTI

3. Symptoms of renal failure: edema, anorexia, nausea, fatigue, difficulty in concentrating. Diabetic nephropathy is the primary cause of end-stage renal failure in the United States.

G. Neuromuscular

1. Neuropathies

2. Symptoms of neuropathies: numbness, tingling, pain, burning

H. GI disturbances

1. Nighttime diarrhea

2. Gastroparesis (faulty absorption)

I. Reproductive

1. Male impotence

2. Vaginal dryness, frequent vaginal infections

3. Menstrual irregularities

J. Psychosocial issues

1. Depression: persons with DM have a high rate of depression. Depression contributes to poor adherence to DM regimens, feelings of helplessness, and poor health outcomes.

2. Increased risk of developing anorexia nervosa and bulimia nervosa in women with type 1 DM.

Nursing Plans and Interventions

A. Determine baseline laboratory data: serum glucose; electrolytes; creatinine; BUN; cholesterol (both LDL and HDL); triglycerides; ABGs (as indicated).

B. Reinforce teaching of injection technique and/or oral medication(s) (Tables 4.25 and 4.26).

1. Identify the prescribed dose and type of insulin.

2. For insulin: lift skin; use 90-degree angle. If very thin or using 5/16-inch or 8-mm needle, may need to use a 45-degree angle.

3. Rotate injection sites.

C. Reinforce teaching about medical nutrition therapy.

1. Work with dietitian to reinforce specific meal plan.

2. Overall goal is to make healthy nutritional choices, eat a varied diet, and maintain an exercise regimen.

3. Encourage carbohydrate counting for those on complex insulin regimens.

4. Remind that meals should be timed according to medication (insulin) peak times.

5. Reinforce knowledge of diet regimen.

a. 45% to 50% carbohydrates

b. 15% to 20% protein

c. 30% or less fat

d. Foods high in complex carbohydrates and fiber and low in fat whenever possible

e. Alcoholic beverages can be included in diet with proper planning

6. Reinforce teaching about managing sick days (illness raises blood glucose).

a. Teach client to keep taking insulin.

b. Monitor glucose more frequently.

c. Watch for signs of hyperglycemia.

D. Reinforce teaching about exercise regimen because exercise decreases blood sugar levels.

1. Exercise after mealtimes; either exercise with someone or let someone know where exercise will take place to ensure safety.

2. A snack may be needed before or during exercise.

3. Monitor blood glucose before, during, and after exercise when beginning a new regimen.

E. Reinforce teaching about signs and symptoms of hyperglycemia and hypoglycemia (Table 4.27, pp. XXX).

F. Reinforce teaching about foot care.

1. Feet should be checked daily for changes; signs of injury and breaks in skin should be reported to HCP.

2. Feet should be washed daily with mild soap and warm water; soaking is to be avoided; feet should be dried well, especially between toes.

3. Feet may be moisturized with a lanolin product, but not between the toes.

4. Well-fitting leather shoes should be worn; going barefoot and wearing sandals should be avoided.

5. Clean socks should be worn daily.

6. Garters and tight elastic-topped socks should never be worn.

7. Corns and calluses should be removed by a professional.

8. Nails should be cut or filed straight across.

9. Warm socks should be worn if feet are cold.

G. Encourage regular health care follow-ups.

1. Ophthalmologist

2. Podiatrist

3. Annual physical examination

H. Teach that immediate attention should be sought if any sign of infection occurs.

I. Refer client to the American Diabetes Association for additional information.

HESI HINT Why do persons with DM have trouble with wound healing? High blood glucose contributes to damage of the smallest vessels—the capillaries. This damage causes permanent capillary scarring, which inhibits the normal activity of the capillary. This phenomenon causes disruption of capillary elasticity and promotes problems such as poor healing of breaks in the skin.

HESI HINT: GLYCOSYLATED HGB Indicates average blood glucose control over previous 2—3 months.

TABLE 4.25　Oral Hypoglycemics

Drugs	Indications	Adverse Reactions	Nursing Implications
• First generation: • Sulfonylureas • Tolbutamide (Orinase) • Chlorpropamide (Diabinese) • Second generation: • Glyburide (Micronase, DiaBeta) • Glipizide (Glucotrol) • Glimepiride (Amaryl)	• Lowers blood sugar by stimulating the release of insulin by the beta cells of the pancreas and causes tissues to take up and store glucose more easily • First generation is low potency and short acting • Second generation is high potency and longer acting	• First generation: • Hypoglycemia • Nausea, heartburn, constipation, anorexia • Agranulocytosis • Allergic skin reactions • Second generation: • Weight gain • Hypoglycemia, particularly in older adults	• First generation: • Responsiveness may decline over time • Given once daily with first meal • Monitor blood sugar • Hard to detect hypoglycemia if older adult or also on beta-blockers • Second generation: • Less likely to interact with other medications
Biguanides Metformin (Glucophage)	• Lowers serum glucose levels by inhibiting hepatic glucose production and increasing sensitivity of peripheral tissue to insulin	• Abdominal discomfort • Diarrhea • Lactic acidosis	• Many drug–drug interactions • Extended-release tablets should be taken with the evening meal • Use cautiously with preexisting renal or liver disease or HF • Discontinue 48 h before and wait 48 h to restart dosage after diagnostic studies requiring IV iodine contrast media • Can lead to vitamin B_{12} deficiency
Alpha-glucosidase inhibitors Acarbose (Precose) Miglitol (Glyset)	• Lowers blood glucose by blunting sugar levels after meals	• Hypoglycemia	• Optimally, must be taken with the FIRST bite of each meal • May be taken with other classes of oral hypoglycemics • Monitor blood sugar • Use is controversial in Inflammatory bowel disease (IBD) client
Thiazolidinediones Rosiglitazone (Avandia) Pioglitazone (Actos)	• Lowers blood sugar by decreasing the insulin resistance of the tissues	• Hypoglycemia • Increased total cholesterol, weight gain • Edema, anemia	• Many drug–drug interactions • Skip dose if meal skipped • No known drug interactions • Monitor liver function • Caution with use in CAD; may precipitate HF
Meglitinides Repaglinide (Prandin) Nateglinide (Starlix)	• Lowers blood sugar by stimulating beta cells in pancreas to release insulin; does this by closing K^+ channels and opening Ca^{++} channels	• Hypoglycemia • Angina, chest pain • Arthralgia, back pain • Nausea and vomiting, dyspepsia, constipation, or diarrhea	• May be used with metformin • Give before meals; if a meal is skipped, skip the dose • Monitor blood sugar
Incretin enhancer Linagliptin (Tradjenta) Saxagliptin (Onglyza) Sitagliptin (Januvia)	• Lowers blood glucose by inhibiting degradation of incretins, which increases insulin secretion	• Hypoglycemia	• Not considered a first-line agent
Combinations Glyburide and metformin (Glucovance) Pioglitazone + metformin (Actoplus Met) Rosiglitazone + glimepiride (Avandaryl) Rosiglitazone + metformin (Advanamet) Glipizide + metformin (Metaglip)	• Lowers blood sugar by combining the advantages of two classes of hypoglycemics	• Note possible adverse reactions to both classes • Hypoglycemia (severe)	• Note implications of both classes of drugs

Second-generation sulfonylureas are much more potent and have fewer drug-to-drug interactions than the first-generation agents.
CAD, Coronary artery disease; *HF,* heart failure; *IV,* intravenous.

TABLE 4.26 Types/Action of Insulin

Type	Name	Onset	Peak Action	Duration	Nursing Implications
• Rapid acting	• Human insulin lispro (Humalog) • Aspart (NovoLog) • Glulisine (Apidra)	• 0.5–1 h • 5–15 min • 25 min	• 2–4 h • 0.75–1.5 h • 1 h	• 4 h • 3–5 h • 2–3 h	• Give within 15 min of a meal (Lispro and Aspart)
• Short acting	• Regular insulin (human) (Humulin R, Novolin R)	• 30–60 min	• 2–3 h	• 5–7 h	• Regular insulin may be given IV
• Intermediate acting	• Isophane insulin (human) (Humulin N, Novolin N)	• 1–2 h	• 6–12 h	• 18–28 h	• Not to be given IV • Mixtures combine rapid-acting regular insulin with intermediate-acting NPH insulin in a 30% regular with 70% NPH proportion or at 50/50 combination
• Long acting	• Glargine (Lantus) • Detemir (Levemir)	• 4–8 h • 1.1 h	• 14–20 h • 5 h (some sources say there is no peak)	• 24 h	• Not to be given IV • Recommended: give once daily, SC, at bedtime. In some cases, given two times a day. Acts as basal insulin. Caution: Solution is clear, but bottle is distinctly different shape from regular insulin. *Do not confuse insulins.* Do not shake solution. Do not mix other insulins with Lantus. Use cautiously if patient is NPO
• Premix	• Humalog 75/25 • Human 70/30 • NovoLog 70/30 • Humalog 50/50				• For all premixes: offer when food readily available • 25% Lispro/75% Humulin N (NPH) • 30% Regular/70% NPH • 30% Aspart/70% NPH

Other Injectable Therapies

Drugs	Action/Indications	Adverse Reaction	Implications and Precautions
Exenatide (Byetta) (Victoza)	Stimulates release of insulin; ↓ glucagon secretion; ↑ satiety; ↓ gastric emptying; may facilitate weight loss (~3–5 kg) Indicated for clients with type 2 DM who are not adequately controlled with oral therapy; not indicated for clients with type 1 DM	Nausea, vomiting, hypoglycemia, diarrhea, headache	Not a substitute for insulin. Not recommended for ESRD, pancreatitis, severe renal impairment, or severe gastrointestinal disease. May slow absorption of other drugs
Pramlintide (Symlin)	Slows gastric emptying time, suppresses the release of glucagon, and appears to suppress appetite. Indicated as adjunct treatment in type 1 DM for clients who have not obtained adequate glycemic control with insulin therapy and for clients with type 2 DM who have not obtained adequate glycemic control with insulin with or without oral therapy	Nausea, vomiting, hypoglycemia, diarrhea, headache	Contraindicated for clients with diabetic gastroparesis. It is also avoided in clients whc have exhibited significant hypoglyceric reactions or who are not able to recognize and manage hypoglycemic reactions

DM, Diabetes mellitus; *IV,* intravenous; *ESRD,* end-stage renal disease.

TABLE 4.27 Comparison Between Hyperglycemia and Hypoglycemia

HYPERGLYCEMIA		HYPOGLYCEMIA	
Signs and Symptoms	**Nursing Action**	**Signs and Symptoms**	**Nursing Actions**

• Polydipsia
• Polyuria
• Polyphagia
• Blurred vision
• Weakness
• Weight loss
• Syncope
	• Encourage water intake
	• Check blood glucose frequently
	• Assess for ketoacidosis:
	  1. Urine ketones
	  2. Urine glucose
	  3. Administer insulin as directed
		• Headache
		• Nausea
		• Sweating
		• Tremors
		• Lethargy
		• Hunger
		• Confusion
		• Slurred speech
		• Tingling around mouth
		• Anxiety, nightmares
			• Usually occurs rapidly and is potentially life-threatening; treat immediately with complex carbohydrates. Example: graham cracker and peanut butter twice, and if no response, seek medical attention
			• Check blood glucose (may seize if less than 40)

HESI HINT: BLOOD GLUCOSE Indicates blood glucose at any one point in time.

HESI HINT: DIABETES SELF-MANAGEMENT EDUCATION The goal is to assist the client to maintain good blood sugar control.

HESI HINT The body's response to illness/stress is to produce glucose. Therefore, any illness or stressor results in hyperglycemia.

HESI HINT If in doubt of whether a client is hyperglycemic or hypoglycemic, treat for hypoglycemia.

HESI HINT: SELF-MONITORING BLOOD GLUCOSE
- Provides data about blood glucose control.
- Good blood glucose control decreases long-term complications.
- Monitoring technique is specific to each meter.
- Monitor before meals, at bedtime, when symptoms occur, or as directed by HCP.
- Record results and report to HCP at time of visit.

❓ REVIEW OF ENDOCRINE SYSTEM

1. What diagnostic test is used to determine thyroid activity?
2. What condition results from all treatments for hyperthyroidism?
3. State three symptoms of hyperthyroidism and three symptoms of hypothyroidism.
4. List five important teaching aspects for clients who are beginning corticosteroid therapy.
5. Describe the physical appearance of clients who are cushingoid.
6. Which type of diabetes always requires insulin replacement?
7. Which type of diabetes sometimes requires no medication?

8. List five symptoms of hyperglycemia.
9. List five symptoms of hypoglycemia.
10. Name the necessary elements to include in teaching the client with newly diagnosed diabetes.
11. A client has purchased a 3-month supply of insulin. Which bottles should be refrigerated?
12. Identify the peak action time of the following types of insulin: rapid-acting regular insulin, intermediate-acting insulin, and long-acting insulin.
13. When preparing the diabetic client for discharge, the nurse teaches the client the relationship between stress, exercise, bedtime snacking, and glucose balance. State the relationship between each of these.
14. When making rounds at night, the nurse notes that an insulin-dependent client is complaining of a headache, slight nausea, and minimal trembling. The client's hand is cool and moist. What is the client most likely experiencing?
15. Identify five foot-care interventions that should be taught to the client with diabetes.
See Answer Key at the end of this text for suggested responses.

MUSCULOSKELETAL SYSTEM

Rheumatoid Arthritis

Description: Rheumatoid arthritis is chronic, systematic, progressive deterioration of the connective tissue (synovium) of the joints characterized by inflammation.
A. The exact cause is unknown, but it is classified as an immune complex disorder.
B. Joint involvement is bilateral and symmetric.
C. Severe cases may require joint replacement (see "Joint Replacement").

HESI HINT A client comes to the clinic complaining of morning stiffness, weight loss, and swelling of both hands and wrists. Rheumatoid arthritis is suspected. Which methods of assessment might the nurse use and which methods would the nurse not use? Use inspection, palpation, and strength testing. Do not use range of motion (ROM). (This activity promotes pain because ROM is limited.)

Nursing Assessment

A. Fatigue

B. Generalized weakness

C. Weight loss

D. Anorexia

E. Morning stiffness

F. Bilateral inflammation of joints with the following symptoms:
1. Decreased ROM
2. Joint pain
3. Warmth
4. Edema
5. Erythema
6. Joint deformity and limitation

> **HESI HINT** In the joint, the normal cartilage becomes soft, fissures and pitting occur, and the cartilage thins. Spurs form and inflammation sets in. The result is deformity marked by immobility, pain, and muscle spasm. The prescribed treatment regimen is corticosteroids for the inflammation; splinting, immobilization, and rest for the joint deformity; and NSAIDs for the pain.

G. Diagnosis confirmed by the following:
1. Elevated erythrocyte sedimentation rate
2. Positive rheumatoid factor
3. Presence of antinuclear anticitrullinated protein antibody (ACPA), antinuclear antibody (ANA), and C-reactive protein (CRP)
4. Joint space narrowing indicated by arthroscopic examination (provides joint visualization)
5. Abnormal synovial fluid (fluid in joint) indicated by arthrocentesis

> **HESI HINT** Synovial tissues line the bones of the joints. Inflammation of this lining causes destruction of the tissue and bone. Early detection of rheumatoid arthritis can decrease the amount of bone and joint destruction. Often the disease will go into remission. Decreasing the amount of bone and joint destruction will reduce the amount of disability.

Nursing Plans and Interventions

A. Implement pain relief measures.
1. Use moist heat: warm, moist compresses; whirlpool baths; hot shower in the morning
2. Use diversionary activities: imaging; distraction; self-hypnosis; biofeedback
3. Administer medications and reinforce teaching about medications (Tables 4.23 and 4.28).

B. Provide periods of rest after periods of activity.
1. Encourage self-care to maximal level.
2. Allow adequate time for the client to perform activities.
3. Perform activities during time of day when client feels most energetic.

C. Do not overexert.

D. Encourage the client to maintain proper posture and joint position.

> **HESI HINT** What activity recommendations should the nurse provide a client with rheumatoid arthritis?
> - Do not exercise painful, swollen joints.
> - Do not exercise any joint to the point of pain.
> - Perform exercises slowly and smoothly; avoid jerky movements.

E. Encourage use of assistive devices.
1. Elevated toilet seat
2. Shower chair
3. Cane, walker, and/or wheelchair
4. Reachers
5. Adaptive clothing with Velcro closures
6. Straight-backed chairs with elevated seat

F. Collaborate with the RN in developing a teaching plan.
1. Medication regimen
2. Need for routine follow-up for evaluation of possible side effects
3. ROM and stretching exercises tailored to specific client needs
4. Safety tips/precautions on equipment use and environment

Lupus Erythematosus

Description: Lupus erythematosus is a systemic, inflammatory connective tissue disorder.

A. There are two classifications of lupus erythematosus:
1. Discoid lupus erythematosus (DLE) affects skin only.
2. Systemic lupus erythematosus (SLE).

B. SLE is more prevalent than DLE.

C. Lupus is an autoimmune disorder.

D. Kidney involvement is the leading cause of death in clients with lupus, followed by cardiac involvement.

> **HESI HINT** Avoiding sunlight is the key in management of lupus erythematosus. This is what differentiates it from other connective tissue diseases.

E. Factors that trigger lupus: sunlight, stress, pregnancy, and drugs

Nursing Assessment

A. DLE: dry, scaly rash on face or upper body (butterfly rash)

B. SLE:
1. Joint pain and decreased mobility
2. Fever
3. Nephritis (hematuria and proteinuria)
4. Pleural effusion
5. Pericarditis
6. Abdominal pain (diarrhea, dysphagia, nausea, and vomiting)

TABLE 4.28 Nonsteroidal Antiinflammatory Drugs

Drugs	Indications	Adverse Reactions	Nursing Implications
• Aspirin (Anacin) • Ibuprofen (Motrin, Nuprin, Advil) • Ketorolac tromethamine (Toradol) • Celecoxib (Celebrex) • Etodolac (Lodine) • Diclofenac potassium (Voltaren) • Naproxen (Anaprox, Naprosyn) • Piroxicam (Feldene)	• Used as antiinflammatory • Antipyretic • Analgesic • Can be used with other agents	• GI irritation, bleeding, nausea, vomiting, constipation • Elevated liver enzymes • Prolonged coagulation time • Tinnitus • Thrombocytopenia • Fluid retention • Nephrotoxicity • Blood dyscrasias	• Reinforce teaching about taking with food or milk to reduce GI symptoms • Monitor serum salicylate level • Reinforce teaching about watching for signs of bleeding • Reinforce teaching about avoiding alcohol • Reinforce teaching about observing for tinnitus • Administer corticosteroids for severe rheumatoid arthritis (see Table 4.23) • NSAIDs reduce the effect of ACE inhibitors in hypertensive clients • Note name similarity of Celebrex with other drugs having one letter difference in spelling • Encourage routine appointments to check liver/renal labs and CBC

ACE, Angiotensin-converting enzyme; *GI,* gastrointestinal; *NSAIDs,* nonsteroidal anti-inflammatory drugs.

7. Photosensitivity
8. Hypertension (stroke, seizures, psychosis, cognitive impairment)
9. Raynaud phenomenon

Nursing Plans and Interventions

A. Reinforce instruction for client to avoid prolonged exposure to sunlight.
B. Reinforce instruction for client to clean the skin with mild soap.
C. Monitor and collaborate with RN to develop and implement a teaching plan for client/family about administration of steroids.
D. Administer medications such as NSAIDs, antimalarials, corticosteroids, immunosuppressive drugs, biologic and targeted therapy agents.

Osteoarthritis

Description: Osteoarthritis (OA) is noninflammatory arthritis. It was formerly known as degenerative joint disease (DJD)
A. OA is characterized by the degeneration of cartilage, a "wear and tear" process.
B. Usually affects one or two joints.
C. Occurs asymmetrically.
D. Obesity and overuse are predisposing factors.

> **HESI HINT** DJD and OA are often described as the same disease, and indeed, they both result in hypertrophic changes in the joints.

Nursing Assessment

A. Joint pain, which increases with activity and improves with rest
B. Morning stiffness

C. Asymmetry of affected joints
D. Crepitus (grating sound in the joint)
E. Limited movement
F. Visible joint abnormalities indicated in x-ray films
G. Joint enlargement and bony nodules

Nursing Plans and Interventions

See Rheumatoid Arthritis.
A. Reinforce weight-reduction diet.
B. Remind client that excessive use of the involved joint aggravates pain and may accelerate degeneration.
C. Collaborate with RN to develop and implement a teaching plan for client/family about:
  1. Correct posture and body mechanics.
  2. Sleep with rolled terry cloth towel under cervical spine if neck pain is a problem.
  3. Encourage the client to relieve pain in fingers and hands, and wear stretch gloves at night.
  4. Keep joints in functional position.

Osteoporosis

Description: Osteoporosis is a metabolic disease in which bone demineralization results in decreased density and subsequent fractures.
A. Many fractures in older adults occur as a result of osteoporosis and often occur before the client falls, rather than the client sustaining a fracture caused by a fall.
B. The etiology of osteoporosis is unknown.
C. Postmenopausal women are at highest risk.

Nursing Assessment

A. Classic dowager hump or kyphosis of the dorsal spine (Fig. 4.8).
B. Loss of height, often 2 to 3 inches.
C. Back pain, often radiating around the trunk.

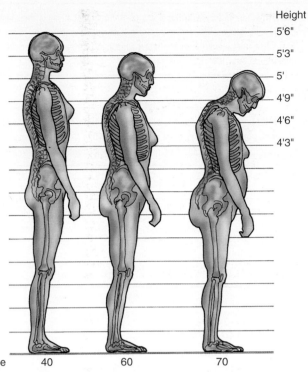

Fig. 4.8 Normal Spine at 40 Years of Age and Osteoporotic Changes at 60 and 70 Years of Age. These changes can cause a loss of as much as 6 inches in height and can result in the so-called dowager hump (far right) in the upper thoracic vertebrae. (Ignatavicius, D. D., Workman, L., & Rebar, C. [2020]. *Medical surgical nursing: Concepts for interprofessional collaborative care* [10th ed.]. St. Louis: Elsevier.)

D. Pathologic fractures, often occurring in the distal end of the radius and the upper third of the femur.

E. Compression fracture of spine can occur: assess ability to void and defecate.

> **HESI HINT** Postmenopausal, thin, white women are at highest risk for development of osteoporosis. Encourage exercise, a diet high in calcium, and supplemental calcium.

Nursing Plans and Interventions

A. Create a hazard-free environment.

B. Keep bed in low position.

C. Encourage client to wear shoes or slippers when out of bed.

D. Encourage environmental safety.
   1. Provide adequate lighting.
   2. Keep floor clear.
   3. Discourage use of throw rugs.
   4. Clean spills promptly.
   5. Keep side rails up at all times.

> **HESI HINT** The main cause of fractures in older people, especially women, is osteoporosis. The main fracture sites seem to be the hip, vertebral bodies, clavicle, and forearm.

E. Provide assistance with ambulation.
   1. May need walker or cane.
   2. May need standby assistance when initially getting out of bed or chair.

F. Reinforce teaching plan regarding regular exercise program.
   1. ROM several times a day.
   2. Ambulate several times a day.
   3. Use of proper body mechanics.
   4. Regular weight-bearing exercises promote bone formation.

G. Provide diet that is high in protein, calcium, and vitamin D; discourage use of alcohol and caffeine.

H. Encourage preventive measures for females.
   1. Estrogen replacement therapy after menopause for some women
   2. High calcium and vitamin D intake beginning in early adulthood
   3. Calcium supplementation after menopause (TUMS is an excellent source of calcium)
   4. Weight-bearing exercise

I. Bone density study as a baseline after menopause, with frequency as recommended by HCP.

J. Administer medications such as estrogen therapy, bisphosphonates, calcium/vitamin D, as prescribed by the HCP.

Fracture

Description: Any break in the continuity of the bone.

A. Fractures are described by type and extent of the break.

B. Fractures are caused by a direct blow, crushing force, sudden twisting motion, or disease such as cancer or osteoporosis.
   1. Complete fracture: break across the entire cross section of the bone.
   2. Incomplete fracture: break occurs across only part of the bone.
   3. Closed fracture: does not produce a break in the skin.
   4. Open fracture: extends through the skin or mucous membranes (much more prone to infection).

C. Five types of fractures
   1. Greenstick: one side of a bone is broken and the other side is bent.
   2. Transverse: break occurs straight across the bone shaft.
   3. Oblique: at an angle across the bone.
   4. Spiral: twisting around the bone.
   5. Comminuted: having more than three fragments.

> **HESI HINT** What type of fracture is more difficult to heal, an extracapsular fracture (below the neck of the femur) or an intracapsular fracture (in the neck of the femur)?

The blood supply enters the femur below the neck of the femur. Therefore, an intracapsular fracture is more difficult to heal and has a greater likelihood of necrosis because it is cut off from the blood supply.

Nursing Assessment

A. Signs and symptoms of fracture
1. Pain, swelling, tenderness
2. Deformity, loss of functional ability
3. Discoloration, bleeding at the site through an open wound
4. Crepitus: crackling sound between two broken bones
B. Fracture evident on x-ray film.
C. Therapeutic management is based on:
1. Reduction of the fracture
2. Maintenance of realignment by immobilization
3. Restoration of function

HESI HINT NCLEX-PN questions focus on safety precautions. Improper use of assistive devices can be risky. When using a nonwheeled walker, the client should lift and move the walker forward, then take a step into it. The client should avoid scooting the walker or shuffling forward into it, which takes more energy and is less stable than a single movement.

D. Observe client's use of assistive devices.
1. Crutches
a. There should be two to three finger widths between axilla and the top of the crutch.
b. Three-point gait is most common. The client advances both crutches and the impaired leg at the same time. The client then swings the uninvolved leg to the crutches.
2. Cane
a. Place on the unaffected side.
b. Top of cane should be parallel to the greater trochanter.
3. Walker
a. Upper extremity and unaffected leg strength assessed and improved with exercises, if necessary, so that upper body is strong enough to use walker.
b. Client lifts and advances the walker and steps forward.
E. See Chapter 5: *Pediatric Nursing* for cast care and care of the client in traction.

HESI HINT The risk of a fat embolism, a syndrome in which fat globules migrate into the bloodstream and combine with platelets to form emboli, is greatest in the first 36 h after a fracture. It is more common in clients with multiple fractures, fractures of long bones, and fractures of the pelvis. The initial symptom of a fat embolism is confusion caused by hypoxemia. If an embolus is suspected, notify HCP STAT, draw blood gases, administer oxygen, and assist with endotracheal intubation.

HESI HINT In clients with hip fractures, thromboembolism is the most common complication. Prevention includes passive ROM exercises, elastic stocking use, and elevation of the foot of the bed 25 degrees to increase venous return, and low-dose heparin therapy.

HESI HINT Clients with fractures, casts, or edema to the extremities need frequent neurovascular assessment distal to the injury. Skin color, temperature, sensation, capillary refill, mobility, pain, and pulses should be assessed.

HESI HINT Assess the "six Ps" of neurovascular functioning: pain, pressure, paresthesia, pulselessness, pallor, and paralysis. Assess for compartment syndrome using "the six Ps." Notify the RN if any of these signs and symptoms are present. Dark reddish-brown urine is released from damaged muscle cells. The HCP must be notified immediately to save the extremity.

Joint Replacement

Description: A surgical procedure in which a mechanical device, designed to act as a joint, is used to replace a diseased joint.
A. Most commonly replaced joints: hip, knee, shoulder, and finger
B. Prostheses may be ingrown or cemented.
C. Accurate fitting is essential.
D. Must have healthy bone stock for adequate healing.
E. Joint replacement provides excellent pain relief in 85% to 90% of the clients who undergo the surgery.
F. Infection is primary concern postoperatively.

Nursing Assessment

A. Joint pathology
1. Arthritis
2. Fracture
B. Pain not relieved with medication.
C. Poor ROM in the affected joint.

Nursing Plans and Interventions

A. Provide postoperative care for wound and joint.
1. Monitor incision site.
a. Monitor for bleeding and drainage.

HESI HINT Orthopedic wounds tend to ooze more than other wounds. A suction drainage device usually accompanies the client to the postoperative floor. Check drainage often.

b. Observe suture line for erythema and/or edema.
c. Determine proper functioning of drainage apparatus.
d. Monitor client for signs of infection.

> **HESI HINT** NCLEX-PN questions about joint replacement focus on complications. A big concern after joint replacement is infection.

2. Monitor functioning of extremity.
   a. Check circulation, sensation, and movement of extremity distal to replacement.
   b. Provide proper alignment of affected extremity (client will return from the operating room with alignment for initial postoperative period).
   c. Provide abductor appliance (hip replacement) or continuous passive motion device as prescribed.
3. Monitor I&O every shift, including suction drainage.

> **HESI HINT** Fractures of bone predispose the client to anemia, especially if long bones are involved. Check Hct every 3—4 days to monitor erythropoiesis.

B. Encourage fluid intake of 3 L/day.
C. Encourage client to perform self-care activities at maximal level.
D. Support the rehabilitation plan: work closely with the health care team to gradually increase client's mobility.
   1. Get client out of bed as soon as possible.
   2. Keep client out of bed as much as possible.
   3. Keep abductor pillow in place while client is in bed (hip replacement) as prescribed.
   4. Use elevated toilet seat and chairs with high seats for those who have had hip or knee replacement (prevents dislocation).
   5. Do not flex hip more than 90 degrees (hip replacement).

> **HESI HINT** Instruct the client not to lift the leg upward from a lying position or to elevate the knee when sitting. This upward motion can pop the prosthesis out of the socket.

> **HESI HINT** Immobile clients are prone to complications: skin integrity problems, formation of urinary calculi (may limit milk intake), and venous thrombosis (may be on prophylactic anticoagulants).

E. Provide discharge planning to include rehabilitation on an outpatient basis as prescribed.

Amputation

Description: Surgical removal of a diseased part or organ.
A. Causes for amputation include the following:
   1. PVD, 80% (75% of these are clients with diabetes)
   2. Trauma
   3. Congenital deformities
   4. Malignant tumors
   5. Infection
B. Amputation necessitates major lifestyle and body image adjustments.

Nursing Assessment

A. Before amputation, symptoms of PVD include:
   1. Cool extremity
   2. Absent peripheral pulses
   3. Hair loss on affected extremity
   4. Necrotic tissue and/or wounds
      a. Blue or blue-gray turning black
      b. Drainage possible, with or without odor
   5. Leathery skin on affected extremity
   6. Decrease of pain sensation in affected extremity
B. Inadequate circulation determined by the following:
   1. Arteriogram
   2. Doppler flow studies
C. Disturbed body image related to…
D. Impaired walking related to…

Nursing Plans and Interventions

A. Provide wound care.
   1. Monitor surgical dressing for drainage.
      a. Mark dressing for bleeding and check marking at least every 8 hours.
      b. Measure suction drainage every shift.
   2. Change dressing as needed (HCP usually performs initial dressing change).
      a. Maintain aseptic technique.
      b. Observe wound color and warmth.
      c. Observe for wound healing.
      d. Monitor for signs of infection: fever, tachycardia, and redness of incision area
B. Maintain proper body alignment in and out of bed.
C. Position client to relieve edema and spasms at residual limb (stump) site.
   1. Elevate residual limb (stump) the first 24 hours postoperatively.

> **HESI HINT** The residual limb (stump) should be elevated on one pillow. If the residual limb (stump) is elevated too high, the elevation can cause a contracture.

   2. Do not elevate residual limb (stump) after 48 hours postoperatively.
   3. Keep residual limb (stump) in extended position and turn prone three times a day to prevent hip flexion contracture.

D. Be aware that phantom pain is *real*, eventually disappears, and responds to pain medication.
E. Handle affected body part gently and with smooth movements.
F. Provide passive ROM until client is able to perform active ROM.
G. Collaborate with rehabilitation team members for mobility improvement.
H. Encourage independence in self-care, allowing sufficient time for client to complete care and to have input into care.

❓ REVIEW OF MUSCULOSKELETAL SYSTEM

1. Differentiate between rheumatoid arthritis and degenerative joint disease in terms of joint involvement.
2. Identify the categories of drugs commonly used to treat arthritis.
3. Identify pain relief interventions for clients with arthritis.
4. What measures should the nurse encourage female clients to take to prevent osteoporosis?
5. What are the common side effects of salicylates?
6. What is the priority nursing intervention used with clients taking NSAIDs?
7. List three of the joints that are most commonly replaced.
8. Describe postoperative residual limb (stump) care (after amputation) for the first 48 hours.
9. Describe nursing care for the client who is experiencing phantom pain after amputation.
10. A nurse discovers that a client who is in traction for a long bone fracture has a slight fever, is short of breath, and is restless. What does the client most likely have?
11. What are the immediate nursing actions if fat embolization is suspected in a fracture/orthopedic client?
12. List three problems associated with immobility.
13. List three nursing interventions for the prevention of thromboembolism in immobilized clients with musculoskeletal problems.

See Answer Key at the end of this text for suggested responses.

NEUROSENSORY SYSTEM

Glaucoma

Description: Chronic open-angle glaucoma, which is also known as simple adult primary glaucoma, and primary open-angle glaucoma (POAG). It is characterized by increased intraocular pressure (IOP).
A. Gradual, painless vision loss (tunnel vision).
B. Acute angle-closure glaucoma signs and symptoms include sudden excruciating pain in or around the eye; nausea and vomiting; colored halos around lights, blurred vision, and ocular redness.
C. Glaucoma may lead to blindness if untreated.
D. Glaucoma is the second leading cause of blindness in the United States.
E. There is an increased incidence in the elderly.
F. Glaucoma usually occurs bilaterally in those who have a family history of the condition.
G. Aqueous fluid is inadequately drained from the eye.

H. Generally asymptomatic, especially in early stages.
I. Tends to be diagnosed during routine visual examinations.
J. Cannot be cured but can be successfully treated pharmacologically and surgically.

Nursing Assessment

A. Early signs
 1. Increase in IOP, greater than 22 mm Hg, in open-angle glaucoma. In acute angle-closure glaucoma, IOP may be greater than 50 mm Hg.
 2. Decreased accommodation or ability to focus.

HESI HINT Glaucoma is often painless and symptom-free. It is usually diagnosed as part of a regular eye examination.

B. Late signs
 1. Loss of peripheral vision
 2. Halos around lights
 3. Decreased visual acuity, not correctable with glasses
 4. Headache or eye pain, which may be so severe as to cause nausea and vomiting (acute closed-angle glaucoma)
C. Diagnostic tests
 1. Tonometer used to measure IOP
 2. Electronic tonometer used to detect drainage of aqueous humor
 3. Gonioscopy used to obtain a direct visualization of the lens
 4. Slit-lamp microscopy
D. Risk factors
 1. Family history of glaucoma
 2. Family history of diabetes
 3. History of previous ocular problems
 4. Medications
  a. Glaucoma is a side effect of many medications (e.g., antihistamines, anticholinergics).
  b. Glaucoma can result from the interaction of medications.

Nursing Plans and Interventions

A. Administer eyedrops as prescribed (Table 4.29).

HESI HINT Eye drops are applied to the affected eye to cause pupil constriction because movement of the muscles to constrict the pupil allows aqueous humor to flow out, thereby decreasing the pressure in the eye. Pilocarpine is often used. Advise the client that vision may be blurred 1–2 h after administration of pilocarpine and that adaptation to dark environments is difficult because of pupillary constriction (desired effect of the drug).

B. Orient client to surroundings.
C. Avoid nonverbal communication that requires visual acuity (e.g., facial expressions).

TABLE 4.29 Treatment of Glaucoma

Drugs	Indications	Adverse Reactions	Nursing Implications

Parasympathomimetics
• Pilocarpine HCL (multiple brands available) 0.5%–0.6% is the drug of choice
	• Enhance papillary constriction (available in drops, gel, and time-release wafer)	• Bronchospasm
		• Nausea, vomiting, diarrhea
		• Blurred vision, twitching eyelids, eye pain with focusing
			• Use cautiously with:
			  1. Pregnancy
			  2. Asthma
			  3. Hypertension
			• Reinforce teaching of proper drop instillation technique
			• Need for ongoing use of the drug at prescribed intervals
			• Blurred vision tends to decrease with regular use of this drug

Beta-Adrenergic Receptor-Blocking Agents
• Timolol maleate optic (Timoptic Solution)
• Carteolol (Ocupress)
• Levobunolol (Betagan)
• Betaxolol (Betoptic S)
• Metipranolol (OptiPranolol)
	• Inhibit formation of aqueous humor	• Side effects are insignificant
		• Hypotension
			• Use cautiously with:
			  1. Hypersensitive
			  2. Asthmatic
			  3. Second- or third-degree heart block
			  4. Heart failure
			  5. Congenital glaucoma
			  6. Pregnancy
			• Reinforce teaching of proper drop instillation technique
			• Need for ongoing use of the drug at prescribed intervals
			• Blurred vision tends to decrease with regular use of this drug

Carbonic Anhydrase Inhibitors • Acetazolamide (Diamox) • Brinzolamide (Azopt) • Dorzolamide (Trusopt)	• Reduce aqueous humor production	• Numbness, tingling hands and feet • Nausea • Malaise	• Administer orally or IV (Diamox) • Produces diuresis • Assess for metabolic acidosis
Alpha Agonists • Brimonidine (Alphagan P) • Apraclonidine (Iopidine)	• Lower intraocular pressure of glaucoma by decreasing fluid produced		Teach to use no more than prescribed Caution with patients who have history of depression, orthostatic hypotension or Reynaud
Prostaglandin Agonists • Latanoprost (Xalatan) • Travoprost (Travatan) • Bimatoprost (Lumigan)	• Lower intraocular pressure of glaucoma by increasing outflow of aqueous humor	• Local irritation • Foreign body sensation • Increased brown pigmentation of iris • Increased eyelash growth	

D. Collaborate with RN and implement a teaching plan.
1. Careful adherence to eyedrop regimen can prevent blindness.
2. Vision already lost cannot be restored.
3. Eye drops are needed for the rest of life.
4. Proper eye-drop installation technique. Obtain a return demonstration.
   a. Wash hands and external eye.
   b. Tilt head back slightly.
   c. Instill drop into lower lid, without touching the lid with the tip of the dropper.
   d. Release the lid and sponge excess fluid from lid and cheek.
   e. Close the eye gently and leave it closed 3 to 5 minutes.
   f. Apply gentle pressure on inner canthus to decrease systemic absorption.

5. Safety measures to prevent injuries
   a. Remove throw rugs.
   b. Adjust lighting to meet client's needs.
6. Avoid activities that may increase IOP.
   a. Emotional upsets
   b. Exertion: pushing, heavy lifting, shoveling
   c. Coughing severely or excessive sneezing; get medical attention before URI worsens
   d. Constrictive clothing: tight collar or tie; belt or girdle too tight
   e. Straining at stool or constipation

> **HESI HINT** There is an increased incidence of glaucoma in the older population.

Nursing Plans and Interventions for the Nonseeing (Blind) Client

A. Upon entering room, announce your presence and identify yourself, address client by name.
B. Do not touch client unless he or she knows you are there.
C. Upon admission to hospital or nursing center, orient client thoroughly to surroundings:
   1. Demonstrate use of the call bell.
   2. Walk client around the room and acquaint him or her with all objects, including chairs, bed, TV, telephone, and bathroom.
D. Guide client when walking.
   1. Walk ahead of client and place his or her hand in the bend of your elbow.
   2. Describe where you are walking. Note if passageway is narrowing or if you are approaching stairs, curb, or an incline.
E. Always raise side rails for the "newly" sightless person, such as postoperative eye patch clients.
F. Assist with meal enjoyment by describing food and its placement in terms of face of a clock—for example, "meat is at 6 o'clock."
G. When administering medications, inform client of number of pills, and give only half a glass of water (to avoid spills).

Cataract

Description: A cataract is a condition characterized by opacity of the lens. Cataracts are the leading cause of blindness in the world.
A. Aging accounts for 95% of cataracts (senile).
B. Remaining 5% are from trauma, toxic substances, or systemic diseases, or are congenital.
C. Safety precautions may reduce incidence of traumatic cataracts.
D. Surgical removal is done when vision impairment interferes with daily activities. Intraocular lens implants may be used.
E. Most surgeries are done under local anesthesia as outpatient surgery.

> **HESI HINT** The lens of the eye is responsible for projecting light, which enters onto the retina so that images can be discerned. Without the lens, which becomes opaque with cataracts, light cannot be filtered, and vision is blurred.

Nursing Assessment

A. Early signs
   1. Blurred vision
   2. Decreased color perception
B. Late signs
   1. Diplopia
   2. Reduced visual acuity progressing to blindness
   3. Clouded pupil, progressing to a milky-white appearance
C. Diagnostic tests
   1. Ophthalmoscope
   2. Slit lamp biomicroscope
   3. Glare testing, keratometry and A-scan ultrasound
D. Ineffective self-health management related

Nursing Plans and Interventions

A. Preoperative: reinforce teaching plan related to eye medication instillation.
B. Reinforce the postoperative teaching plan.
   1. Warn not to rub or put pressure on eye.
   2. Glasses or shaded lens should be worn during waking hours. Eye shield should be worn during sleeping hours.
   3. Avoid lifting objects over 5 pounds, bending, straining, coughing, or any activity that can increase IOP.
   4. Use stool softener to prevent straining at stool.
   5. Avoid lying on operative side.
   6. Keep water from getting into eye while showering or washing hair.
   7. Observe and report signs of increased IOP and infection (e.g., pain, changes in vital signs).
   8. Reinforce RN teaching about new medications that may be prescribed.

> **HESI HINT** When the cataract is removed, the lens is gone, making prevention of falls important. If the lens is replaced with an implant, vision is better than if a contact lens is used (some visual distortion) or if glasses are used (greater visual distortion—everything has a curved shape).

Eye Trauma

Description: Injury to the eye sustained from sharp or blunt trauma, chemicals, or heat.
A. Permanent visual impairment can occur.
B. Every eye injury should be considered an emergency.
C. Protective eye shields in hazardous work environments and during athletic sports may prevent injuries.

Nursing Assessment

A. Determine type of injury and symptoms.
 1. Assess for chemical exposure.
 2. Begin ocular irrigation immediately in case of chemical exposure.
 3. Assess visual acuity.
 4. Do not put pressure on the eye; do not allow client to blow nose.
 5. Stabilize foreign objects.
 6. Cover eyes with dry, sterile patches and protective shields.
 7. Elevate the head of the bed to 45 degrees.
 8. Administer analgesics as prescribed.
B. Diagnostic tests
 1. Slit-lamp examination
 2. Fluorescein dye to detect corneal injury
 3. Visual acuity for medical documentation and legal protection

Nursing Plans and Interventions

A. Position the client relative to the type of injury; sitting position decreases IOP.
B. Remove conjunctival foreign bodies unless embedded.
C. Never attempt to remove a penetrating or embedded object. Do *not* apply pressure.
D. Apply cold compresses to eye contusion.
E. Irrigate the eye with copious amounts of water after chemical injuries.
F. Administer eye medications as prescribed.
G. Explain that an eye patch may be applied to rest the eye. Reading and watching TV may be restricted for 3 to 5 days.
H. Explain that sudden increase in eye pain should be reported.

Detached retina

Description: A hole, tear, or separation of the sensory retina from the pigmented epithelium.
A. Can be a result of increasing age, severe myopia, eye trauma, retinopathy (diabetic), cataract or glaucoma surgery, family or personal history
B. Resealing is done by surgery:
 1. Cryotherapy—freezing
 2. Photocoagulation—laser
 3. Diathermy—heat
 4. Scleral buckling—most often used
 5. Pneumatic retinopexy, vitrectomy

Nursing Assessment

A. Photopsia (light flashes); floaters, cobweb, or ring in the field of vision
B. Painless loss of peripheral or central vision (curtain like)
C. Loss of vision related to area of detachment

Nursing Plans and Interventions

A. Position the client as ordered (thus allowing the agent being used to reattach the retina to the interior surface of the eye).

B. Place eye patch over affected eye.
C. Obtain eye prescription to inhibit accommodation and constriction. Cycloplegics to dilate (mydriatic): homatropine—an anticholinergic.
D. Administer prescribed topical medications such as antibiotics, anti-inflammatory agents, or dilating agents.
E. Postoperative medications for pain—acetaminophen, oxycodone.
F. If gas bubble used (inserted in vitreous), position so bubble can "rise" against area to be reattached.
G. Reinforce client education about no heavy lifting, straining with bowel movement, or vigorous activity for several weeks postoperatively.

Hearing Loss
Conductive Hearing Loss

Description: Hearing loss in which sound does not travel well to the sound organs of the inner ear. The volume of sound is less, but the sound remains clear. If volume is raised, hearing is normal.
A. Hearing loss is the most common disability in the United States.
B. Usually results from cerumen (wax) impaction or middle ear disorders such as otitis media (with effusion): perforation of the tympanic membrane (TM); otosclerosis; and narrowing of the external auditory canal.

HESI HINT The ear consists of three parts: the external ear, the middle ear, and the inner ear. Inner ear disorders, or disorders of the sensory fibers going to the central nervous system (CNS), often are neurogenic in nature and may not be helped with a hearing aid. External and middle ear problems (conductive) may result from trauma, infection, or wax buildup. These types of disorders are treated more successfully with hearing aids.

Sensorineural Hearing Loss

Description: A form of hearing loss in which sound passes properly through the outer and middle ear but is distorted by a defect in the inner ear or damage to cranial nerve (CN) VIII, or both.
A. Perceptive loss, usually progressive and bilateral.
B. Involves damage to the eighth CN.
C. Detected easily by use of a tuning fork.
D. Common causes
 1. Infections such as meningitis and immune diseases
 2. Ototoxic drugs
 3. Trauma
 4. Neuromas
 5. Noise
 6. Aging process
 7. DM; Paget disease of the bone

Nursing Assessment

A. Inability to hear a whisper from 1 to 2 feet away
B. Inability to respond if nurse covers mouth when talking, indicating that client is lip reading
C. Inability to hear a watch tick 5 inches from ear
D. Shouting in conversation
E. Straining to hear
F. Turning head to favor one ear
G. Answering questions incorrectly or inappropriately
H. Raising volume of radio/TV

Nursing Plans and Interventions

A. To enhance therapeutic communication with the hearing-impaired client, the nurse will:
  1. Reduce distraction as much as possible before starting conversation.
  2. Turn the television or radio down or off, close the door, or move to a quieter location.
  3. Devote full attention to the conversation; do not try to do two things at once.
  4. Look and listen during the conversation.
  5. Begin with casual topics and progress to more critical issues slowly.
  6. Avoid switching topics abruptly.
  7. Let the client know if you do not understand.
  8. Face the client directly if he or she is a lip reader.
  9. Speak slowly and distinctly; determine whether you were understood.
  10. Allow adequate time for the conversation to take place; try to avoid hurried conversations.
  11. Use active listening techniques.

HESI HINT NCLEX-PN questions often focus on communicating with older adults who are hearing impaired.
- Speak in a low-pitched voice, slowly, and distinctly.
- Stand in front of the person with the light source behind the client.
- Use visual aids if available.

B. Be sure to inform the health care staff of the client's hearing loss.
C. Helpful aids may include a telephone amplifier, earphone attachments for the radio and TV, and lights or buzzers in the most used rooms of the house that activate when the doorbell is rung.

NEUROLOGIC SYSTEM

Altered State of Consciousness

Nursing Assessment

A. Use agency neurologic vital sign assessment tool. It sometimes contains a scale for scoring, such as the Glasgow Coma Scale (GCS), which objectively documents the client's

TABLE 4.30 Glasgow Coma Scale

Variable	Response	Score
Eye opening	Spontaneously	4
	To verbal command	3
	To pain	2
	No response	1
Motor response	To verbal command	6
	To painful stimuli	
	• Localizes pain	5
	• Flexes/withdraws	4
	• Flexor posturing (decorticate)	3
	• Extensor posturing (decerebrate)	2
	• No response	1
Verbal response	Oriented and converses	5
	Disoriented, converses	4
	Uses inappropriate words	3
	Incomprehensible sounds	2
	No response	1

level of consciousness (Table 4.30). GCS assesses three areas: client's ability to speak, obey commands, and open eyes when a verbal or painful stimulus is applied.
  1. Maximum total is 15 (fully awake), minimum is 3.
  2. GCS of ≥8 generally indicates coma. Clients with lower scores (3 to 4) have poor prognosis and high mortality.
  3. Clients with scores greater than 8 have a good prognosis for recovery.

HESI HINT Use of the GCS eliminates ambiguous terms to describe neurologic status such as *lethargic, stuporous,* or *obtunded.*

B. Neurologic vital sign sheet will also address pupil size (with sizing scale; if intracranial pressure [ICP] increases, both pupils will dilate), shape, movement, and reactivity; limb movement (with scale); and vital signs (BP, temperature, pulse, respirations).
C. Normal reaction is brisk constriction when a light is shone directly into the eye. A sluggish reaction can indicate early pressure on CN III. A fixed pupil unresponsive to light stimulus usually indicates increased ICP. Eye movement, controlled by CN III, IV, and VI is examined in a client who is awake and able to follow commands. Testing cornea reflex gives information about the function of CN V and VII. To test for oculocephalic reflex (doll's eye), turn client's head briskly to the left or right while holding the eyelids open. Normal response is movement of the eyes across the midline in the direction opposite that of the turning. Next, quickly flex and extend the neck. Eye movement should be opposite to the direction of head movement. Monitor skin integrity and corneal integrity.
D. Check bladder for fullness, auscultate lungs, and monitor cardiac status.

E. Identify family's knowledge of client's clinical status, coping skills, and support needs.

F. Assess respiratory status (for example, rate, depth, oxygenation, breath sounds, and sputum).

> **HESI HINT** Clients with an altered state of consciousness are fed by enteral routes because the likelihood of aspiration with oral feedings is great. Residual feeding is the amount of previous feeding still in the stomach. The presence of 100 mL of residual in adults usually indicates poor gastric emptying, and the feeding should be withheld.

> **HESI HINT** Paralytic ileus is common in comatose clients. Gastric tubes aid in gastric decompression.

> **HESI HINT** Any client on bed rest or who is immobilized must have ROM exercises often and very frequent position changes. Do not leave the client in any one position for longer than 2 h. Any position that decreases venous return is dangerous—that is, sitting with dependent extremities for long periods.

Nursing Plans and Interventions

A. Maintain adequate respirations, airway, and oxygenation.
   1. Document and report breathing pattern changes.
   2. Position for maximum ventilation: ¾ prone or semi-prone to prevent tongue from obstructing airway and slightly to one side with arms away from chest wall.
   3. Insert airway if tongue is obstructing or if client is paralyzed.
   4. Prepare for insertion of cuffed endotracheal tube.
   5. Keep airway free of secretions with suctioning (see Table 4.4).
   6. Monitor arterial Po_2 and Pco_2.
   7. Prepare for tracheostomy if prolonged ventilator support is needed.
   8. Provide chest physiotherapy as prescribed by HCP.
   9. Hyperventilate with 100% O_2 before and after suctioning.

B. Provide nutritional and fluid and electrolyte support.
   1. Keep client NPO until responsive, and provide mouth care every 2 to 4 hours and PRN.
   2. Maintain calorie count.
   3. Administer feedings as prescribed (Box 4.1).
   4. Monitor I&O.
   5. Record client's weight (weigh same time each day).

C. Prevent complications of immobility.
   1. Impairment in skin integrity
      a. Turn every 2 hours and assess bony prominences.
      b. Use prescribed airflow therapy beds and mattresses.
      c. Use minimal amount of linens and under pads.
   2. Potential for thrombus formation
      a. Monitor lower extremities for signs of thrombophlebitis.

BOX 4.1 Unconscious Client

Gastric Gavage
- Begin feeding when gastrointestinal peristalsis returns.
- Place client in high Fowler position.
- Place towel over chest.
- Connect gastrostomy tube to funnel or large syringe.
- Check gastric residual to assess absorption and client tolerance; return residual.
- Pour feeding into tilted funnel and unclamp tubing to allow feeding to flow by GRAVITY.
- Regulate flow by raising or lowering container. Feeding too fast causes diarrhea, gastric distention, and pain. Feeding too slowly causes possible obstruction of flow.
- After feeding, irrigate tube with water (tepid) and clamp tube.
- Apply small dressing over tube opening, coil tube, and attach to dressing. May cover with an abdominal binder.
- Get bowel history from reliable source.
- Establish specific time for evacuation. Regularity is essential.
  - An unconscious client can evacuate the bowel after the last tube feeding of day because the gastrocolic and duodenocolic reflexes are active after "meal."
  - Stimulate anorectal reflex with insertion of glycerin suppository 15–30 min before scheduled evacuation time. May need stronger suppository, such as bisacodyl (Dulcolax).
  - Ensure adequate fiber in tube feedings and adequate fluid intake of 2–4 L/day.
  - May apply a rectal pouch to contain fecal material (ostomy bag with seal over anal opening).

b. Perform passive ROM exercises to lower extremities every 4 hours.
   c. Use elastic hose; remove and reapply every 8 hours.
   d. Avoid positions that decrease venous return.
   e. Avoid pillows under knees or gatch bed.
   3. Urinary calculi
      a. Increase fluid intake orally or through gastric tube or IV.
      b. Monitor urine for high specific gravity (dehydration) and balance between I&O.
   4. Contractures/joint immobility
      a. Provide passive ROM every 4 hours.
      b. Sit client up in bed or chair if possible, or use neuro chair if necessary.
      c. Reposition every 2 hours maintaining proper body alignment.
      d. Apply splints or other assistive devices to prevent foot drop, wrist drop, or other improper alignment.

D. Monitor and report the vital sign changes indicating changes in condition.
   1. Pulse: a pulse rate change to less than 60 beats/min can indicate increased ICP. Fast rate (>100 beats/min) can indicate infection, thrombus formation, or dehydration.
   2. BP: rising BP or widening pulse pressure can indicate increased ICP.

3. Temperature: report any abnormalities (temperature elevation can indicate worsening condition, damage to temperature regulating area of brain, and/or infection).
4. Level of consciousness changes: active to somnolent.
5. Pupillary changes: prompt to sluggish, increase in size.

> **HESI HINT** If temperature elevates, take quick measures to decrease it because fever increases cerebral metabolism and can increase cerebral edema.

> **HESI HINT: SAFETY FEATURES FOR IMMOBILIZED CLIENTS**
> - Prevent skin breakdown with frequent turning.
> - Maintain adequate nutrition.
> - Prevent aspiration with slow, small feedings or NG feedings or enteral feedings.
> - Monitor neurologic signs to detect the first signs that ICP may be increasing.
> - Provide ROM exercises to prevent deformities.
> - Prevent respiratory complications—frequent turning and positioning for optimal drainage.

E. Prevent injury/promote safety.
1. Place bed in low position and keep side rails up at all times.
2. Pad side rails if client is agitated or if there is a history of seizure activity.
3. Restrain if client is trying to remove tubes or attempting to get out of bed.
4. Touch gently and talk softly and calmly to the client, remembering that hearing is often intact.

> **HESI HINT** Restlessness may indicate a return to consciousness but can also indicate anoxia, distended bladder, covert bleeding, or increasing cerebral anoxia. Do not oversedate, and report any symptoms of restlessness.

5. Avoid oversedating the client because sedatives/narcotics depress responsiveness and affect pupillary reaction (an important assessment in neurologic vital signs).
6. During all activities, tell the client what you are doing no matter what the client's level of consciousness is.
F. Maintain hygiene/cleanliness.
1. Provide bathing, grooming, and dressing.
2. Provide oral hygiene at least twice daily.
3. Wash hair weekly.
4. Provide nail care within agency guidelines.
G. Observe for bladder elimination problems.
1. Insert indwelling catheter if prescribed.
2. Remove indwelling catheter as soon as possible; use diaper or condom catheter.

H. Document and record bowel movements and report abnormal patterns of constipation or diarrhea.
1. Rapid infusion of tube feedings may cause diarrhea, whereas lack of fiber/inadequate fluids may cause constipation.
2. Initiate bowel program (see Box 4.1).
I. Prevent corneal injury/drying.
1. Remove contact lenses if present.
2. Irrigate eyes with sterile prescribed solution and instill ophthalmic ointment in each eye every 8 hours to prevent corneal ulceration.
J. See Seizures in Chapter 5: *Pediatric Nursing*.

Head Injury

Description: Any traumatic damage to the head.
A. Open head injury occurs when there is a fracture of the skull or penetration of the skull by an object.
B. Closed head injury is the result of blunt trauma (more serious because of the chance of increased ICP in "closed" vault).
C. Increased ICP is the main concern in head injury related to edema, hemorrhage, impaired cerebral autoregulation, and hydrocephalus.

> **HESI HINT** The forces of impact influence the type of head injury. They include acceleration injury, which is caused by the head in motion, and deceleration injury, which occurs when the head stops suddenly. Helmets are a *great* preventive measure for motorcyclists or bicyclists (Fig. 4.9).

Nursing Assessment

Both subjective and objective data for head injury are detailed in Box 4.2.
A. Unconsciousness or disturbances in consciousness
B. Vertigo
C. Confusion, delirium, and/or disorientation
D. Symptoms of increased ICP
1. Change in level of responsiveness is the most important indicator of increased ICP.

> **HESI HINT** Even subtle behavior changes, such as restlessness, irritability, or confusion, may indicate increased ICP.

2. Changes in vital signs
   a. Slowing of respirations or respiratory irregularities
   b. Increase or decrease in pulse
   c. Rising BP or widening pulse pressure
   d. Temperature rise
3. Headache
4. Vomiting (projectile)
5. Pupillary changes reflecting pressure on optic/oculomotor nerves:

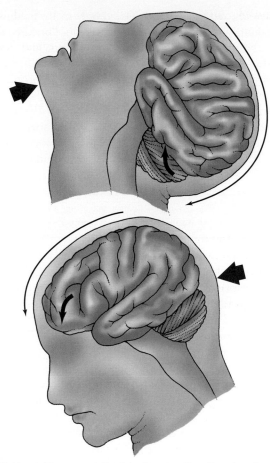

Fig. 4.9 Head Movement During Acceleration-Deceleration Injury. Such movements are typically seen in motor vehicle accidents. (Ignatavicius, D. D., Workman, L., & Rebar, C. [2020]. *Medical-surgical nursing: Concepts for interprofessional collaborative care* [10th ed.]. St. Louis: Elsevier.)

    a. Pupils decrease or increase in size or become unequal

    b. Lack of conjugate eye movement

    c. Papilledema

E. Seizures

F. Ataxia

G. Abnormal posturing (decerebrate or decorticate)

H. Cerebrospinal fluid (CSF) leakage through nose (rhinorrhea) or ear (otorrhea) confirms that a fracture has traversed the dura. Risk of meningitis is high with CSF leak. Usually unilateral.

I. Monitor urine output closely and serum sodium levels because syndrome of inappropriate antidiuretic hormone secretion (SIADH)/diabetes insipidus can be caused by increased ICP.

HESI HINT CSF leakage carries the risk of meningitis and indicates a deteriorating condition. When there is CSF leakage, the usual signs of increased ICP may not occur. To verify the presence of CSF, check drainage with a Dextrostix. The presence of glucose indicates CSF.

BOX 4.2 Nursing Assessment: Head Injury

Subjective Data

Important Health Information

- *Past health history:* Mechanism of injury: motor vehicle collision, sports injury, industrial incident, assault, falls
- *Medications:* Anticoagulant medications

Functional Health Patterns

- *Health perception—health management:* Alcohol or recreational drugs; risk-taking behaviors
- *Cognitive-perceptual:* Headache, mood or behavioral change, mentation changes, aphasia, dysphasia, impaired judgment
- *Coping—stress tolerance:* Fear, denial, anger, aggression, depression

Objective Data

General

- Altered mental status

Integumentary

- Lacerations, contusions, abrasions, hematoma, Battle's sign, periorbital edema and ecchymosis, otorrhea, exposed brain matter

Respiratory

- Rhinorrhea, impaired gag reflex, inability to maintain a patent airway; impending herniation: altered/irregular respiratory rate and pattern

Cardiovascular

- Impending herniation: Cushing's triad (systolic hypertension with widening pulse pressure, bradycardia with full and bounding pulse, irregular respirations)

Gastrointestinal

- Vomiting, projectile vomiting, bowel incontinence

Urinary

- Bladder incontinence

Reproductive

- Uninhibited sexual expression

Neurologic

- Altered level of consciousness, seizure activity, pupil dysfunction, cranial nerve deficit(s)

Musculoskeletal

- Motor deficit/impairment, weakness, palmar drift, paralysis, spasticity, decorticate or decerebrate posturing, muscular rigidity or increased tone, flaccidity, ataxia

Possible Diagnostic Findings

- Location and type of hematoma, edema, skull fracture, and/or foreign body on computed tomography scan and/or magnetic resonance imaging; abnormal electroencephalogram; positive toxicology screen or alcohol level, ↓ or ↑ blood glucose level; ↑ intracranial pressure

From Lewis, S., Dirksen, S., Heitkemper, M., & Bucher, L. (2019). *Medical-surgical nursing: Assessment and management of clinical problems* (11th ed.). St. Louis: Mosby.

J. Computed axial tomography scan or MRI will show lesions such as epidural or subdural hematomas requiring surgery.

K. Electroencephalogram (EEG) determines presence of seizure activity.

L. Other diagnostic studies include positron emission tomography (PET), cervical spine x-ray series, and placement of ICP monitor.

Nursing Plans and Interventions

A. Maintain adequate ventilation/airway.
   1. Monitor Po_2 and Pco_2 for the development of hypoxia and hypercapnia.
   2. Position client semiprone or lateral recumbent to prevent aspiration.
   3. Turn from side to side to prevent lung secretion stasis.
B. Keep the head of the bed elevated 30 to 45 degrees to aid venous return from the neck and decrease cerebral volume.
C. Obtain neurologic vital signs as prescribed (at least every 1 to 2 hours) and maintain a continuous record of observations and GCS ratings.
D. Notify RN and HCP at the *first* sign of deterioration or improvement in condition.
E. Avoid activities that increase ICP.
   1. Change in bed position for caregiving, extreme hip flexion.
   2. Endotracheal suctioning.
   3. Compression of jugular veins (keep head straight and not to one side).
   4. Coughing, vomiting, or straining of any type (no Valsalva: increased intrathoracic pressure increases ICP).
F. If temperature increases, take immediate measures to decrease it (e.g., aspirin, acetaminophen, cooling blanket) because increased temperature increases cerebral blood flow drastically; avoid shivering.
G. Prepare for intracranial monitoring system, if available:
   1. Catheter inserted into lateral ventricle, sensor placed on the dura, or a screw inserted into the subarachnoid space attached to pressure transducer.
   2. Elevations of ICP greater than 20 mm Hg should be reported STAT.
H. Administer and/or monitor medications prescribed by HCP to reduce ICP.
   1. Hyperosmotic agents/diuretics: to dehydrate brain and reduce cerebral edema.
      a. Mannitol (Table 4.31)
      b. Urea

2. Steroids: dexamethasone (Decadron), methylprednisolone sodium/succinate (Solu-Medrol) to reduce brain edema.
3. Barbiturates: to reduce brain metabolism and systemic BP.
4. Paralyzing medicines like Precedex or vecuronium for patients on a ventilator
5. Benzodiazepines for sedation (for example IV propofol).
I. Insert indwelling catheter to prevent restlessness caused by distended bladder and monitor balance between restricted fluid I&O, especially if placed on osmotic diuretics.

> **HESI HINT** Try *not* to use restraints; they only increase restlessness. *Avoid* narcotics because they mask the level of responsiveness.

J. HCP may order passive hyperventilation on ventilator: leads to respiratory alkalosis, which causes cerebral vasoconstriction, decreased cerebral blood flow, and therefore decreased ICP.
K. Continue seizure precautions. The HCP may order prophylactic phenytoin (Dilantin).
L. Prevent complications of immobility (see "*Nursing Plans and Interventions*" for the Unconscious/Immobilized Client).
M. Reinforce teaching plan related to possible aftereffects of head injury.
   1. Posttraumatic syndrome: headache, vertigo, emotional instability, inability to concentrate, impaired memory
   2. Posttraumatic seizure disorder
   3. Posttraumatic neuroses/psychoses

Spinal Cord Injury

Description: Disruption in the nervous system function, which may result in complete or incomplete loss of motor and sensory function. Changes occur in the function of all physiologic systems.
A. Injuries are described by location in the spinal cord. Most common sites are fifth, sixth, and seventh cervical (C-5, C-6, C-7), the twelfth thoracic (T-12), and the first lumbar (L-1).
B. Damage can range from contusion to complete transection.
C. Permanent impairment cannot be determined until spinal cord edema has subsided, usually by 1 week.

TABLE 4.31	Osmotic Diuretic		
Drug	**Indications**	**Adverse Reactions**	**Nursing Implications**
• Mannitol (Osmitrol)	• Acts on renal tubules by osmosis to prevent water reabsorption • In bloodstream, draws fluid from the extravascular spaces into the plasma	• Disorientation, confusion, and headache • Nausea and vomiting • Convulsions and anaphylactic reactions	• Use for short-term therapy ONLY • Never give to clients with cerebral hemorrhage • Intravenous infusion is usually adjusted to urine output—filter and watch for crystals • Never give to clients with no urine output (anuria); if output is less than 30 mL/h, accumulation can cause pulmonary edema and water intoxication

Nursing Assessment

A. Monitor breathing pattern, auscultate lungs.

> **HESI HINT** Physical assessment should concentrate on respiratory status, especially in clients with injury at C-3 to C-5, as the cervical plexus innervates diaphragm. Mechanical ventilation may be required to keep the client alive.

B. Check neurologic vital signs frequently, especially sensory and motor functions. Complete neurologic assessment is required frequently for these patients.

C. Monitor cardiovascular status. Any spinal cord injury above the level of T6 results in bradycardia since this injury decreases the effect of the sympathetic nervous system. Cardiac monitoring is necessary.

D. Monitor abdomen: girth, bowel sounds, and lower abdomen for bladder distention.

E. Observe changes in temperature, remembering hyperthermia often occurs.

F. Identify psychosocial status.

G. Hypotension and bradycardia occur with any injury above T-6 because sympathetic outflow is affected.

H. GI system affected related to hypomotility. There is a high risk for developing paralytic ileus and gastric distention.

I. Urinary retention is a common development in acute spinal injury. Bladder is atonic and becomes overdistended.

J. Skin assessment looking for breakdown over bony prominences.

Nursing Plans and Interventions

A. Acute phase of spinal cord injury
   1. See *Nursing Plans and Interventions* for the Unconscious/Immobilized Client.
   2. Maintain client in an extended position with cervical collar on during any transfer.
   3. Maintain a patent airway—*most important*.
   4. In cervical injuries, skeletal traction is maintained by use of skull tongs or halo ring (Crutchfield tongs or Gardner-Wells fixation device).
   5. High-dose corticosteroids are often given IV to help control edema during the first 8 to 24 hours.
   6. Use a kinetic therapy treatment table, which provides continuous side-to-side motion.
   7. Use Stryker frame or *very firm* mattress with board underneath.
   8. Assess for respiratory failure, especially in clients with high cervical injuries.
   9. Further loss of sensory/motor function below injury can indicate additional damage to cord from edema and should be reported immediately.
   10. Evaluate for presence of spinal shock (a complete loss of all reflex, motor, sensory, and autonomic activity below the lesion). This is a MEDICAL EMERGENCY, which occurs immediately after the injury.

a. Hypotension, bradycardia
b. Complete paralysis and lack of sensation below lesion
c. Bladder and bowel distention

> **HESI HINT** It is imperative to reverse spinal shock as quickly as possible. Permanent paralysis can occur if a spinal cord is compressed for 12–24 h.

   11. Observe for autonomic dysreflexia (exaggerated autonomic responses to stimuli), which occurs in clients with lesions at or above T-6.
   12. Watch for acute paralytic ileus, lack of gastric activity.
       a. Assess bowel sounds frequently.
       b. Initiate gastric suction to reduce distention, prevent vomiting/aspiration.
       c. A rectal tube may be used to relieve gaseous distention.
   13. Suction with caution to prevent vagus nerve stimulation, which can cause cardiac arrest.
   14. Administer high-dose corticosteroids IV to decrease edema and reduce cord damage.

B. Rehabilitative phase
   1. Encourage deep-breathing exercises.
   2. Chest physiotherapy.
   3. Kinetic bed to promote blood flow to extremities.
   4. Antiembolic stockings.
   5. ROM exercises.
   6. Mobilize to chair as soon as possible.
   7. Turn frequently.
   8. Keep the client clean and dry.
   9. Observe for impending skin breakdown.
   10. Reinforce teaching about the importance of impeccable skin care.
   11. Intermittent catheterization every 4 hours. Collaborate with RN to develop and implement client/family teaching plan for catheterization.
   12. Assist with teaching bladder-emptying techniques depending on level of injury and bladder muscle response.
       a. Upper motor neuron (spastic) bladder
       b. Lower motor neuron (flaccid) bladder
   13. Collaborate with RN to develop and implement client/family teaching plan for I&O. Instruct client in I&O.

> **HESI HINT** A common cause of death after spinal cord injury is UTI. Bacteria grow best in alkaline media, so keeping urine dilute and acidic is prophylactic against infection. Also, keeping the bladder emptied assists in avoiding bacterial growth in urine that has stagnated in the bladder.

   14. Reinforce bowel-training program.
   15. Talk with client and family about permanence of disability.
   16. Encourage rehabilitation facility staff to visit client.

17. Encourage client and family to visit the rehabilitation facility.
18. Assist family to find support group, and assist with the referral process for community resources after dismissal from rehabilitation facility.

Brain Tumor

Description: Neoplasm occurring in the brain.
A. Primary tumors arise in any tissue of the brain.
B. Secondary tumors are a result of metastasis from other areas (most often from the lungs, followed by breast metastasis).
C. Without treatment, benign as well as malignant tumors lead to death.

> **HESI HINT** Benign tumors continue to grow and take up space in the confined area of the cranium, causing neural and vascular compromise for the brain, increased ICP, and necrosis of the brain tissue; thus, even benign tumors must be treated because they may have malignant effects.

Nursing Assessment

A. Headache that is more severe may awaken client at night; headache is described as dull, constant, or throbbing
B. Vomiting not associated with nausea
C. Papilledema with visual changes
D. Behavioral and personality changes
E. Seizures
F. Aphasia, hemiplegia, ataxia, and muscle weakness
G. CN dysfunction
H. Abnormal CT, MRI, and PET scans.
I. Hydrocephalus may occur if the tumor obstructs the ventricles or occludes the outlet.

Nursing Plans and Interventions

A. *Nursing plans and interventions* are similar to those implemented for the head injury client with increased ICP. Provide protective measures to prevent self-harm if the client is confused or behaviorally unstable. May need to use prescribed medication, side rails, and restraints as a last resort.
B. Elevate the head of the bed 30 to 40 degrees; maintain head in neutral position.
C. Radiation therapy
  1. Provide skin care with non–oil-based soap and water. Avoid alcohol, powder, or oils on the skin.
  2. Reinforce instructions for client not to wash off the lines drawn by the radiologist.
D. Chemotherapy: medications may be injected intraventricularly or IV.
E. Surgical removal (craniotomy)

1. Preoperative: shave head
2. Postoperative
  a. Frequent neurologic and vital sign assessment.
  b. Position client with the head of the bed elevated 30–45 degrees as per HCP's recommendation. Position client off the operative site.
  c. Monitor dressings for signs of drainage (excess amount of CSF).
  d. Monitor respiratory status to prevent hypoventilation.
  e. Avoid activities that cause increased ICP.
  f. Monitor for seizure activity.
  g. Administer medications (see "Head Injury").

> **HESI HINT: CRANIOTOMY MEDICATIONS**
> - Corticosteroids to reduce swelling
> - Agents (atropine, glycopyrrolate) and osmotic diuretics—for example, mannitol, to reduce secretions
> - Agents to reduce seizures (phenytoin)
> - Prophylactic antibiotics

Multiple Sclerosis

Description: MS is a demyelinating disease resulting in the destruction of the CNS myelin and consequent disruption in the transmission of nerve impulses.
A. Onset is insidious, with 50% of clients still ambulatory 25 years after diagnosis.
B. Diagnosis determined by combination of data:
  1. Presenting symptoms
  2. Increased white matter density on CT scan
  3. Presence of plaques on MRI
  4. Presence of oligoclonal (immunoglobulin G) bands on CSF electrophoresis
C. Current thinking is that MS is autoimmune in origin.

> **HESI HINT** Symptoms involving motor function usually begin in the upper extremities, with weakness progressing to spastic paralysis. Bowel and bladder dysfunction occurs in 90% of the cases. MS is more common in women. Progression is not "orderly."

Nursing Assessment

A. Nursing history of the client
  1. History of symptoms
  2. Progression of illness
  3. Types of treatment received and the response
  4. Additional health problems
  5. Current medications

6. Client's/family's perception of illness
7. Community resources used by the client

B. Physical assessment
    1. Optic neuritis (loss of vision or blind spots)
    2. Visual or swallowing difficulties
    3. Gait disturbances; intention tremors
    4. Unusual fatigue, weakness, and clumsiness; for example, spasms or foot dragging
    5. Numbness, particularly on one side of face, including ataxia, tremor, spasticity, and hyperreflexia
    6. Impaired bladder and bowel control
    7. Speech disturbances
    8. Scotomas (white spots in visual field, diplopia)

Nursing Plans and Interventions

A. Allow hospitalized client to keep own routine.
B. Orient client to environment and teach strategies to maximize vision.
C. Encourage self-care and frequent rest periods.
D. With exercise programs, encourage client to work up to the point just short of fatigue.
E. For muscle spasticity, stretch-hold-relax exercises are helpful, as are riding a stationary bicycle and swimming; use fall precautions.
F. Initially, work with the client on a voiding schedule.
G. As incontinence worsens, the female may need to learn clean self-catheterization; the male may need a condom catheter.
H. Encourage adequate fluid intake, high-fiber foods, and a bowel regimen for constipation problems.
I. Encourage the client and the family to verbalize their concerns with ongoing care issues.
J. Encourage the client to maintain contact with a support group.
K. Assist in the referral process for home health care services.
L. Encourage the client to contact the local MS society for emotional and direct service support.
M. Steroid therapy and chemotherapeutic drugs are administered in acute exacerbations to shorten the length of attack.

HESI HINT Drug therapy for clients with MS: ACTH, cortisone, cyclophosphamide, and other immunosuppressive drugs. Nursing implications for administration of these drugs should focus on prevention of infection. Other prescribed medications include muscle relaxants such as amantadine and CNS stimulants like pemoline to treat fatigue. Anticholinergics to treat bladder symptoms. Antidepressants and antiseizure drugs for chronic pain syndromes. Dalfampridine to improve walking speed. Clients with aggressive forms of MS are given natalizumab and mitoxantrone.

N. Biologic response modifiers such as interferon-beta products have shown recent success in relapsing MS.

Myasthenia Gravis

Description: MG is a disorder affecting the neuromuscular transmission of impulses in the voluntary muscles of the body.

A. Considered an autoimmune disease characterized by presence of acetylcholine receptor antibodies that interfere with neuronal transmission.
B. Usually affects females aged 10 to 40 years and males aged 50 to 70 years.

Nursing Assessment

A. Diplopia (double vision), ptosis (eyelid drooping).
B. Mask-like affect: sleepy appearance because of facial muscle involvement.
C. Weakness of laryngeal and pharyngeal muscles: dysphagia, choking, food aspiration, difficulty speaking.
D. Muscle weakness improved by rest, worsened by activity.
E. Advanced cases have respiratory failure and bladder and bowel incontinence.
F. Myasthenic crisis (attributed to disease worsening) symptoms associated with undermedication. Cholinergic crisis (attributed to anticholinesterase overdosage): diaphoresis, diarrhea, fasciculation, cramps, marked worsening of symptoms from overmedication.

HESI HINT Understand the symptoms associated with anticholinergic agent: impaired vision, dry mouth, dry eyes, orthostatic hypotension, constipation, and urinary retention.

HESI HINT In clients with MG, be alert for changes in respiratory status. The most severe involvement may result in respiratory failure.

Nursing Plans and Interventions

A. If hospitalized, have tracheostomy kit available at bedside for possible myasthenic crisis.
B. Reinforce the teaching plan about the importance of wearing a medical alert bracelet.
C. Administer cholinergic drugs as prescribed (Table 4.32).
D. Schedule nursing activities to conserve energy—that is, complete daily hygiene activities, administration of medications, and treatments all at once, and allow rest periods. Plan activities during high-energy times, often in the early morning.
E. Instruct client to avoid situations that produce fatigue or physical/emotional stress (any type of stress can exacerbate symptoms).

HESI HINT Bed rest often relieves symptoms. Bladder and respiratory infections are often a recurring problem. Remember the need for health promotion teaching and reinforcement of teaching.

TABLE 4.32 Treatment of Myasthenia Gravis

Drug	Indications	Adverse Reactions	Nursing Implications

• Pyridostigmine bromide (Mestinon)	• Inhibits the action of cholinesterase at the cholinergic nerve endings
	• To promote accumulation of acetylcholine at cholinergic receptor sites
		• Cholinergic crisis can occur with overdose	• Atropine is antidote for drug-induced bradycardia
			• Take drug with milk/food to decrease gastrointestinal side effects
			• Dosage regulation required; record keeping; side effects, drug response
			• Observe for symptoms of cholinergic crisis:
			  1. Fasciculations
			  2. Abdominal cramps, diarrhea, incontinence of stool or urine
			  3. Hypotension, bradycardia, respiratory depression
			  4. Lacrimation, blurred vision
			• Drug therapy is lifelong and requires family teaching and support

TABLE 4.33 Comparison of Myasthenic and Cholinergic Crisis

Myasthenic Crisis	Cholinergic Crisis
Causes	
Exacerbation of myasthenia after precipitating factors or failure to take drug as prescribed or drug dose too low	Overdose of anticholinesterase drugs resulting in increased acetylcholine at the receptor sites, remission (spontaneous or after thymectomy)
Differential Diagnosis	
Improved strength after IV administration of anticholinesterase drugs	Weakness within 1 h after ingestion of anticholinesterase
Increased weakness of skeletal muscles manifesting as ptosis, bulbar signs (e.g., difficulty swallowing, difficulty articulating words), or dyspnea	Increased weakness of skeletal muscles manifesting as ptosis, bulbar signs, dyspnea Effects on smooth muscle include pupillary miosis, salivation, diarrhea, nausea or vomiting, abdominal cramps, increased bronchial secretions, sweating, or lacrimation

From Lewis, S., Dirksen, S., Heitkemper, M., & Bucher, L. (2019). *Medical-surgical nursing: Assessment and management of clinical problems* (11th ed.). St. Louis: Mosby.

F. Encourage coughing and deep breathing every 4 to 6 hours. (Muscle weakness limits ability to cough up secretions and promotes URI.)

G. If symptoms worsen, identify type of crisis: myasthenic or cholinergic crisis (Table 4.33).

Parkinson Disease

Description: Parkinson disease is a disorder affecting movement involving the basal ganglia and substantia nigra. It is a chronic, progressive disorder characterized by slowness in the initiation and execution of movement, increased muscle tone (rigidity), tremor at rest, and gait disturbance.

Nursing Assessment

A. Rigidity of extremities (tremor, often the first sign, may be minimal initially but handwriting is affected; tremors more prominent at rest and aggravated by emotional stress or increased concentration

B. Mask-like facial expressions with associated difficulty in chewing, swallowing, and speaking

C. Drooling

D. Stooped posture and slow, shuffling gait (bradykinesia)

E. Tremors at rest, "pill rolling" movement

F. Emotional lability

> **HESI HINT** NCLEX-PN questions often focus on the features of Parkinson disease: tremors (a coarse tremor of fingers and thumb on one hand that disappears during sleep and purposeful activity—also called "pill-rolling"), rigidity, hypertonicity, and stooped posture. Focus: SAFETY!

Nursing Plans and Interventions

A. Schedule activities later in the day to allow sufficient time for client to perform self-care activities without rushing.

B. Encourage activities and exercise. A cane or walker may be needed.

C. Eliminate environmental noise, and encourage the client to speak slowly and clearly, pausing at intervals.

TABLE 4.34 Antiparkinsonian Drugs

Drugs	Indications	Adverse Reactions	Nursing Implications
Anticholinergics (Parasympatholytics)			
• Atropine sulfate (Atropisol) • Benztropine mesylate (Cogentin)	• Used to treat secondary cholinergic symptoms, such as drooling, sweating, tremors	• Increased heart rate • Postural hypotension • Dry mouth • Constipation • Urinary retention	• Review client's history for glaucoma, urinary obstruction • Warn to avoid rapid position changes • Avoid extreme heat • Provide gum, hard candy, and frequent mouth care
Dopamine Agonist			
• Levodopa (Dopar) • Levodopa-carbidopa (Sinemet) • Dopamine-releasing agents • Amantadine HCL (Symmetrel) • Dopamine-receptor agonists • Bromocriptine mesylate (Parlodel) • Pramipexole (Mirapex) • Ropinirole (Requip)	• Stimulate dopamine production or increase sensitivity of dopamine receptors • Newer drugs require lower dosage	• Involuntary movements • Nausea • Vomiting	• Explain drugs may take months to achieve desired effects • Warn to avoid sudden position changes • Avoid foods high in vitamin B_6 (meats, liver—that is, high-protein foods) • If insomnia occurs, suggest taking last dose earlier in day • May initially cause drowsiness; teach to avoid driving until response is determined
Monoamine Oxidase Type B Inhibitor			
• Selegiline (Eldepryl) • Rasaliline (Azilect)	• Used with dopamine agonist when client symptoms do not respond	• Confusion, dizziness • Nausea, dry mouth • Insomnia	• Review drug–drug interaction carefully • Not an option if client on antidepressants (selective serotonin reuptake inhibitors or tricyclics)
Catechol-O-methyl Transferase (COMT) Inhibitor			
• Entacapone (Comtan) • Talcapone (Tasmar)	• Used with levodopa-carbidopa	• May increase levodopa-carbidopa side effects, including dyskinesias	• Levodopa dose may need to be decreased • Combination product may decrease pill burden

D. Serve soft diet that is easy to swallow.

E. Administer antiparkinsonian drugs as prescribed (Table 4.34).

HESI HINT An important aspect of Parkinson treatment is drug therapy. Because the pathophysiology involves an imbalance between acetylcholine and dopamine, symptoms can be controlled by administering dopamine precursor (Levodopa).

Guillain–Barré Syndrome

Description: Guillain–Barré syndrome is a clinical syndrome of unknown origin involving peripheral and cranial nerves. It is characterized by ascending symmetric paralysis that usually affects cranial nerves and the peripheral nervous system.

A. Usually preceded by a viral respiratory or GI infection 1 to 4 weeks before the onset of neurologic deficits.

B. Constant monitoring of clients is required to prevent the life-threatening problem of acute respiratory failure.

C. Full recovery usually occurs within several months to a year after onset of symptoms.

D. About 10% to 20% of those diagnosed with Guillain–Barré syndrome are left with a residual disability. Death occurs in 5%.

Nursing Assessment

A. Paresthesia (tingling and numbness)

B. Most serious complication is respiratory failure, which occurs as the paralysis progresses to the nerves that innervate the thoracic area

C. Muscle weakness (hypotonia) of legs progressing to the upper extremities, trunk, and face

D. Paralysis of the ocular, facial, and oropharyngeal muscles, causing marked difficulty in talking, chewing, and swallowing. Assess for the following:

1. Breathlessness while talking
2. Shallow and irregular breathing
3. Use of accessory muscles while breathing
4. Any change in respiratory pattern
5. Paradoxical inward movement of the upper abdominal wall while in a supine position, indicating weakness and impending paralysis of the diaphragm

E. Autonomic nervous system dysfunction, with manifestations of orthostatic hypotension, hypertension, and abnormal vagal responses (bradycardia, heart block, asystole)

F. Transient hypertension, orthostatic hypotension

G. Possible pain in the back and in calves of legs (described as muscular aches and cramps; the pain appears to be worse at night)

H. Weakness or paralysis of the intercostal and diaphragm muscles may develop quickly

Nursing Plans and Interventions

A. Monitor for respiratory distress and initiate mechanical ventilation if necessary.
B. Monitor vital signs frequently.
C. Provide nutritional needs accordingly.
D. See *Nursing Plans and Interventions* for the Unconscious/Immobilized Client.

Stroke/Brain Attack: Cerebral Vascular Accident (CVA)

Description: Stroke/brain attack: CVA is the sudden loss of brain function resulting from a disruption of the blood supply to a part of the brain. Classified as thrombotic or hemorrhagic.

HESI HINT: CNS INVOLVEMENT RELATED TO CAUSE OF CVA

- Hemorrhagic—caused by a slow or fast hemorrhage into the brain tissue; often related to hypertension or ruptured aneurysm.
- Embolic—caused by a clot that has broken away from some vessel and has lodged in one of the arteries of the brain, blocking the blood supply. It is often related to atherosclerosis and may recur.

A. Risk factors
1. Hypertension
2. Previous transient ischemic attacks
3. Cardiac disease: atherosclerosis, valve disease, history of dysrhythmias (particularly atrial flutter/fibrillation), increased serum cholesterol
4. Nonmodifiable risks: genetic/family history, advanced age, and African American heritage (higher incidence and higher death rate)
5. Diabetes
6. Oral contraceptives and hormone replacement therapy
7. Smoking
8. Alcohol: more than two drinks per day; illicit drug use, such as cocaine

---

HESI HINT Atrial flutter/fibrillation has a high incidence of thrombus formation following dysrhythmia because of the turbulence of blood flow through all valves/heart chambers. Blood pools in the ventricles (due to loss of atrial kick), which allows for clot formation.

B. Diagnosis is made by observation of clinical signs and confirmed by:
1. Cranial CT scan; CT angiography
2. MRI
3. Doppler flow studies
4. Ultrasound imaging

5. Cardiac imaging looking for blood clots, plaque formation, and malformation of vessels
6. Intraarterial digital subtraction angiography

C. Presenting symptoms will relate to the specific area of the brain that has been damaged (Table 4.35).
D. Most common clinical manifestations
1. Motor loss, usually exhibited as hemiparesis or hemiplegia
2. Communication loss exhibited as dysarthria, dysphasia, aphasia, or apraxia
3. Perceptual disturbance that can be visual, spatial, and/or sensory
4. Impaired mental acuity or psychological changes such as decreased attention span, memory loss, depression, lability, and hostility
5. Bladder dysfunction—may be either incontinence or retention
E. Rehabilitation is initiated as soon as the client is stable

---

HESI HINT A client who had a stroke 2 days ago has left-sided paralysis. The client has begun to regain some movement in her left side. What can the nurse tell the family about the client's recovery period? "The quicker movement is recovered, the better the prognosis is for more or full recovery. The client will need patience and understanding from the family while adjusting and trying to cope with the stroke. Mood swings can be expected during the recovery period, and bouts of depression and tearfulness are likely."

TABLE 4.35 Location of Disruption

Feature	Left Hemisphere	Right Hemisphere
• Language	• Aphasia • Agraphia	• May be alert and oriented
• Memory	• No deficit	• Disoriented • Cannot recognize faces
• Vision	• Unable to discriminate words and letters • Reading problems • Deficits in right visual field	• Visual/spatial deficits • Neglect of left visual fields • Loss of depth perception
• Behavior	• Slow • Cautious • Anxious when attempting a new task • Depression or catastrophic response to illness • Sense of guilt • Feeling of worthlessness • Worries over future • Quick anger and frustration	• Impulsive • Unaware of neurologic deficits • Confabulates • Euphoric • Constantly smiles • Denies illness • Poor judgment • Overestimates abilities • Impaired sense of humor
• Hearing	• No deficit	• Loses ability to hear tonal variations

Nursing Assessment

A. Change in level of consciousness
B. Paresthesia, paralysis
C. Aphasia, agraphia
D. Memory loss
E. Vision impairment
F. Bladder and bowel dysfunction
G. Behavioral changes
H. Observe and report client's functional abilities.
   1. Mobility
   2. Activities of daily living (ADLs)
   3. Elimination
   4. Communication
I. Collect data on the client's ability to swallow, eat, and drink without aspiration.

HESI HINT: WORDS THAT DESCRIBE LOSSES FOR CVA

1. **Apraxia:** inability to perform purposed movements in the absence of motor problems
2. **Dysarthria:** difficulty articulating
3. **Dysphasia:** impairment of speech and verbal comprehension
4. **Aphasia:** loss of the ability to speak
5. **Agraphia:** loss of the ability to write
6. **Alexia:** loss of the ability to read
7. **Dysphagia:** dysfunctional swallowing

Nursing Plans and Interventions

A. Control hypertension to help prevent future CVA.
B. Maintain proper body alignment while in bed. Use splints or other assistive devices (including bedrolls and pillows) to maintain functional position.
C. Position client to minimize edema, prevent contractures, and maintain skin integrity.
D. Perform full ROM four times a day. Follow-up with program initiated by other team members.
E. Encourage client to participate in or manage own personal care.
F. Set realistic goals; add new tasks daily.
G. Include self-care activities for the hemiparetic person: bathing; brushing teeth; shaving with electric razor; eating; combing hair
H. Encourage client to assist with dressing activities and modify them as necessary (client will wear street clothes during waking hours).
I. Monitor bladder elimination pattern.
   1. Offer bedpan or urinal according to client's particular pattern of elimination.
   2. Bladder control tends to be regained quickly.
J. Assist with follow-up speech program initiated by the speech/language therapist.
   1. Ensure consistency with this program.
   2. Reassure the client that regaining speech is a very slow process.

K. Do not cause sensory overload for the client—that is, give only one set of instructions at a time.
L. Encourage total family involvement in rehabilitation.
M. Encourage client/family to join a support group.
N. Encourage family members to allow the client to perform self-care activities as outlined by the rehabilitation team.
O. Coordinate outpatient follow-up or home health care.
P. Swallowing modifications may include pureed/soft diet, thickened liquids, and head positioning. Speech therapists should perform a swallowing evaluation before patients are started on oral intake.

HESI HINT Steroids are administered after a stroke to decrease cerebral edema and retard permanent disability. H_2 inhibitors are administered to prevent peptic ulcers. Oral or IV medications to maintain BP within normal to high-normal range.

HESI HINT Patients with arteriovenous malformation or aneurysm can be taken to surgery for clipping the aneurysm or coiling to provide immediate protection against hemorrhage.

HEMATOLOGY/ONCOLOGY

Anemia

Description: Anemia is a deficiency of erythrocytes (RBCs) reflected as decreased Hct, Hgb, and RBCs.

Nursing Assessment

A. Pallor, especially of the face (around the eyes) and nail beds; palmar crease; conjunctiva
B. Fatigue, exercise intolerance, lethargy, orthostatic hypotension
C. Tachycardia, heart murmurs, HF
D. Signs of bleeding such as hematuria, melena, and menorrhagia
E. Dyspnea
F. Irritability, difficulty concentrating
G. Cool skin, cold intolerance
H. Risk factors:
   1. Diet lacking in iron, folate, and/or vitamin B_{12}
   2. Family history of genetic diseases such as sickle cell or congenital hemolytic anemia
   3. Medication history of anemia-producing drugs, such as salicylates, and thiazide diuretics
   4. Exposure to toxic agents such as lead or insecticides
I. Diagnostic tests indicate abnormally low results.
   1. Hgb less than 10 g/dL
   2. Hct less than 36%
   3. RBCs less than 4×10^{12}
   4. Bone marrow aspiration positive for anemia

? REVIEW OF NEUROSENSORY/NEUROLOGIC SYSTEMS

1. What are the classifications of the commonly prescribed eye drops for glaucoma?
2. Identify two types of hearing loss.
3. Write four nursing interventions for the care of the blind person and for the care of the deaf person.
4. In your own words, describe the GCS.
5. List four nursing diagnoses for the comatose client in order of priority. (Remember Maslow's Hierarchy of Needs to help you determine priority.)
6. State four independent nursing interventions to maintain adequate respirations, airway, and oxygenation in the unconscious client.
7. Who is at risk for CVAs?
8. Complications of immobility include the potential for thrombus development. State three nursing interventions to prevent thrombi.
9. List four rationales for the appearance of restlessness in the unconscious client.
10. What nursing interventions prevent corneal drying in a comatose client?
11. When can a comatose client on IV hyperalimentation begin to receive tube feedings instead?
12. What is the most important principle in a bowel management program for a neurologic client?
13. Define CVA.
14. A client with a diagnosis of CVA presents with symptoms of aphasia and right hemiparesis, but no memory or hearing deficit. In what hemisphere has the client suffered a lesion?
15. What are the symptoms of spinal shock?
16. What are the symptoms of autonomic dysreflexia?
17. What is the most important indicator of increased ICP?
18. What vital sign changes are indicative of increased ICP?
19. A neighbor calls the neighborhood nurse stating that he was knocked hard to the floor by his very hyperactive dog. He is wondering what symptoms would indicate the need to visit an emergency room. What should the nurse tell him to do?
20. What activities and situations should be avoided that increase ICP?
21. How do hyperosmotic agents (osmotic diuretics) that are used to treat ICP act?
22. Why should narcotics be avoided in clients with neurologic impairment?
23. Headache and vomiting are symptoms of many disorders. What characteristics of these symptoms would alert the nurse to refer a client to a neurologist?
24. How should the head of the bed be positioned for postcraniotomy clients with infratentorial lesions?
25. Is MS thought to occur because of an autoimmune process?
26. Is paralysis always a consequence of spinal cord injury?
27. What types of drugs are used in the treatment of MG?

See Answer Key at the end of this text for suggested responses.

J. Blood loss, either acute or chronic
K. Medical history of kidney disorders

Nursing Plans and Interventions

A. In accordance with the scope of practice for the PN and agency guidelines, assist RN with administration of blood products as prescribed and monitor client's response to therapy (see Chapter 3: Advanced Clinical Concepts and Table 3.4).
B. Alternate periods of activity with periods of rest.
C. Reinforce diet teaching to include the following:
   1. Instruct in food selection and preparation to maximize intake:
      a. Iron (red meats, organ meats, whole wheat products, spinach, carrots)
      b. Folic acid (green vegetables, liver, citrus fruits)
      c. Vitamin B_{12} (glandular meats, yeast, green leafy vegetables, milk, and cheese)
   2. Reinforce teaching regarding need for vitamin/mineral supplements:
      a. Take iron on an empty stomach to enhance absorption, 1 hour before meals, or 2 hours after meals. Give vitamin C to enhance absorption of iron.
      b. Give liquid iron through a straw, with oral care afterward, to prevent discoloring of teeth.
      c. Inform client that iron (oral) may turn stools black.
D. If parenteral iron is required, use Z-track method for administration to prevent staining of the skin (Table 4.36).
E. Coordinate the referral process for genetic information if client has sickle cell or congenital hemolytic anemia.
F. Sickle cell crisis is precipitated by hypoxia:
   1. Provide pain relief
   2. Provide adequate hydration
   3. Teach client to avoid activities that cause hypoxia
G. Inform the client to report any unusual bleeding to health care professional.

Leukemia

Description: Leukemia is malignant neoplasm of the blood-forming organs.

A. Leukemia is characterized by an abnormal overproduction of immature forms of any of the leukocytes. There is an interference with normal blood production, resulting in decreased erythrocytes and platelets.
   1. Anemia results from decreased RBC production and blood loss.
   2. Immunosuppression occurs because of the large number of immature WBCs or profound neutropenia.
   3. Hemorrhage occurs because of thrombocytopenia (low platelets).
B. Exact etiology of leukemia is unknown, but identified precipitating factors include:
   1. Genetic abnormalities.
   2. Ionizing radiation (therapeutic or atomic).

TABLE 4.36 Administration of Parenteral Iron

Do's	Don'ts
• Use Z-track method of administration. • Use air bubble to avoid withdrawing medication into subcutaneous tissue.	• Do NOT use deltoid muscle. • Do NOT massage injection site.

3. Viral infections (human T cells, leukemia virus).
4. Exposure to certain chemicals or drugs, such as benzene, alkylating chemotherapeutic agents, immunosuppressants, chloramphenicol, and phenylbutazone.

C. Incidence is highest in children aged 3 to 4 years, declines until age 35, and then a steady increase occurs.

D. Diagnosis of leukemia is made by biopsy, bone marrow aspiration, lumbar puncture, and frequent blood counts.

E. Leukemia is treated with antineoplastic chemotherapy.

Types of Leukemia

A. Acute myelogenous leukemia
1. Inability of leukocytes to mature; those that do are abnormal
2. Occurs throughout the life cycle
3. Onset is insidious
4. Prognosis is poor, 5-year survival of 20% overall, 50% for children
5. Cause of death tends to be overwhelming infection

B. Chronic myelogenous leukemia
1. Results from abnormal production of granulocytic cells
2. Is biphasic
3. Chronic stage lasts approximately 3 years
4. Acute phase tends to last 2 to 3 months
5. Occurs in young to middle-aged adults
6. Known causes include:
   a. Ionizing radiation
   b. Chemical exposure
7. Has a poor prognosis, 5-year survival rate of 37%— conservative treatment if no allergenic transplant

C. Acute lymphocytic leukemia
1. Abnormal leukocytes in blood-forming tissue
2. Occurs in children (most common childhood cancer)
3. Favorable prognosis, 80% of children treated live 5 years or longer

D. Chronic lymphocytic leukemia
1. Increased production of leukocytes and lymphocytes and proliferation of cells within the bone marrow, spleen, and liver
2. Occurs after the age of 35, often in older adults
3. Overall 5-year survival rate of 73%
4. Most clients are asymptomatic and are not treated

> **HESI HINT** A 24-year-old woman is admitted with large areas of ecchymosis on both upper and lower extremities. She is diagnosed with acute myelogenous leukemia. What are the expected laboratory findings for this client and what is the expected treatment?
> - *Laboratory:* decreased Hgb, decreased Hct, decreased platelet count, altered WBC (usually quite high)
> - *Treatment:* prevention of infection; prevention and/or control of bleeding; high-protein, high-calorie diet; assistance with ADL; drug therapy

> **HESI HINT** The care of the client with cancer by the PN should be in accordance with the agency policy and scope of practice for the PN.

Nursing Assessment

A. Tendency to bleed
1. Petechiae; nosebleeds; bleeding gums; ecchymosis; non-healing skin abrasions

B. Anemia
2. Fatigue; pallor; headache; bone and joint pain; hepatosplenomegaly

C. Infection
3. Fever; tachycardia; lymphadenopathy (swollen lymph nodes); night sweats; skin infection, poor healing

D. GI distress
4. Anorexia; weight loss; sore throat; abdominal pain; diarrhea; oral lesions, typically thrush

> **HESI HINT** Infection in the immunosuppressed person may not be manifested with an elevated temperature. It is therefore imperative that the nurse performs frequent total and thorough assessments of the client.

Nursing Plans and Interventions for Immunosuppressed Clients and/or Clients With Bone Marrow Suppression

A. Monitor WBC count daily and inform HCP of the count.

B. Routinely examine oral cavity and genital area for signs of yeast infection.

C. Monitor vital signs frequently:
1. Note baseline.
2. Report fever to HCP as requested.
   a. Parameters for reporting tend to be lower than those of postoperative clients.
   b. Usually report temperatures of 100.5°F or above.

D. Administer antibiotics as prescribed, maintaining a strict schedule.

E. Notify HCP if delay in administration occurs.
1. Obtain trough and peak blood levels of antibiotics.
   a. Trough: draw blood sample shortly before administration of antibiotic.
   b. Peak: draw blood sample 30 minutes to 1 hour after administration of drug.
2. Monitor blood levels of antibiotics for therapeutic dose range.

F. Reinforce family/client teaching about the importance of infection control.
1. Wash hands using good handwashing technique.
2. Avoid contact with any infected person.
3. Avoid crowds.
4. Maintain daily hygiene to prevent spread of microorganisms.
5. Avoid eating uncooked foods because they contain bacteria.

6. Avoid water standing in cups, vases, and so forth because these are an excellent source of growth medium for microorganisms (especially mold spores).
7. Neutropenic and reverse isolation precautions PRN.

G. Institute an oral hygiene regimen.
1. Use soft-bristle toothbrush to avoid bleeding gums.
2. Use salt and baking soda mouth rinse.
3. Perform oral hygiene after each meal and at bedtime.
4. Lubricate lips with water-soluble gel.
5. Avoid lemon-glycerin swabs; they dry oral mucosa.

H. Encourage coughing and deep breathing to prevent stasis of secretions in lungs.

I. Avoid rectal thermometers and suppositories, to prevent bleeding.

J. Monitor fluid status and balance; febrile clients dehydrate rapidly.
1. Monitor I&O.
2. Encourage fluid intake of at least 3 L/day.

K. Encourage mobility to decrease pulmonary stasis.

> **HESI HINT** Most oncologic drugs cause immunosuppression. Prevention of secondary infections is vital. Advise client to stay away from persons with known infections such as colds. In the hospital, maintain an environment as sterile and as clean as possible. These persons should not eat raw vegetables or fruits—only those that have been cooked to destroy any bacteria.

L. Protect the client from bleeding and injury.
1. Handle the client gently.
2. Avoid needle sticks. Use smallest-gauge needle possible, and apply pressure for 10 minutes after needle sticks.
3. Encourage use of electric razor only for shaving.
4. Instruct client to avoid blowing or picking nose.
5. Assess for signs of bleeding.
6. Avoid use of salicylates.

Hodgkin Disease

Description: Hodgkin disease is a malignancy of the lymphoid system that initiates in a single lymph node.

A. Hodgkin disease is characterized by a generalized painless lymphadenopathy.
B. Incidence is higher in men and young adults.
C. Etiology is unknown.
D. Prognosis is good, with 5-year survival rate of 90%; however, late recurrences after 5 to 10 years are not uncommon.
E. Diagnosis is made by excision of node for biopsy; characteristic cell called Reed-Sternberg.
F. Determination of stage of disease is done by surgical laparotomy.
1. Stage I: involvement of single lymph node region or a single extra-lymphatic organ or site.
2. Stage II: involvement of two or more lymph nodes on the same side of the diaphragm or localized involvement of an extralymphatic organ or site.
3. Stage III: involvement of lymph node areas on both sides of the diaphragm to localized involvement of one extra-lymphatic organ, the spleen, or both.
4. Stage IV: diffuse involvement of one or more extralymphatic organs with or without lymph node involvement.

G. Treatment
1. Radiotherapy
2. Chemotherapy: nitrogen mustard, Adriamycin, vincristine, prednisone

Nursing Assessment

Enlarged lymph nodes (one or more), usually cervical lymph nodes

A. Anemia, thrombocytopenia, elevated leukocytes, decreased platelets
B. Fever, increased susceptibility to infections
C. Anorexia, weight loss
D. Malaise, bone pain
E. Night sweats
F. Pruritus
G. Pain in the affected lymph node after consuming alcohol

Nursing Plans and Interventions

A. Protect from infection, monitor temperature carefully.
B. Observe for signs of anemia.
C. Provide adequate rest.
D. Provide preoperative and postoperative care for laparotomy and/or splenectomy.
E. Encourage high-nutrient foods.
F. Provide emotional support to the client and family.

> **HESI HINT** Hodgkin disease is one of the most curable of all adult malignancies. Emotional support is vital. Career development is often interrupted for treatment. Chemotherapy renders many male clients sterile. They may bank sperm before treatment, if desired.

General Oncology Content

A. Oncology terms
1. Cancer: disease characterized by uncontrolled growth of abnormal cells
2. Neoplasm: new formation of tissue
3. Carcinoma: malignant tumor arising from epithelial tissue
4. Sarcoma: malignant tumor arising from nonepithelial tissue

5. Differentiation: degree to which neoplastic tissue is different from parent tissue
6. Metastasis: spread of cancer from the original site to other parts of the body
7. Adjuvant therapy: therapy supplemental to the primary therapy
8. Palliative procedure: relieves symptoms without curing the cause

B. Tumors identified by tissue of origin
  1. Adeno: glandular tissue
  2. Angio: blood vessels
  3. Basal cell: epithelium (sun-exposed areas)
  4. Embryonal: gonads
  5. Fibro: fibrous tissue
  6. Lympho: lymphoid tissue
  7. Melano: pigmented cells of epithelium
  8. Myo: muscle tissue
  9. Osteo: bone
  10. Squamous cell: epithelium

C. Seven warning signs of cancer
  1. Change in usual bowel and bladder function
  2. A sore that does not heal
  3. Unusual bleeding or discharge, hematuria, tarry stools, ecchymosis, bleeding mole
  4. Thickening or a lump in the breast or elsewhere
  5. Indigestion or dysphagia
  6. Obvious changes in a wart or mole
  7. Nagging cough or hoarseness

REPRODUCTIVE SYSTEM

Benign Tumors of the Uterus: Leiomyomas (Fibroids, Myomas, Fibromyomas, Fibromas)

Description: Benign tumors arising from the muscle tissue of the uterus.

A. Benign tumors are more common in black women than in white women.
B. Benign tumors are more common in women who have never been pregnant.
C. Most common symptom is abnormal uterine bleeding.
D. Tend to disappear after menopause.

❓ REVIEW OF HEMATOLOGY/ONCOLOGY

1. List three potential causes of anemia.
2. Write two nursing diagnoses for the client suffering from anemia.
3. What is the only IV fluid compatible with blood products?
4. What actions should the nurse take if a hemolytic transfusion reaction occurs?
5. List three interventions for clients with a tendency to bleed.
6. Identify two sites that should be assessed for infection in immunosuppressed clients.
7. Name three food sources of vitamin B_{12}.
8. List three safety precautions for the administration of antineoplastic chemotherapy.
9. Describe the method of collecting the trough and peak blood levels of antibiotics.
10. List four nursing interventions for care of the client with Hodgkin disease.
11. List four topics you would cover when assisting an RN with a teaching plan about infection control for an immunosuppressed client.
See Answer Key at the end of this text for suggested responses.

E. Rarely become malignant.
F. Intervention for severe symptoms is hysterectomy:
  1. Vaginal hysterectomy
  2. Abdominal hysterectomy

Nursing Assessment

A. Menorrhagia (hypermenorrhea: profuse or prolonged menstrual bleeding)
B. Dysmenorrhea (extremely painful menstrual periods)
C. Uterine enlargement
D. Low back pain and pelvic pain

> **HESI HINT** Menorrhagia (profuse or prolonged menstrual bleeding) is the most important factor relating to benign uterine tumors. Assess for signs of anemia.

Uterine Prolapse, Cystocele, and Rectocele

Description: Uterine prolapse is downward displacement of the uterus. Cystocele is the relaxation of the anterior vaginal wall with prolapse of the bladder. Rectocele is the relaxation of the posterior vaginal wall with prolapse of the rectum.

A. Preventive measures
  1. Postpartum perineal exercises
  2. Spaced pregnancies
  3. Weight control
B. Nonsurgical intervention (for uterine prolapse)
  1. Kegel exercises
  2. Knee-chest position
  3. Pessary use
C. Surgical intervention
  1. Hysterectomy for complete prolapse
  2. Anterior and posterior vaginal repair (A&P repair)

> **HESI HINT** What is the anatomic significance of a prolapsed uterus? When the uterus is displaced, it impinges on other structures in the lower abdomen. The bladder, rectum, and small intestine can protrude through the vaginal wall.

Nursing Assessment

A. Predisposing conditions
  1. Multiparity

2. Pelvic tearing during childbirth
3. Vaginal muscle weakness associated with aging
4. Obesity

B. Symptoms associated with uterine prolapse
   1. Dysmenorrhea
   2. Dragging sensation in pelvis and back
   3. Dyspareunia

C. Symptoms associated with cystocele
   1. Incontinence or stress incontinence (dribbling with coughing or sneezing or any activity that increases intra-abdominal pressure)
   2. Urinary retention
   3. Bladder infections (cystitis)

D. Symptoms associated with rectocele
   1. Constipation
   2. Hemorrhoids
   3. Sense of pressure or need to defecate

Nursing Plans and Interventions

A. Provide preoperative and postoperative care (see Perioperative Care in Chapter 3: *Advanced Clinical Concepts*).
B. Administer enema and douche as prescribed preoperatively.
C. Note the amount and character of vaginal discharge. Postoperatively, there should be less than one saturated pad in 4 hours.
D. Avoid rectal thermometers or tubes, especially when A&P repair has been performed.
E. Check extremities for warmth and/or tenderness as indicators of thrombophlebitis.
F. Pain management postoperatively:
   1. Monitor the character of pain and determine appropriate analgesic.
   2. Administer analgesics as needed and determine effectiveness.
G. Encourage ambulation as soon as possible.
H. Monitor urinary output (Foley indwelling urinary catheter is usually inserted in surgery).
I. After catheter removal, monitor voiding patterns, catheterize every 6 to 8 hours if unable to void.
J. Observe incision for bleeding.
K. Abdominal distention may be a sign of gas (flatus) or internal bleeding.
L. Gradually increase diet from liquids to general.
M. Provide stool softeners before first bowel movement and thereafter as needed.
N. Reinforce instructions to client about follow-up care.
   1. Limit tampon use.
   2. Avoid douching.
   3. Refrain from intercourse until approved by HCP (usually 3 to 6 weeks).
   4. Avoid heavy lifting (6 to 8 lb) or heavy housework for 4 to 6 weeks postoperatively.
O. Maintain adequate fluid intake (3 L/day).
P. Notify HCP of complications:
   1. Elevated temperature greater than 101°F
   2. Redness, pain, or swelling of suture line
Q. Encourage verbalization of feelings, especially with significant others.

Cancer of the Cervix

Description: Of cancers occurring in the cervix, 95% are squamous cell in origin. Some cervical cancers are directly linked to the human papillomavirus (HPV). Young women (9 to 26 years of age) are encouraged to be immunized with an intramuscular (IM) injection of quadrivalent HPV (types 6, 11, 16, 18) recombinant vaccine (Gardasil). All women should be tested for HPV.

A. Cancer of the cervix is easily detected early with the Papanicolaou (Pap) test.
B. The precursor to cancer of the cervix is dysplasia.
C. Cancer of the cervix is subdivided into three stages:
   1. Early dysplasia can be treated in a variety of ways.
      a. Cryosurgery
      b. Loop electrocautery excision procedure
      c. Laser
      d. Conization
      e. Hysterectomy

HESI HINT Laser therapy or cryosurgery is used to treat cervical cancer when the lesion is small and localized. Invasive cancer is treated with radiation, conization, hysterectomy, or pelvic exenteration (a drastic surgical procedure where the uterus, ovaries, fallopian tubes, vagina, rectum, and bladder are removed in an attempt to stop metastasis). Chemotherapy is not useful with this type of cancer.

HESI HINT: AMERICAN COLLEGE OF OBSTETRICIANS AND GYNECOLOGISTS (ACOG) 2021 RECOMMENDATIONS FOR PAP SMEARS In women aged 30—65 years, annual cervical cancer screening should not be performed (Level A evidence). Patients should be counseled that annual well-woman visits are recommended even if cervical cancer screening is not performed at each visit. The recommended timeframe for Pap smears is every 3 years. Women aged 30—65 years should have a Pap smear with an HPV test every 5 years. Women over 65 do not need a Pap smear. Pap smears should not be performed for any woman under age 21 regardless of onset of sexual activity.

---

   2. Early carcinoma can be treated with:
      a. Hysterectomy
      b. Intracavity radiation
   3. Late carcinoma (the tumor size and stage of invasion of surrounding tissues increases) treatment often includes:
      a. External beam radiation along with hysterectomy
      b. Antineoplastic chemotherapy is of limited use for cancers arising from squamous cells
      c. Pelvic exenteration

Care of the Client With Radiation Implants

A. Radiation implants are used to treat disease by delivering high-dose radiation seeds directly to the affected tissue.

B. The nurse must take certain precautions for protection of self as well as the client and visitors.

C. Follow specific guidelines provided by the agency. General care guidelines include:
1. Remind the client that she is not radioactive; only the implants contain radioactivity.
2. Remind the client that her isolation time is limited; isolation is not necessarily indefinite.

D. Assign client to a private room and place a "Caution: Radioactive Material" sign on the door.

E. Do not permit pregnant caretakers or pregnant visitors into the room.

F. Discourage visits by small children.

G. Keep a lead-lined container in the room for disposal of the implant, should it become dislodged.

H. Client should remain in bed with as little movement as possible.

I. Be aware that *all* client secretions have the potential of being radioactive.

J. Wear latex gloves when handling potentially contaminated secretions.

K. Wear a radiation badge when providing care to clients with radiation implants.
1. Badge is not to be worn out of doors.
2. Badge is checked at regular intervals by health officials.

L. Provide nursing care in an efficient but caring manner.
1. Plan care to limit overall time in the client's room.
2. When in the room, stand at the greatest distance away from the client to minimize exposure.
3. Stop by to check on the client from the door frequently.

> **HESI HINT** Shielding provides the best protection for nurses providing close care to clients. Time, distance, and shielding are classic precautions for nurses.

M. Keep all supplies and equipment the client might need within reach.

Ovarian Cancer

Description: Cancer of the ovaries can occur at all ages, including infancy and childhood. Early diagnosis is difficult because no useful screening test exists at present. Malignant germ cell tumors are most common in women between 20 and 40 years of age and epithelial cancers occur most often in the perimenopausal age groups.

Nursing Assessment

A. Asymptomatic in early stages.

B. Laparotomy is primary tool for diagnosis and staging of the disease; ovarian cancer is surgically staged, rather than clinically staged.

C. Advanced clinical manifestations include:
1. Pelvic discomfort
2. Low back pain and leg pain
3. Weight change
4. Abdominal pain
5. Nausea and vomiting
6. Increased abdominal girth
7. Constipation
8. Urinary frequency

> **HESI HINT** Ovarian cancer is the leading cause of death from gynecologic cancers in the United States. Growth is insidious, so it is not recognized until it is at an advanced stage.

Nursing Plans and Interventions

A. Care required for any major abdominal surgery following laparotomy.

B. Collaborate with the RN to develop and implement client/family teaching plan about disease and follow-up treatment.

C. Offer supportive care to client and family throughout diagnosis and treatment.

> **HESI HINT** The major emphasis in the nursing management of cancers of the reproductive tract is early detection.

Breast Cancer

Description: Cancer originating in the breast.

A. Breast cancer is the most commonly occurring cancer in women in the United States.

B. One in eight women will develop breast cancer in her lifetime.

C. Early detection is important to successful treatment.

D. Men can develop breast cancer. They account for less than 1% of reported cases.

E. Of all breast cancers, 90% to 95% are discovered through breast self-examination.

F. Risk factors include:
1. Positive family history
2. Menarche before 12 years of age and/or menopause after age 50
3. Nulliparous or those with first child after the age of 30 years
4. History of uterine cancer
5. Daily alcohol intake
6. Highest incidence in those aged 40 to 49 years and over 65 years

G. Breast cancer is generally adenocarcinoma originating in epithelial cells and occurs in the ducts or lobes.

H. Tumors tend to be located in the upper outer quadrant of the breast and more often in the left breast than the right.

I. Early detection is important.
   1. Every woman should perform a breast self-examination monthly, preferably as soon as menstrual bleeding ceases or, if postmenopausal, the same day every month.
   2. Mammography is very helpful with early detection of breast cancer. Recommendations from the American Cancer Society (2015) include:
      a. Women aged 40 to 44 years should have the choice to start annual screening with mammograms if they wish to do so.
      b. Women aged 45 to 54 should get mammograms every year.
      c. Women aged 55 years and older should switch to mammograms every 2 years or can continue yearly screening.
      d. Screening should continue as long as a woman is in good health and is expected to live 10 more years or longer.
      e. Advise not to use lotions, talc powder, or deodorant under arms before procedure (may mimic calcium deposits on x-ray).
   3. Physical examination by a professional skilled in examination of the breast should be done annually.
J. Tumors measuring less than 4 cm are deemed curable.
K. Larger tumors require much more aggressive treatment (cure is difficult).
L. Definitive diagnosis of cancer of the breast is made with biopsy.
M. Common sites of metastasis (spread) are the axillary, supraclavicular, or mediastinal lymph nodes followed by metastases to the lungs, liver, brain, and spine.
N. Bone metastasis is extremely painful.
O. Treatment is dependent on the stage of the disease.
   1. Mastectomy is commonly performed.
   2. Adjuvant treatment consists of radiation (either external beam or implants), antineoplastic chemotherapy, and hormonal therapy.

HESI HINT The presence or absence of hormone receptors is paramount in selecting clients for adjuvant therapy.

Nursing Assessment

A. Hard lump (not freely moveable and not painful)
B. Dimpling of skin
C. Retraction of nipple
D. Alterations in contour of breast
E. Change in the skin color
F. Change in the skin texture (peau d'orange)
G. Discharge from nipple
H. Pain and ulcerations (late signs)
I. Diagnostic tests include:
   1. Mammogram
   2. Biopsy and frozen section

Nursing Plans and Interventions

A. Assess lesion.
   1. Location
   2. Size
   3. Shape
   4. Consistency
   5. Fixation to surrounding tissues
   6. Lymph node involvement
B. Preoperative
   1. Explore client's expectations of surgery and what the surgical site will look like postoperatively.
   2. Discuss skin graft if one is possible and cosmetic reconstruction that might be implemented with mastectomy or at a later time.
C. Postoperative
   1. Monitor bleeding, check under dressing, blood reinfusion system, and under client's back (bleeding will run to back).
   2. Position arm on operative side on a pillow, slightly elevated.
   3. Avoid BP measurements, injections, and venipuncture in the affected arm (side where surgery was performed).
   4. Instruct client to avoid injury such as burns or scrapes to the affected arm.
   5. Encourage hand activity for the side where surgery was performed by squeezing a small rubber ball.
   6. Encourage the client to perform activities that will use arm, such as brushing hair.
   7. Collaborate with RN to develop and implement a teaching plan for client/family about postmastectomy exercises (wall climbing with affected arm and rope turning).
D. Encourage client to verbalize concerns.
   1. Cancer
   2. Death
   3. Loss of breast
E. Encourage client to discuss operation, diagnosis, feelings, concerns, and fears.
F. Be with the client when she first looks at the operative site; offer emotional support.
G. Collaborate with RN and HCP for Reach-to-Recovery visit, Y-me (prescription required).
H. Recognize the grief process.
   1. Allow client to cry, withdraw, and so on.
   2. Help client focus on the future while allowing discussions of loss.
I. If reconstruction was not discussed preoperatively, encourage client to discuss or explore these options postoperatively.
J. Discuss the use of temporary and/or permanent prosthesis.

Testicular Cancer

Description: Cancer of the testes is the leading cause of death from cancer in men aged 15 to 35 years. If untreated, death usually occurs within 2 to 3 years. If detected and treated early, there is a 90% to 100% chance of cure.

Nursing Assessment

A. Early signs are subtle and usually go unnoticed
B. Feeling of heaviness or dragging sensation in the lower abdomen and groin
C. Lump or swelling (painless)
D. Late signs include low back pain, weight loss, and fatigue

> **HESI HINT** Men whose testes have not descended into the scrotum or whose testes descended after age 6 are at high risk for developing testicular cancer. The most common symptom is the appearance of a small, hard lump about the size of a pea on the front or side of the testicle. Testicular self-examination should be done regularly at the same time each month by all men after the age of 14 years. It should be done after a shower by gently palpating the testes and cord to look for a small lump. Swelling may also be a sign of testicular cancer.

Nursing Plans and Interventions

A. Postoperative care after orchidectomy:
   1. Observe for hemorrhage.
   2. Active movement may be contraindicated.
B. Care for clients receiving radiation therapy.
C. Encourage genetic counseling (sperm banking is often recommended before surgery).
D. Reinforce teachings that sexual functioning is usually not affected because the remaining testis undergoes hyperplasia, producing sufficient testosterone to maintain sexual functioning. Although ejaculatory ability may be decreased, orgasm is still possible.

Prostate Cancer

Description: Prostate cancer rarely occurs before 40 years of age, but it is the second leading cause of death from cancer in American men. High-risk groups include those with a history of multiple sexual partners, sexually transmitted diseases (STDs), or certain viral infections, and those with a family history.

Nursing Assessment

A. Asymptomatic if confined to gland
B. Symptoms of urinary obstruction
C. With metastasis: low back pain, fatigue, aching in legs, and hip pain
D. Elevated levels of prostate-specific antigen (PSA)
   1. PSA test should be conducted before a digital rectal examination so that manipulation of the prostate does not give a false-positive reading.
   2. Serial blood screening should be done to observe trends. A rise in PSA or consistently high PSA is more reliable than a single assay.
   3. PSA levels can rise with inflammation, benign hypertrophy, or irritation, as well as in response to cancer.
E. Elevated prostatic acid phosphatase is an indication of metastasis to the bone

F. Digital rectal examination reveals palpable nodule
G. Transrectal ultrasound visualizes nonpalpable tumors
H. Definitive diagnosis is made by biopsy

Nursing Plans and Interventions

A. Reinforce the importance of early detection.
B. Provide preoperative bowel preparation to prevent fecal contamination of operative site.
   1. Enemas and cathartics
   2. Sulfasalazine (Azulfidine) or neomycin
   3. Clear fluids only the day before surgery to prevent fecal contamination of operative site
C. Provide postoperative care.
   1. Monitor for urine leaks, hemorrhage, and signs of infection.
   2. Provide support dressing or supportive underwear to perineal incision.
   3. Use donut cushion to relieve pressure on incision site while sitting.
   4. Avoid rectal manipulation (rectal thermometers, rectal tubes, and hard suppositories).
   5. Provide low-residue diet until wound healing is advanced.
   6. Institute measures to decrease peristalsis in the first postoperative week to prevent contamination of incision.

Sexually Transmitted Infections

Description: Sexually transmitted infections (STIs) are diseases that may be transmitted during intimate sexual contact.
A. STIs are the most prevalent communicable diseases in the United States.
B. Most cases of STIs occur in adolescents and young adults.

> **HESI HINT** STIs in infants and children usually indicate sexual abuse and should be reported. The nurse is legally responsible to report suspected cases of child abuse.

Nursing Assessment

See Table 4.37.

> **HESI HINT** Chlamydia is the most reported communicable disease in the United States.

Nursing Plans and Interventions

A. Use a nonjudgmental approach; be straightforward when taking history.
B. Reassure client that all information is strictly confidential. Obtain a complete sexual history that includes:
   1. The client's sexual orientation
   2. Sexual practices

TABLE 4.37   Sexually Transmitted Infections

Sexually Transmitted Infection	Symptoms	Treatment
Treponema pallidum, Syphilis • Laboratory diagnosis: • VDRL, FTA-ABS	• *Primary (local):* up to 90 days post exposure • Chancre (red, painless lesions with indurated border) • Highly infectious • *Secondary (systemic):* 6 weeks to 6 months postexposure • Influenza-type symptoms • Generalized rash that affects palms of hands and soles of feet • Lesions contagious • *Tertiary:* 10–30 years postexposure • Cardiac and neurologic destruction	• Penicillin G intramuscular (usually 2.4–4.8 million units) • If penicillin allergic (adults), alternatives: tetracycline, doxycycline, or ceftriaxone
Neisseria gonorrhoeae, Gonorrhea • Laboratory diagnosis: • Smears, cultures	• Females: majority are asymptomatic • Males: dysuria, yellowish-green urethral discharge, urinary frequency	• Ceftriaxone sodium plus doxycycline hyclate or azithromycin • Cefixime plus doxycycline or azithromycin
Chlamydia trachomatis, Chlamydia • Laboratory diagnosis: • Tissue culture, Chlamydiazine, MicroTrak	• Females: many asymptomatic, but may exhibit dysuria, urgency, vaginal discharge • Males: leading cause of nongonococcal urethritis	• Doxycycline hyclate • Azithromycin
Trichomonas vaginalis, Trichomoniasis • Laboratory diagnosis: • Wet slide	• Females: green, yellow, or white frothy foul-smelling vaginal discharge with itching • Males: asymptomatic	• Metronidazole (Flagyl) (male partners to be treated to prevent reinfection)
Candida albicans, Candidiasis • Laboratory diagnosis: • Viral culture	• Females: odorless, white or yellow, cheesy discharge with itching • Males: asymptomatic	• Miconazole nitrate (Monistat) • Clotrimazole (Gyne-Lotrimin) • Nystatin (Mycostatin) • Fluconazole (Diflucan) PO single dose

Herpes simplex virus 2, Herpes	• Vesicles in clusters that rupture and leave painful erosions that cause painful urination
	• Characterized by remissions and exacerbations
	• May be contagious even when asymptomatic
		• Acyclovir (Zovirax) partially controls symptoms
		• Famciclovir
		• Valacyclovir
		• Palliative care
		  1. Viscous lidocaine topically to ease pain
		  2. Keep lesions clean and dry

Human papillomavirus (HPV)	• Multiple strains (>70), some of which are implicated in cervical cancer • Alarming rate increase in adolescent population • Lesions may be small, wart-like, or clustered • May be flat or raised	• Routine vaccination is recommended for select populations before onset of sexual activity • Applied medications such as podophyllin (contraindicated in pregnancy) • Trichloroacetic acid (TCA) • Laser • Cryotherapy (freezing)
Human Immunodeficiency Virus (HIV), AIDS	See HIV Infection in Chapter 3: *Advanced Clinical Concepts*	

Continued

Zika Virus

Common Symptoms of Zika (CDC)
- Fever
- Rash
- Joint pain
- Conjunctivitis (red eyes)
- Other symptoms include:
  - Muscle pain
  - Headache
  - Considerations
  - Zika may be sexually transmitted by men or women
  - Zika virus can pass from a pregnant woman to her fetus. Zika is linked to microcephaly,
  - Pregnant women living in an area with Zika, or returning from an area where Zika is present should talk to an health care provider

Data from www.cdc.gov/zika.

 a. Penile-vaginal
 b. Penile-anal
 c. Penile-oral
 d. Oral-vaginal
 e. Anal-oral
 3. Type of protection (barrier) used
 4. Contraceptive practices
 5. Previous history of STIs
C. Collaborate with RN and implement the teaching plan that includes:
 1. Signs and symptoms of STIs.
 2. Mode of transmission of STIs. (Remember, not all persons practice sex in the same manner.)
 3. Sexual contact should be avoided with anyone while infected.
 4. Provide concise written instructions about the treatment; request a return verbalization of these instructions to ensure the client has "heard" the instructions and understands them.
D. Encourage client to provide information regarding *all* sexual contacts.
E. Report incidents of STIs to appropriate health agencies/ departments.
F. Instruct women of childbearing age about risks to newborns.
 1. Gonorrheal conjunctivitis
 2. Neonatal herpes
 3. Congenital syphilis
 4. Oral candidiasis

HESI HINT Pelvic inflammatory disease (PID) involves more than one of the pelvic structures. The infection can cause adhesions and eventually result in sterility. Manage the pain associated with PID with analgesics and warm sitz baths. Bed rest in a semi-Fowler position may increase comfort and promote drainage. Antibiotic treatment is necessary to reduce inflammation and pain.

G. Collaborate with RN to develop and implement a teaching plan about "safer sex."
 1. Reduce the number of sexual contacts.
 2. Avoid sex with those who have multiple partners.
 3. Examine genital area and avoid sexual contact if anything abnormal is present.
 4. Wash hands and genital area before and after sexual contact.
 5. Use a latex condom as a barrier.
 6. Use water-based lubricants rather than oil-based lubricants.
 7. Use a vaginal spermicidal gel.
 8. Avoid douching before and after sexual contact; douching increases risk of infections because the body's normal defenses are reduced or destroyed.
 9. Seek attention from HCP immediately if symptoms occur.

HESI HINT A client comes into the clinic with a chancre on his penis. What is the usual treatment? IM dose of penicillin (such as Benzathine penicillin G 2.4 million units). Obtain a sexual history including the names of his sexual partners so they can receive treatment.

REVIEW OF REPRODUCTIVE SYSTEM

1. What are the indications for a hysterectomy in the client who has fibromas?
2. List the symptoms and conditions associated with cystocele.
3. What are the most important nursing interventions for the postoperative client who has had a hysterectomy with an A&P repair?
4. Describe the priority nursing care for the client who has had radiation implants.
5. What screening tool is used to detect cervical cancer? What are the American Cancer Society's recommendations for women aged 30 to 70 years with three consecutive normal results?
6. Cite two nursing diagnoses for a client undergoing a hysterectomy for cervical cancer.

7. What are the three most important tools for early detection of breast cancer? How often should these tools be used?
8. Describe three nursing interventions to help decrease edema after a mastectomy.
9. Name three priorities to include in a discharge plan for the client who has had a mastectomy.
10. What is the most common cause of nongonococcal urethritis?
11. What is the causative organism for syphilis?
12. Malodorous, frothy, greenish-yellow vaginal discharge is characteristic of which STI?
13. Which STI is characterized by remissions and exacerbations in both men and women?
14. Outline a teaching plan for the client with an STI.
See Answer Key at the end of this text for suggested responses.

BURNS

Description: Tissue injury or necrosis caused by transfer of energy from a heat source to the body.
A. Categories
   1. Thermal
   2. Radiation
   3. Electrical
   4. Chemical
B. Tissue destruction results from:
   1. Coagulation
   2. Protein denaturation
   3. Ionization of cellular contents
C. Critical systems affected include:
   1. Respiratory
   2. Integumentary
   3. Cardiovascular
   4. Renal
   5. GI
   6. Neurologic
D. Severity determined by burn depth (Fig. 4.10)
   1. First degree
      a. Superficial partial-thickness (e.g., sunburn)
      b. Injury to the epidermis
      c. Leaves skin pink or red, but no blisters
      d. Dry
      e. Painful (relieved by cooling)
      f. Slight edema
      g. No scarring; skin grafts are not required
   2. Second degree
      a. Deep partial-thickness destruction of epidermis and upper layers of dermis
      b. Injury to deeper portions of the dermis
      c. Painful (sensitive to touch and cold air)
      d. Appears red or white, weeps fluid, blisters
      e. Hair follicles remain intact—that is, hair does not pull out easily
      f. Very edematous
      g. Blanching followed by capillary refill

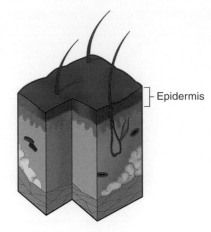

Superficial burns damage only the top layer of the skin—the epidermis. Healing occurs in 3–6 days.

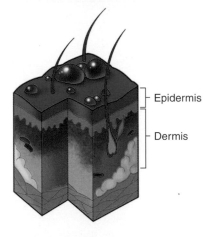

Superficial partial-thickness burns are those in which the entire epidermis and variable portions of the dermis layer of skin are destroyed. Uncomplicated healing occurs in 10–21 days.

Deep partial-thickness burns extend into the deeper layers of the dermis. Healing occurs in 2–6weeks.

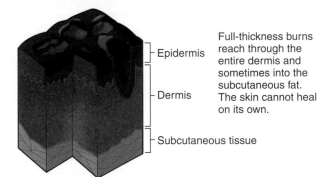

Full-thickness burns reach through the entire dermis and sometimes into the subcutaneous fat. The skin cannot heal on its own.

Fig. 4.10 Tissues Involved in Burns of Various Depths. (Ignatavicius, D. D., Workman, L., & Rebar, C. [2020]. *Medical-surgical nursing: Concepts for interprofessional collaborative care* [10th ed.]. St. Louis: Elsevier.)

      h. Heals without surgical intervention; usually does not scar
   3. Third degree
      a. Deep full-thickness; involves total destruction of dermis and epidermis
      b. Skin cannot regenerate
      c. Requires skin grafting
      d. Underlying tissue (fat, fascia, tendon, bone) may be involved
      e. Wound appears dry and leathery as eschar develops
      f. Painless

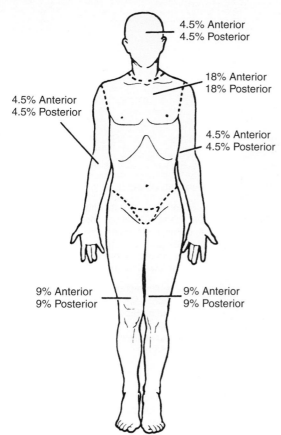

Fig. 4.11 Estimation of Burn Injury in Children and Adults. (Ignatavicius, D. D., Workman, L., & Rebar, C. [2020]. *Medical-surgical nursing: Concepts for interprofessional collaborative care* [10th ed.]. St. Louis: Elsevier.)

4. Severity is determined by the extent of the surface area burned
   a. Rule of nines: head and neck 9%, upper extremities 9% each, lower extremities 18% each, front trunk 18%, back trunk 18%, perineal area 1% (for adults) (Fig. 4.11).
   b. Lund and Browder chart: critical body areas are face, hands, feet, and perineum.
E. Three stages of burn care
  1. Stage I, resuscitative/emergent phase
   a. Begins at the time of injury and concludes with the restoration of normal capillary permeability, which typically reverses 48 to 72 hours after the injury.
   b. Characterized by fluid shift from intravascular to interstitial space and by shock. Focus of care is to preserve vital organ functioning.
   c. Expect to administer large volumes of fluid in this phase based on the client's weight and extent of injury.
   d. Fluid replacement formulas are calculated from the time of injury and not from the time of arrival at the hospital.
  2. Stage II, acute phase
   a. Occurs from beginning of diuresis (48 to 72 hours after injury) to near completion of wound closure.
   b. Characterized by fluid shift from interstitial to intravascular space.

   c. Focus is on infection control, wound care and closure, pain management, nutritional support, and physical therapy.
  3. Stage III, rehabilitation phase
   a. Occurs from major wound closure to return to optimal level of physical and psychosocial adjustment (approximately 5 years).
   b. Characterized by grafting and rehabilitation specific to the client's needs.

Nursing Assessment

Absence of bowel sounds indicating paralytic ileus.
A. Radically decreased urinary output in the first 72 hours after injury with increased specific gravity.
B. Radically increased urinary output (diuresis) 72 hours to 2 weeks after initial injury.
C. Signs of inadequate hydration:
  1. Restlessness
  2. Disorientation
  3. Decreased urinary volume, urinary sodium, and increased urine specific gravity
D. Signs of inhalation burn:
  1. Red or burned face
  2. Singed facial and nasal hairs
  3. Circumoral burns
  4. Conjunctivitis
  5. Sooty nasal mucous or bloody sputum
  6. Hoarseness
  7. Asymmetry of chest movements with respirations and use of accessory muscles indicative of pneumonia
  8. Rales, wheezing, and rhonchi denoting smoke inhalation
  9. Impaired speech and drooling indicating laryngeal edema
E. Description of physiologic responses to burns (Fig. 4.12).
F. Preexisting conditions/illnesses that may influence recovery.

HESI HINT: ABCS OF ASSESSMENT
- Airway
- Breathing
- Circulation

Nursing Plans and Interventions

Emergent phase. Efforts of the health care team are directed toward stabilization with ongoing assessment.

A. Provide admission care.
  1. Extinguish the source of burn (burning may continue with clothing attached to skin).
   a. Thermal: remove clothing, cool burns by immersion in tepid water, apply dry sterile dressings.
   b. Chemical: flush with water or saline.
   c. Electrical: separate client from electrical source.
  2. Provide an open airway; intubation may be necessary if laryngeal edema is a risk.

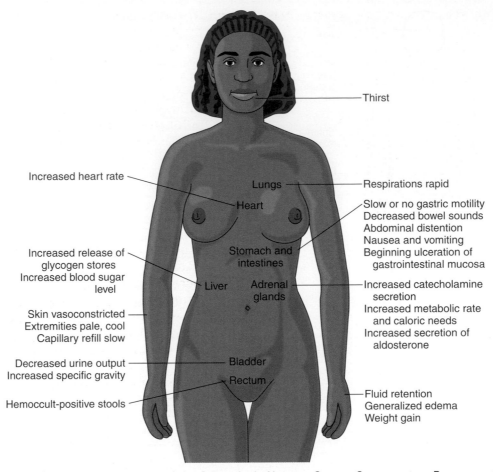

Thirst

Increased heart rate

Lungs

Heart

Respirations rapid

Slow or no gastric motility
Decreased bowel sounds
Abdominal distention
Nausea and vomiting
Beginning ulceration of
gastrointestinal mucosa

Increased release of
glycogen stores
Increased blood sugar
level

Stomach and
intestines

Liver

Adrenal
glands

Increased catecholamine
secretion
Increased metabolic rate
and caloric needs
Increased secretion of
aldosterone

Skin vasoconstricted
Extremities pale, cool
Capillary refill slow

Decreased urine output
Increased specific gravity

Bladder

Rectum

Hemoccult-positive stools

Fluid retention
Generalized edema
Weight gain

Fig. 4.12 The Physiologic Actions of the Sympathetic Nervous System Compensatory Responses to Burn Injury (Early Phase). (Ignatavicius, D. D., Workman, L., & Rebar, C. [2016]. *Medical-surgical nursing: Concepts for interprofessional collaborative care* [9th ed.]. St. Louis: Elsevier.)

3. Determine baseline data: vital signs, blood gases, weight.
4. Determine depth and extent of burn.
5. Administer tetanus toxoid.
6. Initiate fluid and electrolyte therapy; Ringer's lactate with electrolytes and colloids adjusted according to laboratory results and fluid resuscitation formula used.

HESI HINT Massive volumes of IV fluids are given. It is not uncommon to give more than 1000 mL/h during various phases of burn care. Hemodynamic monitoring must be closely observed to ensure that the client is supported with fluid but is not overloaded.

7. Insert NG tube to prevent vomiting, abdominal distention, or gastric aspiration.
8. Monitor client's response to IV pain medication.
B. Monitor hydration status.
   1. Record urinary output hourly (normal range, 30 to 100 mL/h).
   2. Monitor IV fluids and assist the RN in the titration to keep urine output at 30 to 100 mL/h.
   3. Accurately record I&O.
   4. Weigh daily.

5. Observe for signs of inadequate hydration.
   a. Restlessness
   b. Disorientation
   c. Hypothermia
   d. Decreased urine output
C. Monitor respiratory functioning.
   1. Provide care for the intubated client.
   2. Suction endotracheal or nasotracheal.
   3. Monitor ABGs.
   4. Observe for cyanosis, disorientation.
   5. Administer O_2.
   6. Encourage use of incentive spirometer, coughing, and deep breathing.
   7. Elevate the head of the bed to 30 degrees or more for burns of the face and head.
D. Provide wound care.
   1. Use strict aseptic technique.
   2. Debridement and dressing changes according to client's condition.
   3. Change dressings in minimum time (very painful), premedicate.
   4. Maintain room temperature above 90°F, humidified, and free of drafts.

5. Monitor body temperature frequently; have hyperthermia blankets available.
E. Monitor for paralytic ileus.
   1. Absence of bowel sounds
   2. Nausea and vomiting
   3. Abdominal distention
F. Assist with management of pain.
   1. Administer analgesics IV.
   2. Reinforce teaching about distraction/relaxation techniques.
   3. Reinforce teaching about use of guided imagery.
G. Monitor for circulatory compromise in burns that constrict body parts. Prepare client for escharotomy.

> **HESI HINT** Infection is a life-threatening risk for those with burns.

Acute phase. Characterized by fluid shift from interstitial to intravascular (diuresis begins); occurs from 72 hours to 2 weeks after initial injury to near completion of wound closure.

A. Provide infection control, including the following:
   1. Maintain protective isolation of entire burn unit.
   2. Cover hair at all times.
   3. Wear masks during dressing changes.
   4. Use sterile technique for hydrotherapy, dressing change, and debridement.
   5. Monitor client's response to IV antibiotics if indicated.
   6. Live plants and flowers are prohibited.
B. Splint and position client to prevent contractures. Avoid use of pillows with neck burns.
C. Perform ROM exercises; will be painful for client.
   1. Administer pain medication immediately before performing ROM.
   2. Assist client to perform active ROM for 3 to 5 minutes at a time frequently during day.
   3. Mobilize as soon as possible using splints designed for the client.
   4. Encourage active ROM when up and about.
D. Assist the RN in monitoring the client's response to fluid therapy; colloids may be used to keep fluid in vascular space.
   1. Monitor serum chemistries at all times.
   2. Keep an IV site available; a saline lock is helpful.
   3. Maintain strict I&O.
   4. Encourage oral intake of fluids.
E. Provide adequate nutrition.
   1. Provide high-calorie (up to 5000 calories/day), high-protein, and high-carbohydrate diet.

2. Give nutritional supplements via NG tube feeding at night if caloric intake is inadequate.
3. Keep accurate calorie counts.
4. Administer all medications with either milk or juice.
5. Weigh daily.

> **HESI HINT** To ensure electrolyte balance, additional water is not given. These clients need to ingest food products or high-protein drinks with the highest biologic value rather than water.

F. Provide burn/wound care.
   1. Cleansing per agency routine (daily or up to three times a day) in hydrotherapy or shower.
   2. Wet-to-dry dressing changes two to three times a day to remove eschar.
   3. Apply silver sulfadiazine (Silvadene) or mafenide acetate (Sulfamylon) to the burn as prescribed (Table 4.38).
   4. Cover (closed method) or leave open (open method) according to agency policy or HCP's prescription.
   5. Prepare the client for grafting when eschar has been removed.
   6. Prepare the client for autografts (use of client's own skin for grafting).
   7. Use heat lamp to donor site after graft to allow the area to reepithelialize.

> **HESI HINT** Having dressings changed is very painful. Medicate client before procedure.

> **HESI HINT** Preexisting conditions that might influence burn recovery are age, chronic illness (diabetes, cardiac problems, etc.), physical disabilities, disease, medications used routinely, and drug and/or alcohol abuse.

Rehabilitation phase. Characterized by the absence of infection risk.
A. Collaborate with ongoing discharge planning.
B. May return home when the danger of infection has been eliminated.
C. High-protein fluids with vitamin supplement.
D. Pressure dressings or garments may be worn continuously to prevent hypertrophic scarring and contractures.

TABLE 4.38 Topical Antimicrobial Agents

Drugs	Indications	Adverse Reactions	Nursing Implications
• Mafenide acetate (Sulfamylon)	• Treatment of burns • Usually used with OPEN method of wound care	• Painful • Causes mild acidosis	• Administer pain medication before dressing changes • Penetrates wound rapidly
• Silver sulfadiazine (Silvadene)	• Treatment of burns • Usually used with OPEN method of wound care • Used to avoid acid–base complications • Keeps eschar soft making debridement easier	• Penetrates wound slowly	• Administer pain medication before dressing change • Is soothing to the burn

❓ REVIEW OF BURNS

1. List four categories of burns.
2. Burn depth is a measure of severity. Describe the characteristics of superficial partial-thickness, deep partial-thickness, and full-thickness burns.
3. Describe fluid management in the emergent phase, acute phase, and rehabilitation phase of the burned client.
4. Describe pain management of the burned client.
5. Outline admission care of the burned client.

6. Nutritional status is a major concern when caring for a burned client. List three specific dietary interventions used with burned clients.
7. Describe the method of extinguishing each of the following burns: thermal, chemical, and electrical.
8. List four signs of an inhalation burn.
9. Why is the burned client allowed NO "free" water?
10. Describe an autograft.
See Answer Key at the end of this text for suggested responses.

NEXT-GENERATION NCLEX EXAMINATION-STYLE QUESTION

| Health History | Nurses' Notes | Vital Signs | Lab Results |

1400: Client is accompanied by family. Client had been nauseated with vomiting for 4 days. Family states, "Has had a fever has been over 102°F for the last few days and won't eat or drink or take medications." PMH: smoker—1 ppd 40+ years; DM II; CAD; HTN; Hypercholesterolemia; Neuropathy bilat LE.

Home medications
Losartan/HCTZ 100 mg/12.5 mg PO daily
Lovastatin 20 mg PO daily
Pioglitazone 45 mg PO daily
1430: Client is confused AO×2, not oriented to time. Poor skin turgor—2+ tenting.
Weight: 180 lb; Height 5'7"
Vital signs: BP 181/95, HR 110; RR 28; Temp 103.2°F, SPO$_2$ 92% on RA

Laboratory Results
Serum glucose of 650; BNP 32; Na+ 148; K+ 5.0; Serum osmolality 400 mOsm/kg,
Serum ketones 4.1 mmol/L

Ordered Treatments
Started on an insulin drip to be discontinued in 4 hours ago
Start on regular neutral protamine hagedorn (NPH) is An intermediate-acting insulin used in the treatment of diabetes insulin per sliding scale after the insulin drip is stopped

Instructions
Complete the diagram by selecting from the choices below to specify which potential condition the client is most likely experiencing, 2 actions to take, and 2 parameters the nurse would monitor to assess the client's progress.

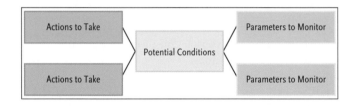

Actions to Take	Potential Conditions	Parameters to Monitor
Administer Acetaminophen 650 mg q 6 h PRN for Fever	Appendicitis	Electrocardiogram (EKG)
Obtain a urine sample for culture	Influenza	Neurologic status
Call laboratory for blood culture draw	Diabetic ketoacidosis	Monitor pulses
Provide K+ as indicated	Food Poisoning	Fall precautions
Reorient client as needed		Blood glucose level

REFERENCES AND BIBLIOGRAPHY

American College of Obstetricians and Gynecologists. (2020). *Updated guidelines for management of cervical cancer screening abnormalities. Practice Advisory.* Washington, DC: American College of Obstetricians and Gynecologists. Available at https://www.acog.org/clinical/clinical-guidance/practice-advisory/articles/2020/10/updated-guidelines-for-management-of-cervical-cancer-screening-abnormalities. Retrieved April 12, 2021.

Arnold, E., & Boggs, K. (2019). *Interpersonal relationships: Professional communication skills for nurses* (8th ed.). St. Louis: Saunders.

Boyles, L., & Baxter, C. (2021). Premenstrual syndrome. *InnovAiT*, *14*(5), 313–317.

Clark, C. (2021). Aromatherapy: Essential oils and nursing: Explore this option for enhancing well-being. *American Nurse Journal, 16*(8), 60–63.

Farrar, A. J., & Farrar, F. C. (2020). Clinical aromatherapy. *Nursing Clinical North America, 55*(4), 489–504. https://doi.org/10.1016/j.cnur.2020.06.015. Published online 2020 Sep 28.

Khardori, R. (2022). *Type 2 Diabetes Mellitus.* https://emedicine.medscape.com/article/117853-overview.

Khardori N. Vaccines and vaccine resistance: Past, present and future. Indian J Med Microbiol. 2022 Apr-Jun;40(2):187-192. https://doi.org/10.1016/j.ijmmb.2021.12.008. Epub 2021 Dec 24. PMID: 34961641.

Puchalski, C., Ferrell, B. R., Borneman, T., DiFrances Remein, C., Haythorn, T., & Jacobs, C. (2022). Implementing quality improvement efforts in spiritual care: Outcomes from the interprofessional spiritual care education curriculum. *Journal of Health Care Chaplaincy, 28*(3), 431−442. https://doi.org/10.1080/08854726.2021.1917168. Epub 2021 Aug 15. PMID: 34396929.

Stussman, B. J., Nahin, R. R., Barnes, P. M., & Ward, B. W. (2020). U.S. Physician recommendations to their patients about the use of complementary health approaches. *Journal of Alternative and Complementary Medicine, 26,* 25−33.

Pediatric Nursing

As a nurse in a pediatric environment the requirements include being able to connect with children in a comforting demeanor. The responsibility encompasses not only the pediatric patient but also the parent/family unit. Understanding the mindset, theoretical stages of development, and the ability to be inclusive of the child and allowing the child to make choices will facilitate a positive interaction. Being a part of the life of a child is a gratifying career choice.

The pediatric nurse encompasses a very different role and cannot be misconstrued as taking care of small adults; this is truly a psychosocial interaction with multiple implications. Conceptually, being involved with a child, infant, or adolescent means being a part of their developmental and psychosocial dynamic, which will require patience and a variety of innovative ideas to accomplish interventions. Generally, the care you provide will be all encompassing including parental education, nutrition, exercise, developmental interactions, and support of a healthy environment. According to the Institute of Pediatric Nursing study 92% (2014) of pediatric nurses said they encourage others to join them in the career because it is a rewarding career to have the opportunity to change the life of a child.

GROWTH AND DEVELOPMENT

A. Nurses need to understand the normal growth and development baselines to be able to assess developmental milestones in all pediatric individuals.
B. Knowledge of psychosocial, cognitive, and moral developmental abilities allows a nurse to adapt teaching to the level of the child.
C. Knowledge of appropriate interests of children at different ages enables the nurse to use innovative interactions to facilitate the child's development and to minimize problems caused by the exposure to a hospitalization and illness.

Theories of Development

A. Erik Erikson was a psychologist who developed one of the most popular and influential theories of development. Erikson's theory centered on psychosocial development.
  1. Stages of Psychosocial Development (Fig. 5.1)
    a. Trust vs. Mistrust
    b. Autonomy vs. Shame
    c. Initiative vs. Guilt
    d. Industry vs. Inferiority
    e. Identity vs. Role Confusion
    f. Intimacy vs. Isolation

  g. Generativity vs. Stagnation
  h. Integrity vs. Despair
B. Piaget Jean Piaget was a Swiss developmental psychologist who studied children in the early 20th century. His theory of intellectual or cognitive development was published in 1936.
  1. Stages of Cognitive Development
    a. Sensorimotor Birth, 18 to 24 months: Motor activity without use of symbols. All things learned are based on experiences, or trial and error.
    b. Preoperational, 2 to 7 years old: Development of language, memory, and imagination. Intelligence is both egocentric and intuitive.
    c. Concrete Operational, 7 to 11 years old: More logical and methodical manipulation of symbols. Less egocentric, and more aware of the outside world and events.
    d. Formal Operational, adolescence to adulthood: Use of symbols to relate to abstract concepts. Able to make hypotheses and grasp abstract concepts and relationships.
C. Lawrence Kohlberg was a developmental theorist of the mid-20th century who is best known for his specific and detailed theory of children's moral development
  1. Moral Development
    a. Naivete and Egocentrism
    b. Punishment-Obedience Orientation
    c. Instrumental Hedonism and Concrete Reciprocity
    d. Good Boy or Good Girl Orientation
    e. Law and Order Orientation
    f. Social Contract Orientation
    g. Personal Principle Orientation
    h. Universal Principle Orientation

Clinical Implications
Birth to 1 Year

A. Developmental milestones
  1. Birth weight doubles by 6 months, triples by 12 months.
  2. Birth length increases by 50% at 12 months.
  3. The infant explores the environment by motor and oral means (Fig. 5.2).
B. Erickson's stage of development
  1. Trust vs. Mistrust
C. Clinical implications
  1. During hospitalization, the infant's emerging skills may disappear.
  2. Infant may be inconsolable due to separation anxiety.

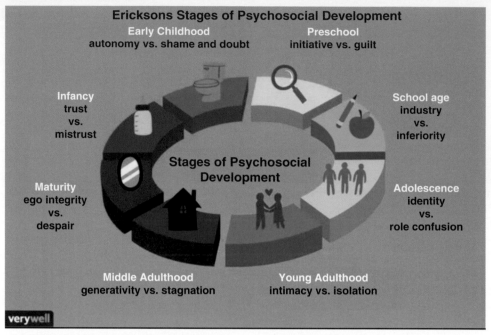

Fig. 5.1 Ericksons Stages of Psychosocial Development (From Verywell/Joshua Seong. Available at: https://www.verywellmind.com/erik-eriksons-stages-of-psychosocial-development-2795740.)

---

3. The practical nurse (PN) should plan and encourage the parents be a part of the infant's care.

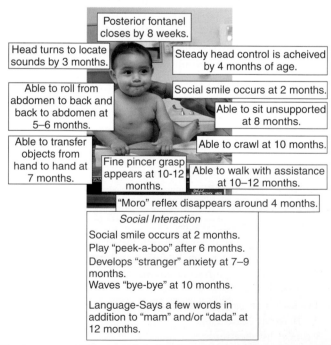

Fig. 5.2 Infant Milestones. (Modified from Hockenberry, M. J. [2019]. *Wong's nursing care of infants and children* [11th ed.]. St. Louis: Elsevier/Mosby.)

4. Encourage the parents to implement a consistent routine when possible.
5. Preparation and teaching should be directed to the family.
6. Always speak to the infant and console the infant, use distraction while performing painful or stressful procedures.
7. Toys for hospitalized infants include mobiles, rattles, squeaking toys, picture books, balls, colored blocks, and activity boxes.

Toddler (1 to 3 Years)

A. Developmental milestones
   1. Birth weight quadruples by 30 months.
   2. Toddler achieves 50% of adult height by 2 years.
   3. Growth velocity slows (Fig. 5.3).
B. Erickson's stage of development
   1. Autonomy vs. Shame
C. Clinical implications
   1. Give simple, brief explanations immediately before procedures, keeping in mind that a 1-year-old does not benefit from the same explanation as that given to a 3-year-old.
   2. During hospitalization, enforced separation from the parents is the greatest threat to the toddler's psychological and emotional integrity.

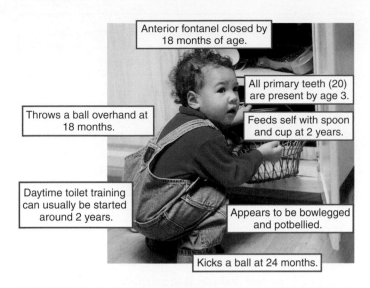

Anterior fontanel closed by 18 months of age.

All primary teeth (20) are present by age 3.

Throws a ball overhand at 18 months.

Feeds self with spoon and cup at 2 years.

Daytime toilet training can usually be started around 2 years.

Appears to be bowlegged and potbellied.

Kicks a ball at 24 months.

Social Interaction:

Two- to three-word sentences are spoken by 2 years.

Three- to four-word sentences are spoken by 3 years.

Own first and last name can be stated by 2½ to 3 years.

Temper tantrums are common.

Safety Issues: Curious about the world around them and like to explore. Poisonous solutions and products need to be kept out of reach from them by being stored away up high and behind locked doors.

Fig. 5.3 Toddler Milestones. (Modified from Perry, S. E., Hockenberry, M. J., Lowdermilk, D. L., et al. [2017]. *Maternal-child nursing* [6th ed.]. St. Louis: Mosby.)

3. Security objects or favorite toys from home should be provided for a toddler.
4. Teach parents to explain their plans to the child (e.g., "I will be back after your nap.").
5. Respect the child's routine and implement whenever possible.
6. Expect regression (e.g., bedwetting).
7. Toys for the hospitalized toddler include a board and mallet, push-pull toys, toy telephones, stuffed animals, and storybooks with pictures. Toddlers benefit from being taken to the hospital playroom because mobility is very important to their development.
8. Toddlers are learning to name body parts and are concerned about their bodies.
9. Very basic explanations should be given to toddlers about procedures.
10. Autonomy should be supported by providing guided choices when appropriate.

Preschool Child (3 to 6 Years)

A. Developmental milestones
   1. Each year, a child gains about 5 pounds and grows 2.5 to 3 inches.

2. The child stands erect, exhibiting a slender posture.
3. The child learns to run, jump, skip, and hop.
4. Handedness is established.
5. The 3-year-old can ride a tricycle.
6. Scissors are used at 4 years.
7. Tying shoelaces is established at 5 years.
8. Colors and shapes are learned.
9. Visual acuity approaches 20/20.
   a. The child learns sexual identity (curiosity and masturbation are common) at 2-3 years.
   b. Imaginary playmates and fears are common at 2-3 years.
   c. Aggressiveness at 4 years is replaced by more independence at 5 years.
B. Erickson's stage of development
   1. Initiative vs. Guilt
C. Piaget's theory: Preoperational thought, intuitive phase = representing things with words and images
D. Clinical implications
   1. Nursing care for hospitalized preschoolers should emphasize an understanding of the child's egocentricity. Explain that he or she did not cause the illness and that painful procedures are not a punishment for misdeeds.
   2. The child's questions should be answered at the child's developmental and learning level. Use simple words that will be understood by the child.
   3. Encourage therapeutic play or medical play that allow the child to act out his or her experiences.
   4. Fear of mutilation caused by procedures is common. A small bandage may be quite helpful in restoring body integrity.
   5. Toys and play for the hospitalized preschooler include coloring books, puzzles, cutting and pasting, dolls, building blocks, clay, and toys that allow the preschooler to work out hospitalization experiences.
   6. The preschooler requires preparation for procedures. He or she should understand what is and what is not going to be "fixed." Simple explanations and basic pictures are helpful. Let the child handle equipment or models of the equipment.

HESI HINT Understanding the developmental stages at the individual ages in planning teaching interventions. Therefore, a 5-year-old child with diabetes could choose the injection sites and provide the child some sense of control.

School-Age Child (6 to 12 Years)

A. Developmental milestones
   1. Each year, a child gains 4 to 6 pounds and about 2 inches in height.
   2. Girls may experience menarche.
   3. Loss of primary teeth and eruption of most permanent teeth occurs.
   4. Fine and gross motor skills mature.

5. Activities include painting, drawing, riding a bicycle, and jumping rope.
B. Erickson's stage of development
   1. Industry vs. Inferiority
C. Piaget's theory: Concrete operations = thinking logically about concrete events and grasping concrete analogies

HESI HINT The NGN-NCLEXPN will test your clinical judgment to differentiate between normal and pathologic based upon the anticipated stages of development and the expectation of the child at the age of intervention. For example, what would be important to children who are school age?

Clinical Implications

A. The hospitalized school-age child may need more support from parents than the child wishes to admit.
B. Maintaining contact with peers and school activities is important during hospitalization.
C. Providing an explanation of all procedures is important. The child can learn from verbal explanations, pictures, and books, as well as by handling equipment.
D. Privacy and modesty are important and should be respected during hospitalization (e.g., close curtains during procedures, allow privacy during baths).
E. Participation in care and planning with staff fosters a sense of involvement and accomplishment.
F. Toys for the school-age child include board games, card games, and hobbies, such as stamp collecting, puzzles, and video games.

HESI HINT Tanner Stages of Pubertal Development (Table 5.1)
Girls: Breast changes, rapid increase in height and weight, growth of pubic hair, appearance of axillary hair, menstruation, abrupt deceleration of linear growth.

Boys: Enlargement of testicles; growth of pubic hair, axillary hair, facial hair, and body hair; rapid increase in height; changes in larynx and voice; nocturnal emissions; abrupt deceleration of linear growth.

Adolescent (12 to 18 Years)

A. Developmental milestones (see Table 5.1).
   1. Girls' growth spurts during adolescence begin earlier than boys' (may begin as early as 10 years for girls).
   2. Boys catch up at around 14 years of age and continue to grow.
   3. Girls finish growth at around age 15, and boys at around age 17.
   4. Secondary sex characteristics develop.
   5. Adult-like thinking begins around age 15. They can problem-solve and use abstract thinking.
   6. Family conflicts develop.
B. Erikson's stage of development
   1. Identity vs. Role Confusion
C. Piaget's theory: Formal operations = thinking about hypothetical scenarios and processing abstract thoughts
D. Immunizations: human papillomavirus (HPV), Meningococcal
E. Clinical implications
   1. Hospitalization of adolescents disrupts school and peer activities; it is important that teens maintain contact with both.
   2. They should share a room with other adolescents.
   3. Illnesses, treatments, and procedures that alter the adolescent's body image can be viewed by the adolescent as devastating.
   4. Teaching about procedures should include time without the parents being present, so that the teen can ask questions that they may not be comfortable asking in front of their parents. It is important to direct questions to the adolescent when the parents are present in order for all involved to hear the same information.

TABLE 5.1 Tanner Stages

Male	Stage	Female
Prepuberty	1	Prepuberty
Enlargement of scrotum and testes and darkening of scrotal sac, scarce light-pigmented pubic hair	2	Breast budding, little amount of breast tissue, enlargement of areola, scarce light pigmented pubic hair
Significant enlargement of penis, further enlargement of testes and darkening of scrotum; increase of pigmentation and amount of pubic hair	3	Further enlargement of breasts, onset of menarche 2% of females; increase of pigmentation and amount of pubic hair
Enlargement of penis, in particular the diameter, development of glands, and further enlargement of testes and darkening of scrotum; pubic hair darkens like an adult, but not as distributed; development of facial hair	4	Breast tissue and areola increase in size and nipple slightly projected; onset of menarche occurs in most females; pubic hair darkens like an adult, but not as distributed; female adult height reached approximately 2 years after onset of menarche
Penis and testes and scrotal sac adult size, continuation of growth of body hair and increase in size of muscles, 20% of males have reached final adult height		Breast tissue adult size and contour, onset of menarche 10% of females; pubic hair pigmented and distributed as an adult

Data from Marshall, W. A., & Tanner, J. M. (1969). Variations in pattern of pubertal changes in girls. *Archives of Disease in Childhood, 44*(235), 291–303; Marshall, W. A., & Tanner, J. M. (1970). Variations in the pattern of pubertal changes in boys. *Archives of Disease in Childhood, 45*(239), 13–23; Sexual Maturity Rating (Tanner Staging) in Adolescents, Copyright © 2010, World Health Organization; Hockenberry, M. J. (2019). *Wong's nursing care of infants and children.* St. Louis: Elsevier.

5. The age of assent for making medical decisions in children and adolescents ranges from 7 to 14 years. Parental consent is also needed for treatment.
6. For prolonged hospitalizations, adolescents need to maintain identity (e.g., have their own clothing, posters, and visitors). A teen room or teen night is very helpful. The adolescent should be part of the decision regarding a parent's rooming-in.
7. When teaching adolescents, the focus should be on the here and now.
   a. "How will this affect me today?"

> **HESI HINT** Clinical judgments are critical during these age categories. Understanding the different concepts of what stage of development changes will occur to know the baseline will be part of the NGN-NCLEXPN exam. Knowing what interventions are necessary if not meeting the baseline will be part of answering the questions for NCLEX

PAIN ASSESSMENT AND MANAGEMENT IN THE PEDIATRIC CLIENT

A. Pediatric pain management may be undertreated, or unrecognized. Untreated pain may lead to complications, such as delayed recovery, change in sleep patterns, and alterations in nutrition.
B. Barriers include unrecognized pain due to different manifestation of pain in the infant and/or toddler who is unable to verbalize the experience of pain and may display pain through actions and mannerisms.
C. Different tools have been developed to help health care providers recognize and identify if the infant or toddler is experiencing pain.
D. Pain assessment encompasses the pain experiences including nature, impact, and context.
E. The multidimensional pain assessment incorporates a clinical assessment on general comfort, treatment effectiveness, pain intensity, activity level, and sleep quality.
F. The tool chosen must be individualized, incorporate child and parental input, developmentally appropriate, valid, and reliable.

Clinical Assessment

A. Obtain a verbal report by the child. Children as young as 3 years of age are able to report the location and degree of pain they are experiencing. The PN collaborates with the registered nurse (RN) to determine the presence of pain and formulates effective interventions to relieve the child's pain.
B. Observe for nonverbal signs of pain, such as grimacing, irritability, restlessness, and difficulty in sleeping or feeding. (This is especially important in nonverbal infants and children.)
C. Include the child's parents in the assessment.

D. Observe for physiologic responses to pain, such as increased heart rate, increased respiratory rate, diaphoresis, and decreased oxygen levels.
E. Physiologic responses to pain are most often seen in response to acute pain rather than in response to chronic pain.

Clinical Judgment

A. Use a pain rating scale appropriate for the child's age and developmental level.
B. *Neonates and infants*
   1. Premature infants, starting around 20 weeks gestation, can perceive and respond to pain. To conserve energy, they frequently show a less-robust physical response compared to full-term infants (for example, they are more likely to close their eyes instead of grimacing and often have lower oxygen saturation levels). This unique response requires a scale specific to premature infants.
   2. The Premature Infant Pain Profile (PIPP), valid only for premature infants ≤37 weeks gestation, is well equipped to measure pain in this patient population. The Neonatal Pain, Agitation and Sedation Scale (N-PASS) includes a sedation assessment so that only one scale is needed for infants 23 weeks gestation through 100 days of life. The N-PASS scores pain/agitation from 0 to 10 and sedation from −10 to 0.
   3. Scales appropriate for full-term and older infants include the Neonatal Infant Pain Scale, the FLACC (Face, Legs, Activity, Cry, Consolability) scale, Child Facial Coding System, CRIES (Crying, requires increased oxygen administration, Increased vital signs, Expression, Sleeplessness) score, Children's Hospital of Eastern Ontario Pain Scale, Riley Infant Pain Scale, and Children and Infants Postoperative Pain Scale.
C. *Toddlers* self-report scales are preferred when children can communicate pain with words (usually by age 3 to 4 years) self-reporting using faces scales.
   1. Faces Pain Scale-Revised (FPS-R) and Wong-Baker FACES pain rating scale. Use the same scale with a child rather than alternating between scales.
D. *School age and adolescents*
   1. Many older children (8 years and older) can self-report pain by using a 0 to 10 scale. Numeric rating scales are easy to use and may be verbal (Verbal Numerical Rating Scale) or written (Visual Analogue Scale) (Fig. 5.4).

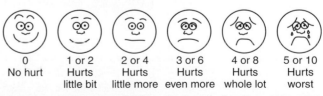

0	1 or 2	2 or 4	3 or 6	4 or 8	5 or 10
No hurt	Hurts little bit	Hurts little more	Hurts even more	Hurts whole lot	Hurts worst

Fig. 5.4 Wong-Baker FACES Pain Rating Scale. (From Wong-Baker FACES Foundation. [2016]. Wong-Baker FACES® Pain Rating Scale. Retrieved June 3, 2016, with permission from http://www.WongBakerFACES.org)

E. *Children with cognitive developmental delays*
1. These children are at increased risk for poor pain assessment and management. Several scales exist, each with varying levels of reliability and validity.
2. The revised FLACC (r-FLACC) has been validated in children from age 4 to 19 years. Using the original FLACC scale as a base, additional indicators (such as head banging and breath holding) were added, along with space for parents to document any features unique to their child. The scale measures Facial expression, Leg movements, Activity, Cry, and Consolability.
3. Another helpful tool is the Individualized Numeric Rating Scale. Caregivers are asked to assign a number to typical pain behavior seen in their child. The scale must be periodically updated because pain signs may change as the child ages.

F. *Intubated and mechanically ventilated children*
1. The COMFORT scale (Van Dijk, et al.) uses six behavioral and two physiological metrics for a total score from 8 to 40.

> **HESI HINT** The American Society of Pain Management Nursing position statement recommends using self-report if possible, evaluating potential sources of pain, assessing patient behaviors, incorporating physiologic measures (keeping in mind that they may not be specific to pain), soliciting input from parents, and assuming pain is present if the child is undergoing a painful procedure or has known reasons for pain (Table 5.2).

2. Nonpharmacologic interventions
   a. Should be used according to the child's age and developmental level
   b. Infants may respond best to pacifiers, holding, and rocking.
   c. Toddlers and preschoolers may respond best to distraction. Distraction may be provided through books, music, television, and bubble blowing.
   d. School-aged children and adolescents may use guided imagery.

TABLE 5.2 Pediatric Pain Management

Age Group	Recommended Pain Scale
Neonates—infants	Premature Infant Pain Profile (PIPP)
	Face, legs, activity, cry, consolability (FLACC)
Toddlers	Numeric rating scales (1—10) or visual analog scales (FACES) or FPS-R (Faces Pain Scale-Revised, p. 134, Fig. 5.1)
School age—adolescents	Numeric rating scales (1—10) or visual analog scales (FACES, FLAAC)
Intubated/mechanical ventilated children	The Comfort Scale (scores 8—40 items on behavioral and physiological/higher score = more discomfort/pain)

Data from Wrona SK, Melnyk BM, Hoying J. Chronic Pain and Mental Health Co-Morbidity in Adolescents: An Urgent Call for Assessment and Evidence-Based Intervention. *Pain Manag Nurs*. 2021 Jun; 22: 252-259.

e. Other interventions may include massage, application of heat or cold, and deep-breathing exercises.
3. Pharmacologic interventions
   a. Before administering a pain medication to a pediatric client, verify that the prescribed dose is safe for the child on the basis of the child's weight (mg/kg).
   b. Monitor the child's vital signs after administration of opioid medications.
   c. Children as young as 5 years of age may be taught to use a patient-controlled analgesia (PCA) pump.
   d. Children may deny pain if they fear receiving an intramuscular (IM) injection.

CHILD HEALTH PROMOTION

Description: Immunization of children against communicable diseases is one of the greatest accomplishments of modern medicine. Childhood mortality and morbidity rates have greatly decreased. Protection against disease should begin in infancy according to the recommendations of the American Academy of Pediatrics and the U.S. Public Health Service (Table 5.3).

Recommendations can be found at: http://www.cdc.gov/vaccines/schedules/hcp/child-adolescent.html, https://www.cdc.gov/vaccines/schedules/hcp/imz/child-adolescent.html#vaccines-schedule, and https://www.cdc.gov/vaccines/schedules/index.html.

A. The nursing care of children with communicable diseases is virtually the same for all, regardless of the particular disease (Table 5.4).

> **HESI HINT** Protection against communicable disease should begin in infancy according to the recommendations of the American Academy of Pediatrics and the U.S. Public Health Service. Recommendations can be found in Table 5.3.

Clinical Care for Children With Communicable Disease

A. Isolate child during period of communicability.
B. Treat fever with *nonaspirin* product.
C. Report occurrence to the health department.
D. Prevent child from scratching skin (e.g., cut nails, apply mittens, and provide soothing baths).
E. Administer diphenhydramine hydrochloride (HCl; i.e., Benadryl) as prescribed for itching.
F. Wash hands after caring for child and handling secretions or child's articles.
G. Administer vaccinations using the recommended Centers for Disease Control and Prevention [CDC] schedule.

> **HESI HINT** Children with communicable disease pose a serious threat to their unborn siblings. The PN should counsel all expectant mothers, especially those with young children, to be aware of the serious consequences of exposure to communicable diseases during pregnancy.

TABLE 5.3   Vaccines

Type of Vaccine	Description
Measles, Mumps, Rubella Vaccine • Measles, mumps, rubella (MMR) • Offers protection against these three diseases	• It is generally administered at 12–15 months of age and repeated at 4–6 years or by 11–12 years. • In times of measles epidemics, it is possible to give measles protection at 6 months and repeat the MMR at 15 months. • Measles vaccine is contraindicated for persons with history of anaphylactic reaction to neomycin or eggs, those with known altered immunodeficiency, and pregnant women. It may be given to those with human immunodeficiency virus (HIV) and to breastfeeding women. • Administer subcutaneously at separate sites. • Child may have a light, transient rash 2 weeks after administration of vaccine.

DTaP Vaccine
• Diphtheria, pertussis, tetanus
• Offers protection against these diseases
	• Beginning at age 2 months, administer three doses at 2-month intervals.
	• Booster doses given at 15–18 months and at 4–6 years.
	• Administer IM (separate site from other vaccine).
	• Not given to children past the seventh birthday; they receive Td, which contains full-strength protection against tetanus and lesser-strength diphtheria protection.
	• When pertussis vaccine is contraindicated, give DT, full-strength diphtheria, and tetanus without pertussis vaccine, until seventh birthday.
	• Contraindications to pertussis vaccine include:
	  • Encephalopathy within 7 days of previous dose of DTaP
	  • History of seizures
	  • Neurologic symptoms after receiving the vaccine
	  • Systemic allergic reactions to the vaccine
	• Parents should be instructed to begin acetaminophen (Tylenol) administration after the immunization (normal dosage is 10–15 mg/kg).
	• Instruct parents to report immediately any side effects of the immunization to the primary caregiver.

Polio Vaccine • Inactive polio vaccine (IPV)	• Recommended for all persons under 18 years. • Administer at 2 months of age and again at 4 months of age. Boosters are given at 6–18 months and at 4–6 years. • Administer IPV subcutaneously or IM at separate site. • IPV is contraindicated for those with history of anaphylactic reaction to neomycin or streptomycin. • May give with all other vaccines.
Hib (*Haemophilus influenzae* Type B) Vaccine • Offers protection against bacteria that cause serious illness (epiglottitis, bacterial meningitis, septic arthritis) in small children and those with chronic illnesses such as sickle cell disease	• Three conjugate vaccines have been recommended for administration to infants: PRP-OPMs can be given beginning as early as 2 months of age; DTaP/Hib combinations should not be used as primary immunizations at ages 2, 4, or 6 months. • Vaccines have different series administration schedules; the schedules cover children through 5 years of age. • Children at high risk who were not immunized previously should be immunized after the age of 5. • Administer IM. • There are no contraindications.
Hepatitis B • Offers protection against hepatitis B • May be given to newborns before hospital discharge • All children up to 18 years of age should be vaccinated.	• Is contraindicated for persons with anaphylactic reaction to common baker's yeast.
Varicella • Offers protection against chickenpox • Is a school entry requirement in almost all states • Is safe for children with asymptomatic HIV infection	• Administer at 12–18 months of age (must be at least 12 months). • Give MMR and varicella on same day or > 30 days apart (separate site).

Continued

TABLE 5.3 Vaccines—cont'd

Type of Vaccine	Description
Tuberculosis (TB) Skin Testing	

• Offers screening for exposure to TB	• Screening is usually done using one of the following:
	  • Mantoux test with PPD (tuberculin purified protein derivative) injected intradermally on the forearm; standard method for identifying infection with *Mycobacterium tuberculosis*
	  • Tine test (OT, old tuberculin), which consists of four prongs pressed into the forearm. These multiple puncture tests are unreliable and should not be used to determine the presence of a TB infection
	• A positive reaction represents exposure to *M. tuberculosis*.
	• Screening can be initiated at 12 months.

Covid-19	• mRNA (Pfizer Biotech)
	  • Age 5 and older
	  • 2 doses, separated by 21 days; both doses must be the appropriate Pfizer-BioNTech vaccine formulations for recipient's age
	  • At least 28 days after completion of the primary series (2nd dose) if 18 or older
	• mRNA (Moderna)
	  • 2 doses, separated by 28 days; both doses must be Moderna vaccine
	  • At least 28 days after completion of the primary series (2nd dose) if 18 or older
	• Viral vector (Janssen, J&J)
	  • 1 dose (18 years & older) mRNA COVID-19 vaccine series is preferred over Janssen COVID-19 vaccine for primary vaccination.

Adapted from https://www.cdc.gov/vaccines/covid-19/downloads/covid19-vaccine-quick-reference-guide-2pages.pdf.

Pediatric Nutritional Assessment

Description: Profile of the child's and family's eating habits

A. Iron deficiency occurs most commonly in children 12 to 36 months old, in adolescent females, and in females during their childbearing years.

The recommended daily amount of vitamin D is 400 international units (IU) for children up to age 12 months, 600 IU for people ages 1 to 70 years, and 800 IU for people over 70 years

  1. If a mother is not taking enough vitamin D, it is recommended that the infant receive an oral dose of 400 IU/daily.

B. The vitamins most often consumed in less-than-appropriate amounts by preschool and school-age children are

  1. Vitamin A
  2. Vitamin C
  3. Vitamin B_6
  4. Vitamin B_{12}

Clinical Interventions

A. Determine dietary history.

  1. The 24-hour recall: Ask the family to recall all food and liquid intake during the past 24 hours.

  2. Food diary: Ask the family to keep a 3-day record (2 weekdays and 1 weekend day) of all food and liquid intake and the amount of each.

  3. Food frequency record: Provide a questionnaire and ask family to record information regarding the number of times per day, week, or month a child consumes items from the four food groups.

B. Perform a clinical assessment or physical exam

  1. Observe the skin, hair, teeth, lips, tongue, and eyes.

  2. Use anthropometry: measurement of height, weight, body mass index (BMI), head circumference in young children, proportion, skinfold thickness, and arm circumference.

    a. Height and head circumference reflect past nutrition.

    b. Weight, skinfold thickness, and arm circumference reflect present nutritional status (especially protein and fat reserves).

    c. Skinfold thickness provides a measurement of the body's fat content (half of the body's total fat stores are directly beneath the skin).

C. Obtain biochemical analysis.

    a. Plasma, blood cells, urine, or tissues from liver, bone, hair, or fingernails can be used to determine nutritional status.

    b. Laboratory testing of hemoglobin (Hgb), hematocrit (Hct), albumin, creatinine, and nitrogen are commonly used to determine nutritional status.

D. Implement appropriate nursing judgment, including client and family teaching, to correct identified nutritional deficits (Table 5.5).

DIARRHEA

Description: Increased number or decreased consistency of stools

A. Diarrhea can be a serious or fatal symptom, especially in infancy.

TABLE 5.4 Communicable Disease in Children

Name of Communicable Disease	Definition	Clinical Transmission	Clinical Symptoms	Clinical Treatment
Rubeola (measles)	A highly contagious viral disease that can lead to neurologic problems or death	Transmitted by direct contact with droplets from infected persons Contagious mainly during the prodromal period Incubation period: 14–21 days	Fever and upper respiratory symptoms including the following: Classic Photophobia Koplik spots	Bed rest Fluids Isolation
Paramyxovirus (mumps)	A viral infection that affects the salivary glands below and in front of the ears. The disease spreads through infected saliva.		Fever, headache, malaise, parotid gland swelling and tenderness; manifestations include submaxillary and sublingual infection, orchitis, and meningoencephalitis	Analgesics are used for pain and antiseptics for fever. Bed rest is maintained until swelling subsides.
Rubella (German measles)	Common viral disease that has teratogenic effects on fetus during the first trimester of pregnancy	Transmitted by droplet and direct contact with infected person	Discrete red maculopapular rash that starts on face and rapidly spreads to entire body Rash disappears within 3 days Fever, headache	Prevention: vaccination

Name of Communicable Disease	Definition	Clinical Transmission	Clinical Symptoms	Clinical Treatment
Varicella (chickenpox)	Viral disease characterized by skin lesions	Transmitted by direct contact, droplet spread, or freshly contaminated objects Communicable prodromal period to the time all lesions have crusted	Lesions that begin on the trunk and spread to the face and proximal extremities Progresses through macular, papular, vesicular, and pustular stages	CDC recommends two doses of varicella vaccine for everyone Children should receive their first dose of varicella vaccine between 12 and 15 months of age and their second dose at 4 to 6 years of age.

TABLE 5.5   Nutritional Assessment

Nutrient	Signs of Deficiency	Food Sources
• Iron	• Anemia • Pale conjunctiva • Pale skin color • Atrophy of papillae on tongue • Brittle, ridged, spoon-shaped nails • Thyroid edema	• Iron-fortified formula • Infant high-protein cereal • Infant rice cereal • Liver • Beef • Pork • Eggs
• Vitamin B_2 (riboflavin)	• Redness and fissuring of eyelid corners; burning, itching, tearing eyes; photophobia • Magenta-colored tongue, glossitis • Seborrheic dermatitis, delayed wound healing	• Prepared infant formula • Liver • Cow's milk • Cheddar cheese • Some green leafy vegetables (broccoli, green beans, spinach) • Enriched cereals
• Vitamin A (retinol)	• Dry, rough skin • Dull cornea; soft cornea; Bitot spots • Night blindness • Defective tooth enamel • Retarded growth; impaired bone formation • Decreased thyroxine formation	• Liver • Sweet potatoes • Carrots • Spinach • Peaches • Apricots
• Vitamin C (ascorbic acid)	• Scurvy • Receding gums that are spongy and prone to bleeding • Dry, rough skin; petechiae • Decreased wound healing • Increased susceptibility to infection • Irritability, anorexia, apprehension	• Strawberries • Oranges and orange juice • Tomatoes • Broccoli • Cabbage • Cauliflower • Spinach
• Vitamin B_6 (pyridoxine)	• Scaly dermatitis • Weight loss • Anemia • Irritability • Convulsions • Peripheral neuritis	• Meats, especially liver • Cereals (wheat and corn) • Yeast • Soybeans • Peanuts • Tuna • Chicken • Bananas

B. Causes include but are not limited to
  1. Infections: bacterial, viral, parasitic
  2. Malabsorption problems
  3. Inflammatory diseases
  4. Dietary factors
C. Conditions associated with diarrhea are
  1. Dehydration
  2. Metabolic acidosis
  3. Shock

Clinical Assessment

A. Usually occurs in infants
B. History of exposure to pathogens, contaminated food, dietary changes

C. Signs of dehydration
  1. Poor skin turgor/tenting of skin
  2. Absence of tears
  3. Dry and sticky mucous membranes
  4. Weight loss (5% to 15%)
  5. Depressed fontanel
  6. Decreased urinary output, increased specific gravity
  7. Acidotic state
D. Laboratory signs of acidosis
  1. Loss of bicarbonate (serum pH <7.35)
  2. Loss of sodium and potassium through stools
  3. Elevated Hct
  4. Elevated blood urea nitrogen (BUN)
E. Signs of shock (late signs)
  1. Decreased blood pressure

2. Rapid, weak pulse
3. Skin: mottled to gray color; cool and clammy to touch
4. Delayed capillary refill greater than (+) 4 seconds
5. Changes in mental status

Clinical Judgment

A. Assess hydration status and vital signs frequently.
B. Monitor intake and output.
C. Do not take temperature rectally.
D. Rehydrate as prescribed with fluids and electrolytes.
E. Collect specimens to aid in diagnosis of cause.
F. Check stools for pH, glucose, and blood.
G. Administer antibiotics as prescribed.
H. Check urine for specific gravity.
I. Institute careful isolation precautions; wash hands with soap and water.
J. Teach home care of child with diarrhea
   1. Provide child with oral rehydration solution such as Pedialyte or Lytren.
   2. Child may temporarily need lactose-free diet.
   3. Children should not receive antidiarrheals (e.g., Imodium A−D).
   4. Do not give child grape juice, orange juice, apple juice, cola, or ginger ale. These solutions have high osmolality.

> **HESI HINT** Antibiotics are not recommended for diarrhea. They are only prescribed if the child has diarrhea caused by a bacterial, fungal, or parasitic infection.

Burns

Description: Tissue injuries caused by heat, electricity, chemicals, or radiation

A. Burns are a major cause of accidental death in children younger than 15 (after automobile accidents).
B. Burns in children are preventable, especially among children under the age of 4 years. The majority of children hospitalized for burns suffer from scald burns (65%) while 20% have contact burns (Johns Hopkins Medicine, 2021, *Burns in Children.*).
C. Scald burns
   1. Children younger than 5 are one of the two highest-risk groups.
   2. Ranked the top cause of burns (accidentally or purposeful) to children younger than 4 years old.
   3. Hot water heater temperature greater than 140 degrees can cause a third-degree burn on a child in 15 seconds and is responsible for 20% of childhood admissions for scald burns.
D. Children younger than age 2 have a higher mortality rate due to
   1. Greater central body surface area. In a child younger than 2, a greater part of the body surface area is concentrated

in the head and trunk compared with an older child or an adult; therefore, the younger child is more likely to have serious effects from burns to the trunk and head (Fig. 5.5)

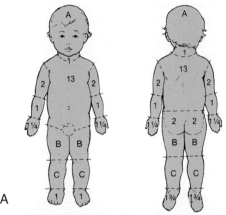

RELATIVE PERCENTAGES OF AREAS AFFECTED BY GROWTH

AREA	BIRTH	AGE 1 YR	AGE 5 YR
A = ½ of head	9½	8½	6½
B = ½ of one thigh	2¾	3¼	4
C = ½ of one leg	2½	2½	2¾

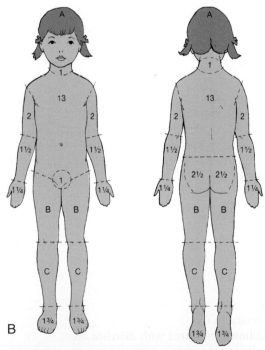

RELATIVE PERCENTAGES OF AREAS AFFECTED BY GROWTH

AREA	AGE 10 YR	AGE 15 YR	ADULT
A = ½ of head	5½	4½	3½
B = ½ of one thigh	4½	4½	4¾
C = ½ of one leg	3	3¼	3½

Fig. 5.5 Estimated Distribution of Burns in Children. (A) Children from birth to age 5 years. (B) Older children. (From Hockenberry, M. J. [2019]. *Wong's nursing care of infants and children* [11th ed.]. St. Louis: Mosby. Betz, C., Sowden, L. [2008]. *Mosby's pediatric nursing reference* [6th ed.]. St. Louis: Mosby.)

2. Greater fluid volume (proportionate to body size)
3. Less effective cardiovascular responses to fluid volume shifts

E. In childhood, a partial-thickness burn is considered a major burn if it involves more than 25% of body surface.

F. A full-thickness burn is considered major if it involves more than 10% of body surface.

G. Because of the changing proportions of the child, especially the infant, the rule of nines cannot be used to assess the percentage of burn (see Fig. 5.5).

H. Fluid needs should be calculated from the time of the burn.

I. The Parkland formula is a commonly used guideline for calculating fluid replacement and maintenance, which is based on the child's body surface area and should include volume for burn losses and maintenance.

J. Adequacy of fluid replacement is determined by evaluating urinary output.

> **HESI HINT** Urinary output for infants and children should be 1 to 2 mL/kg/h.

K. Specific gravity should be less than 1.025.

Non-Accidental Trauma

Description: Non-accidental trauma (NAT) is an injury that is purposefully inflicted upon a child—in other words, child abuse may be intentional or nonintentional, physical and, mental injury, sexual abuse, and emotional and physical neglect of a child. Children under the age of 1 are at the greatest risk of being abused. Often the injury is to the skin and soft tissue, but approximately a third of NATs are fractures. In 2011, 3.4 million instances of NAT were reported to child protection agencies in the U.S. Death from inflicted injury that year was estimated at 2.1 per 100,000 children. All physicians, nurses, and other health care workers are required by law to report suspected abuse. Child neglect is the most common form of abuse (80%).

A. Children under the age of 4 are more at risk for being a victim.

B. Children of special needs are at an increased risk of being abused or neglected.

C. Abused individuals are at an increased risk of becoming a perpetrator of abuse (Weber, 2015a).

Clinical Assessment

A. Most important indicators of NAT
 1. Injuries not congruent with the child's developmental age or skills
 2. Injuries not correlated with the stated cause of injury
  a. Bruises in unusual places and in various stages of healing
  b. Bruises, welts caused by belts, cords, etc.
  c. Burns (cigarette, iron); immersion burns (symmetrical in shape)

  d. Whiplash injuries caused by being shaken
  e. Bald patches where hair was pulled out
  f. Fractures in various stages of healing
 3. Delay in seeking medical care
 4. Failure to thrive (FTT), unattended-to physical problems
 5. Torn, stained, bloody underclothes
 6. Lacerations of external genitalia
 7. Older child bedwetting or soiling
 8. Child with sexually transmitted diseases
 9. Child appearing frightened and withdrawn in the presence of parent or other adult

Clinical Judgment

A. PNs are legally required to report all cases of suspected NAT to the appropriate local or state agency.

B. Take color photographs of injuries.

C. Document factual, objective statements about child's physical condition, child–family interactions, and interviews with family.

D. Establish trust, and care for the child's physical problems; these are the primary and immediate needs of these children.

E. Recognize own feelings of anger toward the parents.

F. Utilize principles of crisis intervention.

G. Assist child and family to develop self-esteem.

H. Teach basic child development and parenting skills to family.

I. Support the need for family therapy.

> **HESI HINT** When NAT is suspected, look for patterns of injury. If getting the patient's history raises concerns, primary care providers should evaluate the patient for cutaneous, cranial, ocular, visceral, and orthopedic injuries (Fig. 5.6).

Poisonings

Every day, over 300 children in the United States ages 0 to 19 are treated in an emergency department, and two children die, as a result of being poisoned. Chemicals in your home marked with clear warning labels can be dangerous to children (Centers for Disease Control and Prevention [CDC], *Poisoning Prevention*, 2019, February 6).

Description: Ingesting, inhaling, or absorbing a toxic substance

A. Poisoning, particularly by ingestion, is a common cause of childhood injury and illness.

B. Poisonings occur in all age groups. However, peak poisonings occur in 1- and 2-year-olds but some poisonings that occur in teens and adults can be more serious (Poison Statistics, 2019 Poison Control).

C. The majority of poisonings (>90%) occur in the home such as in the kitchen, bathroom, or bedroom (Health Resources & Service Administration [HRSA], 2021, *Poison Help and Prevention Tips*).

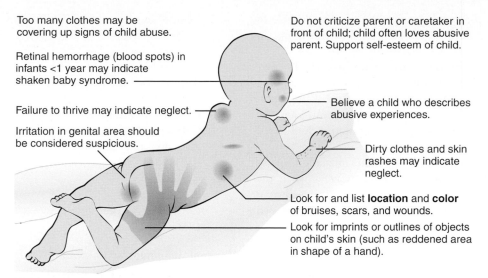

Too many clothes may be covering up signs of child abuse.

Retinal hemorrhage (blood spots) in infants <1 year may indicate shaken baby syndrome.

Failure to thrive may indicate neglect.

Irritation in genital area should be considered suspicious.

Do not criticize parent or caretaker in front of child; child often loves abusive parent. Support self-esteem of child.

Believe a child who describes abusive experiences.

Dirty clothes and skin rashes may indicate neglect.

Look for and list **location** and **color** of bruises, scars, and wounds.

Look for imprints or outlines of objects on child's skin (such as reddened area in shape of a hand).

Divide the body into four planes: front, back, right side, and left side. Injuries occurring in >1 plane should be considered suspicious.

Fig. 5.6 Assessing for Child Abuse. (From Leifer, G. [2014]. *Introduction to maternity and pediatric nursing* [7th ed., pp. 575–576]. St. Louis: Saunders.)

Clinical Assessment

A. Child found near source of poison
B. Gastrointestinal (GI) disturbance: nausea, abdominal pain, diarrhea, vomiting
C. Burns of mouth, pharynx
D. Respiratory distress
E. Seizures, changes in level of consciousness (LOC)
F. Cyanosis
G. Shock

Clinical Judgment

A. Identify the poisonous agent as soon as suspected
B. Observe the child's respiratory, cardiac, and neurologic status.
C. Instruct parent to bring any emesis, stool, etc., to the emergency department.
D. Determine the child's age and weight.

> **HESI HINT** The nationwide poison control center phone number, 1-800-222-1222, on or near every telephone in your home and program it into your cell phone. Call the poison control center if you think a child has been poisoned but they are awake and alert. Call 911 if you have a poison emergency and your child has collapsed or is not breathing.

E. Poison removal and care may require gastric lavage, activated charcoal, N-acetylcysteine, or naloxone HCl.
F. Teach home safety.
   1. Poison-proof and child-proof the home.
      a. Identify location of poisons: under the sink (cleaning supplies, drain cleaners, bug poisons); medicine cabinets; storage rooms (paints, varnishes); garages (antifreeze, gasoline); poisonous plants (philodendron, dieffenbachia).
      b. Put locks on cabinets.
      c. Use safety containers: do not place poisonous materials in non–child-proof containers.
      d. Discard unused medications.
   2. Make sure child is always under adult supervision.
   3. The nationwide poison control center phone number, 1-800-222-1222
   4. Examine the environment from the child's viewpoint (the height to which a 2- to 5-year-old can reach).
   5. Be aware of changes in the child's environment because of house guests or visiting a relative or friends.
G. Contact community health nurse or child welfare agency if necessary.

> **HESI HINT** Common household products that are poisonous to children if ingested include: perfume and aftershave, sunburn relief products, alcohol, cigarettes or any type of tobacco products, and mouthwash.

Lead Poisoning

Description: CDC now uses a blood lead reference value of 5 micrograms per deciliter (µg/dL) to identify children with blood lead levels that are much higher than most children's levels. This new level is based on the U.S. population of children ages 1 to 5 years who are in the highest 2.5% of children when tested for lead in their blood. There is no established "safe" level of lead for children. Every system in the human body can be affected by lead exposure. Lead exposure and elevated levels have been linked to decreased IQs (Centers for Disease Control and Prevention (CDC), 2021, October 27, *Childhood Lead Poisoning Prevention*).

A. Children 6 years of age and younger are most vulnerable to the effects of lead because children tend to put things in their mouths.

B. Though lead can be found in many places in a child's environment, lead exposure is preventable. The key is stopping children from coming into contact with lead. Parents can take simple steps to make their homes more lead-safe. The major cause of lead poisoning is deteriorating lead-based paint.

C. Lead enters the body through ingestion, inhalation, or, in the case of an unborn child, placental transfer when the mother is exposed. The most common route is ingestion either from hand-to-mouth behavior via contaminated hands, fingers, toys, or pacifiers or, less often, from eating sweet-tasting loose paint chips found in a home built before the 1950s or in a play area.

D. The renal, neurologic, and hematologic systems are the most seriously affected by lead.

E. The blood lead level (BLL) test is currently used for screening and diagnosis. BLL testing is currently required at 12 and 24 months for all Medicaid-enrolled children, unless the state has a Centers for Disease Control and Prevention and Centers for Medicare and Medicaid Services (CDC/CMS) waiver indicating that children enrolled in Medicaid are not at higher risk for high BLLs than other children.

Clinical Assessment

A. Screen for lead poisoning using CDC guidelines of blood lead surveillance and other risk factor data collected over time to establish the status and risk of children throughout the state.

B. In areas without available data, universal screening is recommended.
   1. All children should have a BLL test at the ages of 1 and 2 years.
      a. Collect blood in a capillary tube and send to the laboratory.
      b. During collection, avoid contamination of blood specimen and lead on the skin.
   2. Any child between 3 and 6 years of age who has not been screened should also be tested.

C. Obtain a history of possible sources of lead in the child's environment.

D. Physical assessment
   1. General signs/symptoms
      a. Anemia
      b. GI
         1) Acute cramping; abdominal pain
         2) Vomiting
         3) Constipation
         4) Anorexia
      c. Neurologic
         1) Headache
         2) Lethargy
      d. Impaired growth

2. Central nervous system (CNS) signs (early)
   a. Hyperactivity
   b. Aggression
   c. Impulsiveness
   d. Decreased interest in play
   e. Irritability
   f. Short attention span
3. CNS signs (late)
   a. Mental retardation
   b. Paralysis
   c. Blindness
   d. Convulsions
   e. Coma
   f. Death

Clinical Judgment

A. Identify sources of lead in the environment to prevent further exposure.

B. Administer prescribed chelating agents to reduce high BLL levels.

C. Dimercaprol (chelating agent) is contraindicated in patients with a peanut allergy or hepatic insufficiency

D. intramuscular (IM) and intravenous (IV) administration
   1. Calcium disodium ethylenediaminetetraacetic acid (EDTA) is generally administered IM.
   2. Dimercaprol (also called BAL) is given in conjunction with calcium disodium EDTA (may contain peanut oil) to help in efficacy of treatment.
   3. Considerations for administration.
      a. Rotate injection sites if chelating agent is given IM.
      b. Reassure child that injections are a treatment, not a punishment.
      c. Administer the local anesthetic procaine with IM injection of calcium disodium EDTA to reduce discomfort.
      d. Apply eutectic mixture of local anesthetics (EMLA) cream over puncture site 2½ hours before the injection to reduce discomfort.

> **HESI HINT** Monitor client's renal functioning and complete blood count (CBC) while client is receiving chelating agents.

E. Avoid giving iron during chelation because of possible interactive effects.

F. If home oral chelation therapy is used, teach family proper administration of medication.

G. Administer prescribed cleansing enemas or cathartic for acute lead ingestion.

H. Assist family to obtain sources of help for removing lead from the environment.
   1. Do not vacuum hard-surfaced floors or windowsills or window wells in homes built before 1960 because this spreads dust.
   2. Wash and dry child's hands and face frequently, especially before the child eats.

3. Wash toys and pacifiers frequently.
4. Make sure that home exposure is not occurring from parental occupations or hobbies.

RESPIRATORY DISORDERS

Clinical Assessment in Children

A. Normal pulse and respiratory rates (Table 5.6)
B. Signs of respiratory distress in children
   1. Flaring nostrils
   2. Grunting
   3. Retractions
   4. Grunting
   5. Adventitious breath sounds (or absent breath sounds) (Stanford Childrens' Health, 2021, *Signs of Respiratory Distress in Children*).

HESI HINT Symptoms of hypoxia
Early: restlessness, anxiety, tachycardia/tachypnea
Late: bradycardia, extreme restlessness, severe dyspnea
Pediatrics: difficulty feeding, inspiratory stridor, nares flaring, grunting with expirations, sternal retractions

---

C. Clinical judgment

1. Child often goes into respiratory failure before cardiac failure.
2. Identify signs of respiratory distress.

Asthma

Description: Inflammatory reactive airway disease that is commonly chronic

A. The airways become edematous.
B. The airways become congested with mucus.
C. The smooth muscles of the bronchi and bronchioles constrict.
D. Air trapping occurs in the alveoli.
E. Differences with the anatomy in children:
   1. Infants have smaller nares, and are obligate nose breathers (until about 1 to 2 months of age).
   2. Children 8 and younger have immature cartilage, and the epiglottis is more flaccid, making it difficult to completely close.
   3. The trachea has a narrower diameter than an adult's.
   4. Lung tissue develops and grows from birth to about the age of 12.
   5. The alveoli multiply over 10 times the amount an infant is born with.
   6. Children younger than 6 breathe with their abdominal muscles, as there is weak musculature with thoracic muscles (Ward & Hisley, 2011).

Clinical Assessment

A. History of asthma in the family
B. History of allergies and/or eczema
C. Home environment containing pets or other allergens
D. Tight cough (nonproductive cough) usually occurs and/or worsens at nighttime
E. Breath sounds: coarse expiratory wheezing, rales, crackles
F. Chest diameter enlarges (late sign and symptom)
G. Increased number of school days missed during past 6 months
H. Signs of respiratory distress

Clinical Judgment

A. Observe carefully for increasing respiratory distress.
B. Assist RN with the administration of a rapid-acting bronchodilator and steroids for acute attacks.

TABLE 5.6 Normal Pulse and Respiratory Rates for Children

Age	Pulse	Respirations	Nursing Implications
Newborn	100–160	30–60	These ranges are averages only and vary with the sex, age, and condition of the child. Always note whether the child is crying, febrile, or in some distress.
1–11 months	100–150	25–35	
1–3 years (toddler)	80–130	20–30	
3–5 years (preschooler)	80–120	20–25	
6–10 years (school age)	70–110	18-22	
10–16 years (adolescent)	60–90	16-20	

C. Maintain hydration (oral fluids or IV).

D. Monitor blood gas values for signs of respiratory acidosis.

E. Administer oxygen or nebulizer therapy as prescribed.

F. Monitor pulse oximetry as prescribed (usually >95% is normal).

G. Monitor beta-adrenergic agonists, as well as anti-inflammatory corticosteroids, which are commonly used medications (Table 5.7).

H. Teach home care program, including:
   1. Identifying precipitating factors
   2. Eliminating triggers
   3. Reducing allergens in the home
   4. Using metered-dose inhaler/nebulizer
   5. Monitoring peak expiratory flow rate at home
   6. Doing breathing exercises
   7. Monitoring drug actions, dosages, and side effects (Fig. 5.7)
   8. Managing acute episode and when to seek emergency care

I. Refer child and family for emotional and psychological counseling.

Cystic Fibrosis

A. Description: An autosomal-recessive disease caused by a defective gene that inhibits the transport of water and sodium in and out of cells. As a result, secretions become tenacious which causes dysfunction of the exocrine glands. This disease can affect any race, but Caucasians are mostly affected.
   1. Lung insufficiency (most critical problem)
   2. Pancreatic insufficiency
   3. Increased loss of sodium and chloride in sweat

Clinical Assessment

A. Meconium ileus at birth (10% to 20% of cases)

B. Recurrent respiratory infection

C. Pulmonary congestion

D. Steatorrhea (excessive fat, greasy stools)

E. Foul-smelling bulky stools

F. Delayed growth and poor weight gain

G. Skin that tastes salty when kissed (caused by excessive secretions from sweat glands)

H. End stages: cyanosis, nail-bed clubbing, congestive heart failure (CHF)

Clinical Judgment

A. Monitor respiratory status.

B. Observe for signs of respiratory infection.

C. Assist RN with the administration of IV antibiotics as prescribed; manage vascular access.

D. Administer pancreatic enzymes (Cotazym-S, Pancrease: for infants, with applesauce, rice, or cereal; for an older child, with food).

E. Administer fat-soluble vitamins (A, D, E, K) in water-soluble form.

F. Administer oxygen (Box 5.1) and nebulizer treatments (recombinant human deoxyribonuclease or dornase alfa as prescribed).

G. Evaluate effectiveness of respiratory treatments.

H. Teach family percussion and postural-drainage techniques.

I. Teach dietary recommendations: high in calories, high in protein, moderate to high in fat (more calories per volume), and moderate to low in carbohydrates (to avoid an increase in carbon dioxide [CO_2] drive).

J. Provide age-appropriate activities.

K. Refer family for genetic counseling.

HESI HINT Cystic fibrosis is now screened with newborn screening tests performed after birth. The newborn screening test can provide a diagnosis in the child's first month of life before signs and symptoms occur.

Epiglottitis

Description: Severe life-threatening infection of the epiglottis is a medical emergency

A. Epiglottitis progresses rapidly, causing acute airway obstruction.

B. The organism usually responsible for epiglottitis is Haemophilus influenzae (primarily type B).

Clinical Assessment

A. Sudden onset

B. Restlessness

C. High fever

D. Sore throat, dysphagia

E. Drooling

F. Muffled voice

G. Child assuming upright sitting position with chin out and tongue protruding ("tripod position")

Clinical Judgment

A. Encourage prevention with H. influenzae type B (Hib) vaccine.

TABLE 5.7 Adrenergics			
Drugs/Route	**Indications**	**Adverse Reactions**	**Nursing Implications**
• Epinephrine HCl INH, subcutaneous, IM, IV	• Rapid-acting bronchodilator • Drug of choice for acute asthma attack	• Tachycardia • Hypertension • Tremors • Nausea	• Give subcutaneously, IV, via nebulizer • May be repeated in 20 min

Asthma Medicine Plan

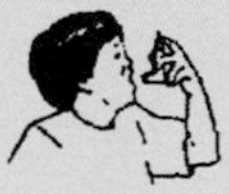

You can use the colors of a traffic light to help learn about your asthma medicines.

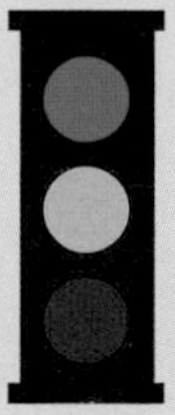

1. **Green** means **Go.**
   Use preventive medicine.

2. **Yellow** means **Caution.**
   Use quick-relief medicine.

3. **Red** means **Stop.**
   Get help from a doctor.

Name: _____

Doctor: _____ Date: _____

Phone for doctor or clinic: _____

Emergency contact phone and name: _____

1. Green — Go

- Breathing is good
- No cough or wheeze
- Can work and play

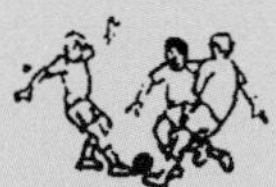

Peak flow number

_____ to _____

Personal best peak flow _____

Use preventive medicine.

Medicine	How much to take	When to take it

5 to 60 minutes before exercise, use this medicine:

_____

2. Yellow — Caution

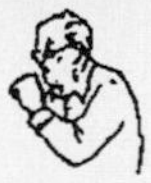

Cough 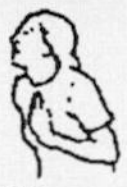   Wheeze 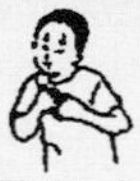   Tight chest

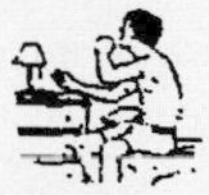

Wake up at night

Peak flow number

_____ to _____

(50 to 80% of my best peak flow)

Take quick-relief medicine to keep an asthma attack from getting bad

Medicine	How much to take	When to take it
(short-acting beta$_2$ agonist)		

If symptoms return to Green Zone after 1 hour of taking above quick-relief medication, take _____ (medicine) and _____ (medicine).

If symptoms **do not** return to Green Zone after 1 hour of taking the quick-relief medication, take _____ (medicine) and add _____ (medicine).
   (short-acting beta$_2$ agonist)   *(oral steroid)*

Call your doctor if symptoms do not improve within _____ hours after taking the oral steroid or if your symptoms are in the Red Zone.

3. Red — Stop — Danger

- Medicine is not helping
- Breathing is hard and fast
- Nose opens wide
- Can't walk
- Ribs show
- Can't talk well

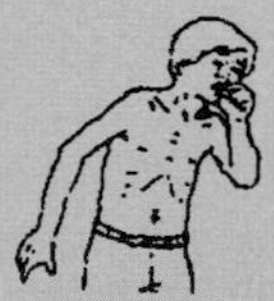

Peak flow number

_____ to _____

(50% or less of personal best)

Get help from a doctor now!
Take these medicines until you talk with the doctor.

Medicine	How much to take	When to take it
(short-acting beta$_2$ agonist)		
(oral steroid)		

Go to the emergency department immediately or call the ambulance if you cannot reach your doctor and you are still in the Red Zone after 15 minutes.

These signs signal **DANGER**:
- Difficulty walking or breathing
- Mental confusion
- Fingernails or lips are blue
Call the ambulance.

Fig. 5.7 **Asthma Action Plan.** (From NIH Publication No. 96-3659A in Hockenberry, M. J., & Wilson, D. [2015]. *Wong's nursing care of infants and children* [10th ed.]. St. Louis: Elsevier/Mosby.)

BOX 5.1   Respiratory Client

Administration of Oxygen

- Oxygen hood: used for infants.
- Nasal prongs: Provide low to moderate concentrations of oxygen (up to 4–6 L).
- Tents: Provide mist and oxygen. Monitor child's temperature. Keep edges tucked in. Keep child dry.

Measurement of Oxygenation

- Pulse oximetry measures oxygen saturation (SaO_2) of arterial Hgb non-invasively via a sensor that is usually attached to the finger or toe, or, in an infant, to sole of foot.
- Nurse should be aware of the alarm parameters signaling decreased SaO_2 (usually <95%).
- Blood gas evaluation is usually monitored in respiratory clients through arterial sampling.
- Norms: PO_2: 80–100 mm Hg; PCO_2: 35–45 mm Hg for children (not infants and newborns)

B. Maintain child in upright sitting position.
C. Prepare for intubation or tracheostomy.
D. Assist with administration of IV antibiotics as prescribed.
E. Prepare for hospitalization in intensive care unit (ICU).
F. Restrain as needed to prevent extubation.
G. Employ measures to decrease agitation and crying.

Bronchiolitis

Description: Viral infection of the bronchioles that is characterized by thick secretions
A. Bronchiolitis is usually caused by respiratory syncytial virus (RSV) and is found to be readily transmitted by close contact with hospital personnel, families, and other children.
B. Bronchiolitis occurs primarily in young infants.

Clinical Assessment

A. History of upper respiratory symptoms
B. Irritable, distressed infant
C. Paroxysmal coughing
D. Poor eating
E. Nasal congestion
F. Nasal flaring
G. Prolonged expiratory phase of respiration
H. Wheezing, rales can be auscultated
I. Deteriorating condition that is often indicated by shallow, rapid respirations

Clinical Judgment

A. Isolate child (isolation of choice for RSV is contact isolation).
B. Observe respiratory status; observe for hypoxia.
C. Clear airway of secretions using a bulb syringe for suctioning.
D. Provide care in mist tent; administer oxygen as prescribed.
E. Maintain hydration (oral and IV fluids).

F. Evaluate response to respiratory therapy treatments.
G. Administer palivizumab to provide passive immunity against RSV in high-risk children (younger than 2 years of age with a history of prematurity, lung disease, or congenital heart disease [CHD]).

Otitis Media

Description: Inflammatory disorder of the middle ear
A. Otitis media may be suppurative or serous.
B. Anatomic structure of the ear predisposes young child to ear infections.
C. The major cause of conductive hearing loss in children is otitis media with effusion.

Clinical Assessment

A. Fever, pain; infant may pull at ear
B. Enlarged lymph nodes
C. Discharge from ear (if drum is ruptured)
D. Upper respiratory symptoms
E. Vomiting, diarrhea

Clinical Judgment

A. Treatment of Acute otitis media (AOM) includes administration of antipyretics and analgesics.
B. Antimicrobial therapy in only select patients
C. Position child on affected side with head of bed elevated.
D. Provide comfort measure: warm compress on affected ear.
E. Collaborate with the RN to enhance and reinforce a teaching plan for home care.
   1. Follow-up visit.
   2. Monitor for hearing loss.
F. Teach preventive care: wash hands and toys frequently to reduce your chances of getting a cold or other respiratory infection.
G. Avoid cigarette smoke.
H. Get seasonal flu shots and pneumococcal vaccines.
I. Breastfeed infants instead of bottle feeding them if possible.
J. If the child has an eustachian tube malfunction leading to chronic infections, then the MD may perform a procedure called a myringotomy with placement of tympanostomy tubes that equalize pressure in the eustachian tubes.

> **HESI HINT** Respiratory disorders are the primary reason most children and their families seek medical care. Therefore, these disorders are frequently tested on the NGN-NCLEX-PN. Knowing the normal parameters of respiratory rates and the key signs of respiratory distress in children is essential!

Tonsillitis

Description: Inflammation of the tonsils
   Pharyngeal tonsils (adenoids) are two glands of tissue visible in the back of the throat. The tonsils function as a part of the immune system protecting the body from infections.

A. Tonsillitis may be viral or bacterial.
B. Tonsillitis may be related to infection by a Streptococcus species.
C. A complication of tonsillitis is a peritonsillar abscess, which happens when the infection spreads behind the tonsils. Early treatment is indicated as it may cause airway obstruction.

Tonsillitis is related to strep, treatment is very important because of the risk for developing. Post-streptococcal glomerulonephritis (PSGN) This may occur which is a rare kidney disease that may develop as a result from group A strep. Best practices include the prevention of streptococcal infections.

Clinical Assessment

A. Sore throat and may have difficulty swallowing that lasts longer than 48 hours
B. Fever
C. Enlarged tonsils (may have purulent discharge on tonsils)
D. Breathing may be obstructed (tonsils touching)
E. Throat culture to determine viral or bacterial cause

Clinical Judgment

A. Collect throat culture if prescribed.
B. Instruct parents in home care.
1. Encourage warm saline gargles.
2. Administer antibiotics if prescribed.
3. Manage fever with acetaminophen.
C. If a tonsillectomy is indicated:
1. Provide preoperative teaching and assessment.
2. Monitor for signs of postoperative bleeding.
   a. Frequent swallowing
   b. Vomiting fresh blood
   c. Clearing throat
3. Encourage soft foods and oral fluids (avoid red fluids, which mimic signs of bleeding); do not use straws.
4. Provide comfort measures: ice collar helps with pain and with vasoconstriction.
5. Provide education Post-tonsillectomy hemorrhage is considered a surgical emergency. Hemorrhage after tonsillectomy can be classified as primary or secondary. If bleeding occurs within the first 24 hours after surgery, it is referred to as a primary hemorrhage. Secondary hemorrhage risk occurs after 24 hours. The risk of primary hemorrhage is 0.2% to 2.2%, and secondary hemorrhage is 0.1% to 4.8%, with an increase in the risk of post-tonsillectomy hemorrhage, including age >5, chronic tonsillitis
6. In children with hemophilia or von Willebrand disease, rates of hemorrhage immediately after tonsillectomy are similar but are substantially higher with delayed hemorrhage.

HESI HINT Teach parents why it is important to administer pain medication as prescribed. Pain medication for this procedure generally has a cough suppressant property to suppress coughing.

Coughing may loosen sutures, or clots, at the surgical site causing active bleeding.

(Table 5.8)

❓ REVIEW OF RESPIRATORY DISORDERS

1. Describe the purpose of bronchodilators.
2. What are the physical assessment findings for a child with asthma?
3. What nutritional support should be provided for a child with cystic fibrosis?
4. Why is genetic counseling important for the family of a child with cystic fibrosis?
5. List signs of respiratory distress in a pediatric client.
6. What position does a child with epiglottitis assume?
7. Why are IV fluids important for a child with an increased respiratory rate?
8. Children with chronic otitis media are at risk for developing what problem?
9. What is the most common postoperative complication after a tonsillectomy? Describe the signs and symptoms of this complication.

See Answer Key at the end of this text for suggested responses.

CARDIOVASCULAR DISORDERS

Congenital Heart Disorders

Description: Heart anomalies that develop *in utero* and manifest at birth or shortly thereafter (Table 5.9)

A. CHDs are the most common birth defects. CHDs occur in almost 1% of births. Approximately 100 to 200 deaths are due to unrecognized heart disease in newborns each year. These numbers exclude those dying before diagnosis. Nearly 40,000 infants in the U.S. are born each year with CHDs (Congenital Heart Disease Facts and Statistics, 2021).
B. We can classify the different types of CHD into several categories in order to better understand the problems your baby may experience. They include:
1. Problems that cause too much blood to pass through the lungs.
2. These defects allow oxygen-rich blood that should be traveling to the body to re-circulate through the lungs, causing increased pressure and stress in the lungs. They include:
   a. Acyanotic
      1) Left-to-right shunts or increased pulmonary blood flow
      2) Obstructive defects

Acyanotic Heart Defects

Ventricular Septal Defect (Increased Pulmonary Blood Flow)

A. In this condition, a hole in the ventricular septum (a dividing wall between the two lower chambers of the heart—the right and left ventricles) occurs. Because of this opening, blood from the left ventricle flows back into the right ventricle, due to higher pressure in the left ventricle. This causes an extra volume of blood to be pumped into the lungs by the right ventricle, often creating congestion in the lungs.

TABLE 5.8 Clinical Judgment Measures: Pediatric Respiratory System

Clinical Judgment Measure	Assessment Characteristics
Recognize Cues	Note any Tachypnea
	Observe for increased heart rate (low oxygen levels may cause an increase in heart rate)
	Color changes: A bluish color seen around the mouth, on the inside of the lips, or on the fingernails, color of the skin may also appear pale or gray
	Grunting
	Nose flaring
	Retractions
	Sweating
	Wheezing
	Stridor
	Accessory muscle use
Analyze Cues	Breathing patterns are consistent with age of patient without (shortness of breath (SOB), confusion, orthopnea)
	Respiratory rate is consistent with age and diagnosis of patient
	Nares clear without mucus
	Productive/non-productive cough
	Either use or no use of accessory muscles
Prioritize Cues	Keep in mind any emergent issue related to: airway, breathing, or circulation (A, B, C)
	Observe for any change in the child's ability to respond to you, needs to be based on the child's age and developmental age
	Note alertness (mentation is what is expected for age and diagnosis)
	Change in skin color (pale, cyanosis)
Solutions	Provide interventions at the level of need
	Remember that hypoxia can manifest differently from infancy to young adult
	Provide oxygen consistent with underlying disease pathology
	Teach family breathing techniques to assure relaxation and to facilitate respirations
	Encourage routine vaccinations that are required for age
Actions	Perform resuscitation as indicated
	Check vital signs for normalcy of age and development
	Note that respiratory rate is within normal limits
	Auscultate lungs for consolidation
	Teach family members to provide rest and exercise consistent with the patient's underlying diagnosis.
Evaluate Outcomes	Respiratory status has improved (respiratory rate normal, color good, use of oxygen properly if ordered for age and patient's diagnosis)
	Response to questions noted by observation if infant, by response if older: Mentation within normal limits (recites date, time, mini-mental exam as an adolescent)
	Respiratory rate consistent with activity (walking, Activities of daily living (ADL))

TABLE 5.9 Congenital Heart Disorders

Congenital Heart Defects	Conditions	Hemodynamics	Classical Symptoms
ACYANOTIC	ASD	Increased pulmonary blood flow	Increase fatigue
L → R shunt	VSD		Murmur
	PDA		Increase risk of endocarditis
	Coarctation/stenosis of aorta	Obstructive pulmonary blood flow	CHF
			Growth retardation
CYANOTIC	Tetralogy of Fallot	Decreased pulmonary blood flow	Squatting
R → L shunt	Transposition of the great vessels (TGV)	Mixed pulmonary blood flow	Cyanosis
			Clubbing
	TA		Syncope

ASD, Atrial septal defect; *CHF*, congestive heart failure; *PDA*, patent ductus arteriosus; *TA*, truncus arteriosus; *VSD*, ventricular septal defect
Created by: Katherine T. Ralph MSN, RN, Curriculum Manager, Elsevier-NHE.

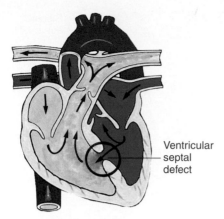

Fig. 5.8 Ventricular Septal Defect. (From Hockenberry, M. J., & Wilson, D. [2011]. *Wong's nursing care of infants and children* [9th ed.]. St. Louis: Mosby.)

B. Oxygenated blood from the left ventricle is shunted to the right ventricle and recirculated to the lungs.

C. Small defects may close spontaneously.

D. Large defects cause Eisenmenger syndrome or CHF and require surgical closures (Fig. 5.8).

Atrial Septal Defect (Increased Pulmonary Blood Flow)

A. In this condition, there is an abnormal opening between the two upper chambers of the heart—the right and left atria—causing an abnormal blood flow through the heart.

B. Oxygenated blood from the left atrium is shunted to the right atrium and lungs.

C. Most defects do not compromise children seriously.

D. Surgical closure is recommended before school age. It can lead to significant problems, such as CHF or atrial dysrhythmias later in life, if not corrected (Fig. 5.9).

Patent Ductus Arteriosus (Increased Pulmonary Blood Flow)

A. Patent ductus arteriosus (PDA): There is an abnormal opening between the aorta and the pulmonary artery. This defect short circuits the normal pulmonary vascular system and allows blood to mix between the pulmonary artery and the aorta. Prior to birth, there is an open passageway between the two blood vessels. This opening closes soon after birth. When it does not close, some blood returns to the lungs. PDA is often seen in premature infants.

B. Usually closes within 72 hours after birth.

C. Remains patent; oxygenated blood from the aorta returns to the pulmonary artery.

D. Increased blood flow to the lungs causes pulmonary hypertension.

E. May require medical intervention with indomethacin (Indocin), Ibuprofen, or Tylenol/Ofirmev administration or surgical closure (Fig. 5.10).

F. Characteristic machine-like murmur

Atrioventricular canal (AVC or AV canal): AVC is a complex heart problem that involves several abnormalities of structures inside the heart, including atrial septal defect (ASD),

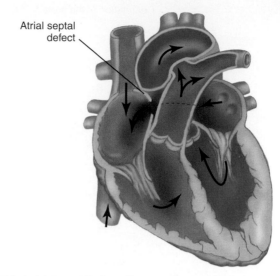

Fig. 5.9 Atrial Septal Defect. (From Hockenberry, M. J., & Wilson, D. [2011]. *Wong's nursing care of infants and children* [9th ed.]. St. Louis: Mosby.)

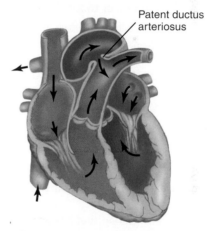

Fig. 5.10 Patent Ductus Arteriosus. (From Hockenberry, M. J., & Wilson, D. [2011]. *Wong's nursing care of infants and children* [9th ed.]. St. Louis: Mosby.)

ventricular septal defect (VSD), and improperly formed mitral and/or tricuspid valves.

Problems that cause too little blood to travel to the body

These defects are a result of underdeveloped chambers of the heart or blockages in blood vessels that prevent the proper amount of blood from traveling to the body to meet its needs. They include:

Coarctation of the Aorta (Obstruction of Blood Flow From Ventricles)

A. In this condition, the aorta is narrowed or constricted, obstructing blood flow to the lower part of the body and increasing blood pressure above the constriction.

B. The most common sites are the aortic valve and the aorta near the ductus arteriosus.

C. A common finding is hypertension in the upper extremities and decreased or absent pulses in the lower extremities.

D. Defect may require surgical correction (Fig. 5.11).

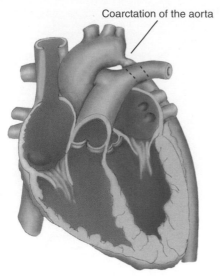

Fig. 5.11 Coarctation of the Aorta. (From Hockenberry, M. J., & Wilson, D. [2011]. *Wong's nursing care of infants and children* [9th ed.]. St. Louis: Mosby.)

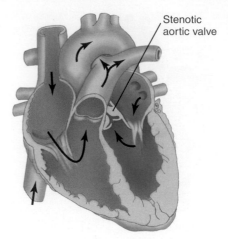

Fig. 5.12 Aortic Stenosis. (From Hockenberry, M. J., & Wilson, D. [2011]. *Wong's nursing care of infants and children* [9th ed.]. St. Louis: Mosby.)

Aortic Stenosis (Obstruction of Blood Flow From Ventricles)

A. In this condition, the aortic valve between the left ventricle and the aorta did not form properly and is narrowed, making it difficult for the heart to pump blood to the body.

B. Oxygenated blood flow from the left ventricle into systemic circulation is diminished.

C. Symptoms are caused by low cardiac output.

D. May require surgical correction (Fig. 5.12).

Hypoplastic left heart syndrome (HLHS): A combination of several abnormalities of the heart and the great blood vessels.

Problems that cause too little blood to pass through the lungs

These conditions allow blood that has not been to the lungs to pick up oxygen to travel to the body. The body does not receive enough oxygen with these heart problems. Babies with these forms of CHD may be cyanotic. These conditions include:

1. Cyanotic
   a. Right-to-left shunts or decreased blood flow
   b. Mixed blood flow

Tetralogy of Fallot (TOF) (Decreased Pulmonary Blood Flow)

A. Tetralogy of Fallot (TOF): This condition is characterized by four defects, including an abnormal opening, or VSD; a narrowing (stenosis) at or just beneath the pulmonary valve that partially blocks the flow of blood from the right side of the heart to the lungs; a right ventricle that is more muscular than normal and often enlarged; and an aorta that lies directly over the VSD.

TOF requires staged surgery for correction (Fig. 5.13).

> **HESI HINT** Hypoplastic left heart syndrome (HLHS): A combination of several abnormalities of the heart and the great blood vessels.

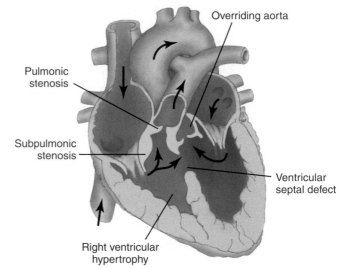

Fig. 5.13 Tetralogy of Fallot. (From Hockenberry, M. J., & Wilson, D. [2011]. *Wong's nursing care of infants and children* [9th ed.]. St. Louis: Mosby.)

Truncus Arteriosus (Mixed Blood Flow)

A. In this condition, the aorta and pulmonary artery start as a single blood vessel, which eventually divides and becomes two separate arteries. Truncus arteriosus (TA) occurs when the single great vessel fails to separate completely, leaving a connection between the aorta and pulmonary artery (Fig. 5.14).

B. One main vessel receives blood from the left and right ventricles together.

C. Blood mixes in right and left ventricles through a large VSD, resulting in cyanosis.

D. Increased pulmonary resistance results in increased cyanosis.

E. This congenital defect requires surgical correction; only the presence of the large VSD allows for survival at birth (Fig. 5.15).

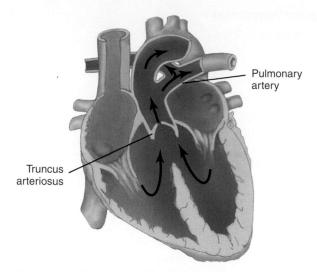

Fig. 5.14 Truncus Arteriosus. (From Hockenberry, M. J., & Wilson, D. [2011]. *Wong's nursing care of infants and children* [9th ed.]. St. Louis: Mosby.)

A.   Common physical characteristics

HEAD

1.   Small head
2.   Flat, wide nasal bridge
3.   Inner epicanthal eye fold
4.   Upward, outward slant of eyes
5.   Brushfield spots on the iris (white spots)
6.   Small, irregularly shaped ears; low-set
7.   Small mouth and protruding tongue

to

8.   Short neck
9.   Short, stubby hands with a single crease in palm (Simian crease)
10. Short arms and legs in comparison to their body
11. Short in stature
12. Hypotonic flexibility
13. Atlantoaxial instability

TOE

14. Short, stubby toes with an enlarged space between the big toe and other toes
15. Hyperextensible and lax joint (hypotonia)

Fig. 5.15 Head to Toe Common Characteristics of Down Syndrome. (From Katherine T. Ralph MSN, RN Elsevier/HESI.)

Transposition of the Great Vessels (Mixed Blood Flow)

A. Transposition of the great arteries (TGA): With this condition, the positions of the pulmonary artery and the aorta are reversed.

B. The great vessels are reversed; the pulmonary artery leaves the left ventricle, and the aorta exits from the right ventricle.

C. The pulmonary circulation arises from the left ventricle, and the systemic circulation arises from the right ventricle.

D. This is incompatible with life unless coexisting VSD, ASD, and/or PDA is present.

E. The diagnosis is a medical emergency. The child is given prostaglandin E (PGE) to keep the ductus open (see Fig. 5.13).

F. Hemodynamic classification may be used.
   1. Increased pulmonary blood flow defects (ASD, VSD, PDA)
   2. Obstructive defects (coarctation of aorta, aortic stenosis [AS])
   3. Decreased pulmonary blood flow defects (TOF)
   4. Mixed defects (TGA, TA)

Care of Children With Congenital Heart Disease
Clinical Assessment

A. Manifestations of CHD
   1. Murmur (present or absent; thrill or rub)
   2. Cyanosis, clubbing of digits
   3. Poor feeding, poor weight gain, failure to thrive
   4. Frequent regurgitation
   5. Frequent respiratory infections
   6. Activity intolerance, fatigue
B. The following are assessed:
   1. Heart rate and rhythm and heart sounds
   2. Respiratory status/difficulty
   3. Pulses (quality and symmetry)
   4. Blood pressure (all 4 extremities)
   5. Feeding difficulties; tires easily

Clinical Judgment

A. Provide care for the child with cardiovascular dysfunction.

> **HESI HINT** Congenital heart problems range from simple to complex. Some heart problems can be monitored and medically managed while others will require heart surgery or cardiac catheterization often in the first few hours after birth (Stanford Childrens' Health, 2021, *Congenital Heart Disease*).

   1. Monitor hydration defects; may cause heart failure (HF)
   2. Maintain neutral thermal environment.
   3. Organize activities to help minimize the child's energy expenditure.
   4. Administer medications as prescribed.
   5. Monitor laboratory data closely
   6. Monitor for signs of deteriorating condition or HF.
   7. Teach family how to monitor for heart failure
B. Assist with diagnostic tests and support family during diagnosis.
   1. Electrocardiogram (ECG)
   2. Echocardiography
C. Prepare family and child for cardiac catheterization (conducted when surgery is probable or as an intervention for certain procedures).

1. Risks of catheterization are similar to those for a child undergoing cardiac surgery:
   a. Arrhythmias
   b. Bleeding
   c. Perforation
   d. Phlebitis
   e. Arterial obstruction at the entry site
2. Child requires reassurance and close monitoring after catheterization:
   a. Vital signs
   b. Pulses
   c. Incision site
   d. Cardiac rhythm
3. Prepare family and child (as able) for surgical intervention if necessary.
D. Prepare child as appropriate for age.
   1. Show ICU.
   2. Explain chest tubes, IV lines, monitors, dressings, and ventilator.
   3. Show family and child waiting area for families.
   4. Use a doll or a drawing for explanations.
   5. Provide emotional support.
   6. Include and incorporate family as much as possible in client teachings.

> **HESI HINT** Basic differences between cyanotic and acyanotic defects:
> - Acyanotic: Has abnormal circulation; however, all blood entering the systemic circulation is oxygenated.
> - Cyanotic: Has abnormal circulation with unoxygenated blood entering the systemic circulation.

Heart Failure

CHF is more often associated with acyanotic defects.

Description: Condition in which the heart is unable to pump effectively the volume of blood that is presented to it (Table 5.10).

> **HESI HINT** CHF is a common complication of CHD. HF reflects the increased workload of the heart caused by shunts or obstructions. The two objectives in treating CHF are to reduce the workload of the heart and increase cardiac output.

Clinical Assessment

A. Edema (face, eyes of infants), weight gain

Clinical Assessment

A. Monitor vital signs frequently and report signs of increasing distress.
B. Maintain neutral thermal environment.
C. Monitor for signs of deteriorating condition or HF.
D. Assess respiratory functioning frequently.
E. Elevate head of bed or use infant seat.
F. Administer oxygen therapy if prescribed.
G. Administer medications as prescribed.
H. Monitor hydration, maintain strict input and output (I&O); defects may cause heart failure (HF) (weigh infant and report unusual weight gains) (Table 5.11)
I. Monitor laboratory data closely
J. Gavage-feed infants if unable to get adequate nutrition by mouth.
K. Teach family how to monitor for heart failure. Organize activities to help minimize the child's energy expenditure.

> **HESI HINT** When frequent weights are required, weigh child on the same scale at the same time of day so that accurate comparisons can be made.

Rheumatic Fever

Description: Rheumatic fever is an inflammatory disease that is a result of exposure to beta-hemolytic streptococcal infection. It is the most common cause of acquired heart disease in children and it affects the heart, joints, brain, and skin. This disease develops when strep throat and scarlet fever infections are not treated properly. Group A Streptococcus causes strep throat and scarlet fever. It usually takes about 1 to 5 weeks after strep throat or scarlet fever for rheumatic fever to develop. Rheumatic fever is thought to be caused by a response of the body's defense system—the immune system. The immune system responds to the earlier strep throat or scarlet fever infection and causes a generalized inflammatory response.

TABLE 5.10	**Congestive Heart Failure Signs and Symptom (pl)**		
	CONGESTIVE HEART FAILURE		
Cardiac	**Pulmonary**	**Gastrointestinal**	**Integumentary**
1. Tachycardia	1. Tachypnea	1. Difficulty feeding	Diaphoresis (especially head)
2. Poor circulation	2. Shortness of breath	2. Hepatomegaly	Edema (face, eyes in infants)
3. Weight gain (excessive fluid)	3. Cyanosis		
	4. Grunting		
	5. Wheezing		
	6. Pulmonary congestion		

TABLE 5.11   Clinical Judgment Measures: Pediatric Cardiovascular

Clinical Judgment Measure	Assessment Characteristics
Recognize Cues	Abnormal heart rate for age/abnormal rhythm if on monitor or during pulse evaluation
	Note paleness/abnormal color/duskiness
	Note tachypnea
	Fatigue or fatigue with exertion even just nippling or eating
	Syncope
	Not on growth curve
	Squatting or leaning forward to breath
	Diaphoresis
	Edema
	Audible wheezing
	Shortness of breath
Analyze Cues	Pulse evaluation abnorml, analyze on monitor
	Saturation monitor
	Tachypnea related to abnormal heart capabilities such as pulmonary edema and congestive heart failure
	Tachypnea, shortness of breath, or audible wheezing, respiratory or cardiac in origin
	Diaphoresis cardiac versus inability to manage heat
	Below growth curve due to fatigue or inability to sustain weight due to work of breathing/cardiac failure
Prioritize Cues	Remember Circulation-Airway-Breathing (CAB) in resuscitation with cardiac failure.
	Analyze rhythm on a monitor for fibrillation; only cure is defibrillation (automated external defibrillator (AED) may be only cure)
	For younger children oxygen may be the initial cure if respiratory system is functional
	Tachypnea relieves work of breathing; oxygen/diuretic may be needed
Solutions	Interventions may vary based on age and underlying conditions.
	Cardiac congenital lesions, cyanotic repaired/single ventricle/pulmonary overload versus need for oxygen
	Pulmonary hypertension requiring need for afterload reduction, evaluating symptoms to clinically intervene
Actions	Evaluate vital signs and intervene as indicated
	Resuscitation based on underlying known cardiac anomaly
	Saturation monitor
	Monitor and/or baseline ECG/AED if indicated
	Auscultate for murmur
	Provide preload support or afterload reduction as indicated
	Teach family home interventions to sustain child
Evaluate Outcomes	Able to sustain vital signs with normal rhythm and saturations.
	Able to sustain caloric intake and maintain and gain weight based on growth curve.
	Respiratory rate is normalized for age
	Diaphoresis is resolved
	Edema is treated
	Color has normalized

> **HESI HINT** People cannot catch rheumatic fever from someone else because it is an immune response and not an infection. However, people with strep throat or scarlet fever can spread group A strep to others, primarily through respiratory droplets.

Inflammatory Disease

A. Rheumatic fever is the most common cause of acquired heart disease in children. It usually affects the aortic and mitral valves of the heart.

B. Rheumatic fever is associated with a Group A Streptococcal (GAS) disease.

C. Rheumatic fever is a collagen disease that injures the heart, blood vessels, joints, and subcutaneous tissue.

Clinical Assessment

A. Chest pain, shortness of breath (pericarditis), heart murmur, cardiomegaly

B. Tachycardia, even during sleep

C. Migratory large-joint pain; painful, tender joints (arthritis), most commonly in the knees, ankles, elbows, and wrists; with nodules under skin near joints

D. Fatigue

E. Chorea (irregular involuntary movements)

F. Rash (erythema marginatum)

G. Fever

H. Laboratory findings
   1. Elevated erythrocyte sedimentation rate (ESR)
   2. C reactive protein

3. Elevated antistreptolysin O (ASO) titer: ASO is an antibody targeted against streptolysin O, a toxic enzyme produced by group A Streptococcus bacteria.
4. Electrocardiogram (ECG or EKG)
5. Echocardiogram

Clinical Interventions

A. Monitor vital signs.
B. Assess for increasing signs of cardiac distress.
C. Encourage bed rest (as needed for fatigue).
D. Assist with ambulation.
E. Reassure child and family that chorea is temporary.
F. Administer prescribed medications.
   1. Penicillin or erythromycin
   2. Aspirin for anti-inflammatory and anticoagulant actions
G. Collaborate with RN to enhance and reinforce a family teaching plan for a home care program.
H. Explain the necessity for prophylactics.
   1. Antibiotics taken either orally or IM
   2. Children given penicillin G benzathine at a dose of 1.2 million U IM q4w
   3. IM penicillin G each month (Table 5.12)
      a. Long-term administration of oral penicillin may be used in lieu of the intramuscular route. Erythromycin or sulfadiazine may be used in patients who are allergic to penicillin.

Pediatric Patients With Congenital Heart Disease

CHD can indicate that prescription of prophylactic antibiotics may be appropriate for children. It is important to note, however, that when antibiotic prophylaxis is called for due to congenital heart concerns, they should only be considered when the patient has:

A. Cyanotic CHD (birth defects with oxygen levels lower than normal), that has not been fully repaired, including children who have had a surgical shunts and conduits.
B. A congenital heart defect that's been completely repaired with prosthetic material or a device for the first 6 months after the repair procedure.
C. Repaired CHD with residual defects, such as persisting leaks or abnormal flow at or adjacent to a prosthetic patch or prosthetic device.
D. Antibiotic prophylaxis is not recommended for any other form of CHD (Graham, 2007).

E. Inform dentist and other health care providers of diagnosis so they can evaluate the necessity for prophylactic antibiotics.
F. Rheumatic fever with carditis and clinically significant residual heart disease requires antibiotic treatment for a minimum of 10 years after the latest episode; prophylaxis is required until the patient is aged at least 40 to 45 years and is sometimes continued for life.
G. Rheumatic fever with carditis and no residual heart disease aside from mild mitral regurgitation requires antibiotic treatment for 10 years or until age 25 years (whichever is longer).
H. Rheumatic fever without carditis requires antibiotic treatment for 5 years or until the patient is aged 18 to 21 years (whichever is longer).

HESI HINT Early diagnosis of these infections and treatment with antibiotics are key to preventing rheumatic fever.

If rheumatic fever is not treated promptly, long-term heart damage (called rheumatic heart disease) may occur. Rheumatic heart disease may require heart surgery since rheumatic heart disease weakens the valves between the chambers of the heart (Centers for Disease Control and Prevention (CDC), 2021, November 27, *Group A Streptococcal [GAS] Disease*).

Kawasaki Disease (Mucocutaneous Lymph Node Syndrome)

Description: Kawasaki disease causes swelling (inflammation) in the walls of medium-sized arteries throughout the body. It primarily affects children. The inflammation tends to affect the coronary arteries, which supply blood to the heart muscle.

Kawasaki disease is sometimes called mucocutaneous lymph node syndrome because it also affects glands that swell during an infection, including lymph nodes, skin, and the mucous membranes inside the mouth, nose, and throat.

Signs of Kawasaki disease, such as a high fever and peeling skin, can be frightening. The good news is that Kawasaki disease is usually treatable, and most children recover from Kawasaki disease without serious problems.

Risk Factors

Three things are known to increase your child's risk of developing Kawasaki disease.
- Age. Children under 5 years old are most at risk of Kawasaki disease.

TABLE 5.12	**Anti-infectives**		
Drugs	**Indications**	**Adverse Reactions**	**Nursing Implications**
Penicillin G	Prophylaxis for recurrence of rheumatic fever	Allergic reactions ranging from rashes to anaphylactic shock and death	• Penicillin G is released very slowly over several weeks, giving sustained levels of concentration • Have emergency equipment available wherever medication is administered. • Always determine existence of allergies to penicillin and cephalosporins; check chart/record and inquire of client/family.

- Sex. Boys are slightly more likely than girls to develop Kawasaki disease.
- Ethnicity. Children of Asian or Pacific Island descent, such as Japanese or Korean, have higher rates of Kawasaki disease.

Complications

Complications include permanent damage to the main arteries of the heart, resulting in the formation of an aneurysm of the coronary artery. Kawasaki disease is a leading cause of acquired heart disease in children (Mayo Clinic, 2021, *Kawasaki Disease*).

Clinical Assessment

Kawasaki disease signs and symptoms usually appear in three phases.

Phase 1. Signs and symptoms of the first phase may include:
- A fever that is often higher than 102.2°F (39°C) and lasts more than three days
- Extremely red eyes without a thick discharge
- A rash on the main part of the body and in the genital area
- Red, dry, cracked lips and an extremely red, swollen tongue
- Swollen, red skin on the palms of the hands and the soles of the feet
- Swollen lymph nodes in the neck and perhaps elsewhere
- Irritability

Phase 2. In the second phase of the disease, your child may develop:
- Peeling of the skin on the hands and feet, especially the tips of the fingers and toes, often in large sheets
- Joint pain
- Diarrhea
- Vomiting
- Abdominal pain

Phase 3. In the third phase of the disease, signs and symptoms slowly go away unless complications develop. It may be as long as 8 weeks before energy levels seem normal again.

Clinical Judgment

A. Treatment of patients who are diagnosed with KD is consistent with American Heart Association (AHA) and American Academy of Pediatrics (AAP) guidelines. The recommended initial therapy includes intravenous immune globulin (IVIG; 2 g/kg) administered as a single infusion over 8 to 12 hours. Assist RN to administer IV immunoglobulin as prescribed.
B. Treatment guidelines also include aspirin (30 to 50 mg/kg daily divided into four doses) with intravenous immunoglobulin (IVIG) as initial treatment of KD.
C. Treat high fevers with acetaminophen as prescribed.
D. Monitor cardiac status by documenting the child's
   1. Intake and output
   2. Daily weights
E. Minimize skin discomfort with lotions and cool compresses.
F. Initiate meticulous mouth care.
G. Monitor intake of clear liquids and soft foods.
H. Support family as they comfort child during periods of irritability.
I. Provide discharge teaching and home referral.

❓ REVIEW OF CARDIOVASCULAR DISORDERS

1. Differentiate between: Problems that cause too much blood to pass through the lungs. Problems that cause too little blood to pass through the lungs. Problems that cause too little blood to travel to the body
2. List the four defects associated with tetralogy of Fallot.
3. List the common signs of cardiac problems in an infant.
4. What are the two objectives in treating CHF?
5. Describe nursing judgment to reduce the workload of the heart.
6. What cardiac complications are associated with rheumatic fever?
7. What medications are used to treat rheumatic fever?

See Answer Key at the end of this text for suggested responses.

NEUROMUSCULAR DISORDERS

Down Syndrome

Description: Most common chromosomal abnormality in children

A. Down syndrome is evidenced by various physical characteristics and by cognitive impairment (see Fig. 5.15).
B. Down syndrome occurs when cell division is abnormal; as a result, there is extra genetic material from chromosome 21 and, in less than 5% of cases, a translocation of chromosome 21.
C. Common associated problems (Fig. 5.16)
   1. Cardiac defects
   2. Respiratory infections
   3. Feeding difficulties
   4. Delayed developmental skills
   5. Low IQ range of 20 to 70
   6. Skeletal defects
   7. Altered immune function
   8. Endocrine dysfunctions; hypothyroidism

Clinical Interventions

A. Assist and support parents during the diagnostic process and management of child's associated problems.
B. Assess and monitor growth and development.
C. Teach use of bulb syringe for suctioning nares.
D. Teach signs of respiratory infection.
E. Assist family with feeding problems.
F. Feed to back and side of mouth.
G. Monitor for signs of cardiac difficulty or respiratory infection.
H. Refer family to early intervention program.
I. Refer to other specialists as indicated: nutritionist, speech therapist, physical therapist, and occupational therapist.

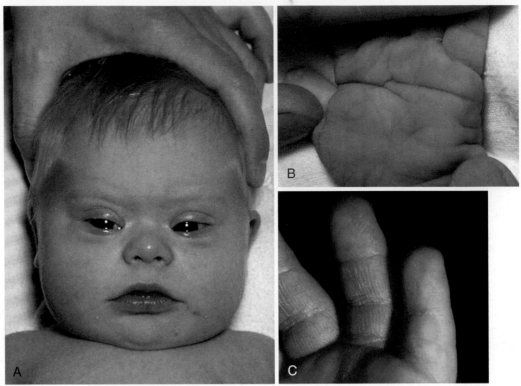

Fig. 5.16 Down Syndrome. (A) The typical facial appearance of an infant with Down syndrome shows the upward slant of the canthal folds of the eyes; protruding tongue; and short, thick neck. (B) The straight simian crease in the palm of the hand is a typical finding in children with Down syndrome. (C) The short fifth finger is a typical finding in children with Down syndrome. The tip of the fifth finger does not extend to the distal joint of the adjoining finger. (From Zitelli, B. L., & Davis, H. W. [2012]. *Atlas of pediatric physical diagnosis* [6th ed.]. St. Louis: Mosby)

HESI HINT The nursing goal in caring for a child with Down syndrome is to help the child reach his or her optimal level of functioning.

Cerebral Palsy

Description: Cerebral palsy (CP) is a nonprogressive injury to the motor centers of the brain causing neuromuscular problems of spasticity or dyskinesia (involuntary movements).

Causes of Cerebral Palsy

A. Anoxic injury before, during, or after birth
B. Kernicterus—excessive bilirubin is deposited in brain cells, affecting neuron function and metabolism.

Risk Factors

A. Low birth weight
B. Maternal infection

Complications of Cerebral Palsy

A. Cognitive impairment
B. Seizure
C. Failure to thrive

Clinical assessment (data collection) of Cerebral Palsy

A. Persistent neonatal reflexes (Moro, tonic neck) after 6 months
B. Delayed developmental milestones
C. Apparent early preference for one hand
D. Poor suck, tongue thrust
E. Spasticity (may be described as "difficulty with diapering" by mother or caregiver) legs are extended and crossed over each other; feet are plantar flexed.
F. Scissoring of legs is a common characteristic of spastic CP
G. Involuntary movements
H. Seizures

Clinical Interventions

A. Observe for CP through follow-up of high-risk infants such as premature infants
B. Coordinate with community-based agencies
C. Coordinate with physical therapist, occupational therapist, speech therapist, nutritionist, orthopedic surgeon, and neurologist
D. Support family through grief process at diagnosis and throughout the child's life. Caring for severely affected children can be very challenging for the family.

HESI HINT Feed an infant or child with CP using nursing judgment aimed at preventing aspiration. Position child upright and support the lower jaw.

E. Administer anticonvulsant medications such as phenytoin (Dilantin) if prescribed (Table 5.13).

F. Administer diazepam (Valium) for muscle spasms if prescribed.

Attention-Deficit/Hyperactivity Disorder

Description: Attention-deficit/hyperactivity disorder (ADHD) is one of the most common neurodevelopmental disorders of childhood. It is usually first diagnosed in childhood and often lasts into adulthood. Children with ADHD may have trouble paying attention, controlling impulsive behaviors, or be overly active (see Chapter 7, Psychiatric Nursing).

There are three different types of ADHD, depending on which types of symptoms are strongest in the individual:

A. Predominantly Inattentive Presentation: It is hard for the individual to organize or finish a task, to pay attention to details, or to follow instructions or conversations. The person is easily distracted or forgets details of daily routines.

B. Predominantly Hyperactive-Impulsive Presentation: The person fidgets and talks a lot. It is hard to sit still for long (e.g., for a meal or while doing homework). Smaller children may run, jump, or climb constantly. The individual feels restless and has trouble with impulsivity. Someone who is impulsive may interrupt others a lot, grab things from people, or speak at inappropriate times. It is hard for the person to wait their turn or listen to directions. A person with impulsiveness may have more accidents and injuries than others.

TABLE 5.13 Anticonvulsants

Drugs/Routes	Indications	Adverse Reactions	Nursing Implications
• Phenobarbital PO, IM, IV	• Tonic-clonic and partial seizures • Is the longest acting of common barbiturates • Usually combined with other drugs	• Drowsiness • Nystagmus • Ataxia • Paradoxic excitement	• Therapeutic levels: 15.40 mcg/mL • Avoid rapid IV infusion. • Monitor blood pressure during IV infusion.
• Phenytoin PO, IV	• Tonic-clonic and partial seizures	• Gingival hyperplasia • Dermatitis • Ataxia • Nausea, anorexia • Bone marrow depression • Nystagmus	• Therapeutic levels: 10–20 mcg/mL • Monitor any drug interactions. • Do not administer with milk. • Ensure meticulous oral hygiene. • Monitor CBC. • Report to physician if any rash develops. • For IV administration, flush IV line before and after with normal saline only.
• Fosphenytoin sodium IM, IV	• Generalized convulsive status epilepticus • Prevention and treatment of seizures during neurosurgery • Short-term parenteral replacement for phenytoin oral (Dilantin)	• Rapid IV infusion can cause hypotension. • Severe: ataxia, CNS toxicity, confusion, gingival hyperplasia, irritability, lupus erythematosus, nervousness, nystagmus, paradoxic excitement, Stevens-Johnson syndrome, toxic epidural necrosis	• Use for short-term parenteral use (IV infusion or IM injection) only. • Should always be prescribed and dispensed in phenytoin sodium equivalents (PEs) • Before IV infusion, dilute in D₅W or NS to administer. • Infuse at IV rate of no more than 150 mg PE/min.
• Valproic acid PO	• Absence seizures • Myoclonic seizures	• Hepatotoxicity, especially in children less than 2 years • Prolonged bleeding times • GI disturbances	• Monitor liver function. • Potentiates phenobarbital and Dilantin, altering blood levels • Therapeutic levels: 50–100 mEq/mL
• Carbamazepine PO	• Tonic-clonic, mixed seizures • Drowsiness • Ataxia	• Hepatitis • Agranulocytosis	• Monitor liver function while on therapy. • Therapeutic levels: 6–12 mcg/mL
• Lamotrigine PO	• Partial seizures • Tonic-clonic seizures • Absence seizures	• Dizziness • Headache • Nausea • Rash	• Withhold drug if rash develops. • Do not discontinue abruptly.
• Clonazepam PO	• Absence seizures • Myoclonic seizures	• Drowsiness • Hyperactivity • Agitation • Increased salivation	• Therapeutic levels: 20–80 mcg/mL • Do not abruptly discontinue drug. • Monitor liver function, CBC, and renal function periodically.

C. Combined Presentation: Symptoms of the previous two types are equally present in the person.

Symptoms can change over time; the presentation may change over time as well. In most cases:

A. ADHD is best treated with a combination of behavior therapy and medication.

B. For preschool-aged children (4 to 5 years of age) with ADHD, behavior therapy, particularly training for parents, is recommended as the first line of treatment before medication is tried.

C. What works best can depend on the child and family. Good treatment plans will include close monitoring, follow-ups, and making changes, if needed, along the way.

D. In addition to behavioral therapy and medication, having a healthy lifestyle can make it easier for your child to deal with ADHD symptoms. Here are some healthy behaviors that may help:

E. Developing healthy eating habits such as eating plenty of fruits, vegetables, and whole grains and choosing lean protein sources

F. Participating in daily physical activity based on age

G. Limiting the amount of daily screen time from TVs, computers, phones, and other electronics

H. Getting the recommended amount of sleep each night based on age (Centers for Disease Control and Prevention [CDC], 2021, September 23, *Attention Deficit Hyperactivity Disorder*).

Spina Bifida

Spina Bifida, also known as neural tube defect (NTD). When the neural tube doesn't close all the way, the backbone that protects the spinal cord doesn't form and close as it should. Spina bifida might cause physical and intellectual disabilities that range from mild to severe. The severity depends on:

• The size and location of the opening in the spine.

• Whether part of the spinal cord and nerves are affected.

Description: Malformation of the vertebrae and spinal cord; can happen anywhere along the spine if the neural tube does not close all the way, which causes damage to the spinal cord and nerves, resulting in varying degrees of disability and deformity depending on the location of the malformation (Fig. 5.17)

Types of Spina Bifida

A. Spina bifida occulta—there is a small gap in the spine, but no opening or sac on the back. The spinal cord and the nerves usually are normal and may not be discovered until late childhood or adulthood. This type of spina bifida usually does not cause any disabilities.

B. Meningocele—there is a sac of fluid that comes through an opening along the back; it contains only meninges and spinal fluid, but the spinal cord is not in this sac. There is usually little or no nerve damage and this type of spina bifida can cause minor disabilities.

C. Myelomeningocele is the most serious type of spina bifida. A sac of fluid comes through an opening in the back. Part of the spinal cord and nerves are in this sac and are damaged. This type of spina bifida causes moderate to severe disabilities, causing incontinence, parathesis, and paralysis.

Prevention

A. Women in childbearing years before and during pregnancy should consume a minimum of 400 mcg of folic acid daily.

Clinical Assessment

A. Spina bifida occulta: dimple with or without hair tuft at base of spine

B. Presence of sac in myelomeningocele.

C. Paralysis and parathesis below the defect

D. Head circumference at variance with norms on growth grids

E. Associated problems
   1. Hydrocephalus (90% with myelomeningocele)
   2. Neurogenic bladder, poor anal sphincter tone

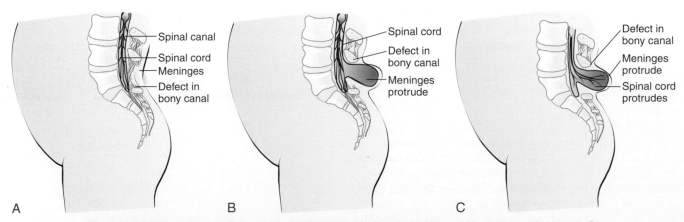

Fig. 5.17 Midline Defects of Osseous Spine With Varying Degrees of Neural Herniations. (A) Normal. (B) Spina bifida occulta. (C) Meningocele. (D) Myelomeningocele. (From Hockenberry, M. J., & Wilson, D. [2011]. *Wong's nursing care of infants and children* [9th ed.]. St. Louis: Mosby.)

3. Congenital dislocated hips
4. Club feet
5. Skin problems associated with parathesis below the defect
6. Scoliosis
7. Avoid latex in children with spina bifida.

Clinical Judgment

A. Preoperative: Place infant in prone position.
1. Keep sac free of stool and urine.
2. Cover sac with moist sterile dressing.
3. Position child on abdomen, legs in natural position.
4. Measure head circumference at least every 8 hours or every shift; check fontanel.
5. Observe neurologic function.
6. Monitor for signs of infection.
7. Catheterize routinely (usually every 6 hours).
8. Promote parent–infant bonding.
B. Postoperative: Place infant in prone position.
1. Make same observation as preoperatively.
2. Observe incision for drainage and infection.
3. Monitor head circumference.
4. Assess neurologic function.
C. Long-term care.
1. Collaborate with RN to teach family catheterization program.
2. Older children to learn self-catheterization.
3. Collaborate with RN to enhance and implement a bowel program.
   a. High-fiber diet
   b. Increased fluids
   c. Regular fluids
   d. Suppositories as needed
4. Observe skin condition frequently.
5. Assist with range-of-motion (ROM) exercises, ambulation, and bracing as indicated by physical therapy and occupational therapy.
6. Coordinate with team members: neurologist, orthopedist, urologist, physical therapist, occupational therapist, and nutritionist.
D. Support independent functioning of child.
E. Assist family to make realistic developmental expectations of child (Centers for Disease Control and Prevention [CDC], 2020, September 3, *What Is Spina Bifida?*).

Hydrocephalus

Description: Condition characterized by an abnormal accumulation of cerebrospinal fluid (CSF) within the ventricles of the brain that does not drain properly from the cranium.

The two major types of hydrocephalus are called communicating hydrocephalus and non-communicating hydrocephalus (U.S. Department of Health and Human Services, 2020, May 13, *Hydrocephalus Fact Sheet*) (Box 5.2).
A. Caused by an obstruction in the flow of CSF between the ventricles.

B. Results in enlargement of the ventricles, which causes pressure on the brain tissue.

Hydrocephalus is most often associated with spina bifida; it can be a complication of meningitis.

> **HESI HINT** Infants with hydrocephalus have enlarged head circumference as a result of widening fontanels that compensate for accumulating cerebral spinal fluid and relieve pressure of the developing brain.

Clinical Assessment

A. Toddlers and older children show classic signs of intracranial pressure (ICP).
1. Change in LOC
2. Irritability
3. Vomiting
4. Headache on awakening
5. Motor dysfunction
6. Unequal pupil response
7. Seizures
8. Decline in academics
9. Change in personality
B. Signs of increased ICP in infants
1. Irritability, lethargy
2. Increasing head circumference
3. Bulging fontanels
4. Widening suture lines
5. "Sunset" eyes
6. High-pitched cry
7. Feeding difficulties
8. Decreased muscle tone and strength

Clinical Judgments

A. Prepare infant and family for diagnostic procedures.
B. Monitor for signs of increased ICP.
C. Maintain seizure precautions.
D. Elevate head of bed.
E. Prepare parents for surgical procedure (e.g., ventricular shunt placement).
F. Purpose of the shunt is to drain the excess fluid off the brain.
G. Postoperative care

BOX 5.2 Hydrocephalus

- Communicating hydrocephalus occurs when the flow of cerebrospinal fluid (CSF) is blocked after it exits the ventricles. This form is called communicating because, since the CSF flows between the ventricles, the passages remain open. Reduced flow and absorption of CSF into specialized blood vessels called arachnoid villi can also result in a buildup of CSF in the ventricles and communicating hydrocephalus.
- Non-communicating hydrocephalus: the flow of CSF is blocked along one or more of the narrow passages connecting the ventricles.

Adapted from https://www.ninds.nih.gov/Disorders/Patient-Caregiver-Education/Fact-Sheets/Hydrocephalus-Fact-Sheet

1. Assess for signs of shunt malfunction.
   a. Infant
      1) Change in size, signs of bulging, tenseness in fontanels, and separation of suture lines
      2) Irritability, lethargy, or seizure activity
      3) Altered vital signs and feeding behavior
   b. Older child: Increase in ICP
      1) Change in LOC
      2) Complaint of headache
      3) Changes in customary behavior (sleep patterns, developmental capabilities)
2. Assess for signs of infection (meningitis).
   a. Increase fever greater than 38.6°C (100.5°F).
   b. Shunt tract may appear erythemic, tender, and swollen; drainage may be present.
   c. Decrease feeding/increase vomiting
   d. Stiff neck and headache
3. Monitor I&O closely.
4. Assess surgical sites (head and abdomen).
H. Collaborate with RN to enhance and reinforce a family teaching plan for a home care program.
   1. Teach to watch for signs of increased ICP or infection.
   2. Follow up appointments for shunt function and potential need for shunt revision.
   3. Provide anticipatory guidance for potential problems with growth and development.

Seizures

Description: Uncontrolled electrical discharges of neurons in the brain which may be caused by:

- An imbalance of nerve-signaling brain chemicals (neurotransmitters)
- Genetics
- Brain tumor
- Stroke
- Brain damage from illness or injury, including those at birth
- Medicines or illegal drugs
- Immaturity of the CNS, fever, infection, neoplasms, cerebral anoxia, and metabolic disorders.

In most cases, the cause of a seizure can't be found.

A. Seizures are categorized as generalized or partial/focal.

A generalized seizure occurs in both sides of the brain causing loss of consciousness and a postictal state. Types of generalized seizures include:

1. Absence seizure. This is also called petit mal seizure. This seizure causes a brief changed state of consciousness, staring, and posturing with twitching and possibly rapid blinking. The seizure usually lasts no longer than 30 seconds. Usually, no recall of what just occurred and may go on with activities as though nothing happened. These seizures may occur several times a day. Absence seizures almost always start between ages 4 and 12.
2. Atonic seizure. A sudden loss of muscle tone and may fall from a standing position or suddenly drop his or her head. During the seizure child will be limp and unresponsive.

3. Generalized tonic-clonic seizure (GTC)/grand mal seizure which has 5 distinct phases:
   a. body, arms, and legs will flex (contract)
   b. stiffness of entire body (Tonic)
   c. extend (straighten out), and tremor (shake)
   d. followed by contraction and relaxation of the muscles (clonic period)
   e. Postictal period/sleepy and possible problems with vision or speech, subsequent bad headache, fatigue, or body aches. (Not all of these phases occur in everyone)
4. Myoclonic seizure. Quick movements or sudden jerking of a group of muscles. These seizures tend to occur in clusters. This means that they may occur several times a day, or for several days in a row.

Focal seizures take place when abnormal electrical brain function occurs in one or more areas of one side of the brain. Before a focal seizure, some may experience an aura, or signs that a seizure is about to occur which is more common with a complex focal seizure. The most common aura involves feelings, such as déjà vu, impending doom, fear, or euphoria. There may also be visual changes, hearing abnormalities, or changes in sense of smell.

The two types of focal seizures are:

1. Simple focal seizure. The symptoms depend on which area of the brain is affected. If the abnormal electrical brain function occurs in occipital lobe which involves vision, then sight may be altered. More often, muscles are affected, and the seizure activity is limited to an isolated muscle group such as fingers, or larger muscles in the arms and legs. There may be sweating, nausea, or paleness, but no loss of consciousness.
2. Complex focal seizure. This type of seizure often occurs in the temporal lobe which controls emotion and memory function causing altered consciousness or loss of consciousness or just stop being aware of surroundings and still look awake but have a variety of unusual behaviors including but not limited to gagging, lip smacking, running, screaming, crying, or laughing and then move to postictal period.

Clinical Assessment

A. Generalized
   1. Aura (a warning sign of impending seizure)
   2. LOC
   3. Generalized stiffness of entire body
   4. Apnea, cyanosis
   5. Spasms followed by relaxation
   6. Pupils dilated and nonreactive to light
   7. Incontinence
   8. Postictal, disoriented, sleepy
B. Absence seizures (petit mal)
   1. Onset between 4 and 12 years of age
   2. Lasts 5 to 10 seconds
   3. Child appears to be inattentive, daydreaming
   4. Poor performance in school

> **HESI HINT** Medication noncompliance is the most common cause of increased seizure activity.

Clinical Judgment

A. Maintain airway during seizure: Turn client on side to aid ventilation.

B. Do not restrain client.

C. Protect client from injury during seizure and support head (avoid neck flexion).

D. Document seizure, noting all data in assessment.

E. Maintain seizure precautions.
1. Reduce environmental stimuli as much as possible.
2. Pad side rails or crib rails.
3. Have suction equipment and oxygen quickly accessible; set up at the bedside/crib side. Tape oral airway to the head of the bed.

> **HESI HINT** Do not use tongue blade, padded or not, during a seizure as this may cause traumatic damage to the oral cavity.

A. Support during diagnostic tests: electroencephalogram (EEG), computed tomography (CT) scan

B. Support during workup for infections such as meningitis

C. Administer anticonvulsant medications as prescribed (see Table 5.13).
1. For tonic-clonic seizures: Carbamazepine, Phenytoin, Valproic acid, Oxcarbazepine, Lamotrigine Gabapentin, Topiramate, Phenobarbital.
2. For focal seizures: Carbamazepine, Oxcarbazepine, Lacosamide
3. For absence seizures: ethosuximide or valproate

D. Monitor therapeutic drug levels.

E. Teach family about drug administration: dosage, action, and side effects.

F. Consider Ketogenic diet

G. Vagus nerve stimulator

H. Possible surgical interventions

For more information, see "Epilepsy and Seizures in Children" (Stanford Children's Health, 2021).

Bacterial Meningitis

Bacterial meningitis is very serious, and death can occur in a few hours. Most will recover but may have permanent disabilities (such as brain damage, hearing loss, and learning disabilities).

Description: Bacterial inflammatory disorder of the meninges that cover the brain and spinal cord

- Meningitis is usually caused by:
  - *Streptococcus pneumoniae*
  - Group B Streptococcus
  - *Neisseria meningitidis*
  - *Haemophilus influenzae*
  - *Listeria monocytogenes*

These bacteria can also be associated with another serious illness, sepsis, which is extreme response to infection. Without timely treatment, sepsis can quickly lead to tissue damage, organ failure, and death.

Causes

Usual Source: Bacterial invasion from the middle ear, nasopharynx, and wounds including fractures of the skull, lumbar punctures, and shunts.

A. Exudate covers brain and cerebral edema occurs.

B. Lumbar puncture shows
1. Increased white blood cells (WBCs)
2. Decreased glucose
3. Elevated protein
4. Increased ICP
5. Positive culture for meningitis

Clinical Assessment

A. Older children
1. Classic signs of increased ICP (see the section "Hydrocephalus" earlier)
2. Fever, chills
3. Neck stiffness, opisthotonos
4. Photophobia
5. Positive Kernig sign (inability to extend leg when thigh is flexed anteriorly at hip)
6. Positive Brudzinski sign (neck flexion causing adduction and flexion movements of lower extremities)

B. Infants and young children (3 months to 2 years old)
1. Absence of classic signs demonstrating generalized symptoms
2. Poor feeding with vomiting, irritability
3. Bulging fontanel (an important sign)
4. Seizures

C. Neonates (birth to 2 months)
1. Very difficult to diagnose
2. Temperature nonspecific: may be normal, hypothermia, or hyperthermia
3. Symptoms can appear a few days after birth.
4. Infant has difficulty eating and refuses to eat when prompted.
5. Weak cry
6. Vomiting and diarrhea may be present.
7. Movement decreases, along with tone
8. Restless, sleep pattern changes
9. Late sign: bulging and tense fontanel

Clinical Interventions

A. Administer antibiotics (may be ampicillin, and appropriate cephalosporin) and antipyretics as prescribed.
B. Isolate for at least 24 hours.
C. Monitor vital signs and neurologic signs.
D. Keep environment quiet and darkened to prevent overstimulation.
E. Implement seizure precautions.
F. Position for comfort: head of the bed slightly elevated, with client on side if prescribed.
G. Measure head circumference daily in infants.
H. Monitor I&O closely.

> **HESI HINT** With meningitis, there may be inappropriate antidiuretic hormone (ADH) secretions causing fluid retention (cerebral edema) and dilutional hyponatremia.

I. Administer Hib vaccine to protect against *H. influenzae* infection (see Table 5.3).

Reye Syndrome

Description: Reye syndrome is an acute encephalopathy and hepatic dysfunction. Disease is staged by the clinical manifestations to reflect the severity of the condition.

Causes

A. Influenza
B. Varicella virus (chickenpox)
C. Aspirin usage

Risk factors of Reyes Syndrome

A. Aspirin use to treat viral infections
B. School age

Clinical Assessment (Data Collection) of Reye Syndrome
Diagnostics

A. Elevated aspartate transaminase (AST), alanine transaminase (ALT), lactate dehydrogenase, serum ammonia, decreased prothrombin time (PT)

Signs and symptoms

A. Lethargy rapidly progressing to deep coma (marked cerebral edema)
B. Vomiting
C. Hypoglycemic

Clinical Interventions

A. Assist with critical care early in syndrome

B. Monitor neurologic status: frequent noninvasive assessments and invasive ICP monitoring
C. Maintain ventilation
D. Monitor cardiac parameters
E. Monitor I&O
F. Care for Foley catheter
G. Provide emotional support to family.

Brain Tumors

Description: Brain tumor is the second most common cancer in children. Most pediatric brain tumors are infratentorial, making them difficult to excise surgically. Tumors usually occur close to vital structures. Gliomas are the most common childhood brain tumors.

Causes of brain tumor

A. Genetics
B. Radiation exposures

Complication of brain tumor

A. Neurological damage
B. Infection
C. Bleeding

Clinical Assessment

A. Headache

> **HESI HINT** Many children with a brain tumor experience headaches before their diagnosis

B. Vomiting and nausea
C. Loss of concentration
D. Change in behavior or personality
E. Balance issues
F. Vision, hearing, and speech changes, tilting of the head
G. Seizures
H. In infants: widening sutures, increasing frontal occipital circumference, tense fontanel

Clinical Interventions

A. Identify baseline neurologic functioning.
B. Support child and family during diagnostic workup and treatment.
C. If surgery is treatment of choice, provide preoperative teaching.
  1. Explain changes including that head will be shaved and describe ICU, dressings, IV lines, etc.
  2. Identify child's developmental level and plan teaching accordingly.

3. Radiation to the tumor site is sometimes performed before surgical excision of the tumor, in attempt to shrink the size of the tumor and to save as much brain tissue as possible.

D. Assess family's response to the diagnosis and treat family appropriately.

E. After surgery, position client as prescribed by the health care provider.

F. Postoperatively, after the operation to remove the tumor, the child may have a drain coming out of the incision that allows excess CSF to drain from the skull. Other tubes may be placed to allow blood that builds up after surgery to drain from under the scalp.

> **HESI HINT** Most postoperative clients with infratentorial tumors are prescribed to lie flat or turn to either side. A large tumor may require that the child not be turned to the operative side.

G. Monitor IV fluids and output carefully. Overhydration can cause cerebral edema and increased ICP.

H. Steroids and osmotic diuretics may be prescribed.

I. Brain tumors are treated with surgery, radiation, and chemotherapy. The specific treatment and prognosis depend on the type, grade, and location of the tumor. Depending on the type of tumor and the promptness of diagnosis, the 5-year survival rate is 40% to 80%. Long-term management of brain cancer survivors is complex and requires a multidisciplinary approach.

J. Support child and family to promote optimum functioning postoperatively.

Muscular Dystrophy

Muscular dystrophies are a group of genetic disorders that result in muscle weakness over time. Each type of muscular dystrophy is different and has no cure but acting early may help an individual with muscular dystrophy get the services and treatments he or she needs to lead a full life.

Description: Inherited disease of the muscles, causing muscle atrophy and weakness

A. Duchenne muscular dystrophy (DMD) and Becker muscular dystrophy (BMD) can have the same symptoms and are caused by mutations in the same gene. BMD symptoms can begin later in life and be less severe than DMD. However, because these two kinds are very similar, they are often studied and referred to together (DBMD).

B. DMD is a rare muscle disorder but it is one of the most frequent genetic conditions affecting approximately 1 in 3500 male births worldwide and is usually recognized between three and six years of age. DMD is characterized by weakness and atrophy of the muscles of the pelvic area followed by the involvement of the shoulder muscles. As the disease progresses, muscle weakness and atrophy spread to affect the trunk and forearms and gradually progress to involve additional muscles of the body. The disease is progressive and most affected individuals require a wheelchair by the teenage years. Serious life-threatening complications may ultimately develop including cardiomyopathy and respiratory difficulties.

C. DMD is caused by mutations of the DMD gene on the X chromosome. The gene regulates the production of a protein called dystrophin that is found in association with the inner side of the membrane of skeletal and cardiac muscle cells. Dystrophin is thought to play an important role in maintaining the membrane (sarcolemma) of muscle cells (National Organization of Rare Diseases [NORD], 2021). For further information, see https://rarediseases.org/rare-diseases/duchenne-muscular-dystrophy/.

Clinical Assessment

A. Waddling gait, lordosis

B. Increasing clumsiness, muscle weakness

C. Gowers sign: difficulty rising from a squatting position; has to use arms and hands to "walk" up legs to stand erect

D. Pseudohypertrophy of muscles (especially noted in calves) due to fat deposits

E. Muscle degeneration, especially the thighs, and fatty infiltrates (detected by muscle biopsy); cardiac muscle also involved

F. Delayed cognitive development, severity of the cognitive impairment varies

G. Later in disease: scoliosis, respiratory difficulty, and cardiac difficulties

H. Eventual wheelchair dependency, confinement to bed

Clinical Interventions

A. Provide supportive care.

B. Provide exercises (active and passive).

C. Prevent exposure to respiratory infection.

D. Encourage a balanced diet to avoid obesity.

E. Support family's grieving process.

F. Support participation in the Muscular Dystrophy Association: https://www.mda.org/

G. Coordinate with health care team: physical therapist, occupational therapist, nutritionist, neurologist, orthopedist, and geneticist.

> **HESI HINT** Encourage the parents of children who are diagnosed with any type of neuromuscular disease to allow the child to do as much as possible as an effort to try to maintain muscle function and independence.

❓ REVIEW OF NEUROMUSCULAR DISORDERS

1. What are the physical features of a child with Down syndrome?
2. Describe scissoring.
3. What are two priorities for a newborn with myelomeningocele?
4. List the signs and symptoms of increased intracranial pressure in older children.
5. What teaching should parents of a newly shunted child receive?
6. State the three main goals in providing care for a child experiencing a seizure.
7. What are the side effects of Dilantin?
8. Describe the signs and symptoms of a child with meningitis.
9. What antibiotics are usually prescribed for bacterial meningitis?
10. What increases intracranial pressure?
11. Describe the mechanism of inheritance of Duchenne muscular dystrophy.
12. What is the Gowers sign?

See Answer Key at the end of this text for suggested responses.

Renal Disorders

Post-Streptococcal Glomerulonephritis

Description: Acute glomerulonephritis (AGN) is an immune complex response to an antecedent beta-hemolytic streptococcal infection of the skin or pharynx. Antigen-antibody complexes become trapped in the membrane of the glomeruli, causing inflammation and decreased glomerular filtration.

Causes of AGN

A. Infection
B. Autoimmune disease
C. Vasculitis

Risk factors for AGN

A. Infection
B. Autoimmune disease

Complications of AGN

A. Kidney disease/failure
B. Hypertension
C. Nephrotic syndrome
Clinical assessment
Diagnostics.
A. Elevated antistreptolysin (ASO) titer
B. Elevated Blood urea nitrogen (BUN) and creatinine

Signs and symptoms.
A. Recent streptococcal infection
B. Mild to moderate edema (often confined to face)
C. Irritable, lethargic
D. Dark-colored urine (hematuria)
E. Proteinuria

Clinical interventions.
A. Provide supportive care
B. Monitor vital signs (especially BP) frequently
C. Monitor I&O
D. Weigh daily

E. Provide low-sodium diet with no added salt; low-potassium diet, if oliguric.
F. Encourage bed rest during acute phase (usually 4 to 10 days).
G. Administer antihypertensives if prescribed.
H. Monitor for seizures (hypertensive encephalopathy).
I. Monitor for signs of CHF.
J. Monitor for signs of renal failure (uncommon).

Nephrotic Syndrome

Description: Childhood nephrotic syndrome is not a disease in itself; rather, it is a group of symptoms that indicate kidney damage—particularly damage to the glomeruli that results in the release of too much protein from the body into the urine causing protein albumin, normally found in the blood, will leak into the urine.

A. The two types of childhood nephrotic syndrome are
   1. Primary—the most common type of childhood nephrotic syndrome, which is idiopathic, or unknown begins in the kidneys and affects only the kidneys.
   2. Secondary—the syndrome is caused by other diseases

Clinical Assessment

A. Edema that begins insidiously becomes severe and generalized.
B. Lethargy
C. Anorexia
D. Pallor
E. Urine
   1. Frothy-appearing urine
   2. Massive proteinuria
F. Laboratory findings
   1. Hypoproteinemia
   2. Hypercholesterolemia

Clinical Judgment

Congenital Nephrotic Syndrome: Researchers have found that medications are not effective in treating congenital nephrotic syndrome, and that most children will need a kidney transplant by the time they are 2 or 3 years old.

In order to attempt to sustain a child until transplant:
- albumin injections to make up for the albumin lost in urine
- diuretics
- antibiotics to treat the first signs of infection
- growth hormones to promote growth and help bones mature
- removal of one or both kidneys to decrease the loss of albumin in the urine
- dialysis to artificially filter wastes from the blood if the kidneys fail

A. Provide supportive care.
B. Monitor temperature; assess for signs of infection.
C. Protect from persons with infections.

D. Provide skin care, specifically of vulnerable edematous areas.

E. Maintain bed rest during edematous phase.

F. Administer medications as ordered.

G. Monitor I&O.

H. Teach dietary changes.
1. limiting the amount of sodium, often from salt, they take in each day
2. reducing the amount of liquids they drink each day
3. eating a diet low in saturated fat and cholesterol to help control elevated cholesterol levels

I. Collaborate with RN to enhance and reinforce a family teaching plan for a home care program.
1. Instruct to weigh child daily.
2. Train to prevent infection.

Secondary childhood nephrotic syndrome is treated by knowing the underlying cause of the primary illness by treating the underlying cause of the primary illness.

J. Prescribing antibiotics for an infection

K. Adjusting medications to treat lupus, HIV, or diabetes

L. Changing or stopping medications that are known to cause secondary childhood nephrotic syndrome

Urinary Tract Infection

Description: Bacterial infection most common is Escherichia coli (E. coli) bacteria. A urinary tract infection (UTI) is not common in children younger than age 5. A UTI is much more common in girls, due to a shorter urethra. A UTI can occur in boys if part of the urinary tract is blocked. Uncircumcised boys are more at risk for a UTI than circumcised boys. A child with a part or full blockage in the urinary tract is more likely to develop a UTI.

Clinical Assessment

A. In infants
1. Vague symptoms
2. Fever
3. Irritability
4. Poor food intake
5. Diarrhea, vomiting, jaundice
6. Foul smelling urine
7. Signs of sepsis

B. In older children
1. Urinary frequency
2. Hematuria
3. Enuresis
4. Dysuria
5. Fever
6. Signs of sepsis, fever chills

Clinical Interventions

A. Suspect and assess for UTI in infants who are ill.

B. Assess for recurrent UTI. In infants and young boys, UTI may indicate structural abnormalities of the urinary system.

C. Collect clean voided or catheterized specimen, as prescribed (Table 5.14).

D. Administer antibiotics as prescribed.

E. Collaborate with RN to enhance and reinforce a family teaching plan for a home care program.
1. Finish all prescribed medication.
2. Follow-up specimens may be indicated.
3. Increase oral fluids.
4. Instruct to void frequently and fully empty bladder.
5. Teach females to clean genital area from front to back.
6. Note symptoms of recurrence (Johns Hopkins Medicine, 2021).

Vesicoureteral Reflex

Description: Result of valvular malfunction and backflow of urine into the ureters (and higher) from the bladder (severe cases are associated with hydronephrosis).

Primary vesicoureteral reflex (VUR) is when children are born with an abnormal ureter and the valve between the ureter and the bladder does not close therefore urine comes back up the ureter toward the kidney. VUR unilateral reflux is when only one ureter and one kidney are affected. Primary VUR can get better or go away. As a child grows the entrance of the ureter into the bladder matures and the valve works.

Children have secondary VUR for many reasons, including a blockage or narrowing in the bladder neck or urethra. The blockage prevents some of the urine from leaving the body, so the urine is retrograde into the urinary tract. Secondary VUR may also be due to the nerves in the bladder not working. The nerve problems can prevent the bladder from relaxing and contracting normally to release urine. Secondary VUR is often bilateral reflux. Secondary VUR is sometimes diagnosed in utero (National Institute of Diabetes and Digestive and Kidney Diseases, 2018).

Clinical Assessment

A. Recurrent UTI

B. Reflux (common with neurogenic bladder)

C. Reflux noted on voiding cystourethrogram (VCUG)

D. VUR is graded 1 through 5. Grade 1 is the mildest form of the condition, and grade 5 is the most serious.

Clinical Interventions

A. Teach home program for prevention of UTI.

B. Teach family the importance of medication compliance, which usually leads to resolution of mild cases.

C. Provide support for children and families requiring surgery.

D. Surgery to remove a blockage

E. Antibiotics to prevent or treat UTIs

F. Surgery to correct an abnormal bladder or ureter

G. Intermittent urinary catheterization

H. Monitor postoperative urinary drainage.
1. Measure output.
2. Assess dressing and incision for drainage.

I. Maintain hydration with IV or oral fluids.

J. Manage pain relief postoperatively.

TABLE 5.14 Clinical Judgment Measures: Pediatric Neuromuscular

Clinical Judgment Measure	Assessment Characteristics
Recognize Cues	Lethargy
	Hyperactivity
	Aggression
	Impulsiveness
	Decreased interest in play
	Irritability
	Short attention span
	Stiff muscles (spasticity)
	Uncontrollable movements (dyskinesia)
	Poor balance and coordination (ataxia)
Analyze Cues	Headache
	Hydrocephalus, measure head circumference
	Neurogenic bladder, catheterize routinely
	Full fontanel check fontanel
	Evaluate neurologic function
	Monitor for signs of infection
	Brain tumor
	Stroke
	Brain damage from illness or injury, including those at birth
	Medicines or illegal drugs
	Immaturity of the central nervous system (CNS)
Prioritize Cues	Keep in mind any emergent issue related to: airway, breathing, or circulation (A, B, C).
	Observe for any change in the child's ability to respond to you, needs to be based on the child's age and developmental age. (Tanner Stages)
	Note alertness (mentation is what is expected for age and diagnosis)
	Change in skin color (pale, cyanosis)
Solutions	Normalize vital signs
	Position for comfort: head of the bed slightly elevated
	Manage pain
	Control Fever
	Control Seizures
	Promote parent—infant bonding.
Actions	Treat fever
	Evaluate for infection, neoplasms, cerebral anoxia, and metabolic disorders
	Identify baseline neurologic functioning.
	Monitor vital signs and neurologic signs.
	Keep environment quiet and darkened to prevent overstimulation.
	Implement seizure precautions.
	Measure head circumference daily in infants.
	Monitor I&O closely
Evaluate Outcomes	Coordinate with team members: neurologist, orthopedist, urologist, physical therapist, occupational therapist, and nutritionist
	Coordinate with genetics if indicated
	Refer to community-based agencies

1. Surgical pain
2. Bladder spasms

For more information, see https://www.niddk.nih.gov/health-information/urologic-diseases/hydronephrosis-newborns/vesicoureteral-reflux.

Wilms Tumor (Nephroblastoma)

Description: Malignant renal tumor. Wilms tumor is the most frequent tumor of the kidney in infants and children. Wilms tumor typically develops in otherwise healthy children without any predisposition to developing cancer; however, approximately 10% of children with Wilms tumor have been reported to have a congenital anomaly. Children with Wilms tumor may have associated hemihyperplasia and urinary tract anomalies, including cryptorchidism and hypospadias. Children may have recognizable phenotypic syndromes such as overgrowth, aniridia, genetic malformations, and others. These syndromes have provided clues to the genetic basis of the disease.

A. Wilms tumor is embryonic in origin.

B. The tumor tends to be encapsulated and vascularized.

C. Occurs most often in children 3 to 4 years of age and is much less common after age 5.

D. Can affect one or both kidneys

E. It is important to recognize that the absolute risk of Wilms tumor varies with the underlying condition or anomaly (National Cancer Institute, 2021).

Clinical Assessment

A. A lump, swelling, or pain in the abdomen. Most children present with an asymptomatic mass that is noted when they are bathed or dressed. Abdominal pain is present in 40% of children.

B. Blood in the urine. Gross hematuria occurs in about 18% of children with Wilms tumor at presentation, and microscopic hematuria is seen in 24% of patients.

C. Hypertension. About 25% of children have hypertension at presentation, which is attributed to activation of the renin-angiotensin system.

D. Hypercalcemia. Symptomatic hypercalcemia can sometimes be seen at presentation of rhabdoid tumors.

E. Constitutional symptoms such as fever, anorexia, and weight loss occur in 10% of cases (National Cancer Institute, 2021).

Clinical Interventions

A. Support family during diagnostic period.

B. Protect child from injury; place a sign on bed stating "no abdominal palpation" (to prevent accidental fragmentation and dislodging of tumor pieces into the abdominal cavity).

C. Prepare family and child for possible surgery.

D. Provide postoperative care.
1. Monitor for increased blood pressure.
2. Monitor kidney function: I&O, urine specific gravity.
3. Plan care for abdominal surgery.
   a. Maintain nasogastric tube.
   b. Check for bowel sounds.
4. Support child and family during interventions.

Hypospadias

Description: Congenital defect of urethral meatus in males; urethra opens on ventral side of penis behind the glans.

Clinical Assessment

A. Abnormal placement of meatus

B. Altered voiding stream

C. Presence of chordee

D. Undescended testes and inguinal hernia (may occur concurrently)

Clinical Judgments

A. Prepare child and family for surgery (no circumcision before surgery).

B. Assess circulation to tip of penis postoperatively.

C. Monitor urinary drainage after urethroplasty.
1. Plan for possible tubes and drains post op.

D. Maintain hydration (IV and oral fluids).

E. Collaborate with RN to enhance and reinforce a family teaching plan for a home care program.
1. Teach care of drains and tubes.
2. Instruct to increase oral fluids.
3. Describe signs of infection.

❓ REVIEW OF RENAL DISORDERS

1. Compare the signs and symptoms of post-streptococcal glomerulonephritis (PSGN) with those of nephrosis.
2. What antecedent event occurs with PSGN?
3. Compare the dietary interventions for PSGN and nephrosis.
4. What is the physiologic reason for the laboratory finding of hypoproteinemia in nephrosis?
5. Describe safe monitoring of prednisone administration and withdrawal.
6. What interventions can be taught to prevent UTIs in children?
7. Describe the pathophysiology of vesicoureteral reflux.
8. What are the priorities for children with a Wilms tumor?
9. Explain why hypospadias correction is performed before the child reaches preschool age.

See Answer Key at the end of this text for suggested responses.

GASTROINTESTINAL DISORDERS

Cleft Lip or Palate

Description: Malformations of the face and oral cavity that seem to be multifactorial in hereditary origin (Fig. 5.18)

A. Cleft lip is readily apparent.

B. Cleft palate may not be identified until the infant has difficulty with feeding.

C. Initial surgical closure of cleft lip is performed ~3 months of age.

D. Surgical closure of palate defect is usually performed at ~10 to 12 months of age.

Clinical Assessment

A. Failure of fusion of the lip, palate, or both

B. Difficulty sucking and swallowing

C. Parent reaction to facial defect

Clinical Judgment Measures

A. Promote family bonding.

B. Discuss surgical options.

C. In newborn period, assist with feeding.
1. Feed in upright position.
2. Feed slowly, with frequent burping.
3. Use appropriate nipples and speech therapy.
4. Support mother's breastfeeding if possible.

D. Provide postoperative care.
1. Maintain patent airway and proper positioning.
2. Sutures are self-dissolving.
3. Provide soft foods.
4. Use special sleeves ("no-nos") that prevent the elbows from bending

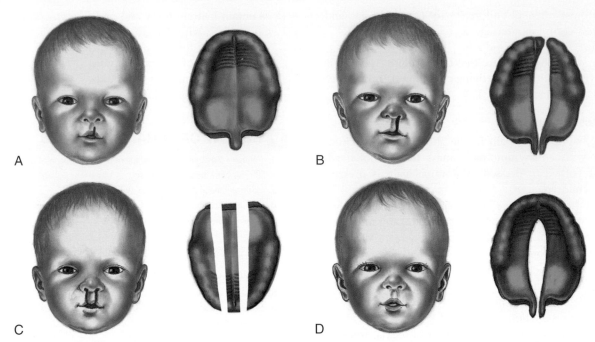

Fig. 5.18 Variations in Clefts of Lip and Palate at Birth. (A) Notch in vermilion border. (B) Unilateral cleft lip and cleft palate. (C) Bilateral cleft lip and cleft palate. (D) Cleft palate. (From Hockenberry, M. J., & Wilson, D. [2011]. *Wong's nursing care of infants and children* [9th ed.]. St. Louis: Mosby.)

5. Remove oral secretions carefully
6. Protect surgical site

> **HESI HINT** The surgical closure for repair of the cleft lip will occur at ~3 months for cleft lip and ~10–12 months for palate.

7. Provide age-appropriate stimulation.
8. Feeding as prescribed. Cleanse suture site with sterile water after feeding.
9. Teach family care and feeding. https://kidshealth.org/en/parents/cleft-palate-cleft-lip.html
10. Usually for cleft palate: Coordinate long-term care with other team members: plastic surgeon, ear/nose/throat (ENT) specialist, nutritionist, speech therapist, orthodontist, pediatrician, nurse (Nemours Kids Health, 2021, *Cleft Palate with Cleft Lip*) (see Fig. 5.18).

> **HESI HINT** Typical parent and family reactions to a child with an obvious malformation such as cleft lip or palate are guilt, disappointment, grief, sense of loss, and anger. Therefore, it is helpful for the families to be provided pictures of before and after surgical repair of children with cleft lip or cleft palate.

Esophageal Atresia With Tracheoesophageal Fistula

Description: Congenital anomaly in which the esophagus does not fully develop (Most common: upper esophagus ends in a blind pouch, and the lower part of the esophagus is connected to the trachea.

A. This condition is a clinical and surgical emergency.

Clinical Assessment

A. Three Cs of tracheoesophageal fistula (TEF) in the newborn
1. Choking
2. Coughing
3. Cyanosis
   a. Excess salivation
   b. Respiratory distress
   c. Aspiration pneumonia

Clinical Judgment Measures

A. Provide preoperative care.
1. Monitor respiratory status.
2. Remove excess secretions (suction is usually continuous due to the blind pouch).
3. Provide oxygen if needed.
4. Maintain nothing by mouth (NPO).
5. Administer IV fluids as prescribed.
B. Provide postoperative care.
1. Maintain NPO.
2. Administer IV fluids.
3. Monitor I&O.
4. Provide tube feedings as prescribed.
5. Provide pacifier to meet developmental needs.

6. Monitor child for postoperative stricture of the esophagus.
   a. Poor feeding
   b. Dysphagia
   c. Drooling
   d. Regurgitating undigested food
C. Promote parent—infant bonding for high-risk infant.

Pyloric Stenosis

Description: In pyloric stenosis, the pylorus muscles thicken and become abnormally large, blocking food from reaching the small intestine, which is an uncommon condition in infants. Pyloric stenosis can lead to forceful vomiting, dehydration, and weight loss. Babies with pyloric stenosis may seem to be hungry all the time. Surgery cures pyloric stenosis.

Clinical Assessment

A. Vomiting after feeding (projectile vomiting). Vomiting might be mild at first and gradually become more severe as the pylorus opening narrows.
B. Persistent hunger
C. Stomach contractions (peristalsis) that ripple across upper abdomen
D. Dehydration subsequent lethargy
E. Changes in bowel movements/constipation
F. Weight loss
G. Usually occurs in first-born males.
H. Hunger
I. Metabolic alkalosis (decreased serum chloride, increased pH and bicarbonate or CO_2 content)
J. Palpable olive-shaped mass in upper-right quadrant of the abdomen

Clinical Judgment Measures

A. Preoperative care
   1. Assess for dehydration.
   2. Administer IV fluids and electrolytes as prescribed.
   3. Weigh daily; monitor I&O.
B. Prepare family for surgery by teaching that
   1. The hypertrophied wall is surgically corrected to allow proper drainage from the stomach into the small intestines.
C. Postoperative care
   1. Observe for dehydration and monitor IV fluids as prescribed.
   2. Provide small oral feedings with electrolyte solutions or glucose as ordered.
   3. Position on right side in semi-Fowler position after feeding.
   4. Burp frequently to avoid stomach becoming distended and putting pressure on surgical site.
   5. Weigh daily; monitor I&O (Mayo Clinic, 2021, *Pyloric Stenosis*).

Intussusception

Description: Telescoping of one part of the intestine into another part of the intestine, usually the ileum into the colon (called ileocolic). Most common cause for bowel obstruction in children under 3 years old. Intussusception more often affects boys.

- Abnormal intestinal formation at birth. Intestinal malrotation: the intestine does not develop or rotate correctly, which increases the risk of intussusception.
- Certain condition: cystic fibrosis, Henoch-Schoenlein purpura (also known as IgA vasculitis), Crohn disease, and celiac disease—can increase the risk of intussusception
A. Partial to complete bowel obstruction occurs.
B. Blood vessels become trapped in the telescoping bowel, causing necrosis.

Clinical Assessment

A. Acute, intermittent abdominal pain
B. Screaming, with legs drawn up to abdomen
C. Vomiting
D. "Currant jelly" stools (mixed with blood and mucus)/diarrhea
E. Sausage-shaped mass in upper right quadrant and lower-right quadrant is empty

Clinical Judgment

A. Monitor carefully for shock and bowel perforation.
B. Report decreased BP, increased pulse, and increased respirations to RN.
C. Monitor I&O.
D. Prepare family for emergency intervention.
E. Assist with preparation of child for barium enema (which provides hydrostatic reduction). Two of three cases respond to this treatment; if not, surgery is necessary.
F. Provide postoperative care for clients who require abdominal surgery.

> **HESI HINT** Nutritional needs and fluid and electrolyte balance are key problems for children with GI disorders. The younger the child, the more vulnerable to fluid and electrolyte imbalances, which increases the need for the caloric intake required for growth.
> Certain condition: cystic fibrosis, Henoch-Schoenlein purpura (also known as IgA vasculitis), Crohn disease, and celiac disease—can increase the risk of intussusception

Congenital Aganglionic Megacolon (Hirschsprung Disease)

Description: Congenital absence of autonomic parasympathetic ganglion (HSCR). This disorder is characterized by the absence of particular nerve cells (ganglions) in a segment of the bowel in an infant. The absence of ganglion cells causes the muscles in the bowels to lose their ability to move stool through the intestine (peristalsis). In the newborn period, failure to pass a meconium for 24 to 48 hours is suggestive of HSCR.

HSCR can sometimes lead to a condition called enterocolitis, which is inflammation of the small intestines and colon. This is often referred to as Hirschsprung-associated enterocolitis. Hirschsprung-associated enterocolitis is the most frequent complication of HSCR occurring in 30% to 40% of individuals with HSCR.

Untreated Hirschsprung-associated enterocolitis may develop sepsis, which also can lead to toxic megacolon.

Approximately 90% of initial HSCR diagnoses in the United States are made within the first year of life. Most of the remaining 10% are made in early childhood.

A. There is a lack of peristalsis in the area of the colon where the ganglion cells are absent.
B. Fecal contents accumulate above the aganglionic area of the bowel.
C. Correction may involve several surgical procedures.
   1. A temporary colostomy with reanastomosis and closure of the colostomy

Clinical Assessment

A. Suspicion in newborn who fails to pass meconium within 24 hours
B. Distended abdomen, chronic constipation alternating with diarrhea
C. Nutritionally deficient child
D. Enterocolitis that occurs as an emergency event
E. Ribbonlike stools in the older child

Clinical Judgment

A. Provide preoperative care.
   1. Begin preparation for abdominal surgery.
   2. Provide bowel-cleansing program as prescribed.
   3. Observe for symptoms of bowel perforation.
      a. Abdominal distention (measure abdominal girth)
      b. Vomiting
      c. Increased abdominal tenderness
      d. Irritability
      e. Dyspnea and cyanosis
   4. Initiate preoperative teaching regarding colostomy.
B. Provide postoperative care.
   1. Check vital signs, axillary temperature.

HESI HINT In the newborn period, failure to pass a meconium for 24–48 hours is suggestive of HSCR.
   HSCR can sometimes lead to a condition called enterocolitis, which is inflammation of the small intestines and colon.

---

https://rarediseases.org/rare-diseases/hirschsprungs-disease/

   2. Assist with IV fluids as prescribed.
   3. Monitor I&O.

   4. Care for nasogastric tube with connection to intermittent suction.
   5. Check abdominal and perineal dressings.
   6. Assess bowel sounds and bowel function.
C. Collaborate with RN to enhance and reinforce a family teaching plan for a home care program.
   1. Teach care of temporary colostomy.
   2. Teach skin care.
   3. Refer family to enterostomal therapist, GI specialist, nutritionist, OT/PT, and speech therapy and social services.
D. Prepare child and family for closure of temporary colostomy.
E. After closure, encourage family to be patient with child when toileting.
F. Teach family to begin toilet training after age 2.

Anorectal Malformations

A. Overview of anorectal malformations
   1. An anorectal malformation is a congenital malformation of the anorectal section of the GI tract (imperforate anus); it is often associated with a fistula.
   2. The type and level of rectal anomaly determines the surgical procedure and degree of bowel control possible.
B. Causes of anorectal malformation
   1. Digestive system issues
   2. Urinary tract issues
   3. Spinal issues
   4. Down syndrome
   5. Townes-Brock syndrome
C. Risk factors for anorectal malformation
   1. Maternal fever
   2. Maternal obesity
   3. Teratogens
   4. Occupational toxins
D. Complications of anorectal malformation
   1. Intestinal perforation
   2. Postoperative sepsis
   3. Death
E. Nursing assessment (data collection) of anorectal malformation
   1. Unusual-appearing anal dimple.
   2. Newborn who does not pass meconium stool within 24 hours.
   3. Meconium appearing from perineal fistula or in urine.
F. Nursing plans and interventions for anorectal malformation
   1. Determine the newborn's first temperature; axillary or tympanic temperature is used for first reading unless hospital policy indicates otherwise.
   2. Observe the newborn for passage of meconium.
   3. Assist the family's ability to cope with diagnosis.
   4. Provide preoperative care to the infant.
      a. Assess vital signs.
      b. Monitor I&O.
   5. Provide postoperative care for anal reconstruction.
      a. Keep the perineal site clean.

b. Position the child in the side-lying prone position with the hips elevated (decreased pressure on perineal sutures).

c. Provide colostomy care if needed.

d. Avoid postoperative rectal temperatures.

6. Assist with home care.

a. Collaborate with the RN to enhance and reinforce a family teaching plan for home care of the colostomy if necessary.

b. With high-level defects, long-term follow-up is required.

c. Toilet training is delayed, and full continence may not be achieved.

Appendicitis

A. Overview of appendicitis
  1. Appendicitis is inflammation of the vermiform appendix.
B. Causes of appendicitis
  1. Obstruction of the lumen of the appendix that causes hardened fecal matter
C. Risk factors for appendicitis
  1. Age range 10 to 30 years
D. Complications of appendicitis
  1. Rupture
  2. Abscess
E. Nursing assessment (data collection) of appendicitis
  1. Colicky, crampy abdominal pain
  2. Pain at McBurney point
  3. Fever
  4. Perforation
    a. Temporary relief of pain occurs after rupture.
F. Nursing plans and interventions for appendicitis
  1. Surgical removal of the appendix requires:
    a. Pain management
    b. Ambulation
    c. NPO status until bowel sounds return
    d. Antibiotics as prescribed
  2. If the appendix ruptures, do the following:
    a. Maintain NG tube for decompression.
    b. Maintain NPO status until tube removal.
    c. Monitor vital signs for signs of abscesses.

❓ REVIEW OF GASTROINTESTINAL DISORDERS

1. Describe feeding techniques for a child with cleft lip or palate.
2. List the signs and symptoms of esophageal atresia with tracheoesophageal fistula (TEF).
3. What actions are initiated for the newborn with suspected esophageal atresia with TEF?
4. Describe the postoperative care for an infant with pyloric stenosis.
5. Describe the preoperative care for a child with Hirschsprung disease.
6. What care is needed for a child with a temporary colostomy?
7. What are the signs of anorectal malformation?
8. What are the priorities for a child undergoing abdominal surgery?

See Answer Key at the end of this text for suggested responses.

HEMATOLOGIC DISORDERS

Iron Deficiency Anemia

Description: Hgb levels below normal range because of the body's inadequate supply, intake, or absorption of iron

A. Iron deficiency anemia is the leading hematologic disorder in children.
B. The need for iron is greater in children than in adults because of accelerated growth.
C. Anemia may be caused by the following:
  1. Inadequate stores during fetal development
  2. Deficient dietary intake
  3. Chronic blood loss
  4. Poor utilization of iron by the body

Clinical Assessment

A. Pallor, paleness of mucous membranes
B. Tiredness, fatigue
C. Usually seen in infants 6 to 24 months old (times of growth spurt); toddlers and female adolescents most affected
D. Dietary intake low in iron
E. Pica habit (eating nonfood substances)
F. Laboratory values
  1. Decreased Hgb
  2. Low serum iron level
  3. Elevated total iron binding capacity (TIBC)

HESI HINT Remember the Hgb norms:
- Newborn: 14–24 g/dL
- Infant: 9.5–14 g/dL
- Child: 10.5–15 g/dL

Clinical Judgment Measures

A. Support child's need to limit activities.
B. Provide rest periods.
C. Administer oral iron (ferrous sulfate) as prescribed.

HESI HINT Teach the family about administration of oral iron:
- Give on empty stomach (as tolerated, for better absorption).
- Give with citrus juices (vitamin C) for increased absorption.
- Use dropper or straw to avoid discoloring teeth.
- Teach that stools will become tarry.
- Teach that iron can be fatal in severe overdose; keep away from other children.
- Do not give with any dairy products.

D. Assist the RN by enhancing and reinforcing a family teaching plan concerning iron deficiency.
  1. Teach about dietary sources of iron.
    a. Meat
    b. Green, leafy vegetables

c. Fish
d. Liver
e. Whole grains
f. Legumes
g. For infants: iron-fortified cereals and formula
2. Teach about appropriate nutrition for child's age.
E. Be aware of family's income and cultural food preferences.
F. Refer family to nutritionist.
G. Refer to Women, Infants, and Children's (WIC) nutrition program, if available to family.

Hemophilia

Description: Inherited bleeding disorder

Causes of Hemophilia

A. Transmitted by an X-linked recessive chromosome. (The mother is the carrier; her sons may express the disease.)
B. A normal individual has between 50% and 200% factor activity in the blood, the hemophiliac has from 0% to 25% activity.
C. The affected individual usually is missing either factor VIII (classic, 75% of cases) or factor IX.

Risk Factors for Hemophilia

A. Family history

Complication of Hemophilia

A. Deep internal bleeding
B. Joint damage
C. Infection
D. Adverse reaction to clotting factor treatment

Clinical Assessment (Data Collection) of Hemophilia

A. Diagnostics
B. Partial thromboplastin time (PTT) is prolonged
C. Factor assays are less than 25%
D. Male child: first "red flag" may be prolonged bleeding after circumcision or after vitamin K injection
E. Prolonged bleeding with minor trauma
F. Hemarthrosis (most frequent site of bleeding)
G. Spontaneous bleeding into muscles and tissues (less severe cases have fewer bleeds)
H. Loss of motion in joints
I. Pain

Clinical Judgment

A. RN administers infusions, which help to replace the clotting factors that are omit mission or low, as prescribed HCP.
B. Administer pain medication as prescribed (analgesics containing no aspirin).

C. Collaborate with RN to enhance and reinforce a family teaching plan for home care.
1. Recognize early signs of bleeding into joints.
2. Local treatment for minor bleeds (pressure, splinting, ice).
3. Administration of factor replacement
4. Dental hygiene: soft toothbrushes
5. Protective care: soft toys, padded bed rails
6. Wear medic alert identification.
7. Support family seeking genetic counseling.
D. Support the child and family during periods of growth and development when increased risk for bleeding occurs (i.e., learning to walk, tooth loss).

HESI HINT Inherited bleeding disorders (hemophilia and sickle cell disease [SCD]) are often used to test knowledge of genetic transmission patterns. Remember:
- Autosomal recessive: Both parents must be heterozygous, or carriers of the recessive trait, for the disease to be expressed in their offspring. With each pregnancy, there is a one in four chance that the infant will have the disease. However, all children of such parents can get the disease—not just 25% of them. This is the transmission pattern of SCD, cystic fibrosis, and phenylketonuria (PKU).
- X-linked recessive trait: The trait is carried on the X chromosome; therefore, it usually affects male offspring, as in hemophilia. With each pregnancy of a woman who is a carrier, there is a 25% chance of having a child with hemophilia. If the child is male, he has a 50% chance of having hemophilia. If the child is female, she has a 50% chance of being a carrier.

Sickle Cell Disease

Description: Sickle cell anemia is one of a group of disorders known as sickle cell disease (SCD). Sickle cell anemia is an inherited red blood cell disorder without enough healthy red blood cells to carry oxygen throughout the body. Flexible, round red blood cells move easily through blood vessels. In sickle cell anemia, the red blood are shaped like sickles or crescent moons. These rigid, sticky cells can get stuck in small blood vessels, which can slow or block blood flow and oxygen to parts of the body.

Genetics: both parents must carry a sickle cell gene. In the United States, sickle cell anemia most commonly affects black people. There is no cure for sickle cell anemia, usually diagnosed after 6 months of age.
A. Hemoglobin S (HgbS) replaces all or part of the normal Hgb, which causes the red blood cells (RBCs) to sickle when oxygen is released into the tissues.
1. Sickled cells cannot flow through capillary beds (Fig. 5.19).
2. Dehydration promotes sickling.
3. Increased sickling episodes occur with cold because cold causes constriction of the vessels (Mayo Clinic, 2021, *Sickle Cell Anemia*).

A Normal red blood cells

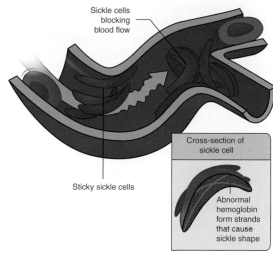

Normal
red blood
cell (RBC)

RBCs flow freely
within blood vessel

Cross-section of RBC

Normal
hemoglobin

B Abnormal, sickled, red blood cell
(sickle cells)

Sickle cells
blocking
blood flow

Sticky sickle cells

Cross-section of
sickle cell

Abnormal
hemoglobin
form strands
that cause
sickle shape

Fig. 5.19 Normal Red Cells and Sickle Red Cells. (A) Normal red blood cells flowing freely in a blood vessel. The inset image shows a cross-section of a normal red blood cell with normal Hgb. (B) Abnormal, sickled red blood cells blocking blood flow in a blood vessel. The inset image shows a cross-section of a sickle cell with abnormal (sickle) Hgb forming abnormal stiff rods. (From NIH. *National heart, lung, and blood institute.* Retrieved from http://www.nhlbi.nih.gov/health/health-topics/topics/sca)

HESI HINT Hydration is very important in the treatment of sickle cell disease because it promotes hemodilution and circulation of red cells through the blood vessels.
 Tissue ischemia causes widespread pathologic changes in spleen, liver, kidney, bones, and the central nervous system .

HESI HINT Important terms:
• Heterozygous gene (HgbAS)—sickle cell trait
• Homozygous gene (HbSS)—sickle cell disease
• Abnormal hemoglobin (HgbS)—disease and trait

Clinical Assessment

A. Children of African descent, usually over 6 months of age
B. Parents with sickle cell trait or SCD
C. Laboratory diagnosis: Hgb electrophoresis (differentiates trait from disease)
D. Frequent infections (nonfunctional spleen)
E. Fatigue
F. Chronic hemolytic anemia
G. Delayed physical growth
H. Vasoocclusive crisis; the classic signs include the following:
  1. Fever
  2. Severe abdominal pain
  3. Hand–foot syndrome (infants); painful edematous hands and feet
  4. Arthralgia
I. Leg ulcers (adolescents)
J. Cerebrovascular accidents (increased risk with dehydration)

Clinical Judgment Measures

A. Collaborate with RN to enhance and reinforce the family and client teaching plan for the prevention of crisis.
B. Teach family that to prevent crisis (hypoxia), they should
  1. Keep child from exercising strenuously.
  2. Keep child away from high altitudes.
  3. Avoid letting child become infected and seek care at first sign of infection.
  4. Keep child well hydrated.
  5. Do not withhold fluids at night because enuresis is a complication of both the disease and the treatment.
C. For a child hospitalized with a vasoocclusive crisis
  1. Monitor IV fluids and electrolytes, as prescribed, to increase hydration and treat acidosis.
  2. Monitor I&O.
  3. Administer blood products as prescribed.
  4. Administer analgesics, including parenteral morphine for severe pain, as prescribed.
  5. Use warm compresses (not ice).
  6. Administer prescribed antibiotics to treat infection.
D. Administer pneumococcal vaccine, meningococcal vaccine, and Hib vaccine as prescribed.
E. Administer hepatitis B vaccine as prescribed.
F. Refer family for genetic counseling.
G. Support child and family experiencing chronic disease.

HESI HINT Supplemental iron is not given to clients with SCD. The anemia is not caused by iron deficiency. Folic acid is given orally to stimulate RBC synthesis.

Acute Lymphocytic Leukemia

Description: Cancer of the blood and bone marrow. The most common subtype, acute lymphoblastic (also termed lymphocytic or lymphoid) leukemia (ALL), accounts for 75% to 80% of all cases of childhood leukemia, whereas acute myeloid (also termed myelocytic, myelogenous, or non-lymphoblastic) leukemia (AML) comprises approximately 20%.

A. ALL is a type of cancer in which the bone marrow makes too many immature lymphocytes (type of WBC).

B. Leukemia may affect red blood cells, WBCs, and platelets.

C. It is noted for the presence of lymphoblasts (immature lymphocytes), which replace normal cells in the bone marrow.

D. Blast cells are also seen in the peripheral blood.

E. Acute lymphocytic leukemia is classified according to whether it involves

　1. B lymphocytes that make antibodies to help fight infection

　2. T lymphocytes that help B lymphocytes make the antibodies that help fight infection.

　3. Natural killer cells that attack cancer cells and viruses

F. ALL has increased stem cells that become lymphoblasts, B lymphocytes, or T lymphocytes/leukemia cells, which do not function as normal lymphocytes and do not fight infection. Also, as the number of leukemia cells increases in the blood and bone marrow, there are less healthy WBCs, red blood cells, and platelets, causing infection, anemia, and easy bleeding.

G. Treatment can be divided into four phases.

　1. First phase—induction chemotherapy.

　2. Second phase—consolidation chemotherapy.

　3. Third phase—maintenance chemotherapy.

　4. Fourth phase—CNS prophylaxis

Clinical Assessment

A. Pallor, tiredness, weakness, lethargy

B. Petechia, bleeding, bruising

C. Infection

D. Bone joint pain

E. Enlarged lymph nodes; hepatosplenomegaly

F. Headache and vomiting (signs of CNS involvement)

G. Anorexia, weight loss

H. Laboratory data: A diagnosis of ALL generally requires that at least 20% of the cells in the bone marrow are blasts.

I. A bone marrow aspiration and biopsy is the only definitive way to diagnose leukemia.

Clinical Judgment Measures

A. Isolation if prescribed. Or recommend private room if possible.

B. Provide child with age-appropriate explanations for diagnostic tests, treatments, and care.

C. Examine child for infection of skin, needle-stick sites, and dental problems.

D. Assist with administration of blood products as prescribed.

E. Assist with administration of antineoplastic chemotherapy.

F. Monitor for side effects of chemotherapeutic agents.

G. Provide care directed toward managing side effects and toxic effects of antineoplastic agents.

> **HESI HINT** Corticosteroids are often given with chemotherapy to help destroy leukemia cells or to reduce allergic reactions to some chemotherapy drugs. The most commonly used steroids for ALL include prednisolone and dexamethasone.

　1. Administer antiemetics as prescribed.

　2. Monitor fluid balance.

　3. Monitor for signs of infection.

　4. Monitor for signs of bleeding.

　5. Monitor for cumulative toxic effects of drugs: hepatic toxicity, cardiac toxicity, renal toxicity, and neurotoxicity.

　6. Provide oral hygiene.

　7. Provide small, appealing meals; increase calories and protein; refer to nutritionist.

　8. Promote self-esteem and positive body image if child has alopecia, severe weight loss, or other disturbance in body image.

　9. Provide care to prevent infection.

　10. Provide emotional support for family in crisis.

　11. Encourage family's and child's input and control in determining plans and treatment.

❓ REVIEW OF HEMATOLOGIC DISORDERS

1. Describe the information families should be given when a child is receiving oral iron preparations.
2. List dietary sources of iron.
3. What is the genetic transmission pattern of hemophilia?
4. Describe the sequence of events in a vasoocclusive crisis in sickle cell disease (SCD).
5. Explain why hydration is a priority in treating SCD.
6. What should families and children do to avoid triggering sickling episodes?
7. Interventions and treatments for a child with leukemia are based on what three physiologic problems?

See Answer Key at the end of this text for suggested responses.

METABOLIC AND ENDOCRINE DISORDERS

Congenital Hypothyroidism

Description: Congenital condition resulting from inadequate thyroid tissue development *in utero*. Cognitive impairment and growth failure occur if it is not detected and treated in early infancy.

Clinical Assessment

A. Newborn screening (NBS) reveals low thyroxine (T_4) and high thyroid-stimulating hormone (TSH).

B. Symptoms in the newborn

1. Long gestation (>42 weeks)
2. Large hypoactive infant
3. Delayed meconium passage
4. Feeding problems (poor suck)
5. Prolonged physiologic jaundice
6. Hypothermia

C. Symptoms in early infancy if untreated with T_4
1. Large, protruding tongue
2. Coarse hair/hairline will appear low.
3. Lethargy, sleepiness
4. Flat expression
5. Constipation
6. Hypotonia
7. Large soft spots of the skull
8. Hoarse cry
9. Distended stomach with outpouching of the belly button (umbilical hernia)
10. Feeding problems, including needing to be awakened for feedings and difficulty swallowing
11. "Floppy" (poor muscle tone, also called hypotonia)
12. Delay of serum phenylalanine testing will lead to CNS damage, delays in learning.

D. Prognosis is good if the condition is recognized and treated. The infant's development is usually not affected if treatment is initiated within the first month of life.

> **HESI HINT** Congenital hypothyroidism is a condition resulting from inadequate thyroid tissue development in utero. Cognitive impairment and growth failure occur if it is not detected and treated in early infancy. Testing includes a newborn screen based on state requirements which will reveal low thyroxine (T_4) and high thyroid-stimulating hormone (TSH).

Clinical Judgment Measures

A. Perform NBS programs per state regulations.
B. Assess newborn for signs of congenital hypothyroidism.
   Once identified, teach family about replacement therapy with thyroid hormone.
C. Treatment involves monitoring of blood thyroid hormone levels (TSH and free T4) to make sure that the amount of medication is adjusted to keep up with how fast the baby is growing. Generally, blood tests are checked every 1 to 2 months up to 6 months of age and then every 2 to 3 months thereafter.
D. Collaborate with RN to enhance and reinforce a family teaching plan for replacement therapy with thyroid hormone.
1. Explain that child will have a lifelong need for the therapy.
2. Tell parents to give child a single dose in the morning.
3. Signs of overdose include rapid pulse, irritability, fever, weight loss, and diarrhea.
4. Signs of underdose include lethargy, fatigue, constipation, and poor feeding.

5. Periodic thyroid testing is necessary (American Thyroid Association [ATA], 2021, *Congenital Hypothyroidism*)

Phenylketonuria

Description: Rare autosomal-recessive disorder in which the body cannot metabolize the essential amino acid phenylalanine, which accumulates in the blood after the infant begins consuming breast milk or formula and is in all foods containing protein. PKU can cause intellectual and developmental disabilities (IDDs) if not treated. High phenylalanine will damage the brain. Children and adults who are treated early and consistently develop normally.

All children born in U.S. hospitals are tested routinely for PKU soon after birth, making it easier to diagnose and treat affected children early.

Clinical Assessment (If Undetected and/or Untreated)

A. NBS using the Guthrie test; positive result; serum phenylalanine level of 4 mg/dL
B. Frequent vomiting, failure to gain weight
C. Irritability
D. Musty odor of urine
1. Delayed growth and development
2. Signs of FTT
3. Unpleasant peculiar body odor and urine
4. In the United States, PKU is most common in people of European or Native American ancestry. It is much less common among people of African, Hispanic, or Asian ancestry.
5. May have microcephaly
E. Mothers diagnosed with PKU disease who do not maintain a low-phenylalanine diet during pregnancy can cause problems for their children who do inherit PKU. Those infants are at risk for:
1. Cognitive impairment
2. Microcephaly
3. Birth weight below 2500 g
4. Disrupted growth and development
5. Congenital heart anomalies

> **HESI HINT** Early detection of hypothyroidism and PKU is essential for preventing cognitive impairment in infants. Knowledge of normal growth and developmental patterns is important because a lack of attainment can be used to detect the presence of a disease and to evaluate the treatment's effects.

Clinical Interventions

A. Perform NBS based on state requirements. Obtain a subsequent sample as notified by NBS. Screen infants born at home who have no hospital contact, as well as infants adopted internationally.
B. Collaborate with RN to enhance and reinforce a family teaching plan and dietary management.
1. Stress the importance of strict adherence to prescribed low-phenylalanine diet.

2. Instruct family to provide special formulas for infant.
3. Teach family to avoid foods high in phenylalanine (that is, high-protein foods) and encourage family to work with nutritionist.
4. Refer for genetic counseling.

For more information, see https://www.nichd.nih.gov/health/topics/pku/conditioninfo/default

> **HESI HINT** Assure family is educated regarding a low-phenylalanine diet.

Insulin-Dependent Diabetes Mellitus or Type 1 Diabetes

Description: Metabolic disorder in which the insulin-producing cells (beta cells) of the pancreas are nonfunctioning as a result of some insult. The child's body no longer produces the hormone (insulin) and may be the result of an autoimmune reaction.

Causes

A. Heredity, viral infections, and autoimmune processes are implicated in diabetes mellitus (DM).

Risk Factors for Type 1 Diabetes

A. Infancy
B. School-age children

Complications of Type 1 Diabetes

A. Altered carbohydrate, protein, and fat metabolism

Clinical Assessment

A. Classic three Ps:
   1. Polydipsia
   2. Polyphagia
   3. Polyuria, enuresis (bedwetting) in previously continent child
B. Unintentional weight loss
C. Fatigue
D. Irritability or behavior changes
E. Fruity-smelling breath
F. Abdominal complaints, nausea, and vomiting
G. Usually occurs in school-age children but can occur even in infancy.

> **HESI HINT** DM in children was typically diagnosed as insulin-dependent diabetes (type 1) until recently. A marked increase in type 2 DM (noninsulin-dependent DM [NIDDM]), known as type 2, has occurred in the United States, particularly among Native American, African American, and Hispanic children and adolescents. Average age at diagnosis is 13.7 years, with overweight or obesity being a major concern.

Clinical Judgment Measures

A. If a child is in ketoacidosis, provide care in collaboration with the RN and other HCPs for the seriously ill child (may be unconscious).
   1. Monitor vital signs and neurologic status.
   2. Monitor blood glucose, pH, and serum electrolytes.
   3. Observe hydration status.
   4. Maintain strict I&O.
B. Reinforce home-teaching program with child and family.
   1. Medications
      a. Type 1 insulin administration, either two or more injections per day or insulin pump
      b. Type 2: oral medication or insulin or a combination of the two.
   2. Dietary management (carbohydrate counting preferred).
      a. Meals and snacks
      b. Growth and exercise needs
      c. Basic four food groups, no concentrated sweets
      d. Refer to a nutritionist
   3. Exercise.
      a. Regular, planned activities
      b. Diet modification; snacks before or during exercise
   4. Home glucose monitoring and urine testing
   5. Medical management and follow-up as needed
   6. Ensure that the parents involve the school nurse and/or daycare in daily management.
D. Reinforce a teaching program for the school-aged.
   1. Identify issues specific to school.
      a. Physical education class and exercise
      b. Scheduled times for meals and snacks
      c. Need to be like peers
   2. Teach that a school-age child should be responsible for most management.
   3. Wear a medical alert ID.

https://www.mayoclinic.org/diseases-conditions/type-1-diabetes-in-children/symptoms-causes/syc-20355306

❓ REVIEW OF METABOLIC AND ENDOCRINE DISORDERS

1. How is congenital hypothyroidism diagnosed?
2. What are the symptoms of congenital hypothyroidism in early infancy?
3. What are the outcomes of untreated congenital hypothyroidism?
4. What are the metabolic effects of phenylketonuria?
5. List food types high in phenylalanine.
6. What are the three classic signs of diabetes?
7. Differentiate the signs of hypoglycemia and hyperglycemia.
8. Describe the care of a child with ketoacidosis.
9. Describe developmental factors that would affect the school-age child with diabetes.
10. What is the relationship between hypoglycemia and exercise?

See Answer Key at the end of this text for suggested responses.

SKELETAL DISORDERS

Fractures

Description: Traumatic injury to bone. Younger children diagnosed with fractures may be at risk for child abuse. 4.4 million child maltreatment referral reports received. Child abuse reports involved 7.9 million children. 45.4% of children who die from child abuse are under one year. Boys had a higher child fatality rate than girls. The history of the incident matches the physical injury and sounds feasible (American Society for Preventive Care of Children, 2021, *Children Maltreatment*).

A. Fractures can be classified according to type. Pediatric fractures often have distinct fracture patterns due to the unique properties of growing bones. The periosteum in growing bones is thicker and stronger than in adult bones, which is why children are more prone to more incomplete fractures, such as the greenstick fracture or torus fracture.

In addition, periosteum is metabolically active. This feature also explains why childhood fractures heal faster than fractures in adults.

B. Salter-Harris fractures are fractures of the epiphyseal plate of long bones. These fractures only arise in children and adolescents whose skeletal growth is not yet complete. Salter-Harris fractures are classified into 5 types (Type I—V with V) according to the extent of damage to the growth plate and joint involvement.

C. Open fracture (compound fracture): The bone pokes through the skin and can be seen. Or a deep wound exposes the bone through the skin. Closed fracture (simple fracture). The bone is broken, but the skin is intact.
1. Complete fractures: Bone fragments are completely separate.
2. Incomplete fractures: Bone fragments remain attached (e.g., greenstick, bowing, buckles).
3. Comminuted fractures: Bone fragments from the fractured shaft break free and lie in the surrounding tissue; usually associated with high impact and trauma.
4. Spiral fractures: Fracture line results from twisting force; forms a spiral encircling the bone (*Pediatric fractures—knowledge @ amboss.* ambossIcon).

HESI HINT Fractures in older children are common because they fall during play and are involved in motor vehicle accidents.
- Spiral fractures (caused by twisting) and fractures in infants may be related to child abuse.
- Fractures involving the epiphyseal plate (growth plate) can have serious consequences in terms of the growth of the affected limb.

Clinical Assessment

A. General condition
1. Visible bone fragments
2. Misalignment of the limb
3. Pain
4. Swelling

5. Contusions
6. Child guarding or protecting the extremity
7. Limited range of motion

B. The five Ps are a late indication of compartment syndrome:
1. Pain
2. Pallor
3. Pulselessness
4. Paresthesia
5. Paralysis

Clinical Interventions

A. Obtain baseline data and frequently perform neurovascular assessments.
1. Pulses: Check pulses distal to the injury to assess circulation.
2. Color: Check injured extremity for pink, brisk, capillary refill.
3. Movement and sensation: Check injured extremity for nerve impairment; compare for symmetry with uninjured extremity (child may guard injury).
4. Temperature: Check extremity for warmth.
5. Swelling: Check for an increase in swelling. Elevate extremity to prevent swelling.
6. Pain: Monitor for severe pain that is not relieved by analgesics.
7. Newly fractured sites are generally splinted and braced until swelling goes down. Once the swelling has subsided, a cast is applied to the affected extremity.

B. Report abnormal neurovascular assessments promptly!

HESI HINT Compartment syndrome is a progressive decrease of tissue perfusion occurring as a result of increased pressure from edema or swelling that presses on the tissues and vessels. Compromised circulation with abnormal neurovascular checks is the result of compartment syndrome. If compartment syndrome occurs and is not treated immediately with a fasciotomy, it can result in permanent nerve and vasculature damage, possibly leading to amputation of the limb.

C. Maintain traction if prescribed. Note bed position, type of traction, weights, pulleys, pins, pin sites, adhesive strips, Ace wraps, splints, and casts.
1. Skin traction: Force is applied to skin.

HESI HINT Skin traction for fracture reduction should not be removed unless the health care provider prescribes its removal.

---

   a. Buck extension traction: lower extremity, legs extended, no hip flexion
   b. Dunlop traction: two lines of pull on the arm
   c. Russell traction: two lines of pull on the lower extremity, one perpendicular, one longitudinal
   d. Bryant traction: both lower extremities flexed 90 degrees at hips (rarely used because extreme elevation of lower extremities causes decreased peripheral circulation)
2. Skeletal traction: Pin or wire applies pull directly to the distal bone fragment.

a. Ninety-degree traction: 90-degree flexion of hip and knee; lower extremity is in a boot cast; can also be used on upper extremities.

b. Dunlop traction: may be used as skeletal traction

> **HESI HINT** Pin sites can be a source of infection. Monitor for signs of infection. Cleanse and dress pin sites as prescribed.

> **HESI HINT** When moving the client in bed, with either skin or skeletal traction, it is necessary for someone to hold and move the weights of the traction as the client changes position to avoid additional tension on the traction and fracture sites.

A. Maintain child in proper body alignment; restrain if necessary.

B. Monitor for problems of immobility.

C. Provide age-appropriate play and toys.

D. Prepare child for cast application; use age-appropriate terms when explaining procedures.

E. Provide routine cast care after application; petal cast edges.

F. Collaborate with RN to enhance and reinforce a family teaching plan for home cast care to family, including

1. Neurovascular assessment of casted extremity
2. Not to get cast wet
3. Teach that, in the presence of a hip spica, family may use a Bradford frame under a small child to help with toileting; they must not use an abduction bar to turn child.
4. Teach to seek follow-up care with health care provider.

> **HESI HINT** Skeletal disorders affect the infant's or child's physical mobility, and typical NGN-NCLEX-PN questions focus on appropriate toys and activities for the child who is confined to bed rest and who is immobilized.

Developmental Dysplasia of Hip

Description: Abnormal development of the femoral head in the acetabulum, usually diagnosed at birth. Although developmental dysplasia of hip (DDH) is most often present at birth, it may also develop during a child's first year of life. Recent research shows that babies whose legs are swaddled tightly with the hips and knees straight are at a notably higher risk for developing DDH after birth. As swaddling becomes increasingly popular, it is important for parents to learn how to swaddle their infants safely, and to understand that when done improperly, swaddling may lead to problems like DDH.

In all cases of DDH, the socket (acetabulum) is shallow, meaning that the ball of the thighbone (femur) cannot firmly fit into the socket. Sometimes, the ligaments that help to hold the joint in place are stretched. The degree of hip looseness, or instability, varies among children with DDH.

- Dislocated: In the most severe cases of DDH, the head of the femur is completely out of the socket.

- Dislocatable: In these cases, the head of the femur lies within the acetabulum, but can easily be pushed out of the socket during a physical examination.

- Subluxatable: In mild cases of DDH, the head of the femur is simply loose in the socket. During a physical examination, the bone can be moved within the socket, but it will not be dislocated.

Contributing factors: DDH tends to run in families and can be present in either hip and in any individual. It usually affects the left hip and is predominant in:

- Girls
- Firstborn children
- Babies born in the breech position (especially with feet up by the shoulders). The American Academy of Pediatrics now recommends ultrasound DDH screening of all female breech babies.
- Family history of DDH (parents or siblings)
- Oligohydramnios

A. Treatment

1. When DDH is detected at birth, it can usually be corrected with the use of a harness or brace. If the hip is not dislocated at birth, the condition may not be noticed until the child begins walking. At this time, treatment is more complicated, with less predictable results.

2. Newborns. The baby is placed in a soft positioning device, called a Pavlik harness, for 1 to 2 months to keep the thighbone in the socket. This special brace is designed to hold the hip in the proper position while allowing free movement of the legs and easy diaper care. The Pavlik harness helps tighten the ligaments around the hip joint and promotes normal hip socket formation.

3. 1 month to 6 months. Similar to newborn treatment, a baby's thighbone is repositioned in the socket using a harness or similar device. This method is usually successful, even with hips that are initially dislocated.

4. 6 months to 2 years. Older babies are also treated with closed reduction and spica casting. In most cases, skin traction may be used for a few weeks prior to repositioning the thighbone. Skin traction prepares the soft tissues around the hip for the change in bone positioning. It may be done at home or in the hospital.

Clinical Assessment

A. *Infant*

1. Positive Ortolani sign ("clicking" with abduction; is the sound heard when the health care provider maneuvers the femoral head and it slips back into the acetabulum)

2. Positive Barlow maneuver ("feel" the dislocation as the femur leaves the acetabulum when the health care provider adducts and extends the hips while stabilizing the pelvis) (Fig. 5.20)

B. *Older child*

1. Limp on affected side
2. Trendelenburg sign
https://orthoinfo.aaos.org/en/diseases–conditions/developmental-dislocation-dysplasia-of-the-hip-ddh/

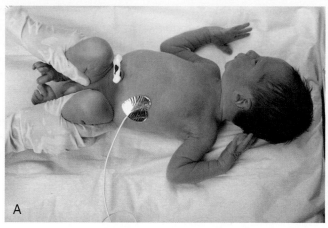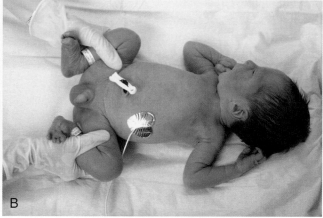

Fig. 5.20 Assessment of the Hips. (A) Barlow test: adduct the hips and apply gentle pressure down and back with the thumbs. In hip dysplasia, the examiner can feel the femoral head move out of the acetabulum. (B) Ortolani test: abduct the thighs and apply gentle pressure forward over the greater trochanter. A "clunking" sensation indicates a dislocated femoral head moving into the acetabulum. A hip click is normal from ligament movement. (From McKinney, E. S., James, S. R., Murray, S. S., Nelson, K. A., & Ashwill, J. W. [2013]. *Maternal-child nursing* [4th ed.]. St. Louis: Saunders.)

> **HESI HINT** A positive Trendelenburg sign usually indicates weakness in the hip abductor muscles: gluteus medius and gluteus minimus.

Clinical Judgment Measures

A. Perform newborn assessment at birth.

B. Apply abduction device or splint (Pavlik harness) as prescribed. Therapy involves positioning legs in flexed abducted position.

C. Collaborate with RN to enhance and reinforce a family teaching plan for home care.
 1. Teach application and removal of device (worn 24 hours a day).
 2. Teach skin care and bathing (physician may allow parents to remove device for bathing).
 3. Teach that follow-up care involves frequent adjustments because of growth.

D. Teach how to provide care for an infant if splinting is ineffective.
 1. Instruct to monitor circulation to feet.
 2. Instruct to meet developmental needs of an immobilized infant.
 3. Incorporate family in care.
 4. Prepare family for spica cast application.

E. Provide care for a child requiring surgical correction.
 1. Perform preoperative teaching of child and family, including cast application.
 2. Perform postoperative care.
  a. Assess vital signs.
  b. Check cast for drainage and bleeding.
  c. Perform neurovascular assessment of extremities.
  d. Promote respiratory hygiene.
  e. Administer narcotic analgesics as prescribed.
  f. Teach family cast care when child gets home, including checking the cast for "hot spots" (possibly indicative of infection).

Scoliosis (Idiopathic, Congenital, and Neuromuscular)

Description: Lateral curvature of the spine that generally occurs during rapid growth spurts in adolescents. Hereditary conditions, neuromuscular diseases, congenital spinal defects, and trauma or infections to the spine may factor in the development of scoliosis. Treatment depends on the curvature of the spine.

Idiopathic scoliosis, which means the exact cause is not known, is a condition that causes the spine to curve sideways. Idiopathic scoliosis curves vary in size, and mild curves are more common than larger curves. If a child is still growing, a scoliosis curve can worsen rapidly during a growth spurt. Although it can develop in toddlers and young children, idiopathic scoliosis most often begins during puberty. Both boys and girls can be affected; however, girls are more likely to develop larger curves that require medical care.

Congenital scoliosis. Problems in the spine sometimes develop before a baby is born. Babies with congenital scoliosis may have spinal bones that are not fully formed or are fused together.

Neuromuscular scoliosis. Medical conditions that affect the nerves and muscles, such as muscular dystrophy or cerebral palsy, can lead to scoliosis. These types of neuromuscular conditions can cause imbalance and weakness in the muscles that support the spine.

Clinical Assessment

A. Occurs most commonly in adolescent females (10 until fully grown)
 1. Elevated shoulder or hip
 2. Head and hips not aligned
 3. While child is bending forward, a rib hump is apparent. (Ask child to bend forward from the hips with arms hanging free, and examine child for a curve of the spine, rib hump, and hip asymmetry.)

Clinical Judgment Measures

A. Assist the RN with screening all adolescent children, especially females, during growth spurt.

B. Prepare child and family for conservative treatment, such as the use of a brace.

C. Observation. If spinal curve is less than 25 degrees or if almost full-grown, monitor the curve to make sure it does not get worse, including a recheck about every 6 to 12 months and schedule follow-up x-rays until child is fully grown.

D. Bracing. If the spinal curve is between 25 and 45 degrees and is still growing, bracing may be recommended. Although bracing will not straighten an existing curve, it often prevents it from getting worse to the point of requiring surgery. Braces are underarm braces that are custom-made to fit the child's body comfortably.

E. Spinal Fusion for a curve that is greater than 45 to 50 degrees or if bracing did not stop the curve from reaching this point. Severe curves that are not treated could eventually worsen to the point where they affect lung function. This will straighten the curve and then fuse the vertebrae together so that they heal into a single, solid bone. This will stop growth completely in the part of the spine affected by scoliosis. Metal rods are typically used to hold the bones in place until the fusion happens. The rods are attached to the spine by hooks, screws, and/or wires.

   1. Suggest clothing modifications to camouflage brace.
   2. Reinforce prescribed exercise regimen for back and abdominal muscles.
   3. Plan ways of improving self-concept with the adolescent.
   4. Teach family that severe, untreated scoliosis can cause respiratory difficulty.
   5. A brace does not correct the spine's curve in a child with scoliosis; it only stops or slows the progression.

F. Prepare child and family for surgical correction if required.

   1. Teach child and family log-rolling technique.
   2. Teach how to practice respiratory hygiene.
   3. Orient child to ICU.
   4. Discuss possible postoperative tubes.
   5. Describe postoperative pain management; PCA may be used.
   6. Obtain a baseline neurologic assessment.

G. Provide postoperative care.

   1. Perform frequent neurologic assessments.
   2. Log-roll for 5 days.
   3. Monitor IV fluids and analgesics as prescribed.
   4. Perform oral hygiene.
   5. Assist with ambulation.
   6. Encourage child's participation in care to promote self-esteem.
      https://orthoinfo.aaos.org/en/diseases–conditions/idiopathic-scoliosis-in-children-and-adolescents/

Juvenile Arthritis or Juvenile Idiopathic Arthritis

Description: Juvenile arthritis affects nearly 300,000 kids and teens in the United States.

Juvenile arthritis (JA), also known as pediatric rheumatic disease, is an umbrella term to describe the inflammatory and rheumatic diseases that develop in children under the age of 16.

Causes

Most kinds of JA are autoimmune or autoinflammatory diseases. The immune system is confused and releases inflammatory chemicals that attack healthy cells and tissue. In most JA cases this causes joint inflammation, swelling, pain, and tenderness, but some types of JA have few or no joint symptoms or only affect the skin and internal organs.

The exact causes of JA are unknown, but researchers believe that certain genes may cause JA when activated by a virus, bacteria, or other external factors. There is no evidence that foods, toxins, allergies, or lack of vitamins cause the disease.

Juvenile idiopathic arthritis. Juvenile idiopathic arthritis is the most common form of juvenile arthritis and includes six types: oligoarthritis, polyarthritis, systemic, enthesitis-related, juvenile psoriatic arthritis, and undifferentiated.

Signs of JA include limited range of motion, rash, eye symptoms, and joint swelling, tenderness, and pain. Laboratory tests that look for inflammatory markers and imaging tests (x-rays, CT scans, MRIs) to look for signs of joint damage can also help rule out other causes like trauma or infection.

Treatment

There is no cure for JA, but with early diagnosis and aggressive treatment, remission is possible.

Chronic inflammatory disorder of the joint synovium is considered one of the most common rheumatoid conditions occurring in children under the age of 17. JIA is diagnosed when the client presents with the following symptoms for a minimum of 6 weeks:

A. Continuous arthritic pain in single or multiple joints

B. Repetitive fevers up to 39.44°C (103°F)

C. Systematic indications appearing as pinkish/reddish rash on the legs, arms, and trunk

D. The exact cause is unknown; the child's immune system attacks the synovial lining of the joints

Clinical Assessment

A. Joint swelling and stiffness (usually large joints)

B. Painful joints

C. Generalized symptoms: fever, malaise, and rash

D. Periods of exacerbations and remissions

E. Varying severity: mild and self-limited or severe and disabling

Clinical Judgment Measures

A. A well-rounded plan includes medication, physical activity, complementary therapies (acupuncture, massage, mind-body therapies), and healthy eating habits.

B. Medications: Drugs that control disease activity include corticosteroids and disease-modifying antirheumatic drugs (DMARDs).

C. Support the maintaining of school schedule and activities appropriate for age.

D. Encourage periodic eye examinations for early detection of iridocyclitis (inflammation of the iris) to prevent vision loss.

> **HESI HINT** A well-rounded plan includes medication, physical activity, complementary therapies (acupuncture, massage, mind-body therapies), and healthy eating habits.

⚡ REVIEW OF SKELETAL DISORDERS

1. List normal findings in a neurovascular assessment.
2. What is compartment syndrome?

3. What are the signs and symptoms of compartment syndrome?
4. Why are fractures of the epiphyseal plate a special concern?
5. How is skeletal traction applied?
6. What discharge instructions should be included concerning a child with a spica cast?
7. What are the signs and symptoms of congenital dislocated hip in infants?
8. How would the nurse conduct a scoliosis screening?
9. What instructions should a child with scoliosis receive about a skeletal brace?
10. What care is indicated for a child with juvenile rheumatoid arthritis?

See Answer Key at the end of this text for suggested responses.

For more review, go to http://evolve.elsevier.com/HESI/RN for HESI's online study examinations.

NEXT-GENERATION NCLEX EXAMINATION-STYLE QUESTIONS

Orders

O₂ oxygen at 2 L, chest x-ray, IV 1000 NS @60 cc/h. routine laboratory, hourly I & O, silver nitrate to open skin, dressing changes q.8 h. V.S. q. 30 min; safety parameters.

Health History	Nurses' Notes	Vital Signs	Lab Results

Ms. Carol James, a 21-year late adolescent, has run into the emergency room stating that her 2-year-old daughter fell into their home jacuzzi. You notice that the child's respiratory rate is rapid and labored and that there are burns to about 25% of the child's face and front and back torso. She is screaming in pain and she has an oozing wound to her L arm. Her mother states her daughter was playing near her; however, when her telephone rang she began talking to a friend without paying attention to her daughter. When she got off the phone she called out to her daughter and found her on the patio in the jacuzzi. When she reached down to pull her child out, her daughter began to scream and cry immediately. Ms. James picked up her child, ran to her car, and drove to the emergency room.

Instructions

Complete the diagram by selecting from the choices below to specify what potential condition the client is most likely experiencing, 2 actions to take, and 2 parameters the nurse would monitor to assess the client's progress.

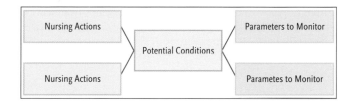

Nursing Actions	Potential Conditions	Parameters to Monitor
Obtain post-op orders	Fracture to left ribs and thoracic cage	60 cc hour up to 1000 cc per IV fluid per day
Contact social services for child abuse assessment	Exacerbated respiratory syndrome	Monitor ECG and heart rate
Initiate physical therapy treatment	First- and second-degree burns	Oriented to time, person, and place
Monitor I&O	Acute skin abrasions secondary to fall	Assess pain level
separate the mom from her daughter		have the doctor order a MRI

REFERENCES AND BIBLIOGRAPHY

American Society for Preventive Care of Children. (2021). *Children maltreatment.* Retrieved December 4, 2021, from https://americanspcc.org/child-abuse-statistics/.

American Thyroid Association (ATA). (2021). *Congenital hypothyroidism.* Retrieved October 21, 2021, from https://www.thyroid.org/congenital-hypothyroidism/.

Centers for Disease Control and Prevention (CDC). (2019, February 6). *Poisoning prevention.* Centers for Disease Control and Prevention. Retrieved October 8, 2021, from https://www.cdc.gov/safechild/poisoning/index.html.

Graham, L. (2007). AHA Releases updated guidelines on prevention of Infective Endocarditis. *American Family Physician, 77*(4), 538–545. Retrieved October 2021, http://circ.ahajournals.org/cgi/content/full/116/15/1736.

Health Resources & Service Administration (HRSA). (2021). *Poison Help and Prevention Tips.* Retrieved October 10, 2021, from https://poisonhelp.hrsa.gov/what-you-can-do/prevention-tips.

Hirschsprung disease. (2017, February 1). *NORD (National Organization for Rare Disorders).* Retrieved October 8, 2021, from https://rarediseases.org/rare-diseases/hirschsprungs-disease/.

Kim, A. H., & Erby, M. (2020). *Physical abuse (non-accidental trauma).* PM&R KnowledgeNow. Retrieved October 8, 2021, from https://now.aapmr.org/physical-abuse-nonaccidental-trauma/.

National Cancer Institute. (2021). *Wilms tumor and other childhood kidney tumors treatment (PDQ®)—health.* Retrieved October 30, 2021, from https://www.cancer.gov/types/kidney/hp/wilms-treatment-pdq.

Nemours Kids Health. (2021). *Cleft palate with cleft lip.* Retrieved November 10, 2021, from https://kidshealth.org/en/parents/cleft-palate-cleft-lip.html.

National Organization of Rare Diseases (NORD). (2021). *Duchenne muscular dystrophy.* Retrieved October 8, 2021, from https://rarediseases.org/rare-diseases/duchenne-muscular-dystrophy/.

Stanford Childrens' Health. (2021). *Congenital heart disease.* Retrieved November 8, 2021, from https://www.stanfordchildrens.org/en/topic/default?id=signs-of-respiratory-distress-in-children-90-P02960.

Stanford Childrens' Health. (2021). *Epilepsy and seizures in children.* Retrieved November 20, 2021, from https://www.stanfordchildrens.org/en/topic/default?id=seizures-and-epilepsy-in-children-90-P02621.

Stanford Childrens' Health. (2021). *Signs of respiratory distress in children.* Retrieved November 8, 2021, from https://www.stanfordchildrens.org/en/topic/default?id=congenital-heart-disease-90-P02346.

U.S. Department of Health and Human Services. (2020, May 13). *Hydrocephalus fact sheet.* National Institute of Neurological Disorders and Stroke. Retrieved October 8, 2021, from https://www.ninds.nih.gov/Disorders/Patient-Caregiver-Education/Fact-Sheets/Hydrocephalus-Fact-Sheet.

Ward, S., & Hisley, S. (2016). *Maternal-child nursing care with the women's health companion: optimizing outcomes for mothers, children and families* (pp. 54–66). Philadelphia, PA: F.A. Davis. ISBN-13: 978-0-8036-2813-7.

Weber, L. (2015a). *Guidelines for non-accidental trauma pediatric perspectives.* Retrieved October 8, 2021, from https://www.gillettechildrens.org/assets/uploads/for-medical-professionals/Guidelines_for_Non-Accidental_Trauma_Pediatric_Perspectives_Vol._24_No.2.pdf.

Weber, L. (2015b). Practical guidelines for identifying non-accidental trauma in children. *A Pediatric Perspective, 24*(2), 144–146.

Wrona, S. K., Melnyk, B. M., & Hoying, J. (2021). Chronic pain and mental health Co-Morbidity in adolescents: An urgent call for assessment and Evidence-Based Intervention. *Pain Manag Nurs, 22,* 252–259.

Maternity Nursing

THE MENSTRUAL CYCLE

Menarche

Description: Menarche is defined as the onset of menstruation. Menarche usually occurs between 11 and 13 years with a median age of 12.8 years, or 2 to 3 years after breast budding (thelarche). The first menstrual cycles are typically anovulatory, often irregularly spaced, and can produce heavy bleeding. Regularity and predictability of cycles generally occur within 3 years of menarche. While ovulation can occur at the time of menarche, it most often takes several months to establish regular ovulatory patterns. However, while most women will have ovulatory cycles within 2 years of menarche, young women should be aware that pregnancy can occur after the onset of menarche.

Menarche is viewed very differently among different cultures; some celebrate the event and others treat it as taboo. Providing education about menarche can increase the comfort of young women. It signifies an important transition into adulthood for young women.

The complete menstrual cycle is under physiological control of the hypothalamic-pituitary ovarian (H-P-O) axis. The HPO axis releases hormones in a pulsatile fashion and triggers changes on both the uterine endometrium (endometrial cycle) and the ovaries (ovarian cycle); whatever happens in the endometrium during the menstrual cycle matches with ovarian activities.

The hypothalamus initially releases gonadotropin-releasing hormone (GnRH). GnRH then stimulates the pituitary gland to produce luteinizing hormone (LH) and follicle-stimulating hormone (FSH), along with several other thyroid, adrenal, and pancreatic hormones. LH and FSH in turn stimulate ovarian production of estrogen and progesterone. LH and FSH regulate the activities of the menstrual cycle through a complex system of negative and positive feedback loops. These feedback loops work synergistically to control functional changes to the endometrial lining and ovulation from the ovaries.

The normal menstrual cycle length is approximately 21 to 35 days. The menstrual cycle can be further defined through ovarian activities and endometrial changes.

Ovarian Cycle

There are three phases in the ovarian cycle.

A. **Follicular phase**: Begins the first day of menstruation (day 1) through day 14 of a typical 28-day cycle. In this preovulatory phase, FSH is secreted by the anterior pituitary and rises triggering one dominant follicle to emerge. As the dominant follicle further develops it moves toward the surface of the ovary in anticipation of the LH surge.

B. **Ovulatory phase**: Ovulation is the process that releases the mature ovum from the dominant follicle. About 34 to 36 hours prior to ovulation, there is a marked rise in LH that prompts the final maturation of the ovum and its release. The ovum is picked up by the fimbriated end of the fallopian tube and transported to the uterus.
1. Indications of ovulation. A slight drop in temperature occurs 1 day before ovulation (basal body temperature may be less than 37°; a rise of 0.5 to 1° in temperature occurs at ovulation). Temperature remains elevated for approximately 10 to 12 days. Preovulatory and postovulatory mucus is thick, but at ovulation, cervical mucus is abundant, watery, thin, and clear (it resembles egg white, called spinnbarkeit). The cervical os dilates slightly, softens, and rises in the vagina. Some women have localized abdominal pain (mittelschmerz) that coincides with ovulation. Ferning can be seen microscopically.

C. **Luteal phase**: begins immediately after ovulation and ends with initiation of menstruation. This phase is relatively constant at 14 days. The influence of LH helps form the corpus luteum. The corpus luteum secretes progesterone and some estrogen to start the negative feedback loop to the HPO axis and prevents further ovulation in the current cycle. Corpus luteum reaches its peal of functional activity 8 days after ovulation. If conception occurs, the fertilized ovum is implanted in the prepared endometrium. In the absence of implantation, the corpus luteum regresses, estrogen and progesterone levels decrease, and the endometrium is shed via menstruation.

Endometrial Cycle

There are four phases of the endometrial cycle (Fig. 6.1).

A. **Menstrual phase**: Begins with initiation of menses. Periodic vasoconstriction in the upper layers of the endometrium initiates shedding of functional 2/3 of the endometrium. Menses, or menstrual flow, typically lasts 3 to 5 days but normal variations are noted with as little as 2 days up to 7 days of flow. The average amount of flow ranges from 35 to 80 mL with an average of 50 mL.

B. **Proliferative phase**: Primarily influenced by estrogen. Typically begins on day 4 to 5 and replenishes the endometrium after menses. This phase lasts about 10 days.

C. **Secretory phase**: Primarily influenced by progesterone. Begins at ovulation, usually day 15, and lasts through day 28. During this phase, the endometrium becomes thick and nutritive as it prepares for implantation of a fertilized ovum. Implantation of a fertilized ovum usually occurs about 7 to 10 days after ovulation. If fertilization and

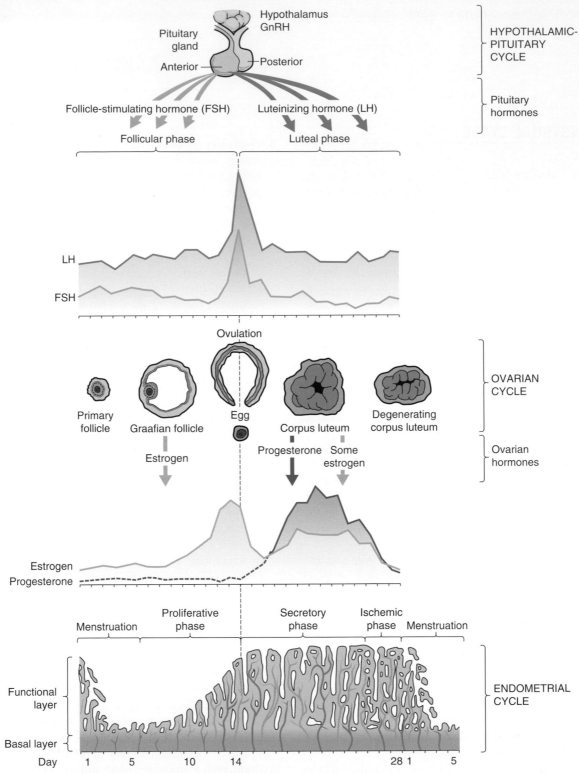

Fig. 6.1 Menstrual Cycle: Hypothalamic-pituitary, Ovarian, and Endometrial. *GnRH,* Gonadotropin releasing hormone. (From Lowdermilk, D. L., Perry, S. E., Cashion, K., Alden, K., & Olshansky, E. [2020]. *Maternity and women's health care* [12th ed., 10]. St. Louis, MO: Elsevier.)

implantation do not occur, the corpus luteum regresses and a rapid decrease in progesterone and estrogen occurs.

D. **Ischemic phase:** Blood supply to the superficial endometrial layers decreases to the superficial endometrial layers causing ischemia and triggering menses. Newer literature suggests that estrogen-progesterone withdrawal prompts enzymatic autodigestion of the endometrium and initiates menses.

> **HESI HINT** To avoid pregnancy, a woman should abstain from unprotected sexual intercourse during her fertile days. The fertile period begins 4–5 days prior to ovulation and ends 24–48 h after ovulation. A couple should not engage in unprotected intercourse before an anticipated ovulation and for approximately 3 days after ovulation to prevent a mistimed pregnancy.

Conception

The union of a single egg and sperm.

Fertilization

Description: The process of fusing the sperm and the ovum (23 chromosomes each) to create a diploid cell with 46 chromosomes. Fertilization usually occurs in 18 to 24 hours and takes place in ampulla (outer third) of the fallopian tube. The zygote is formed. Mitotic cellular replication begins within 30 hours after fertilization. Three to four days later, the zygote has traveled into the uterus and gone through rapid cell division to create additional cells becoming a morula (12 to 16 cells) and then a blastocyst. Implantation then occurs approximately 7 to 10 days post-conception. Some women may experience slight bleeding at the time of implantation.

Embryo and fetal development

A. **Embryo.** The embryonic period lasts between 2 and 8 weeks following fertilization. At the end of this stage, the embryo is approximately 3 cm.
   1. During this period of organogenesis, the embryo is most vulnerable to teratogens (viruses, drugs, radiation, or infections), which can cause major congenital anomalies.
B. **Fetus.** The fetal period lasts from 9 weeks until birth. The age of the fetus is measured in gestational weeks and refers to the number of weeks after fertilization (Fig. 6.2).

MATERNAL PHYSIOLOGIC CHANGES DURING PREGNANCY

Signs of Pregnancy

A. **Presumptive (subjective):** Fatigue, amenorrhea, nausea and vomiting, urinary frequency, breast changes, quickening
B. **Probable (objective):** Hegar sign (softening of the isthmus of cervix), Goodell sign (softening of cervix at approximately 4 weeks gestation), Chadwick's sign (bluish-violet color of cervix and vagina at approximately 6 to 8 weeks gestation), positive pregnancy test.
C. **Positive (objective):** Fetal heart tones, visualization of fetus on ultrasound

Pregnancy Testing

A. **Blood or urine testing:** Recognizes or measures human chorionic gonadotropin (hCG) or a beta subunit of hCG (B-hCG).
   1. hCG levels can be detected as soon as 7 to 8 days before expected menses, usually double every 2 days for the first 4 weeks of pregnancy and peak at about 60 to 70 days.
B. **Gestational age.** Most women do not know the exact date of fertilization, so historically the estimated due date is calculated as 280 days (40 weeks) from the first day of her last menstrual period (LMP). This is approximately 266 days (38 weeks) from ovulation.
   1. Naegele's rule estimates the due date. To calculate, 7 days are added to the LMP and then 3 months are subtracted. This is based on a 28-day cycle.
C. **The prenatal period is divided into three trimesters each lasting about 12 to 13 weeks**
   1. First trimester: From the first day of LMP through 12 weeks
   2. Second trimester: 13 weeks through 27 weeks
   3. Third trimester: 28 to 40 weeks

Maternal Physiological Adaptations to Pregnancy and Nurse's Clinical Response

First Trimester

A. **Maternal Adaptations**
   1. Uterus begins to change from pear shape to globular (ball) shape. Size remains below symphysis pubis.
   2. There is often no noticeable weight gain.
   3. Vaginal discharge may start to increase (Leukorrhea)
   4. Breast tenderness is often present
   5. Urinary frequency is noticeable
   6. Weight gain is 2 to 4 lb during the first trimester
B. **Clinical Judgment Measures**
   1. Common discomforts of pregnancy
      a. Nausea may be relieved by eating small, frequent meals, avoiding fried fatty foods with strong odors, avoiding skipping meals. Antiemetic medications may be prescribed by obstetric provider.
      b. Breast tenderness may be lessened by wearing a supportive bra.
      c. Constipation may occur secondary to effects of first trimester progesterone changes. Increase fluids, drink warm liquids, eat foods with natural fiber, and avoid castor oil.
      d. Fatigue may improve with regular, approved exercise and increased rest
      e. Urinary frequency is common in first trimester but monitor for signs of a urinary tract infection.

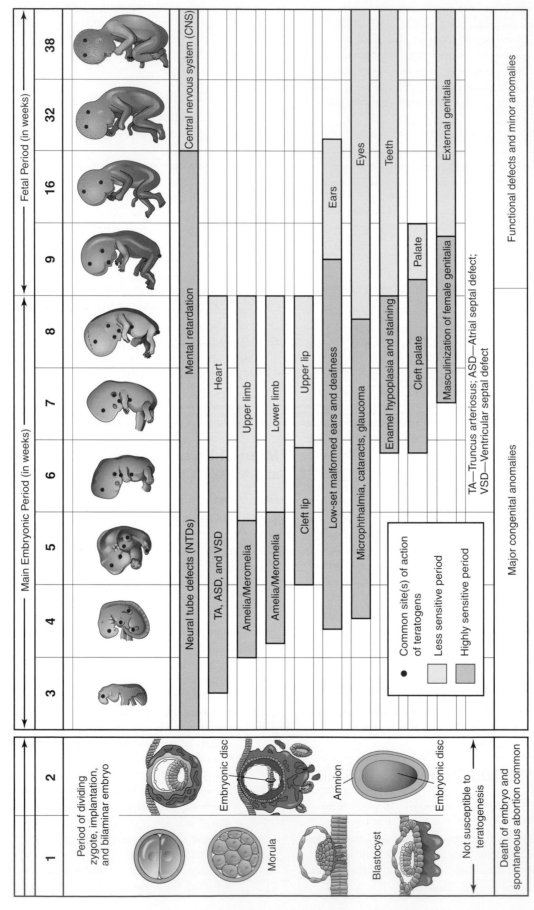

Fig. 6.2 Critical Periods in Human Prenatal Development. Purple denotes highly sensitive periods; green indicates stages that are less sensitive to teratogens. (From Moore, K. L., Persaud, T. V. N., & Torchia, M. G. [2016]. *Before we were born: Essentials of embryology and birth defects* [9th ed.]. Philadelphia: Elsevier.)

2. Safety
   a. Avoid hot tubs, saunas, and steam rooms throughout pregnancy (may increase risk for neural tube defects [NTD] in first trimester; hypotension may cause fainting).
   b. Avoid known teratogens like alcohol, tobacco/nicotine, and substances of abuse
   c. Report any unusual pain or vaginal bleeding throughout pregnancy
   d. Report persistent nausea and vomiting or inability to keep any food and fluids down
   e. Report urinary tract infection (UTI) symptoms throughout pregnancy
   f. Screen for intimate partner violence
   g. Educate about perinatal mental health (especially depression and anxiety)
3. Preparation for pregnancy.
   a. Orient to schedule of prenatal care visits and cost of prenatal care and birth.
   b. Discuss choice of obstetric provider.
   c. Discuss early pregnancy classes that focus on what to expect during pregnancy.
   d. Provide information about childbirth preparation classes.
   e. Include partner and family in preparation for childbirth (Table 6.1).

> **HESI HINT** For many women, intimate partner violence or perinatal intimate partner violence (emotional and/or physical abuse) begins during pregnancy. Women should be assessed for abuse in private, away from the partner, by a nurse who is familiar with local resources and can offer information about available services.

Second Trimester

A. Maternal Adaptations
1. Uterus rises above pelvic brim. Fundus reaches level of umbilicus by approximately 20 weeks. Two to four fingerbreadths above the umbilicus by 24 weeks, and is halfway between umbilicus and xiphoid process by the end of 27 weeks.
2. Areolas darken and superficial veins noted.
3. Colostrum may be present from the nipples by 16 weeks.
4. Striae gravidarum (stretch marks) may become more noticeable.
5. Quickening, the mother's first perception of fetal movement, may be noted between 16 and 20 weeks.
6. Varicose veins may begin to develop.
7. Glomerular filtration rate increases by 50% over pre-pregnant levels and peaks at 12 weeks.
8. Placenta is fully functioning and producing hormones.
9. Amniotic sac holds approximately 400 mL of fluid. (Average amount is 700 to 800 mL at term.)
10. Postural hypotension may occur. Blood pressure decreases gradually from pre-pregnancy values reaching its nadir in the second trimester then gradually increases at 24 to 32 weeks and returns to pre-pregnancy levels by term.

TABLE 6.1 Clinical Judgment Measures: First Trimester Common Discomforts

Clinical Judgment Measure	Assessment Characteristics
Recognize Cues	Nausea
	Breast tenderness
	Vaginal spotting
	Fatigue
	Mild cramping
Analyze Cues	Determine frequency of nausea, ability to hold down food, fluids
	Determine when breast tenderness began, unilateral or bilateral
	Determine characteristics of vaginal bleeding: amount, color, time of occurrence, associated pain
	Discuss fatigue noting onset, alleviating factors
	Verify constitution of cramping (location, frequency, degree of intensity)
Prioritize Cues	Determine last menstrual period, possible date of conception, date of first positive pregnancy test, gestational age
	Verify obstetric history and determine risk factors for ectopic pregnancy or spontaneous abortion
	Determine ability to hold down food and fluids
Solutions	Discuss possible reasons for vaginal spotting in first trimester
	Discuss potential lab work, US to further evaluate vaginal spotting
	Provide information about small frequent meals to treat nausea, when to contact provider for additional evaluation of nausea
	Teach to wear a supportive bra to help alleviate breast tenderness
	Encourage frequent rest periods

11. Serum cholesterol increases from 16 to 32 weeks of pregnancy and remains at this level until after birth.
12. Insulin resistance begins as early as 14 to 16 weeks of gestation and continues to rise until it stabilizes during the last few weeks of pregnancy.
13. Approximate weight gain of 1 lb per week beginning in the second trimester and continuing until delivery.

B. Clinical Judgment Measures
1. Common discomforts of pregnancy
   a. Flatulence and gas may be improved with approved exercise.
   b. Nasal congestion may be relieved with humidifier. Best to avoid nasal sprays with epinephrine
   c. Round ligaments increase in length and stretch as uterus rises in abdomen and may cause pain. May change position to lessen tension on round ligament or wear maternity abdominal supports as directed by provider.
   d. Remaining active may help with constipation, fatigue.
   e. Lower extremity edema. Elevate feet when possible. Avoid prolonged sitting and crossing legs. Teach about use of support stockings if directed.

f. Suggest that cool-air vaporizer or saline nasal spray may help with nasal stuffiness.

g. Lower back pain may start to increase. Encourage proper body mechanics.

h. Dyspareunia may be present. Positional changes to accommodate enlarging uterus may help. Report any unusual vaginal discharge or odor.

i. Mild dyspnea may be noticeable by end of second trimester and continue to increase. Educate about expected physiologic changes and warning signs.

2. Safety

a. Review diet and exercise.

b. Teach prevention of UTIs.

c. Remind of importance of dental care throughout pregnancy as needed.

d. Report leg cramps.

e. Report heart palpitations.

f. Report any unresolved nausea or vomiting.

g. Report any vaginal bleeding or cramping, unusual back pain, or discomfort.

h. Be aware of signs of intimate partner violence.

i. Review body mechanics to avoid increased back discomfort.

3. Preparation for pregnancy

a. Discuss nutrition and regular exercise (Box 6.1).

b. Discuss possible effects of pregnancy on sexual relationship. Recognize partner's role as partner learns to incorporate the parental role into self-identity.

c. Discuss screening and diagnostic rests for fetal aneuploidy or carrier testing for cystic fibrosis, hemoglobinopathies, spinal muscular atrophy. Typically performed in first or second trimester. May include ultrasound and blood tests, chorionic villus sampling (CVS) testing for nuchal translucency/thickness (NT) or open neural tube defects (ONTD). Maternal serum markers or noninvasive prenatal testing may be options.

1) Maternal serum alpha-fetoprotein (AFP) screens for NTD

a) Performed between 15 and 20 weeks of gestation, 16 to 18 weeks ideal

b) Elevated levels associated with open NTD

c) Low levels associated with Down syndrome

d) Abnormal levels are confirmed with additional testing

2) Multiple-marker screens for fetal chromosomal abnormalities, particularly trisomy 21 (Down syndrome) and NTDs. Can be performed in place of maternal serum alpha-fetoprotein test (MSAFP). Includes serum levels of hCG, AFP, estriol, inhibin A

a) May be performed in first trimester with serum testing and ultrasound or performed in second trimester as "quad screen" at 16 to 18 weeks.

b) Elevated levels of AFP associated with risk for NTD

c) Low levels of AFP associated with Down syndrome and other chromosomal abnormalitie

d) Elevated levels of hCG and inhibin A associated with risk for Down syndrome

e) Low levels of estriol associated with risk for Down syndrome

3) Explain screening for gestational diabetes that is usually done between 24- and 28-weeks' gestation.

4) Sign up for prepared childbirth classes if desired.

5) Adoula is a trained labor support person who may be contracted by the mother to provide emotional and physical support during labor and postpartum.

6) Discuss desire to breastfeed or bottle feed and provide education accordingly.

Third Trimester

A. **Maternal Adaptations**

1. Fundus is halfway between umbilicus and xiphoid process at 28 weeks, is about 3 to 4 fingerbreadths below xiphoid process at 32 weeks, and 1 fingerbreadth below xiphoid process at 36 to 38 weeks. If lightening occurs, may be 2 to 3 fingerbreadths below xiphoid process.

2. Thoracic breathing replaces abdominal breathing.

3. Cardiac output increases by 30% to 50% and peaks at about 30 weeks. Blood volume increases by 40% to 50% over the pregnancy reaching a maximum at about 32 weeks.

4. Heartburn may begin.

5. Hemorrhoids may develop.

6. Urinary frequency may increase and nocturia become more prevalent throughout remainder of pregnancy.

7. Breasts are full and tender. Colostrum may be present.

8. Swollen ankles may occur.

9. Sleeping problems may develop.

10. Dyspnea may be more noticeable and persist until delivery.

BOX 6.1 Iron Supplementation

- Iron supplements should be taken upon the recommendation of the health care provider.
- A diet rich in vitamin C (in citrus fruits, tomatoes, melons, and strawberries) and heme iron (in meats) increases the absorption of the iron supplement; therefore, include these in the diet often.
- Bran, tea, coffee, milk, oxalates (in spinach and Swiss chard), and egg yolk decrease iron absorption. Avoid consuming them at the same time as the supplement.
- Iron is absorbed best if it is taken when the stomach is empty; that is, take it between meals with a beverage other than tea, coffee, or milk.
- Iron can be taken at bedtime if abdominal discomfort occurs when it is taken between meals.
- If an iron dose is missed, take it as soon as it is remembered if that is within 13 h of the scheduled dose. Do not double up on the dose.
- Keep the supplement in a childproof container and out of the reach of any children in the household.
- The iron may cause stools to be black or dark green.
- Constipation is common with iron supplementation. A diet high in fiber with adequate fluid intake is recommended.

From Lowdermilk, D. L., Perry, S. E., Cashion, K., Alden, K., & Olshansky, E. (2020). *Maternity and women's health care* (12th ed.). St. Louis, MO: Elsevier.

11. Lightening may occur. Around 36 weeks and on.
12. Backaches may increase.
13. Braxton Hicks contractions may be more noticeable.

B. Clinical Judgment Measures

1. Common discomforts of pregnancy
   a. Discuss eating small, frequent meals, avoiding fatty foods, avoiding laying down after meals to help with heartburn. Review medications and over-the-counter treatments as prescribed.
   b. Educate about any prescribed interventions for hemorrhoids like stool softeners or topical agents.
   c. Encourage to wear a well-fitting bra.
   d. Teach measures to decrease lower leg edema and encourage leg elevation one or 2 times per day. Report any varicosities.
   e. Encourage sleeping on side for comfort during rest and to help prevent symptoms of supine hypotensive syndrome.
   f. Encourage proper posture and review correct body mechanics.
2. Safety
   a. Encourage to report any vaginal bleeding, loss of fluid, unusual back pain.
   b. Discuss third trimester warning signs of pre-eclampsia:
      1) Visual disturbances
      2) Swelling of face, fingers, or sacrum
      3) Severe, continuous headache
      4) Persistent vomiting
      5) Epigastric pain
   c. Discuss signs of Infection
      1) Chills
      2) Temperature over 38°C
      3) Dysuria. Pain in abdomen
   d. Report any change in fetal movement. Review fetal movement kick counting.
   e. Reviews signs of labor. Report any preterm labor symptoms. Discuss when to notify obstetric provider about onset of labor symptoms.

> **HESI HINT** Daily fetal movement counting (Kick counting) is done by the mother at home. The presence of fetal movements is a generally reassuring sign of fetal health.

3. Preparation for labor, delivery, and parenthood.
   a. Discuss mother's and support person's expectations of labor and delivery (L&D). Assess partner's role during childbirth.
   b. Encourage woman to start childbirth-preparation classes.
   c. Discuss location of delivery, i.e., birth center, hospital, homebirth plans; and tour of area.
   d. Encourage review of any birth plans with obstetric provider.
   e. Encourage to pack supplies for hospital or birth center.

TABLE 6.2 Clinical Judgment Measures: Third Trimester Common Discomforts

Clinical Judgment Measure	Assessment Characteristics
Recognize Cues	Low back pain
	Mild abdominal cramping
	History of preterm labor
	Frequent voiding
Analyze Cues	Determine where pain is located
	Verify constitution of pain (constant, intermittent, only with voiding, increasing in intensity)
	Ascertain ability to stop pain with activity (change of position alleviates discomfort or worsens it)
	Determine frequency of voiding and characteristics
	Clarify gestational age
Prioritize Cues	Determine risk factors for preterm labor
	Verify normalcy of voiding patterns in pregnancy
	Clarify any loss of fluids
	Establish fetal well-being (FHR, movement)
Solutions	Teach about preterm labor symptoms, Braxton Hicks contractions, and differences between true labor and false labor
	Provide guidelines for when to contact obstetric provider with concerns
	Prevent UTIs with adequate hydration, frequent voiding, and fully emptying of bladder
	Teach clients about proper body mechanics, appropriate exercises and activity, and adequate rest after activity
	Teach clients to assess for fetal well-being through fetal kick counting

FHR, Fetal heart rate.

f. Answer questions regarding breastfeeding.
g. Discuss postpartum choices and decisions: circumcision, rooming-in, initiation of breastfeeding or bottle feeding, support partner's role, cultural beliefs and practices, plans for discharge. If adoption is anticipated, discuss postpartum plans.
h. Review signs of postpartum blues, postpartum depression.
i. Review expected postpartum changes and discomforts like vaginal bleeding, any incisional or episiotomy pain, care for vaginal health, voiding and changes to bowel movements.
j. Review postpartum warning signs for UTIs, preeclampsia, unusual vaginal bleeding, development of blood clots (DVT, PE).
k. Confirm choice and provide education for any desired contraception (Table 6.2).

PSYCHOSOCIAL RESPONSES TO PREGNANCY

Description: Adaptation to pregnancy is a complex process for the mother, the father or the non-pregnant partner, and the entire family. It is influenced by culture, societal trends, family beliefs, and available supports. Adaptation will vary with each pregnancy and with every person involved. There is no one perfect pathway but there are similar steps in the process as each person accepts the pregnancy, identifies with their emerging roles, adapts to changing personal relationships (including a relationship with the fetus), and prepares for the birth.

Examples of Psychosocial Responses

A. First trimester
1. Ambivalence: Whether pregnancy is planned or mistimed, ambivalence is normal and discussions may include attitudes toward pregnancy and desire to continue pregnancy.
2. Financial worries about increased responsibility and care of an infant are often experienced.
3. Career concerns may arise.

B. Second trimester
1. Quickening occurs and fetal movement is experienced by the mother and her partner. Pregnancy may feel more "real" and prompt acceptance of pregnancy.
2. There may still be some ambivalence toward the pregnancy and the mother and partner may still be considering parenting or other options like adoption.

C. Third trimester
1. The pregnant person may appear more introverted or self-absorbed as she contemplates delivery, parenting.
2. Pregnant woman and partner may feel strain in the relationship or experience differing views on delivery, postpartum recovery, and changing roles as each plan for transition into parenthood individually and as a couple.

ANTEPARTUM NURSING CARE

Description: The antepartum period (pregnancy) is a time of physical and psychological preparation for the birth. The routine prenatal visit schedule typically includes a first visit within the first trimester of pregnancy, monthly visits during weeks 16 to 28, visits every 2 weeks from weeks 29 to 36, and weekly visits until birth.

The First Prenatal Visit

A. Obtain history
1. Medical history
   a. Family history
   b. Social history
   c. Mental health screening (i.e., history of mood and anxiety disorders)
   d. Substance use screening
   e. Sexual health screening: STDs, TORCH infections (See Chapter 4)
   f. IPV screening
2. Obstetrical history. Pregnancy count can be determined by two common methods.
   a. Two digits: G/P only records the gravida and para of a client.

1) Gravida refers to the number of times a woman has been pregnant (regardless of the duration or outcome). The count includes the current pregnancy.
2) Para refers to the number of times a woman has given birth to a fetus of at least 20 weeks or greater gestation (viable or nonviable). Multiple births count as one birth

   b. Five digits nomenclature (GTPAL) provides more detailed information about the client's obstetrical history.
   1) Gravida—total number of pregnancies, including current pregnancy
   2) Term—total number of pregnancies that reached 37 0/7 weeks gestation or greater
   3) Preterm—total number of pregnancies that were 20 0/7 weeks gestation to 36 6/7 weeks gestation regardless of fetal outcome or number of fetuses
   4) Abortions—total number of spontaneous and induced abortions prior to 20 0/7 weeks.
   5) Living Children—total number of living children. This usually equals the total of term and preterm numbers but may be greater if woman has had multiples or less if any children have died.
   c. History and status of current pregnancy. Including presumptive, probable, and positive signs of pregnancy.

> **HESI HINT** Practice determining gravidity and parity. A woman who is 6 weeks pregnant has the following maternal history:
> - She has healthy 2-year-old male fraternal twins.
> - She had a miscarriage at 22 weeks.
> - She had an induced abortion at 6 weeks, 5 years earlier.
> - G/P: Gravida 4, Para 2.
> - GTPAL: 4 1-1-1-21 (G-4 pregnancies [twins, miscarriage, induced abortion, current pregnancy]): T-1 (twins count as one birth); P-1 (22-week miscarriage); A-1 (induced abortion at 6 weeks); L-2 (twins).

> **HESI HINT** Practice calculating estimated date of birth using Naegele's rule. The first day of a woman's last normal menstrual period was December 9. What is her EDB?
> Answer: September 16. Count back 3 months and add 7 days (always give February 28 days).

B. Assist with physical examination
1. Vital signs (T, P, R, BP), height and weight
   a. BP: Systolic: Slight or no decrease from pre-pregnancy level. Diastolic: Slight decrease to mid-pregnancy (24 to 32 weeks) and gradual return to pre-pregnancy levels by end of pregnancy
   b. Heart rate: Increases 15 to 20 beats/min
2. Abdominal exam (including auscultation of fetal heart tones and fundal height measurement as applicable)
3. Pelvic exam (may include pelvimetry, pap testing, sexually transmitted infection [STI] testing, vaginal discharge screening)

HESI HINT Some women may decline a pelvic exam for cultural, religious, or personal reasons. Pelvic and/or breast exams may trigger adverse emotions if the woman has experienced sexual abuse or is currently experiencing abuse.

C. Routine laboratory data (see Appendix A).

1. Complete blood count
   a. Hemoglobin (Hgb): values during pregnancy greater than 1 at least 11 g/dL first trimester and 10.5 g/dL second trimester
   b. Hematocrit (Hct): values during pregnancy greater than 33% first and third trimesters and at least 32% in second trimester
   c. MCV
   d. Platelets
2. Human immunodeficiency virus (HIV)
3. Hepatitis B (HBsAg)
4. Hepatitis C (if high risk)
4. Rubella titer (>1:10 = immunity)
5. Syphilis (rapid plasma regain [RPR], Venereal Disease Research Laboratory [VDRL])
6. Blood type, RH, antibody screen
7. Varicella immunity (if applicable)
8. Hgb electrophoresis (sickle cell) (if applicable)
9. Pap smear (if applicable)
10. Additional STI screening
    a. Gonorrhea
    b. Chlamydia
11. Tuberculin skin testing (if applicable)
12. Urinalysis and culture
13. Genetic Testing, Carrier Screening, Fetal Aneuploidy Screening as applicable and desired.

Subsequent Antepartum Visits

A. Vital Signs
B. Check urine

1. Albumin: No more than a trace is a normal finding (related to preeclampsia)
2. Glucose: No more than 1+ is a normal finding (related to gestational diabetes)
3. Protein: A trace amount of protein may be present in the urine; a higher presence may indicate contamination by vaginal secretions, kidney disease, or preeclampsia.

C. Graph weight gain.

1. Two to four lb weight gain in the first trimester is recommended.
2. 1 lb per week weight gain thereafter is recommended.
3. Total weight gain during the pregnancy for a woman with a pre-pregnancy normal body mass index (BMI) should be approximately 25 to 35 lb.

D. Check fundal height (Fig. 6.3)
E. Check fetal heart rate (FHR)

1. 10 to 12 weeks: detectable by using Doppler
2. 15 to 20 weeks: detectable by using fetoscope
3. 110 to 160 beats/min: normal FHR range.

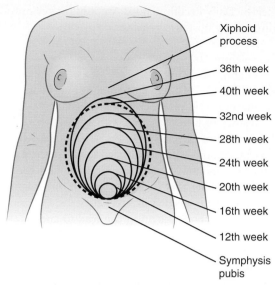

Fig. 6.3 Fundal Height Assessment.

Xiphoid process
36th week
40th week
32nd week
28th week
24th week
20th week
16th week
12th week
Symphysis pubis

HESI HINT The normal baseline FHR is 110–160 beats/min. Changes in FHR are often the first and most important indicators of compromised blood flow to the fetus.

F. Screen for and address psychosocial concerns: i.e., depression, IPV, substance use.

Prenatal Nutrition

A. Diet

1. Use a questionnaire to determine routine dietary habits, individual deficiencies, vegetarian needs, current food aversions, and any subsequent nausea and/or vomiting.
2. Determine food insecurity.
3. Any symptoms of pica (this should be an ongoing assessment)
4. Review foods that are less safe during pregnancy and should be avoided.
   a. Unpasteurized cheeses
   b. Raw eggs, meat, fish
   c. Fish containing high levels of mercury
5. Determine BMI.
   a. Weight (those who weigh <100 lb or >200 lb may be at higher risk)
6. Note symptoms of malnutrition.
   a. Glossitis
   b. Cracked lips
   c. Dry, brittle hair

B. Determine history of dental care, dental caries, periodontitis
C. Educate about increased nutritional needs in pregnancy

1. Increase intake by about 340 to 450 calories per day (starting in the second trimester) for women carrying one fetus.
2. Have a minimum of 60 g of protein a day.

3. Review Daily Recommended Amounts of key nutrients as directed by obstetric provider. Typically:
   a. Iron—27 mg
   b. Calcium 1000 mg
   c. Vitamin A—770 µg
   d. Folic acid—600 µg. This amount may be increased by the obstetric provider if the pregnant woman has a history of having a child with an NTD.
5. Review use of prenatal vitamins. A balanced diet typically provides all the nutrients needed for a healthy pregnancy, however, many women in the United States consume an inadequate diet that does not provide the vitamins and micronutrients needed in pregnancy.
6. Explain that poor nutrition can lead to anemia, preterm labor, obesity, and intrauterine growth restriction (IUGR).
7. Drink 8 to 10 glasses of water per day.
8. Provide a copy of daily food guide for quick reference. Consider cultural food patterns in choices given. Include the following:
   a. 3 servings from dairy group (milk, cheese)
   b. 3 servings of protein (meats, eggs, legumes)
   c. 4 to 5 servings of vegetables (green and deep yellow vegetables are good sources of vitamin C)
   d. 9 to 11 servings of breads or cereals
   e. 3 to 4 servings of fruit.

? REVIEW OF ANATOMY AND PHYSIOLOGY OF REPRODUCTION AND ANTEPARTUM NURSING CARE

1. State the objective signs that signify ovulation.
2. Ovulation occurs how many days before the next menstrual period?
3. State three ways to identify the chronological age of a pregnancy (gestation).
4. Name the major discomforts of the first trimester and one suggestion for amelioration of each.
5. At 20 weeks' gestation, the fundal height would be _____.
6. State three principles relative to the pattern of weight gain in pregnancy.
7. FHR can be auscultated by Doppler at _____ weeks' gestation.
8. Describe the schedule of prenatal visits for a low-risk pregnant woman.

See Answer Key at the end of this text for suggested responses.

ANTEPARTUM FETAL AND MATERNAL ASSESSMENTS

Description: Assessments to obtain data regarding fetal and maternal physiologic status.

A. Assess maternal risk factors which include but are not limited to
1. Age under 17 or over 34 years
2. High parity (>5)
3. Recent pregnancy history including recent pregnancy loss (3 months or less since last delivery)
4. Hypertension, preeclampsia in current pregnancy
5. Anemia, history of hemorrhage, or current hemorrhage
6. Multiple gestations
7. Rh incompatibility
8. History of dystocia or previous operative delivery
9. A height of 60 inches (5 feet) or less
10. Malnutrition (15% under ideal weight) or extreme obesity (20% over ideal weight)
11. Medical disease during pregnancy (diabetes, hyperthyroidism, hyperemesis, clotting disorders)
12. Infection in pregnancy: **T**oxoplasmosis, **O**ther agents, **R**ubella, **C**ytomegalovirus, **H**erpes simplex (**TORCH** diseases); influenza; HIV; STIs *(chlamydia or gonorrhea)*; human papillomavirus (HPV)
13. History of family violence, lack of social support
14. History of assisted reproductive technology

B. Various examinations used to determine fetal and maternal well-being.

Ultrasonography

Description: High-frequency sound waves are used to produce an image of the fetus and surrounding structures to record the fetus's location, size, and biophysical status. Used in first trimester to determine number of fetuses, presence of fetal cardiac movement and rhythm, uterine abnormalities, gestational age. Used in second and third trimesters to determine fetal viability and gestational age, size—date discrepancies, amniotic fluid volume (AFV), placental location and maturity, uterine anomalies, and abnormalities, cervical length, and status, and during amniocentesis.

A. Ultrasound Findings
1. Fetal heart activity is apparent as early as 6 to 7 weeks' gestation.
2. Serial evaluation of biparietal diameter and limb length can differentiate between wrong dates and true IUGR.
3. A biophysical profile (BPP) is made to ascertain fetal well-being. It uses both ultrasound and a non-stress test.
   a. Five variables are assessed: Fetal breathing movements (FBM), gross body movements (FM), fetal tone (FT), reactivity of FHR (FHR typically assessed over 20 minutes), and AFV and index.
   b. A score of 2 or 0 can be obtained for each variable. An overall score of 8 to 10 designates that the fetus appears well on the day of the examination.

B. Clinical Judgment Measures
1. Explain procedure.
2. Instruct the woman to drink 3 to 4 glasses of water before coming for examination and not to urinate. In the first and second trimesters the client's bladder must be full during the examination in order for the uterus to be supported for imaging. (A full bladder is not needed if ultrasound is done transvaginally instead of abdominally.)
3. Position the woman with pillows under neck and knees to keep pressure off bladder; late in the third trimester, place wedge under right hip to displace uterus to the left.

4. Position display so woman can watch if she wishes.
5. Have bedpan or bathroom immediately available.

C. Complications
   1. There are no known complications or risks to mother or fetus.
   2. There is controversy regarding routine use of ultrasound in pregnancy.

Chorionic Villi Sampling

Description: Chorionic villi sampling (CVS) is the collection of placental tissue between 10 and 12 weeks' gestation. It is collected transcervically or transabdominally under ultrasound guidance.

A. Findings
   1. The test determines genetic karyotyping for detection of aneuploidy during the first trimester.

B. Clinical Judgment Measures
   1. Have informed consent signed before any procedure.
   2. Assist with confirmation of gestational age prior to procedure. (Documented risk of limb reduction birth defects if performed at an earlier age.)
   3. Collect appropriate medical history, including blood type and Rh.
   4. Warn of slight sharp pain upon catheter insertion.

C. Complications
   1. Slightly higher risk of spontaneous abortion over average risk
   2. Risk of infection, cramping, bleeding, leaking of amniotic fluid
   3. Risk for fetal limb loss
   4. Risk for Rh sensitization

Amniocentesis

Description: Removal of amniotic fluid sample from the uterus for testing or treatment. Typically performed between 15 and 20 weeks. Procedure is used to determine fetal genetic and chromosomal testing, assess for NTDs (usually in the second trimester), fetal lung maturity (last trimester), fetal well-being, uterine infection, Rh disease, may be used for follow up after abnormal maternal serum screening tests.

A. Findings
   1. Genetic disorders
      a. Karyotype: determines Down syndrome (trisomy 21), other trisomies, and sex-linked disorders
      b. Biochemical analysis: determines more than 60 types of metabolic disorders (Tay-Sachs)
      c. AFP: Elevations may be associated with neutral tube defects; low levels may indicate trisomy 21
   2. Fetal lung maturity
      a. L/S ratio: 2:1 ratio indicates fetal lung maturity unless mother is diabetic or has Rh disease or fetus is septic.
      a. Presence of blood or meconium in the sample can alter the result
      b. L/S ratio and presence of phosphatidylglycerol (PG): Most accurate determination of fetal maturity. PG is present after 35 weeks' gestation.

c. Lung maturity is the best predictor of extrauterine survival.
   3. Fetal well-being
      a. Analysis of amniotic fluid for bilirubin (usually collected after 28 weeks' gestation) is helpful to evaluate severity of hemolytic disease of a newborn.
      b. Meconium in amniotic fluid may indicate fetal distress.

B. Clinical Judgment Measures
   1. Obtain and document baseline vital signs and FHR before procedure.
   2. Collect appropriate medical history, including blood type and Rh.
   3. Explain procedure and obtain informed consent.
   4. Have client empty bladder.
   5. Place client in supine position.
   6. Provide emotional support and stay with the client. Monitor vital signs, FHR, contractions throughout procedure.
   7. After specimen is drawn, wash abdomen; assist woman to empty bladder. A full bladder can irritate the uterus and cause contractions.
   8. Monitor vital signs, FHR, contractions for 30 minutes to 1 hour after procedure.
   9. Administer Rho(D) immune globin to mother if Rh-negative.
   10. Instruct woman to report any contractions, change in fetal movement, or fluid leaking from vagina, vaginal bleeding for symptoms of infection (chills, fever).

C. Complications
   1. Risk of spontaneous abortion (1%)
   2. Fetal injury
   3. Infection
   4. Bleeding or leaking of amniotic fluid from puncture site or vagina
   5. Preterm labor

Nonstress Test

Description: Noninvasive test to determine fetal well-being. The FHR is recorded for 20 minutes but by may be extended to 40 minutes if needed.

A. Findings
   1. A healthy fetus will usually respond to its own movement by means of an FHR acceleration of 15 beats/min, lasting for at least 15 seconds after the movement, twice in a 20-minute period.
   2. The fetus that responds with the 15/15 acceleration within a 20-minute tracing is considered "reactive" and healthy.

B. Clinical Judgment Measures
   1. Apply fetal monitor, ultrasound, and tocodynamometer to maternal abdomen.
   2. Mother placed in semi-recumbent or side lying position.
   3. Give mother handheld event marker and instruct her to push the button whenever fetal movement is felt. Monitor client for 20 minutes, observing for reactivity.

4. Vibroacoustic stimulation (VAS) may be used to elicit an acceleration, increase FHR variability, or change the fetal wake/sleep cycle during a nonstress test (NST). After obtaining a 5-minute baseline, the artificial larynx is placed near fetal head and stimulus applied for 1 to 3 seconds and fetal response is observed.
   a. Do not use VAS during episodes of bradycardia or during a deceleration.

Contraction Stress Test or Oxytocin Challenge Test (OCT)

Description: The purpose of test is to detect late decelerations with uterine contractions which are due to uteroplacental insufficiency (UPI). Contractions can be induced by nipple stimulation or by infusing a dilute solution of oxytocin.

A. Findings
1. The contraction stress test (CST) is positive if fetus has late decelerations with at least 50% of contractions in 10 minutes. A negative test suggests fetal well-being (i.e., no occurrence of late decelerations).

B. Clinical Judgment Measures
1. Assess for contraindications: prematurity, preterm labor, placenta previa, multiple gestation, previous uterine classical scar, previous uterine rupture, preterm rupture of membranes (ROM).
2. Explain procedure. Place mother in semi-Fowler's position. Place external monitors on abdomen (FHR ultrasound monitor and tocodynamometer).
3. Record a 20-minute baseline strip to determine fetal well-being (reactivity) and presence or absence of contractions.
4. To assess for fetal well-being, a recording of at least three contractions in 10 minutes must be obtained.
5. If no spontaneous contractions are noted, nipple stimulation is attempted. Patient may brush, massage, or roll one nipple for 10 minutes. A warm, wet washcloth may be applied to nipples prior to massaging. If contractions do not begin in 10 minutes, may proceed with oxytocin infusion to stimulate uterine contractions.

HESI HINT With nipple stimulation, there is no control of the "dose" of oxytocin delivered by the posterior pituitary. The chance of hyperstimulation or tachysystole (5 contractions within 10 min or contractions lasting longer than 90 s) may be increased. The test should be discontinued if this occurs.

Biophysical Profile

Description: Combines real-time ultrasonography with an NST to evaluate fetal health by assessing FBM, gross body movement, FT, AFV, and FHR reactivity. Each variable receives 2 points for a normal response or 0 points for an abnormal or absent response.

A. Findings
1. A score of 8 to 10 indicates fetal well-being.

B. Clinical Judgment Measures
1. Prepare client for procedure.
2. Inform client of purpose of examination.
3. Provide psychological support, especially if testing will continue throughout the pregnancy.
4. Advise client that a low score indicates fetal compromise that would warrant more detailed investigation.
5. A score of 8 to 10 indicates fetal well-being.

HESI HINT Percutaneous umbilical blood sampling (PUBS) is the removal of fetal blood from the umbilical cord. It can be done during pregnancy (usually second trimester) under ultrasound for prenatal diagnosis and therapy. Hemoglobinopathies, infections, fetal karyotyping, metabolic disorders can be done using this method.

? REVIEW OF FETAL AND MATERNAL ASSESSMENT TECHNIQUES

1. Name five maternal variables associated with diagnosis of a high-risk pregnancy.
2. What does the biophysical profile determine?
3. List necessary nursing actions before an ultrasound examination for a woman in the first trimester of pregnancy.
4. State the advantage of chorionic villus sampling over amniocentesis.
5. Why are serum or amniotic alpha-fetoprotein levels done prenatally?
6. What is an important determinant of fetal maturity for extrauterine survival?
7. What is a reactive nonstress test?
8. What are the dangers of the nipple-stimulation stress test?

See Answer Key at the end of this text for suggested responses.

ANTEPARTUM COMPLICATIONS

Spontaneous Abortion

Description: A pregnancy that ends through natural causes before 20 weeks of gestation and a fetal weight less than 500 g. It is also referred to as a miscarriage. About 80% of spontaneous abortions occur before 12 weeks' gestation and are not clinically recognized. Ten percent to 15% of clinically recognized pregnancies will end in spontaneous abortion. Possible causes include chromosomal abnormalities, various medical disorders (especially if poorly controlled), substance use, environmental toxins, or trauma.

Types of Spontaneous Abortions

1. Threatened: painless vaginal bleeding without cervical changes; uterine size is equal to dates.
2. Inevitable: moderate vaginal bleeding, uterine cramping, and cervical dilation and/or ROMs; uterine size is equal to dates.
3. Incomplete: moderate to heavy vaginal bleeding, uterine cramping with passage of some fetal or placental tissue through the dilated cervix.

4. Complete: spontaneous expulsion of all fetal and placental tissue from uterine cavity; uterus is pre-pregnancy size, cervix may be closed or dilated.

5. Missed: nonviable products of conception are retained; vaginal bleeding may be present or has occurred, then stopped and reoccurred. Possible history of uterine cramping.

6. Recurrent: three or more spontaneous abortions occurring consecutively.

A. Common symptoms

1. Uterine cramping
2. Backache
3. Pelvic pressure
4. Abnormal uterine bleeding
   a. May be bright-red, dark maroon, scant or heavy, intermittent, or continuous

B. Clinical Judgment Measures

1. Care of the woman will vary by type of spontaneous abortion. Provider may advise expectant management at home (threatened) or follow up treatment if symptoms worsen and progress. Fifty percent to 85% of spontaneous abortions will complete with expectant management. Medical or surgical management may also be ordered (incomplete or missed abortion). The nurse must assess client's and family's emotional status, needs, and support systems regardless of type of abortion.

C. Labs

1. Pregnancy test (usually serum, quantitative hCG)
2. WBC
3. Hgb/Hct
4. Confirmation of maternal blood type and Rh factor ($Rh_o(D)$ immune globin may be ordered for women who are Rh-negative)

D. Diagnostic assessment

Provider may order US and see the client for a physical exam with cervical assessment

E. Expectant Management

1. Teach client to notify provider of:
   a. Temperature above 38°C
   b. Foul-smelling vaginal discharge
   c. Bright-red bleeding accompanied by any tissue larger than a dime; client should also monitor amount and color of bleeding
   d. Worsening cramping or unmanaged pain
2. Acetaminophen-based analgesics may be ordered
3. Avoid sexual intercourse, inserting anything into vagina, or tub baths
4. Discuss follow up with provider as directed. Follow up hCG tests or US may be ordered.

F. Medical or surgical management (D&C) if pregnancy loss confirmed (incomplete, missed)

1. Nurse should follow admission protocols and assessments, monitor vital signs, assure intravenous (IV) access, educate woman and support persons about treatment.
2. Post-medical or post-surgical care will include monitoring vital signs, administering medications if ordered

(oxytocin, antibiotics, Rh(D) immune globin), providing compassionate psychosocial care that addresses perinatal loss. Families are often provided with an opportunity to see the fetus or products of conception.

3. Educate on follow-up care.

Hyperemesis Gravidarum

Description: The inability to control nausea and vomiting during pregnancy. Hyperemesis gravidarum is characterized by excessive vomiting that causes weight loss, electrolyte imbalance, nutritional deficiencies, and ketonuria. It occurs in up to 3% of pregnancies. Pregnancy and nonpregnancy risk factors include first pregnancy, younger maternal age, multifetal gestation, gestational trophoblastic disease (GTD), chronic medical conditions (asthma, DM is (diabetes mellitus), hyperthyroid disorders), and history of this condition.

A. Symptoms

1. Excessive vomiting
2. Weight loss
3. Dehydration
4. Dry mucous membranes, poor skin turgor
5. Low BP, increased pulse

B. Clinical Judgment Measures

1. Assess frequency, severity, duration of vomiting
2. Monitor I&O
3. Monitor vital signs
4. Establish and maintain IV access, IV fluids as ordered
5. Administer antiemetics, antihistamines as ordered.
6. Provide emotional support

C. Labs

1. Chemistry panel
2. Urinalysis
3. CBC mean corpuscular volume (size of red blood cells)

D. Discharge

1. Discuss advancement of diet once vomiting has stopped.
2. Review medications as prescribed.
3. Review follow-up care and importance of regular prenatal assessment of maternal weight gain, fetal growth, and well-being.

Molar Pregnancy (Hydatidiform Mole)

Description: Proliferative growth of placental trophoblast where chorionic villi develop into edematous, cystic, transparent vesicle; appear as a grapelike cluster. Embryo is not viable. The molar pregnancy is a form of GTD that can be associated with pregnancy-related cancers. Cause is unknown but risk is higher for those who have had a previous molar pregnancy and those at extreme ages for reproduction; occurs in 1 in 1000 pregnancies. May be complete (absence of fetal tissue) or partial (nonviable fetal tissue).

A. Symptoms

1. Vaginal bleeding; dark red or brown, may be intermittent
2. Abdominal tenderness
3. Severe nausea and vomiting persisting beyond 12 weeks
4. Uterus may be larger than expected by dates.
5. Fatigue

6. Woman may pass vesicles.
7. Early symptoms of preeclampsia may present.

B. Clinical Judgment Measures
  1. Assess vital signs, vaginal discharge, uterine cramping.

C. Labs
  1. Serum B-hCG levels are ordered (typically high or rising)

D. Diagnostics
  1. US ordered

E. Surgical intervention (D&C) likely
  1. Provide preoperative and postoperative education and care.

F. Provide discharge instructions
  1. Follow up care includes frequent physical exams.
  2. Teach to report signs of complications to obstetric provider immediately.
     a. Bright-red, frank vaginal bleeding
     b. Temperature spike over 100.4°F
     c. Foul-smelling vaginal discharge
  3. Weekly, then monthly serum B-hCG levels are usually monitored for 6 to 12 months to assure B-hCG levels return to normal. Rising B-hCG levels and an enlarging uterus may indicate malignancy.

G. Refer to community resources for grief and loss

Ectopic Pregnancy

Description: Fertilized ovum is implanted outside the uterine cavity, about 90% are located in a fallopian tube. Occurs in about 2% of pregnancies and carries increased risk for pregnancy loss, tubal rupture, excessive blood loss, and possible future infertility. Potential risk factors include previous history of ectopic pregnancy, previous tubal surgeries, pelvic infections, use of intrauterine contraceptive devices. It is considered a medical emergency.

A. Symptoms
  1. The three most classic symptoms include abdominal pain (dull to colicky and progresses to constant and severe), delayed menses or may report a very light or irregular menses, abnormal vaginal bleeding (dark brown or red or intermittent spotting).
  2. May report full feeling in lower abdomen, lower quadrant tenderness
  3. Referred shoulder pain

B. Clinical Judgment Measures
  1. Provide admission care including education, psychological support, and preparation for surgery.
  2. Assess vital signs every 15 minutes and as needed.
  3. Start IV to administer fluids.
  4. Assess for active bleeding (associated with tubal rupture). A vaginal exam or abdominal palpation should only be done with caution.

C. Labs
  1. Serum pregnancy test (quantitative B-hCG). When B-hCG levels are greater than 1500 to 2000 milli International Units/mL, a normal intrauterine pregnancy should be visible on transvaginal US.
  2. Progesterone

  3. CBC
  4. Blood type and Rh

D. Diagnostics
  1. Transvaginal US

E. Medical or surgical intervention likely
  1. Those with early diagnosis of ectopic pregnancy may be treated with methotrexate
  2. Surgical management depends on location of ectopic pregnancy, extent of tissue involved, woman's desires for future pregnancies. Salpingectomy or salpingostomy are options.

F. Post-treatment care
  1. May include serial B-hCG levels (after methotrexate) and physical exam.
  2. Education should include discussion of contraceptive options as pregnancy should be delayed for at least 3 months. Future fertility should be discussed.

HESI HINT Suspect ectopic pregnancy in any woman of childbearing age who presents at an emergency department, clinic, or office with unilateral or bilateral abdominal pain.

Abruptio Placentae and Placenta Previa

Description: Two of the major causes of bleeding in late pregnancy are abruptio placentae and placenta previa. It is important to rapidly assess and intervene with these two conditions to prevent both maternal and fetal morbidity and mortality (Tables 6.3—6.5).

HESI HINT A client who is at 32 weeks' gestation calls the health care provider because she is experiencing dark-red vaginal bleeding. She is admitted to the emergency department, where the nurse determines the FHR to be 100 beats/min. The client's abdomen is rigid and boardlike, and she is complaining of severe pain. Which actions should the nurse take?
1. Differentiate between abruptio placentae (this client) and placenta previa (painless bright-red bleeding occurring in the third trimester).
2. Notify the health care provider.
3. Do not perform any abdominal or vaginal manipulation or examinations.
4. Administer O$_2$ by facemask.
5. Monitor for bleeding at IV sites and gums because of the increased risk for Disseminated intravascular coagulation (DIC).
6. Prepare for emergency cesarean section because uteroplacental perfusion to the fetus is being compromised by early separation of the placenta from the uterus.

HESI HINT DIC is a syndrome of abnormal clotting that is systematic and pathologic. Large amounts of clotting factors, especially fibrinogen, are depleted, causing widespread external, and internal bleeding. DIC is related to fetal demise, infection and sepsis, gestational hypertension, preeclampsia, and abruptio placentae. (DIC is discussed in greater detail in Chapter 3: Advanced Clinical Concepts.)

TABLE 6.3 Major Causes of Late Pregnancy Bleeding: Abruptio Placentae Versus Placenta Previa

Abruptio Placentae	Placenta Previa
A. Partial or complete premature detachment of the placenta from its site of implantation in the uterus, a medical emergency	A. Abnormal implantation of placenta in lower uterine segment near or over the cervical os
B. Occurs in 1 of 80–250 pregnancies	B. Occurs in 1 of 200 pregnancies
C. Usually occurs in third trimester or in labor	C. Bleeding usually occurs in the second or third trimester
D. Classification of abruption	D. Classification of previas
1. Retroplacental: blood collection between placenta and uterine wall	1. Incomplete (Partial): Placenta lies over part of cervical os.
2. Subchorionic: bleeding between placenta and membranes	2. Complete: Placenta lies over entire cervical os.
3. Preplacental: blood collection between placenta and amniotic fluid (within the amnion and chorion)	3. Marginal: Edge of placenta 2.5 cm or closer to the cervical os.
E. Associated with	4. Low lying: Placenta implants in lower uterine segment with a placental edge lying near the cervical os, extent not determined.
1. Hypertensive disorders	E. Associated with
2. High gravidity	1. Previous uterine scars
3. Blunt, external abdominal trauma (MVA or intimate partner violence [IPV])	2. Surgery, cesarean birth
4. Short umbilical cord	3. Smoking
5. Substance use (i.e., cocaine)	4. History of previa

TABLE 6.4 Symptoms of Abruptio Placentae and Placenta Previa

Abruptio Placentae	Placenta Previa
A. Symptoms vary with degree of separation	A. Painless, bright-red vaginal bleeding in second or third trimester
B. Vaginal bleeding, dark red	B. Uterus soft, nontender
C. Uterine tenderness, often a sudden onset	C. Vital signs usually normal, unless significant blood loss
D. Persistent abdominal pain	D. Placenta in lower uterine segment (indicated by ultrasound)
E. Contractions; may have a rigid, boardlike abdomen (hypertonicity)	E. FHR is usually reassuring
F. FHR abnormalities	

FHR, Fetal heart rate.

HYPERTENSIVE DISORDERS OF PREGNANCY

Classification

A. **Gestational Hypertension:** Onset of hypertension without proteinuria or other systemic findings after 20 weeks' gestation in a previously normotensive woman; resolves after birth.

B. **Preeclampsia:** Pregnancy specific condition; hypertension and proteinuria developed after 20 weeks' gestation in a previously normotensive woman. In the absence of proteinuria, preeclampsia may be diagnosed when hypertension is accompanied by multisystem changes as follows. Can also develop in early postpartum period.
  1. Occurs in 2% to 8% of all pregnancies.
  2. There is no known cause of preeclampsia. Pathophysiology is characterized by
     a. Generalized vasospasm and vasoconstriction leading to vascular damage, poor tissue perfusion to major organs, intravascular protein and fluid loss, and less plasma volume

  3. Preeclampsia is characterized by:
     a. BP of ≥140/90 mm Hg on two occasions at least 4 hours apart after 20 weeks of gestation in a woman with a previously normal blood pressure OR
     b. Systolic blood pressure of ≥160 mm Hg or diastolic blood pressure of 110 mm Hg, AND
     c. Concomitant evidence of proteinuria.
     d. OR, in the absence of proteinuria, hypertension with any of the following is diagnostic:
        1. Thrombocytopenia
        2. Renal insufficiency
        3. Pulmonary edema
        4. Impaired liver function
     e. Woman may present with visual changes, RUQ pain or epigastric pain, nausea, central nervous system (CNS) symptoms (headache, irritability), edema (especially around eyes, face, and fingers), reflexes may be normal or 2+, weight gain.
     f. Risk factors include nulliparity, maternal age ≥35 years, previous hypertension or previous pregnancy with preeclampsia, diabetes, thrombophilia, multifetal gestation, autoimmune disorders, family history of preeclampsia.

C. **Clinical Judgment Measures**

Nursing care will vary based on time of diagnosis during the antepartum, intrapartum, or postpartum period.

A. **Antepartum**
  1. Expectant management: If symptoms are mild in women less than 34 0/7 weeks, home management may be an option and guidelines will be established by obstetric provider. If symptoms progress, hospitalization may be necessary and nursing actions will be implemented.
  2. Upon hospital admission:
     a. Monitor level of consciousness
     b. Frequent vital signs (correct BP monitoring is critical)

TABLE 6.5 Clinical Judgment Measures for Abruptio Placentae Versus Placenta Previa

Abruptio Placentae	Placenta Previa
A. Institute bed rest with *no* vaginal or rectal examinations, no internal monitoring, and notify obstetric provider immediately.	A. Do not perform vaginal examination, rectal examination, or internal monitoring, notify obstetric provider.
B. Monitor vital signs frequently.	B. Expectant management: Initial hospitalization with bed rest to extend the period of gestation, continuous external fetal and uterine monitoring. Home care may be a later option if stable.
C. Apply continuous, external uterine and fetal monitoring.	
D. Assess ongoing vaginal bleeding. Serial fundal height measurements may be ordered (increasing fundal height indicates concealed bleeding).	C. If previa determined during labor, institute bed rest immediately and notify obstetric provider.
E. Start and maintain large bore IV access; administer IV fluids, medications, blood products as ordered.	D. Monitor vital signs frequently.
F. Labs: CBC, coagulation studies, blood type and screen; Kleihauer-Betke test may be ordered.	E. Start and maintain large bore IV access.
G. US and BPP may be ordered.	F. Labs: blood type and screen, CBC, coagulation studies.
H. Watch for signs of DIC (can be associated with moderate to severe abruption).	G. If less than 34 weeks, corticosteroids may be ordered.
1. Bleeding from three unrelated sites; spontaneous nosebleed	H. Continuous assessment of blood loss.
2. Petechiae	I. Prepare client and family for probable cesarean birth emergently if indicated or at 36 weeks or beyond 36 weeks if stabilized.
3. Ecchymosis	
4. Hypotension	
5. Tachycardia	
6. Abnormal coagulation tests	J. Provide emotional support and appropriate teaching regarding usual management and outcomes of placenta previa.
I. Prepare for immediate birth (vaginal or cesarean).	
J. Expectant management is usually only implemented if both woman and fetus are stable and fetus is between 20 and 34 weeks.	
K. Provide emotional support; teach regarding usual management and expected outcomes of abruption.	

BPP, Biophysical profile.

   c. Assess deep tendon reflexes (DTRs) frequently for evidence of clonus

   d. Oxygen status

   e. Measure input and output, daily weights.

   f. Assess for vaginal bleeding and abdominal pain.

   g. Maintain large bore IV access.

   h. Typically bedrest with left side-lying position

   i. Administer antihypertensive medications if ordered.

   j. Nifedipine, hydralazine, methyldopa, or labetalol are common choices (Table 6.6).

   k. Administer magnesium sulfate if ordered.

     1) Magnesium sulfate (IV) is the medication of choice for preventing and treating seizure activity.

     2) Must be aware of risk of magnesium toxicity (absent DTRs, decreased respiratory rate, decreased level of consciousness); if suspected, infusing should be discontinued immediately. Calcium gluconate is the antidote.

     3) Never abbreviate magnesium sulfate as $MgSO_4$ in documentation as it is a high-alert medication.

 3. Obtain fetal assessment continuously; apply external fetal monitor.

 4. Assess lab findings daily (Table 6.7).

 5. Prepare client for delivery if symptoms worsen, mother or fetus are showing evidence of complications, labor begins.

   a. Imminent or actual eclampsia

   b. Uncontrolled hypertension

   c. Placental abruption

   d. DIC

   e. Non-reassuring fetal status

B. Intrapartum

 1. Continue same, frequent assessments as noted in antepartum care.

 2. Have emergency medications, oxygen, and suction equipment available.

 3. Control the amount of stimulation in the labor room.

   a. Keep nurse-to-client ratio at 1:1.

   b. If possible, put client in darkened, quiet private room.

   c. Keep client on absolute bed rest, side-lying and with side rails up.

   d. Disturb client as little as possible with nursing interventions.

   e. Have client choose support person to stay with her and limit other visitors.

 4. Continuously explain rationale for procedures and care.

 5. Ongoing assessment of labor status and progress

   a. Promptly identify FHR abnormalities.

   b. Ongoing assessment of maternal central nervous, cardiovascular, pulmonary, hepatic, and renal systems

 6. If seizures occur

   a. Stay with client, summon help, and contact obstetric team immediately.

   b. Turn client onto side to prevent aspiration.

   c. Do *not* attempt to force objects inside mouth or put fingers into woman's mouth.

   d. Administer oxygen and have suction available.

TABLE 6.6   Pharmacologic Control of Hypertension in Pregnancy

Action	Target Tissue	Maternal Effects	Fetal Effects	Nursing Actions
Hydralazine (Apresoline, Neopresol)				
Arteriolar vasodilator	Peripheral arterioles: to decrease muscle tone, decrease peripheral resistance; hypothalamus and medullary vasomotor center for minor decrease in sympathetic tone	Headache, flushing, palpitations, tachycardia, some decrease in uteroplacental blood flow, increase in heart rate and cardiac output, increase in oxygen consumption, nausea and vomiting	Tachycardia; late decelerations and bradycardia if maternal diastolic pressure <90 mm Hg	Assess for effects of medication; alert woman (family) to expected effects of medication; assess blood pressure frequently because precipitous drop can lead to shock and perhaps placental abruption; if giving multiple doses, wait at least 20 min after the first dose is given to administer an additional dose to allow time to assess the effects of the initial dose; assess urinary output; maintain bed rest in lateral position with side rails up; use with caution in presence of maternal tachycardia.
Labetalol Hydrochloride (Normodyne, Trandate)				
Combined alpha- and beta-blocking agent causing vasodilation without significant change in cardiac output	Peripheral arterioles (see Hydralazine)	Lethargy, fatigue, sleep disturbances; Minimal: flushing, tremulousness, orthostatic hypotension; minimal change in pulse rate	Minimal, if any. May be associated with small-for-gestational-age infant	See hydralazine; less likely to cause excessive hypotension and tachycardia; less rebound hypertension than hydralazine. Do not use in women with asthma, heart disease, or congestive heart failure. Do not exceed 80 mg in a single dose. Do not give more than 300 mg total in a 24-h period.
Methyldopa (Aldomet)				
Maintenance therapy if needed: 250—500 mg orally every 8 h (α_2-receptor agonist)	Postganglionic nerve endings: interferes with chemical neurotransmission to reduce peripheral vascular resistance; causes CNS sedation	Sleepiness, postural hypotension, constipation, hepatic dysfunction and necrosis, hemolytic anemia; rare: drug-induced fever in 1% of women and positive Coombs test result in 20% of women	After 4 months of maternal therapy, positive Coombs test result in infant	See Hydralazine.
Nifedipine (Adalat, Procardia)				
Calcium channel blocker	Arterioles: to reduce systemic vascular resistance by relaxation of arterial smooth muscle	Headache, flushing, tachycardia; may interfere with labor	Minimal	See Hydralazine. Avoid concurrent use with magnesium sulfate because skeletal muscle blockade can result. Avoid immediate release or sublingual form due to increased risk for profound maternal hypotension

CNS, Central nervous system.From Lowdermilk, D. L., Perry, S. E., Cashion, K., Alden, K., & Olshansky, E. (2020). *Maternity and women's health care* (12th ed.). St. Louis, MO: Elsevier. Data from Harvey, C., & Sibai, B. (2013). Hypertension in pregnancy. In N. Troiano, C. Harvey, & B. Chez (Eds.), *AWHONN's high risk and critical care obstetrics* (3rd ed.). Philadelphia: Wolters Kluwer/Lippincott Williams & Wilkins; Poole, J. H. (2014). Hypertensive disorders of pregnancy. In K. R. Simpson & P. Creehan (Eds.), *AWHONN's perinatal nursing* (4th ed.). Philadelphia: Lippincott Williams & Wilkins; Sibai, B. (2017). Preeclampsia and hypertensive disorders. In S. G. Gabbe, J. R. Niebyl, & J. L. Simpson, et al. (Eds.), *Obstetrics: Normal and problem pregnancies* (7th ed.). Philadelphia: Elsevier; Witcher, P. M. (2017). Caring for the laboring woman with hypertensive disorders complicating pregnancy. In B. B. Kennedy & S. M. Baird (Eds.), *Intrapartum management modules: A perinatal education program* (5th ed.). Philadelphia: Wolters Kluwer.

TABLE 6.7	Common Laboratory Changes in Preeclampsia		
	Normal Nonpregnant	**Preeclampsia**	**HELLP**
Hemoglobin, hematocrit	12–16 g/dL, 37%–47%	May ↑	↓
Platelets (cells/mm^3)	150,000–400,000/mm^3	<100,000/mm^3	<100,000/mm^3
Prothrombin time (PT), partial thromboplastin time (PTT)	12–14 s, 60–70 s	Unchanged	Unchanged
Fibrinogen	200–400 mg/dL	300–600 mg/dL	↓
Fibrin split products (FSPs)	Absent	Absent or present	Present
Blood urea nitrogen (BUN)	10–20 mg/dL	↑	↑
Creatinine	0.5–1.1 mg/dL	>1.1 mg/dL	↑
Lactate dehydrogenase (LDH)[a]	45–90 units/L	↑	↑ (>600 units/L)
Aspartate aminotransferase (AST)	4–20 units/L	↑	↑ (>70 units/L)
Alanine aminotransferase (ALT)	3–21 units/L	↑	↑
Creatinine clearance	80–125 mL/min	130–180 mL/min	↓
Burr cells or schistocytes	Absent	Absent	Present
Uric acid	2–6.6 mg/dL	>5.9 mg/dL	>10 mg/dL
Bilirubin (total)	0.1–1 mg/dL	Unchanged or ↑	↑ (>1.2 mg/dL)

[a]LDH values differ according to the test or assays being performed.
From Lowdermilk, D. L., Perry, S. E., Cashion, K., Alden, K., & Olshansky, E. (2020). *Maternity and women's health care* (12th ed.). St. Louis, MO: Elsevier. Data from American College of Obstetricians and Gynecologists (ACOG). (2002). *Practice bulletin no. 33: Diagnosis and management of preeclampsia and eclampsia.* Washington, DC: ACOG; American College of Obstetricians and Gynecologists. (2013). Executive summary: Hypertension in pregnancy. *Obstetrics & Gynecology, 122*(5), 1122–1131; Dildy, G. (2004). Complications of preeclampsia. In G. Dildy, M. Belfort, & G. Saade, et al. (Eds.), *Critical care obstetrics* (4th ed.). Malden, MA: Blackwell Science; Witcher, P. M., & Shah, S. S. (2019). Hypertension in pregnancy. In N. H. Troiano, P. M. Witcher, & S. M. Baird (Eds.), *AWHONN's high risk and critical care obstetrics* (4th ed.). Philadelphia: Wolters Kluwer.

C. Immediate Postpartum

Nurse should continue to monitor for signs and symptoms of preeclampsia. Preeclampsia usually resolves within 48 hours after birth.

1. Ongoing, frequent assessment of vital signs, I&O, DTRs, and level of consciousness
2. Magnesium sulfate infusion is typically continued for first 24 hours postpartum.
   a. Continue to monitor for side effects and toxicity.
3. Carefully assess uterine tone and fundal height for uterine atony.
4. Monitor for blood loss.
5. Instruct client to report headache, visual disturbances, or epigastric pain.
6. Check with the health care provider before administration of *any* ergot derivatives.
7. Upon discharge, client and support persons should be educated about symptoms of preeclampsia in the postpartum recovery period and be advised to report any new or ongoing symptoms to obstetric provider immediately or return to the hospital. Home BP monitoring may be ordered and antihypertensive medications may be restarted or ordered and directions should be followed as ordered.

D. Eclampsia: Onset of seizures or coma in a woman with preeclampsia who has no history of preexisting seizure pathology; life-threatening complication of preeclampsia.

E. Hemolysis, Elevated Liver enzymes and Low Platelets (HELLP) syndrome: Severe form of preeclampsia associated with increased maternal morbidity and mortality. HELLP stands for hemolysis (H), elevated liver enzymes (EL), and low platelets (LP).

Gestational Diabetes Mellitus

Description: Impaired glucose tolerance that occurs during pregnancy. Occurs in about 10% of pregnancies. Risk factors include family history, personal history of gestational diabetes mellitus (GDM) in previous pregnancy, previous pregnancy that ended in stillbirth, previous delivery of a macrosomic infant, obesity, hypertension (HTN). Associated with increased incidence of macrosomia, birth trauma, neonatal hypoglycemia, and hydramnios.

Women with GDM typically fall into one of two classes:

1. Class A1: Two or more abnormal values on oral glucose tolerance test (OGTT) but fasting and postprandial glucose values are diet controlled
2. Class A2: Not known to have diabetes prior to pregnancy but requires either insulin or oral hypoglycemic mediation for blood glucose control (see Diabetes Mellitus in Chapter 4)

A. Symptoms

1. May be asymptomatic or describe similar symptoms to diabetes mellitus
   a. The three Ps: **p**olyphagia, **p**olydipsia, and **p**olyuria.

B. Clinical Judgment Measures

1. Educate about physiological changes of blood glucose and insulin needs during pregnancy and pathology of GDM
   a. Hypoglycemia risk in first trimester
   b. Hyperglycemia risk in second and third trimesters: maternal nutrient ingestion contributes to greater and sustained level of blood glucose; maternal insulin resistance increases. If woman unable to compensate for insulin resistance, GDM can result.

2. Educate about risks and adverse outcomes associated with GDM.
3. Explain screening for GDM and lab testing procedures.

C. Labs
1. Early prenatal screening may be done for women considered high risk.
2. Routine screening typically done between 24 and 28 weeks' gestation.
   a. Two-step screening: (non-fasting) 50-g oral glucose load followed by plasma glucose measurement 1 hour later
   b. Value of 130 to 140 mg/dL or higher considered positive screen; follow up step of a fasting 3-hour OGTT: fasting glucose level obtained, followed by a 100-g oral glucose load, and then plasma glucose levels obtained at 1-, 2-, and 3-hour intervals.

D. Education
1. If woman determined to have GDM, educate on prescribed medications, diet, exercise.
   a. Refer client to dietitian for individualized diet management.
2. Explain self-monitoring of blood glucose levels.
3. Educate on increased fetal surveillance like NSTs, BPPs, amniocentesis.
4. Teach fetal kick counting.
5. Teach client signs and symptoms of ketoacidosis and to seek immediate assistance should it occur.
6. Discuss possibility of scheduled induction between 38 and 40 weeks' gestation, dependent on maternal-fetal well-being.

E. Intrapartum Care for Client with GDM
1. Establish IV access. Client may need IV insulin and maintenance fluids (once in active labor, or if glucose levels fall below 70 mg/dL, client may need fluids containing 5% dextrose.
2. Monitor glucose levels per orders.
3. Check urine for ketones.
4. Monitor fetus continuously (FHR).
5. Prepare for complications at birth like dystocia, macrosomic infant, or need for cesarean birth.

F. Postpartum Care for Client with GDM
1. Insulin administration and maintenance fluids may be continued until stable. Monitor glucose levels per orders and observe for symptoms of hypoglycemia or hyperglycemia.

2. Check for urine ketones.
3. Monitor for complications.
   a. Preeclampsia
   b. Postpartum hemorrhage (PPH) (postpartum uterine atony associated with uterine overdistension)
   c. Infection
4. Encourage breastfeeding.
5. Postpartum education should include guidelines for glucose monitoring, continuation of any insulin or oral hypoglycemic medications, and follow-up care.

> **HESI HINT** Insulin requirements decrease during the first 24 h after delivery and can drop precipitously; therefore, clients should be monitored closely.

Anemia

Description: A decrease in the O_2-carrying capacity of blood. Occurs in 20% to 50% of pregnant women; often related to iron deficiency. Risk factors include diet low in iron, shortened interval between pregnancies. Associated with increased incidence of preterm birth and low-birth-weight infants. Sickle cell anemia can be reviewed in Chapter 5.

A. Symptoms
1. Fatigue
2. Pallor
3. Weakness
4. Pica

B. Clinical Judgment Measures
1. Dietary history
2. Educate about maternal and fetal concerns associated with iron deficiency anemia.
3. Discuss labs.

C. Labs
A. Hgb and Hct
   1. Hgb <11 g/dL, Hct <37% in first, third trimesters
   2. Hgb <10.5 g/dL, Hct <35% in second trimester
   3. Hct <33%

D. Medical treatment
1. Oral iron supplementation is often ordered (Table 6.8).

Infections

Description: Maternal infection during pregnancy can cause significant concerns for both the woman and the fetus. The

TABLE 6.8 **Iron**			
Drug	**Indications**	**Adverse Reactions**	**Nursing Implications**
Ferrous sulfate	Iron deficiency anemia	• Constipation • Diarrhea • Gastric irritation • Nausea or vomiting	• Iron is best absorbed on an empty stomach. • To be taken with vitamin C source such as orange juice to increase absorption • Should not be taken with cereal, eggs, or milk, which decrease absorption • Should be taken in the evening if problem exists with morning sickness • Stools will turn dark green to black. • Laboratory values should be checked for increased reticulocytes and rising hemoglobin and hematocrit.

woman is typically screened for STDs at her first antepartum appointment and as needed during the remainder of the pregnancy. (See Chapter 4 for review of STIs and HIV/AIDS.)

A. Symptoms

Description: Maternal and fetal symptoms will vary with each disease process.

Sexually Transmitted Infections

STIs can cause significant maternal and fetal morbidity. Many can be vertically transmitted to the fetus during pregnancy or through the birth canal in labor (Table 6.9).

TORCH Infections

Description: TORCH is a collective acronym for toxoplasmosis, other infections (hepatitis), rubella, cytomegalovirus (CMV), and herpes simplex. These infections can cause significant maternal and fetal morbidity (Table 6.10).

Group B Streptococcus

Description: Group B streptococcus (GBS) can be found in normal vaginal flora and will be present in about 25% of pregnant women. While many women with GBS will be asymptomatic or experience mild symptoms, this infection can cause significant neonatal morbidity and mortality.

Pregnant women with GBS may experience UTIs, develop uterine infections like chorioamnionitis or postpartum endometritis, sepsis, or experience a stillbirth. GBS can cause preterm labor and birth, preterm ROM, or cause intrapartum maternal fever. At birth, GBS infection can cause the neonate to have a fever, difficulty feeding, be irritable or lethargic, or have difficulty breathing.

HIV/AIDS

Description: Women should be universally screened for HIV early in pregnancy, and again in the third trimester for those who are considered to be high risk, so that treatment can be started expeditiously, and the likelihood of perinatal transmission can be reduced. Women with HIV may be asymptomatic, or laboratory studies may reveal leukopenia, thrombocytopenia, anemia, or an elevated erythrocyte sedimentation rate (see Chapter 4). Decisions to proceed with a vaginal birth or a cesarean birth will depend on the degree of the maternal viral load. In the United States, women with HIV are advised not to breastfeed their infants.

OTHER VAGINAL INFECTIONS

Bacterial Vaginosis

Description: The most common vaginal infection in women of childbearing age. Bacterial vaginosis (BV) can be sexually associated but it is not an STI. It occurs secondary to a reduction in the normal lactobacilli found in vaginal flora. Characteristically, women will complain of vaginal discharge

TABLE 6.9	Maternal and Fetal Effects of Common Sexually Transmitted Infections	
Infection	**Maternal Effects**	**Fetal Effects**
Chlamydia	Prelabor rupture of membranes	Low birth weight
	Preterm labor	
	Postpartum endometritis	
Gonorrhea	Miscarriage	Preterm birth
	Preterm labor	IUGR
	Prelabor rupture of membranes	
	Chorioamnionitis	
	Postpartum endometritis	
	Postpartum sepsis	
Group B streptococcus	Urinary tract infection	Preterm birth
	Chorioamnionitis	
	Postpartum endometritis	
	Sepsis	
	Meningitis (rare)	
Herpes simplex virus	Intrauterine infection (rare)	Congenital infection (rare)
Human papillomavirus	Dystocia from large lesions	None known
	Excessive bleeding from lesions after birth trauma	
Syphilis	Miscarriage	IUGR
	Preterm labor	Preterm birth
		Stillbirth
		Congenital infection
Trichomoniasis	Yellow-green vaginal discharge; may be frothy and mucopurulent. Often copious amounts	Preterm labor and birth
		Premature rupture of membranes
	Cervix and vaginal walls may have tiny petechiae (strawberry spots)	

IUGR, Intrauterine growth restriction. Adapted from Lowdermilk, D. L., Perry, S. E., Cashion, K., Alden, K., & Olshansky, E. (2020). *Maternity and women's health care* (12th ed.). St. Louis, MO: Elsevier. Data from Gilbert, E. (2011). *Manual of high risk pregnancy & delivery* (5th ed.). St. Louis, MO: Mosby; Duff, P., Sweet, R., & Edwards, R. (2013). Maternal and fetal infections. In R. K. Creasy, R. Resnik, J. D. Iams, C. J. Lockwood, T. R. Moore, & M. F. Greene (Eds.), *Creasy and Resnik's maternal-fetal medicine: Principles and practice* (7th ed.). Philadelphia: Saunders.

TABLE 6.10   TORCH Infections: Maternal and Fetal

Infection	Maternal Effects	Fetal Effects	Counseling: Prevention, Identification, and Management
Toxoplasmosis (protozoa)	Most infections asymptomatic Acute infection similar to mononucleosis Woman immune after first episode (except in immuno-compromised clients)	Congenital infection is most likely to occur when maternal infection develops during the third trimester. The risk of fetal injury, however, is greatest when maternal infection occurs during the first trimester.	Good handwashing technique should be used. Eating raw or rare meat and exposure to litter used by infected cats should be avoided; *Toxoplasma* titer should be checked if there are cats in the house. If titer is rising during early pregnancy, therapeutic abortion may be considered an option.
Other Infections			
Hepatitis A (infectious hepatitis) (virus)	Liver failure (extremely rare) Low-grade fever, malaise, poor appetite, right upper quadrant pain and tenderness, jaundice, and light-colored stools	Perinatal transmission virtually never occurs.	Spread by fecal-oral contact especially by culinary workers; gamma globulin can be given as prophylaxis for hepatitis A. Hepatitis A vaccine is available.
Hepatitis B (serum hepatitis) (virus)	May be transmitted sexually Approximately 10% of clients become chronic carriers. Some people with chronic hepatitis B eventually develop severe chronic liver disease, such as cirrhosis or hepatocellular carcinoma.	Infection occurs during birth. Maternal vaccination during pregnancy should present no risk for fetus; however, data are not available.	Generally passed by contaminated needles, syringes, or blood transfusions; also can be transmitted PO or by coitus (but incubation period is longer); hepatitis B immune globulin can be given prophylactically after exposure. Hepatitis B vaccine recommended for populations at risk
Rubella (3-day or German measles) (virus)	Rash, fever, mild symptoms such as headache, malaise, myalgias, and arthralgias; postauricular lymph nodes may be swollen; mild conjunctivitis.	Approximately 50%–80% of fetuses exposed to the virus within 12 weeks after conception will show signs of congenital infection. Very few fetuses are affected if infection occurs after 18 weeks of gestation. The most common fetal anomalies associated with congenital rubella syndrome are deafness, eye defects (e.g., cataracts or retinopathy), central nervous system defects, and cardiac defects.	Vaccination of pregnant women is contraindicated; nonimmune women should be vaccinated in the early postpartum period; pregnancy should be prevented for 1 month after vaccination. Women may breastfeed after vaccination and the vaccine can be administered along with immunoglobulin preparations such as Rh immune globulin.
Cytomegalovirus (CMV) (a herpesvirus)	Most adults are asymptomatic or have only mild influenza-like symptoms. The presence of CMV antibodies does not totally prevent reinfection.	The fetus can be infected transplacentally. Infection is much more likely with a primary maternal infection. The most common indications of congenital infection include hepatosplenomegaly, intracranial calcifications, jaundice, growth restriction, microcephaly, chorioretinitis, hearing loss, thrombocytopenia, hyperbilirubinemia, and hepatitis.	The virus is transmitted by transplantation of an infected organ, transfusion of infected blood, sexual contact, or contact with contaminated saliva or urine. Virus may be reactivated and cause disease *in utero* or during birth in subsequent pregnancies; fetal infection may occur during passage through infected birth canal. Prevention includes use of CMV-negative blood products if transfusion of pregnant women is necessary and teaching all women to wash hands carefully after handling infant diapers and toys.
Herpes Genitalis (herpes simplex virus, type 1 or type 2 [HSV-1 or HSV-2])	Primary infection with painful blisters, tender inguinal lymph nodes, fever, viral meningitis (rare). Recurrent infections are much milder and shorter.	Transplacental infection resulting in congenital infection is rare and usually occurs with primary maternal infection. The risk mainly exists with infection late in pregnancy.	As many as two-thirds of women with HSV-2 antibodies acquired the infection asymptomatically; however, asymptomatic women can give birth to seriously infected neonates. Risk of transmission is greatest during vaginal birth if woman has active lesions; thus cesarean birth is recommended. Acyclovir can be used to treat recurrent outbreaks during pregnancy or as suppressive therapy late in pregnancy to prevent an outbreak during labor and birth.

TORCH, Toxoplasmosis, other infections, rubella, cytomegalovirus, herpes genitalis. From Lowdermilk, D. L., Perry, S. E., Cashion, K., Alden, K., & Olshansky, E. (2020). *Maternity and women's health care* (12th ed.). St. Louis, MO: Elsevier. Data from Duff, P., Sweet, R., & Edwards, R. (2013). Maternal and fetal infections. In R. K. Creasy, R. Resnik, J. D. Iams, C. J. Lockwood, T. R. Moore, & M. F. Greene (Eds.), *Creasy and Resnik's maternal-fetal medicine: Principles and practice* (7th ed.). Philadelphia: Saunders.

that is milky, white, or grayish and is accompanied by a fishy odor. BV can cause preterm labor and birth.

Candidiasis

Description: This is sometimes known as a "yeast infection" or vulvovaginal candidiasis and is the second most common type of vaginal infection in the United States. Predisposing factors include antibiotic therapy, diabetes, obesity, and immunosuppressed states. Vaginal discharge is often thick, white, clumpy or cottage cheese-like, and accompanied by vaginal and vulvar itching. It may be connected to oral thrush in the neonate.

A. **Clinical Judgment Measures**
 1. All pregnant clients should be screened for risk factors for infections.
 2. All prenatal clients should be screened for symptoms of infections.
 3. A thorough sexual history should include asking about Partners, Practices, Protection from STDs, Past history of STDs, Prevention of pregnancy (prior to conception and postpartum plans).
 4. Educate the mother about infections, possible maternal and fetal effects, and treatment options.
 5. Administer medications as prescribed.

B. **Labs**
 1. May include serology (HIV, syphilis, TORCH), endocervical swabs (chlamydia, gonorrhea), vaginal and rectal swabs (GBS), urine, vaginal, or anal cultures, pap testing, antibody titers.
 2. Labs are typically completed at the first prenatal appointment, repeated as applicable, and third trimester screening is recommended for women who continue to be at high risk.

C. **Diagnostics**
 1. May include additional fetal surveillance, i.e., US, if mother is positive for infection and fetal growth appears to be impacted or there is concern of congenital anomalies or infection.

Substance Use Disorders (see Chapter 7)

All women should be universally screened for substance use and substance use disorders (SUDs) during pregnancy and in the postpartum period. SUDs can contribute to significant maternal morbidity and mortality as well as obstetric complications. They can impact fetal growth and development. Treatment options that are safe for both the mother and infant are available during the perinatal period.

💡 REVIEW OF ANTEPARTUM COMPLICATIONS

1. What instructions should the nurse give the woman with a threatened abortion?
2. Identify the nursing plans and interventions for a woman hospitalized with hyperemesis gravidarum.
3. Describe discharge counseling for a woman after hydatidiform mole evacuation by D&C.
4. What condition should the nurse suspect if a woman of childbearing age presents to an emergency department with bilateral or unilateral abdominal pain, with or without bleeding?

5. List three symptoms of abruptio placentae and three symptoms of placenta previa.
6. All pregnant women should be taught preterm labor recognition. Describe the warning symptoms of preterm labor.
7. List the factors predisposing a woman to preterm labor.
8. Magnesium sulfate is used to treat preeclampsia.
   A. What is the purpose of magnesium sulfate?
   B. What is the main action of magnesium sulfate?
   C. What is the antidote for magnesium sulfate?
   D. List the three main assessment findings indicating toxic effects of magnesium sulfate.
9. What are the major symptoms of preeclampsia?
10. A woman on the oral hypoglycemic tolbutamide asks the nurse if she can continue this medication during pregnancy. How should the nurse respond?
11. Name three maternal and three fetal complications of gestational diabetes.
12. State three priority nursing actions in the postdelivery period for the client with preeclampsia.
13. What are the two most difficult times for control in the pregnant diabetic?
14. Why is regular insulin used in labor?
15. List three conditions clients with diabetes mellitus are more prone to developing.

See Answer Key at the end of this text for suggested responses.

INTRAPARTUM NURSING CARE

Description: The process of labor and birth. Five key factors affect the process of labor and birth. They are noted as the 5 P's:
1. **Passengers (fetus and placenta)**
2. **Passageway (birth canal)**
3. **Powers (contractions)**
4. **Position of the mother**
5. **Psychologic response**

Stages of Labor

A. First stage of labor: From the beginning of regular contractions to 10 cm dilatation and 100% effacement
 1. Latent phase: 0 to 3 cm
 2. Active phase: 4 to 7 cm
 3. Transition phase: 8 to 10 cm (Table 6.11)
B. Second stage of labor: 10 cm to delivery of the fetus
C. Third stage of labor: From delivery of the fetus to delivery of the placenta. Typically the shortest phase of labor
D. Fourth stage of labor: About 1 to 2 hours after delivery of the placenta (immediate recovery)

True or False Labor

A. True labor
 1. Pain accompanied by rhythmic contractions that become stronger, longer, and more regular
 2. Contractions that intensify with ambulation or activity change
 3. Progressive cervical softening, dilatation, and effacement

TABLE 6.11	**First Stage of Labor**	
Phase	**Description**	**Psychological and Physical Responses**
Latent	From beginning of true labor until 3—4 cm cervical dilatation	• Mildly anxious, conversant • Able to continue usual activities • Contractions mild, initially 10—20 min apart, 15—20 s duration; later 5—7 min apart, 30—40 s duration
Active	From 4—7 cm cervical dilatation	• Increased anxiety • Increased discomfort • May not want to be left alone • Contractions moderate to severe, 2—3 min apart, 30—60 s duration

Transition	From 8—10 cm cervical dilatation	• Changed behavior:
		  • Sudden nausea, hiccups
		  • Increased irritability, may not want to be touched, although desirous of companionship and support
		  • Contractions severe, 1½ min apart, 60—90 s duration

B. False labor
   1. Discomfort may be localized in abdomen
   2. Contractions decrease in intensity or frequency with ambulation or changing position
   3. No cervical change in dilation or effacement
C. Impending labor signs may include the following:
   1. Lightening (fetal presenting part drops into true pelvis)
   2. Braxton Hicks contractions (irregular contractions)
   3. Lower back pain
   4. Increase in vaginal discharge, bloody show, or expulsion of mucous
   5. Burst of energy, "nesting instinct"

Initial Nursing Assessment of Client Presenting in Labor

Interview to determine reason client is presenting for care
A. Triage for obstetrical emergencies (i.e., vaginal bleeding, no fetal movement, ROMs, trauma, abnormal vital signs) (Fig. 6.4)
B. Client report of status of membranes
C. Pain assessment
D. Review of prenatal records, obstetric problems (i.e., diabetes mellitus, gestational hypertension), pertinent laboratory and diagnostic test results
   1. Gravidity and parity
   2. Gestational age
E. Psychosocial assessment
   1. General appearance and behavior
   2. Presence of support person
F. Physical examination
   1. General systems assessment with vital signs
      a. Laboratory and diagnostic tests as ordered, i.e., urinalysis, blood tests (Hct, CBC, ABO typing, and Rh-factor), GBS status if not known
   2. Fetal assessment
      a. Leopold's maneuvers: Abdominal palpation to determine which fetal part is in the fundus, where the fetal back is located, and what is the presenting part.

Leopold's may help determine the number of fetuses (Box 6.2 and Fig. 6.5).
      b. **Fetal lie:** The relationship of the long axis (spine) of the fetus to the long axis (spine) of the mother. It can be longitudinal (up and down), transverse (perpendicular), or oblique (slanted; see Fig. 6.6).
      c. **Fetal presentation:** The part of the fetus that presents to the inlet (see Fig. 6.6)
         1) Cephalic (Vertex, face brow)
         2) Shoulder (acromion)
         3) Breech (buttocks)
      d. **Fetal position:** Determine location of fetal back. The location of the back in the anterior, lateral, or posterior portion of the abdomen also helps determine the variety (position). Fetal small parts (hands, feet, knees) should be opposite the fetal back. The relationship of the point of reference (occiput, sacrum, acromion) on the fetal presenting part (cephalic, breech, shoulder) to the mother's pelvis. Most common is left occiput anterior (LOA). The point of reference on the vertex (occiput) is pointed up toward the symphysis and directed toward the left side of the maternal pelvis (Fig. 6.7, pp. XXX).
      e. **Fetal station:** Relationship of presenting part to an imaginary line drawn between the maternal ischial spines. Measures degree of descent of presenting fetal part through birth canal. Expressed as cm above or below the ischial spines. Best assessed as part of the vaginal exam and should be determined when labor begins so that rate of fetal descent can be assessed regularly and accurately (Fig. 6.8, pp. XXX).
         1) Station 0 is engaged.
         2) Negative stations are above the ischial spines.
         3) Positive stations are below the ischial spines
      f. Fetal attitude:
         1) Relationship of the fetal parts to one another
         2) Flexion or extension
         3) Flexion is desirable so that the smallest diameters of the presenting part move through the pelvis.

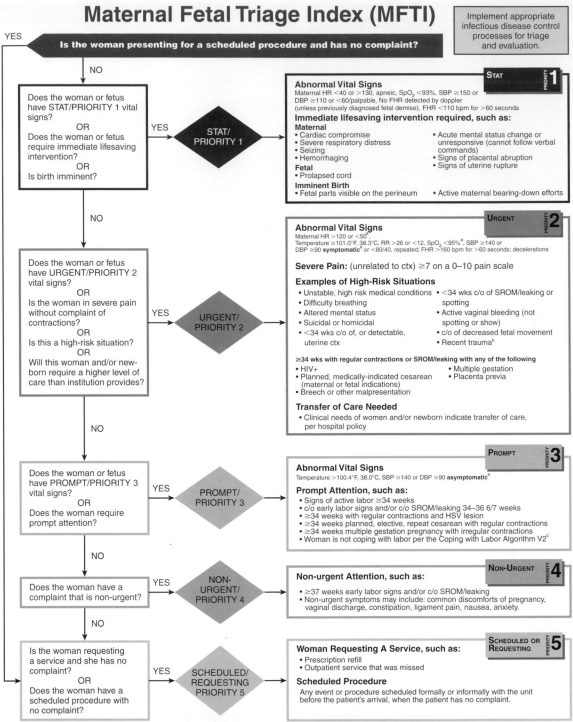

Maternal Fetal Triage Index (MFTI)

Implement appropriate infectious disease control processes for triage and evaluation.

YES

Is the woman presenting for a scheduled procedure and has no complaint?

NO

Does the woman or fetus have STAT/PRIORITY 1 vital signs?
OR
Does the woman or fetus require immediate lifesaving intervention?
OR
Is birth imminent?

YES → STAT/ PRIORITY 1 →

STAT PRIORITY 1

Abnormal Vital Signs
Maternal HR <40 or >130, apneic, SpO₂ <93%, SBP ≥150 or DBP ≥110 or <60/palpable, No FHR detected by doppler (unless previously diagnosed fetal demise), FHR <110 bpm for >60 seconds

Immediate lifesaving intervention required, such as:
Maternal
- Cardiac compromise
- Severe respiratory distress
- Seizing
- Hemorrhaging
- Acute mental status change or unresponsive (cannot follow verbal commands)
- Signs of placental abruption
- Signs of uterine rupture

Fetal
- Prolapsed cord

Imminent Birth
- Fetal parts visible on the perineum
- Active maternal bearing-down efforts

NO

Does the woman or fetus have URGENT/PRIORITY 2 vital signs?
OR
Is the woman in severe pain without complaint of contractions?
OR
Is this a high-risk situation?
OR
Will this woman and/or newborn require a higher level of care than institution provides?

YES → URGENT/ PRIORITY 2 →

URGENT PRIORITY 2

Abnormal Vital Signs
Maternal HR >120 or <50ᵃ, Temperature ≥101.0°F, 38.3°C, RR >26 or <12, SpO₂ <95%ᵃ, SBP ≥140 or DBP ≥90 **symptomatic**ᵃ or <80/40, repeated; FHR >160 bpm for >60 seconds; decelerations

Severe Pain: (unrelated to ctx) ≥7 on a 0–10 pain scale

Examples of High-Risk Situations
- Unstable, high risk medical conditions
- Difficulty breathing
- Altered mental status
- Suicidal or homicidal
- <34 wks c/o of, or detectable, uterine ctx
- <34 wks c/o of SROM/leaking or spotting
- Active vaginal bleeding (not spotting or show)
- c/o of decreased fetal movement
- Recent traumaᵇ

≥34 wks with regular contractions or SROM/leaking with any of the following
- HIV+
- Planned, medically-indicated cesarean (maternal or fetal indications)
- Breech or other malpresentation
- Multiple gestation
- Placenta previa

Transfer of Care Needed
- Clinical needs of women and/or newborn indicate transfer of care, per hospital policy

NO

Does the woman or fetus have PROMPT/PRIORITY 3 vital signs?
OR
Does the woman require prompt attention?

YES → PROMPT/ PRIORITY 3 →

PROMPT PRIORITY 3

Abnormal Vital Signs
Temperature >100.4°F, 38.0°C, SBP ≥140 or DBP ≥90 **asymptomatic**ᵃ

Prompt Attention, such as:
- Signs of active labor ≥34 weeks
- c/o early labor signs and/or c/o SROM/leaking 34–36 6/7 weeks
- ≥34 weeks with regular contractions and HSV lesion
- ≥34 weeks planned, elective, repeat cesarean with regular contractions
- ≥34 weeks multiple gestation pregnancy with irregular contractions
- Woman is not coping with labor per the Coping with Labor Algorithm V2ᶜ

NO

Does the woman have a complaint that is non-urgent?

YES → NON- URGENT/ PRIORITY 4 →

NON-URGENT PRIORITY 4

Non-urgent Attention, such as:
- ≥37 weeks early labor signs and/or c/o SROM/leaking
- Non-urgent symptoms may include: common discomforts of pregnancy, vaginal discharge, constipation, ligament pain, nausea, anxiety.

NO

Is the woman requesting a service and she has no complaint?
OR
Does the woman have a scheduled procedure with no complaint?

YES → SCHEDULED/ REQUESTING PRIORITY 5 →

SCHEDULED OR REQUESTING PRIORITY 5

Woman Requesting A Service, such as:
- Prescription refill
- Outpatient service that was missed

Scheduled Procedure
Any event or procedure scheduled formally or informally with the unit before the patient's arrival, when the patient has no complaint.

ᵃ High Risk and Critical Care Obstetrics, 2013
ᵇ Trauma may or may not include a direct assault on the abdomen. Examples are trauma from motor vehicle accidents, falls, and intimate partner violence.
ᶜ Coping with Labor Algorithm V2 used with permission.
The HFTI is exemplary and does not include all possible patient complaints or conditions. The MFTI is designed to guide clinical decision-making but does not replace clinical judgement. Vital signs in the MFTI are suggested values. Values appropriate for the population and geographic region should be determined by each clinical team, taking into account variables such as altitude.
©2015 Association of Women's Health, Obstetric and Neonatal Nurses. For permission to use the MFTI or integrate the MFTI into the Electronic Medical Record contact permissions@awhonn.org.

Fig. 6.4 Maternal Fetal Triage Index (MFT). (From Lowdermilk, D. L., Perry, S. E., Cashion, K., Alden, K., & Olshansky, E. [2020]. *Maternity and women's health care* [12th ed., 10]. St. Louis, MO: Elsevier. Reprinted with permission from the Association of Women's Health, Obstetric and Neonatal Nurses (AWHONN) (www.awhonn.org). AWHONN Maternal Fetal Triage Index. Copyright AWHONN. To access the full PDF version of the MFTI Index for clinical use, email requests to permissions@awhonn.org)

3. FHR and pattern assessment
   a. FHR best heard over fetal back (see Fig. 6.5 and Box 6.2)
   b. Assessment of uterine contractions (Fig. 6.9, pp. XXX)
      1) Frequency. Time contractions from beginning of one contraction to the beginning of the next (measured in minutes apart).
      2) Duration. Time the length of the entire contraction (from beginning to end).
      3) Strength. Assess the intensity of strongest part (peak) of contraction. It is measured by clinical estimation of the indentability of the fundus through palpation (use gentle pressure of fingertips to determine it).
         a) Very indentable (mild)
         b) Moderately indentable (moderate)
         c) Unindentable (firm)

> **HESI HINT** Internal electric monitoring with an intrauterine pressure catheter is the most accurate way to assess uterine contraction intensity and uterus resting tone.

BOX 6.2 Leopold Maneuvers

Description: Abdominal palpations used to determine fetal presentation, lie, position, and engagement
A. With client in supine position, place both cupped hands over fundus and palpate to determine whether breech (soft, immovable, large) or vertex (hard, movable, small).
B. Place one hand firmly on side and palpate with other hand to determine presence of small parts or fetal back. (Fetal heart rate is heard best through fetal back.)
C. Facing client, grasp the area over the symphysis with the thumb and fingers and press to determine the degree of descent of the presenting part. (A ballotable or floating head can be rocked back and forth between the thumb and fingers.)
D. Facing the client's feet, outline the fetal presenting part with the palmar surface of both hands to determine the degree of descent and attitude of the fetus. (If cephalic prominence is located on the same side as small parts, assume the head is flexed.)

4. Sterile vaginal examination (performed only when indicated by the status of the client and the fetus). Nurse should obtain permission to touch the woman prior to the exam.
   a. Sterile gloves are worn.
   b. Examinations are not done routinely. They are sharply curtailed after membranes rupture to prevent infection.
   c. Vaginal exams should not be performed with active vaginal bleeding.
      1) Possible placenta previa, placental abruption, fetal vessels may be lying over the cervical os
   d. Vaginal examinations are performed before analgesia and anesthesia, to determine the progress of labor, to determine whether second-stage pushing can begin.
   e. Cervical assessment:
      1) Cervical dilation: Cervix opens from 0 to 10 cm.
      2) Cervical effacement: Cervix is taken up into the upper uterine segment; expressed in percentages from 0% to 100%.
      3) Cervical position: Cervix can be directly anterior and palpated easily, or can be posterior and difficult to palpate.
      4) Cervical consistency: It is firm to soft.
   f. Status of membranes (ruptured, bulging, or intact)
      1) Determined by vaginal exam or obvious leaking of fluid
      2) Microscopic examination of vaginal fluid for ferning
      3) Nitrazine paper turns black or dark blue with presence of amniotic fluid.
      4) Chart time of rupture, fetal response, and any describing characteristics (color, odor, clarity) including evidence of meconium

Electronic Fetal Monitoring
Variables Measured by Fetal Monitoring
A. Contractions
   1. Beginning, peak (acme), and end of each contraction
   2. Duration: Length of each contraction from beginning to end
   3. Frequency: Beginning of one contraction to beginning of the next (three to five contractions must be measured)

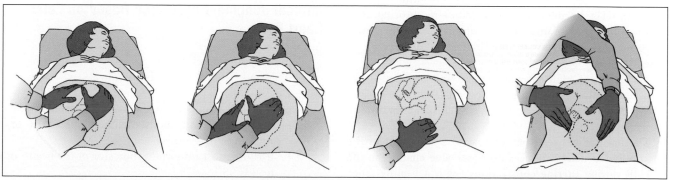

Fig. 6.5 Leopold Maneuvers. (From Lowdermilk, D. L., Perry, S. E., Cashion, K., Alden, K., & Olshansky, E. [2020]. *Maternity and women's health care* [12th ed., 10]. St. Louis, MO: Elsevier.)

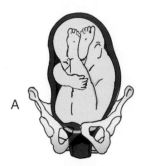

Frank breech

Lie: Longitudinal or vertical
Presentation: Breech (incomplete)
Presenting part: Sacrum
Attitude: Flexion, except for legs at knees

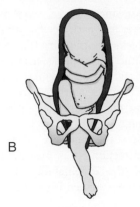

Single footling breech

Lie: Longitudinal or vertical
Presentation: Breech (incomplete)
Presenting part: Sacrum
Attitude: Flexion, except for one leg extended
at hip and knee

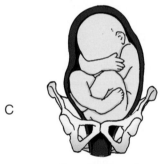

Complete breech

Lie: Longitudinal or vertical
Presentation: Breech (sacrum and feet presenting)
Presenting part: Sacrum (with feet)
Attitude: General flexion

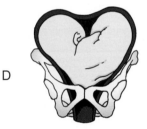

Shoulder presentation

Lie: Transverse or horizontal
Presentation: Shoulder
Presenting part: Scapula
Attitude: Flexion

Fig. 6.6 Fetal Presentations. (A–C) Breech (sacral) presentation. (D) Shoulder presentation. (From Lowdermilk, D. L., & Perry, S. E. [2010]. *Maternity nursing* [9th ed.]. St. Louis, MO: Mosby.)

4. Intensity: Measured not by external monitoring but in mm Hg by internal (intrauterine) monitoring after amniotic membranes have ruptured; ranges from 30 mm Hg (mild) to 70 mm Hg (strong) at peak

B. Baseline FHR
  1. The range of FHR (average 110 to 160 beats/min) between contractions, monitored over a 10-minute period. The baseline segment should be greater than 2 minutes of tracing.
  2. The balance between parasympathetic and sympathetic impulses usually produces no observable changes in the FHR during uterine contractions (with a healthy fetus, a healthy placenta, and good uteroplacental perfusion; Fig. 6.10).

Clinical Judgment Measures Based on Fetal Heart Rate

A. Baseline FHR
  1. Normal rhythmicity
  2. Average FHR 110 to 160 beats/min
  3. Description
     a. The FHR results from the balance between the parasympathetic and the sympathetic branches of the autonomic nervous system.
     b. It is the most important indicator of the health of the fetal CNS.
B. Variability (Fig. 6.11, pp. XXX)

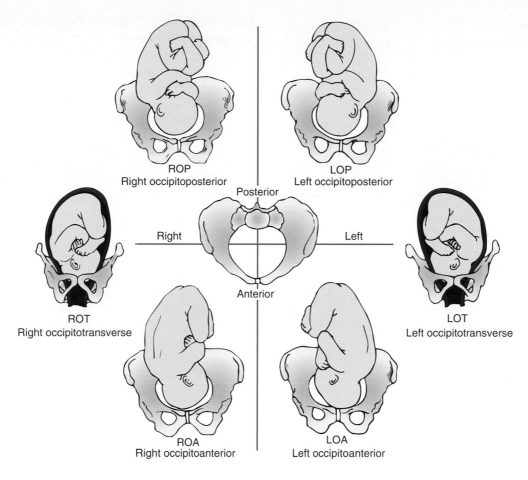

ROP
Right occipitoposterior

LOP
Left occipitoposterior

Posterior

Right   Left

Anterior

ROT
Right occipitotransverse

LOT
Left occipitotransverse

ROA
Right occipitoanterior

LOA
Left occipitoanterior

Lie: Longitudinal or vertical
Presentation: Vertex
Reference point: Occiput
Attitude: General flexion

Fig. 6.7 Fetal Positions. Examples of fetal vertex (occiput) presentations in relation to front, back, or side of maternal pelvis. (From Lowdermilk, D. L., & Perry, S. E. [2010]. *Maternity nursing* [9th ed.]. St. Louis, MO: Mosby.)

1. A characteristic of the baseline FHR and described as normal irregularity of the cardiac rhythm. Moderate variability signifies that the fetus does not have ischemia.
2. There are four categories of variability.
   a. Absent: Amplitude range undetectable
   b. Minimal: Amplitude range detectable up to and including 5 beats/min
   c. Moderate: amplitude range of 6 to 25 beats/min
   d. Marked: amplitude range greater than 25 beats/min
C. Clinical Judgment Measures
   1. Assess contractions using monitor strip.
   2. Assess FHR for normal baseline range and variability.
D. Periodic changes
   1. FHR changes in relation to uterine contractions (Fig. 6.12)
   2. Description
      a. Accelerations: abrupt increase in FHR of at least 15 beats/min and lasting 15 seconds or more above baseline

   1) Caused by sympathetic fetal response
   2) Occur in response to fetal movement
   3) Indicative of a reactive, healthy fetus
   b. Early decelerations: a gradual decrease in FHR, at least 30 seconds to lowest part of deceleration (nadir) (Fig. 6.13)
      1) Benign pattern caused by parasympathetic response, i.e., head compression
      2) Heart rate slowly and smoothly decelerates at beginning of contraction and returns to baseline at end of contraction
      3) Often appear in active labor
3. Nursing interventions for early decelerations
   a. No nursing interventions are required except to monitor the progress of labor.
   b. Document the processes of labor.

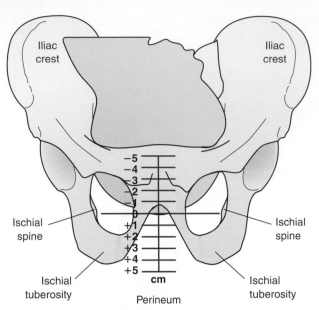

Fig. 6.8 Fetal Stations. Stations of presenting part, or degree of descent. The lowermost portion of the presenting part is at the level of the ischial spines, station 0. (From Lowdermilk, D. L., & Perry, S. E. [2010]. *Maternity nursing* (9th ed.). St. Louis, MO: Mosby.)

Fetal Heart Rate Patterns Requiring Clinical Judgment Measures

A. Decreased Variability (see Fig. 6.11)
1. Absent or minimal. Interpretation based on presence or absence of accelerations or recurrent decelerations.
2. Causes
   a. Hypoxia (asphyxia)
   b. Acidosis
   c. Maternal drug ingestion (opiates, CNS depressants such as magnesium sulfate, beta adrenergic agents [Terbutaline])
   d. Fetal rest cycles; typically last 20 to 40 minutes
3. Nursing Intervention
   a. Change maternal position, left-lateral
   b. Stimulate fetal scalp if indicated
   c. Discontinue oxytocin if infusing
   d. Assist provider with application of scalp electrode for internal fetal monitoring
B. Bradycardia
1. Baseline FHR is below 110 beats/min (assessed between contractions) for 10 minutes (as differentiated from a periodic change).

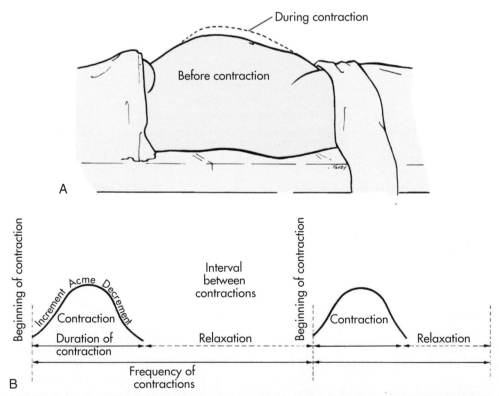

Fig. 6.9 Assessment of Uterine Contractions. (A) Abdominal contour before and during uterine contraction. (B) Wavelike pattern of contractile activity. (From Lowdermilk, D. L., Perry, S. E., Cashion, K., Alden, K., & Olshansky, E. [2020]. *Maternity and women's health care* (12th ed., p. 388, 10). St. Louis, MO: Elsevier. Courtesy Julie Perry Nelson, Loveland, CO.)

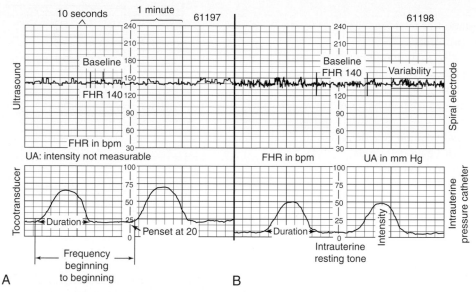

Fig. 6.10 Display of Fetal Heart Rate and Uterine Activity on Chart Paper. (A) External mode with ultrasound and tocotransducer as signal course. (B) Internal mode with spiral electrode and intrauterine catheter as signal source. Frequency of contractions is measured from the beginning of one contraction to the beginning of the next. Peak-to-peak measurement is sometimes used when electronic uterine activity monitoring is done. (From Miller, L., Miller, D. A., & Tucker, S. M. [2013]. *Pocket guide to fetal monitoring and assessment* [7th ed.]. St. Louis, MO: Mosby.)

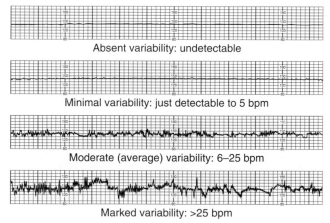

Absent variability: undetectable

Minimal variability: just detectable to 5 bpm

Moderate (average) variability: 6–25 bpm

Marked variability: >25 bpm

Fig. 6.11 Classification of Variability. (From Miller, L., Miller, D. A., & Tucker, S. M. [2013]. *Pocket guide to fetal monitoring and assessment* [7th ed.]. St. Louis, MO: Mosby.)

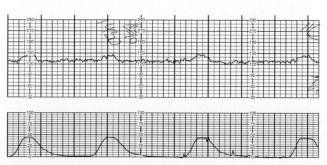

Fig. 6.12 Periodic Accelerations with Uterine Contractions. (From Miller, L., & Tucker, S. M. [2013]. *Pocket guide to fetal monitoring and assessment* [7th ed.]. St. Louis, MO: Mosby.)

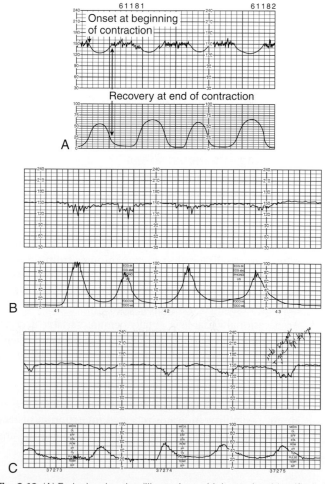

Fig. 6.13 (A) Early deceleration (illustration, with key points identified). (B and C) Early decelerations (actual tracings). (From Miller, L., & Tucker, S. M. [2013]. *Pocket guide to fetal monitoring and assessment* [7th ed.]. St. Louis, MO: Mosby.)

2. Causes
   a. Late manifestation of fetal hypoxia
   b. Fetal cardiac problems
   c. Maternal hypoglycemia, hypothermia
   d. Prolonged umbilical cord compression or head compression during rapid descent
3. Nursing interventions dependent on cause. Possible actions:
   a. Change maternal position to side-lying
   b. Stop oxytocin (if being delivered)
   c. Administer maternal oxygen
   d. Notify provider
C. Tachycardia
   1. Baseline FHR is above 160 beats/min (assessed between contractions) for 10 minutes
   2. Causes
      a. Early sign of fetal hypoxia
      b. Fetal infection
      c. Maternal infection, maternal fever
      d. Maternal hyperthyroidism
      e. Medication induced (atropine, terbutaline, hydroxyzine) or illicit drugs
      f. Rare: fetal anemia, acute fetal blood loss (placental abruption)
      g. Mild tachycardia common in fetus less than 28 weeks' gestation
   3. Nursing interventions dependent on cause. Possible actions:
      a. Reduce maternal fever; administer antipyretics as prescribed
      b. Administer maternal oxygen
      c. Consider IV fluid bolus
      c. Notify provider

Nonreassuring (Ominous) Signs

A. Variable deceleration pattern (Fig. 6.14, pp. XXX)
   1. It is the most common variant pattern. May occur episodically (random) or periodically (with each contraction). Visually abrupt decrease in FHR below baseline of at least 15 beats/min or more, lasting at least 15 seconds, returns to baseline in less than 2 minutes from onset.
   2. It occurs in 45% to 75% of all labors and is caused mainly by cord compression but can also indicate rapid fetal descent, nuchal cord, or short cord.
   3. An occasional variable is usually benign. Variable decelerations that return to baseline in less than 60 seconds with associated normal baseline and moderate variability are not usually associated with fetal acidemia.
   4. If recurrent or if FHR below 70 beats/min lasting longer than 30 to 60 seconds, and accompanied by minimal or absent variability, indicates repeated interruption of fetal oxygen supply and requires urgent evaluation and consideration of action.

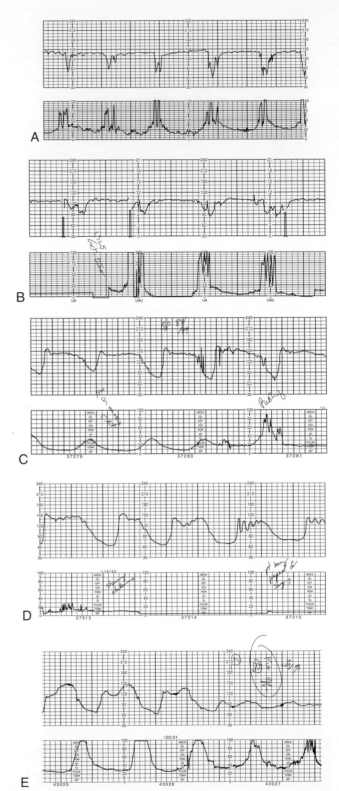

Fig. 6.14 Variable Decelerations. Note the progression in severity from panel (A) to panel (E) with overshoots and decreasing variability and eventually a prolonged and smooth deceleration (actual tracings). (From Miller, L., & Tucker, S. M. [2013]. *Pocket guide to fetal monitoring and assessment* [7th ed.]. St. Louis, MO: Mosby.)

5. Clinical Judgment Measures for variable decelerations
   a. Discontinue oxytocin if infusing.
   b. Change maternal position.
   c. Administer oxygen at 10 L by facemask.
   d. Notify provider.
   e. Assist with vaginal or speculum examination.
   f. Assist with amnioinfusion if ordered.
   g. Prepare for delivery if pattern cannot be corrected.

B. Late decelerations (Fig. 6.15)
   1. A visually apparent, gradual decrease in and return to baseline FHR. Associated with contractions. Deceleration begins after contraction starts and lowest point of deceleration occurs after contraction peak. Does not return to baseline until after contraction is over. The shape is uniform. The depth of the deceleration does not necessarily indicate severity; may become progressively deeper as fetal acidemia worsens.
      a. The situation is ominous and requires immediate intervention when deceleration patterns are recurrent and associated with decreased or absent variability and tachycardia.
   2. Indicative of UPI
      a. Late decelerations indicate UPI and are associated with conditions such as post-maturity, uterine tachysystole, maternal supine hypotension, epidural or spinal anesthesia, placental previa or abruption, maternal hypertensive disorders, diabetes mellitus, cardiac disease, and IUGR (Fig. 6.16B).
      b. A decrease in uteroplacental perfusion results in late decelerations with cord compression resulting in a pattern of variable decelerations (see Fig. 6.16C).
   3. Clinical Judgment Measures
      a. Discontinue oxytocin (Pitocin) if infusing.
      b. Immediately turn client to lateral, side-lying position.
      c. Administer oxygen at 10 L by nonrebreather facemask.
      d. Correct maternal hypotension by elevating legs.
      e. Maintain IV line, IV fluids.
      f. Palpate uterus to assess for tachysystole.
      g. Determine presence of FHR variability.
      h. Notify health care provider.
      i. Consider preparation for internal fetal monitoring.
      j. Prepare to assist with birth if pattern cannot be corrected.

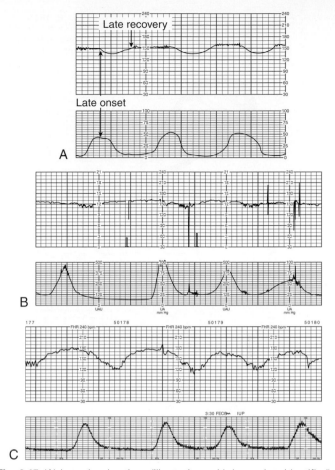

Fig. 6.15 (A) Late decelerations (illustration, with key points identified). (B and C) Late decelerations (actual tracings). (From Miller, L., & Tucker, S. M. [2013]. *Pocket guide to fetal monitoring and assessment* [7th ed.]. St. Louis, MO: Mosby.)

HESI HINT Check for labor progress if early decelerations are noted (see Fig. 6.13A). Early decelerations caused by head compression and fetal descent usually occur in the second stage of labor between 4 and 7 cm dilation.

HESI HINT If cord prolapse is detected, call for assistance immediately. The examiner should position the mother to relieve pressure on the cord (i.e., knee-chest position, extreme Trendelenburg) and using two gloved fingers (one on either side of the cord) push the presenting part off the cord to relieve compression and do not move hand. Notify obstetric provider immediately!

LABOR AND DELIVERY PREPARATION

Once determined that client is in labor, the registered nurse (RN) and practical nurse (PN) continues to regularly assess the client.

First Stage of Labor

Description: Begins from the onset of regular uterine contractions and ends with full dilation and effacement of cervix

Clinical Judgment Measures

A. Identify presence of support person.
B. Explain all activities and procedures to mother and support person.
C. Discuss birth plan.
   1. Analgesia and anesthesia are often offered and/or needed during the active phase of labor. If pharmacologic methods are used too early, they may slow the progress of labor; if used too close to delivery, narcotics increase the risk of neonatal respiratory depression. Common causes of

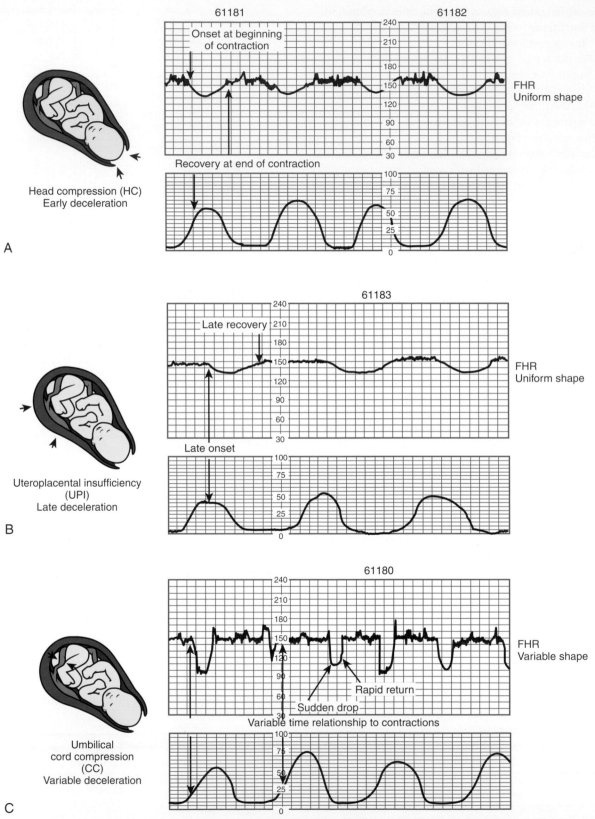

Fig. 6.16 Review of Fetal Variability. (A) Early decelerations caused by head compression. (B) Late decelerations caused by uteroplacental insufficiency. (C) Variable decelerations caused by cord compression. (From Miller, L., & Tucker, S. M. [2013]. *Pocket guide to fetal monitoring and assessment* [7th ed.]. St. Louis, MO: Mosby.)

first-stage pain: dilation, effacement, stretching of cervix, contractions, distention of lower uterine segment
2. Postpartum preferences, i.e., cutting umbilical cord, rooming in, feeding choice
3. Cultural considerations for birth and postpartum care

D. Assess maternal vital signs (BP, P, respirations).
1. Take BP *between* contractions, every 30 to 60 minutes in early labor and every 15 to 30 in active labor unless abnormal or maternal appearance changes (Lowd, 385).
2. Take temperature every 4 hours until membranes rupture, then every 2 hours (Lowd, 385).

E. Ongoing FHR assessment
1. External fetal monitoring
2. Low Risk: Assess FHR every 30 minutes in active phase and at least every 15 minutes during second stage
3. Higher Risk: Assess FHR at least every 15 minutes in active phase and at least every 5 minutes during second stage
4. Assess contractions when assessing FHR.
5. Vaginal exams as needed to identify labor progress

> **HESI HINT** Meconium-stained fluid is yellow-green or gold-yellow and may indicate fetal stress.

F. Palpate for bladder distention and encourage regular voiding at least every 2 hours during labor (a full bladder can impede labor progress).
G. Oral intake: It is becoming more common practice for clients to have clear liquids during labor, however, nurses should follow obstetric provider orders. Provide mouth care as needed for dry mouth. IV intake may be needed if client is not permitted oral intake during labor.
H. Assist woman with use of psychoprophylactic coping techniques, such as breathing exercises and effleurage (abdominal massage).
1. Breathing techniques, such as deep chest, accelerated, and cued, are not prescribed by the stage and phase of labor but by the discomfort level of the laboring woman. If coping is decreasing, switch to a new technique.
2. Hyperventilation results in respiratory alkalosis that is caused by blowing off too much carbon dioxide (CO_2). Symptoms include
   a. Dizziness
   b. Tingling of fingers
   c. Stiff mouth
3. Have woman breathe into her cupped hands or a paper bag in order to rebreathe CO_2.
I. Encourage ambulation if membranes are intact, after ROM only if fetal presenting part is engaged and if client has not received pain medication. If unable to ambulate, encourage frequent position changes while lying in bed (every 30 to 60 minutes).
J. Maintain asepsis in labor by means of frequent perineal care, changing linen and under pads.
K. Notify obstetric provider if any of the following occurs:
1. Labor progress slows or stops.

2. Maternal vital signs are abnormal, uterine activity changes (tachysystole, abrupt cessation), pain is not controlled with prescribed measures.
3. Fetal distress is noted.

Labor with Analgesia or Anesthesia
Nonpharmacologic Pain Reduction Strategies
Description: Methods are simple and inexpensive with rare to any side adverse reactions. They can be used throughout labor and include cutaneous stimulation (effleurage, counterpressure, walking, rocking, water therapy), sensory stimulation (aromatherapy, breathing techniques, music), and cognitive strategies (childbirth education and hypnosis).

Pharmacologic Pain Reduction Strategies
Description: Pharmacologic pain management options are often used with nonpharmacologic strategies and typically implemented in the active phase of labor. Anesthesia includes analgesia, amnesia, relaxation, and reflex activity. Analgesia alleviates the sensation of pain without loss of consciousness. Use of either method is determined by the stage of labor and the method of birth planned by the woman

A. Sedatives (barbiturates)
1. May be used in early or latent phases to relieve anxiety and help with sleep.
2. Should be avoided if birth anticipated within 12 to 24 hours, therefore not used often.

B. Systemic analgesia (opioid agonists, opioid agonist-antagonists)
1. Provides sedation and euphoria. Pain relief is temporary, generally more effective in early, active labor.
2. Administered intramuscular (IM), intravenous (IV) and Patient controlled analgesic (PCA).
3. Most serious side effect is respiratory depression. Others include nausea/vomiting, dizziness, altered mental status, decreased gastric motility, urinary retention.
4. Cross the placenta and can cause changes to FHR variability during labor, neonatal respiratory depression after birth.
5. Common drugs include: meperidine, fentanyl, nalbuphine.
6. Naloxone (opioid antagonist) can promptly reverse CNS depressant effects.

> **HESI HINT** Opioid agonist-antagonist and antagonist analgesics should not be used in women with opioid dependence as they could precipitate withdrawal symptoms.

Clinical Judgment Measures for Pain Reduction
A. Administration of analgesic medications in labor
1. Determine client's desires regarding analgesics. Educate about the purpose and effects of medication options.

2. Document baseline maternal vital signs and FHR before administration of analgesics/narcotics (Table 6.12).
3. Assess phase and stage of labor.
4. Obtain provider's order for medication.
5. Do *not* give PO medications. Labor retards gastrointestinal activity and absorption.
6. Administer medications IV when possible, IM if necessary.
   a. IV administration of analgesics is preferred to IM administration for a client in labor because the onset and peak occur more quickly, and the duration of the drug is shorter. Typical IV administration: Onset: 5 minutes, Peak: 30 minutes
   b. Typical IM administration: Onset: within 30 minutes, Peak: 1 to 3 hours after injection

B. After medication administration
   1. Record the woman's response and level of pain relief.
   2. Monitor maternal vital signs, FHR, and characteristics of uterine contractions every 15 minutes for 1 hour after administration.
   3. Monitor bladder for distention and retention (medication can decrease perception of bladder filling).
   4. Decrease environmental stimuli: Darken room, reduce number of visitors, turn off TV.

5. Note on delivery record the time between drug administration and birth. If delivery occurs during peak drug absorption time, notify pediatrician or neonatologist for delivery room assistance and possible use of naloxone (Narcan) for neonate.

Nerve Block Analgesia and Anesthesia

Description: Causes a temporary interruption of nerve impulses (pain relief and motor blockade) over a specific body area.

A. Local anesthesia
   1. Used for pain relief during episiotomy and perineal laceration repair
   2. Lidocaine is commonly used.
B. Regional Block Anesthesia (pudendal, epidural, spinal)
   1. Used for relief of perineal and uterine pain
   2. Types of regional blocks
      a. Pudendal block: Given in second stage (episiotomy, forceps, or vacuum assisted delivery)
         1) Has no effect on pain of uterine contractions, relieves pain in lower vagina, vulva, perineum.
      b. Epidural block: Given in first or second stage of labor. Local anesthetic alone or in combination with opioid agonist analgesic. Common medications include

TABLE 6.12 Analgesics

Drugs	Indications	Adverse Reactions	Nursing Implications
• Fentanyl Citrate	• Opioid agonist analgesic used for moderate to severe labor pain, or postoperative pain (cesarean delivery)	• Sedation • Nausea and vomiting • Respiratory distress • Fetal distress • Hypotension	• Record use accurately. • Implement safety measures • Have naloxone available as an antidote • Monitor respirations, pulse, BP closely
• Meperidine Hydrochloride	• Opioid agonist analgesic used for moderate to severe labor pain, or post-operative pain (cesarean delivery)	• Tachycardia • Sedation • Nausea and vomiting • Altered mental status • Decreased gastric motility, delayed gastric emptying • Urinary retention	• Implement safety measures • Do not give if birth is expected to occur within 1—4 h after administration (may cause neonatal respiratory depression) • Monitor respirations, pulse.
• Nalbuphine Hydrochloride	• Opioid agonist-antagonist analgesic used for moderate to severe labor pain, or post-operative pain (cesarean delivery)	• Sedation • Nausea and vomiting • Dizziness • Respiratory depression • May cause temporary absent or minimal FHR variability	• May precipitate withdrawal symptoms in opioid-dependent woman and newborn • Assess maternal vital signs, pain level, FHR, uterine activity prior to and after administration • Observe for respiratory depression • Encourage voiding, palpate for bladder distention
• Naloxone Hydrochloride	• Opioid antagonist used to reverse opioid-induced respiratory depression in mother or newborn	• Maternal hypotension or hypertension • Tachycardia • Hyperventilation • Nausea and vomiting	• Do not administer if woman is opioid dependent as may cause abrupt withdrawal • Duration of action is shorter than most opioids, monitor closely for return of opioid depression when effects of naloxone are gone, may need to readminister • Pain may return suddenly

FHR, Fetal heart rate.

bupivacaine, fentanyl. Injection between L4 and L5 relieves labor and vaginal birth pain through a block from T10 to S5. For cesarean birth, block from T8 to S1 needed.

    1) May be given in single dose or continuously through catheter threaded into epidural space

    2) Is moderately associated with hypotension, which can cause maternal and fetal distress

    3) Epidural block can be associated with prolonged second stage due to decreased effectiveness of pushing.

  c. Spinal block: given in second stage of labor. Local anesthetic alone or in combination with opioid agonist analgesic. Injection through L3, L4, or L5 lumbar interspace into subarachnoid space to relieve vaginal birth pain from T10 (hips) to feet. When used for cesarean birth, provides anesthesia from T6 (nipple) to feet.

    1) Rapid onset, but highly associated with maternal hypotension, which can cause maternal and fetal distress

    2) Client must remain flat for 6 to 8 hours after delivery.

  d. Epidural block: injection of local anesthetic agent and opioid analgesic into epidural space to relive pain from T10 to S5. Most common effective pharmacologic pain relief method in labor.

    1) Contraindications to epidural and spinal blocks

      a) Client's refusal or fear

      b) Anticoagulant therapy or presence of bleeding disorder

      c) Presence of antepartum hemorrhage causing acute hypovolemia

      d) Infection or tumor at injection site

      e) Allergy to -caine medications

      f) CNS disorders, previous back surgery, or spinal anatomic abnormality.

C. Clinical Judgment Measures for Nerve Block Analgesia and Anesthesia

  1. Ensure that the health care provider has explained the procedures, risks, benefits, and alternatives. Encourage woman to empty her bladder.

  2. Obtain maternal vital signs and a 20- to 30-minute electronic fetal monitoring strip to assess FHR and contractions prior to anesthesia. After anesthesia, maternal vital signs and FHR and pattern should be assessed and documented every 5 to 10 minutes.

  3. Fluid balance is assessed. Bolus of 500 to 1000 mL IV fluid (Lactated Ringers or normal saline) is infused 15 to 30 minutes before initiation of anesthetic. This IV fluid preload reduces the frequency of maternal hypotension after spinal anesthesia.

  4. The client sits or lies on her side with back curved to widen intervertebral space; head is flexed.

  5. A test dose of medication may be given prior to administering a bolus dose or drip in epidurals. Ask client to describe symptoms after test dose.

    a. Metallic taste in mouth and ringing in ears denote possible injection of medication into bloodstream.

    b. Nausea and vomiting are among the first signs of hypotension.

    c. The first sign of a block's effectiveness is usually warmth and tingling in the buttocks or legs, feet, or toes.

  6. Determine maternal vital signs every 5 minutes for the first half hour after administration of anesthetic drug and initiate continuous fetal monitoring. Maternal vitals should then be monitored every 10 minutes for the second half hour after administration and then every 30 minutes. Monitor for hypotension (20% decrease from preblock baseline level of ≤100 mm Hg systolic), fetal bradycardia, absent or minimal FHR variability.

  7. If hypotension occurs:

    a. Immediately turn client onto lateral position.

    b. Maintain IV infusion rate as specified or increase per hospital protocol.

    c. Begin O$_2$ at 10 to 12 L/min by nonrebreather facemask.

    d. Elevate legs.

    e. Notify obstetric and anesthesia health care provider.

    f. Have vasopressor at bedside and administer per protocol if previous measures have been ineffective.

  8. Assess maternal vital signs and FHR every 5 minutes until stable or per orders.

  9. Assist client to keep bladder empty. Catheterization may be needed.

  10. Assess level of pain relief.

  11. Report return of pain sensation, incomplete anesthesia, or uneven anesthesia to anesthesiologist.

  12. Because the woman is unable to sense contractions, assist client in the pushing technique once complete dilatation has been achieved.

D. General anesthesia is rarely used but may be needed because of a delivery complication, emergency delivery, or when regional block anesthesia is contraindicated.

E. Clinical Judgment Measures with general anesthesia

  1. Make sure client is NPO.

  2. Monitor maternal vital signs and FHR and pattern.

  3. Ensure IV is in place.

  4. Administer drugs to reduce gastric secretions (e.g., famotidine or clear [nonparticulate]), antacids to neutralize gastric acid.

  5. Place wedge under one of client's hips; helps to displace uterus.

  6. General anesthesia is associated with postpartum uterine atony. Assess closely for uterine atony; check fundal firmness and uterine contractions (Table 6.13).

TABLE 6.13 Clinical Judgment Measures: First Stage of Labor Pain Management

Clinical Judgment Measure	Assessment Characteristics
Recognize Cues	Note contraction pattern, frequency
	Note labor progress (cervical dilation, effacement, station)
	Review mother's birth plan; especially consider plan for pain management, analgesia, anesthesia
Analyze Cues	Determine mother's ability to manage pain without medication (breathing pattern, relaxation between contractions, activity with contractions, requests for pain medication)
	Identify effectiveness of support person during contractions
	Assess maternal VS
	Note fetal response to labor (heart rate decelerations, ominous fetal heart rate patterns)
Prioritize Cues	Note irregular BP, P, respirations, or temperature (dizziness, tingling of fingers, (resp. alkalosis), acute escalation of pain symptoms
	Report changes in fetal heart rate
	Report any stalling of labor progress to obstetric provider
	Report any changes in maternal pain tolerance (unable to relax between contractions, hyperventilation, verbal report of pain or request for additional pain management)
	Note any unusual vaginal bleeding, change in fetal presentation, cord prolapse
Solutions	Review birth plan; if mother and fetus are stable, and mother desires unmedicated birth, consider additional pain management options:
	Assist with position changes, walking if applicable, breathing techniques, use of tub (if applicable) to support non-medication pain management options as desired
	Assist support person with coaching during delivery
	If mother wishes to explore use of analgesia or anesthesia, discuss options
	Contact obstetric provider for orders

Second Stage of Labor

Description: Begins with full cervical dilation (10 cm) and complete effacement (100%) and ends with the birth. The length of second stage varies and is affected by parity, use of epidural anesthesia, woman's age, BMI, emotional state and adequacy of support, level of fatigue, fetal size, position, and often presentation (Fig. 6.17). Second stage is comprised of the latent phase (passive descent) and the active pushing phase.

> **HESI HINT** The Ferguson reflex is activated when presenting part presses on stretch receptor of pelvic floor and triggers a strong, involuntary urge to bear down.

Clinical Judgment Measures

A. Assess and document maternal BP, pulse, respirations every 15 minutes between contractions.
B. Check FHR with each contraction or by continuous fetal monitoring.
  1. External fetal monitoring
    a. Low Risk: Assess FHR and pattern at least every 15 minutes during second stage
    b. Higher Risk: Assess FHR and pattern at least every 5 minutes during second stage
C. Observe perineal area for increase in bloody show, signs of fetal descent (bulging perineum and anus, visibility of the presenting part)
D. Palpate bladder for distention.
E. Assess amniotic fluid for color and consistency.
F. Comfort measures: Continue mouth care, assist with position changes, help with pain relief, provide breathing instruction and support and positive reinforcement of pushing efforts.
G. Teach mother positions for pushing such as squatting, side-lying, or high-Fowler/lithotomy and encourage open-glottis pushing (bearing down while exhaling) followed by a cleansing breath after each contraction.
H. Set up delivery table, including bulb syringe, cord clamp, and sterile supplies.
I. Perform perineal cleansing if directed.
J. Make sure client and support person can visualize delivery if they desire. A mirror can be offered. If siblings are present, make sure they are closely attended to by support person explaining that their mom is all right.
K. Record *exact* delivery time (complete delivery of baby).

Third Stage of Labor

Description: From birth of the fetus to complete expulsion of the placenta. Typically the shortest stage of labor with an average length of 5 to 15 minutes.

Clinical Judgment Measures

> **HESI HINT** Oxytocin (Pitocin) is typically administered after the placenta is delivered because the drug will cause the uterus to contract. If the oxytocic drug is administered before the placenta is delivered, it may result in a retained placenta, which predisposes the client to hemorrhage and infection.

1. Assess maternal BP, pulse, and respirations every 15 minutes.
2. Assess for signs of placental separation: lengthening of umbilical cord outside vagina, gush of blood, change in uterus shape from oval (discoid) to globular, vaginal fullness on exam. Assist mother to bear down to facilitate expulsion of placenta when directed to do so.
3. After placenta is expelled, uterine fundus is massaged and oxytocic medication is administered as ordered.
4. Administer analgesics as ordered.

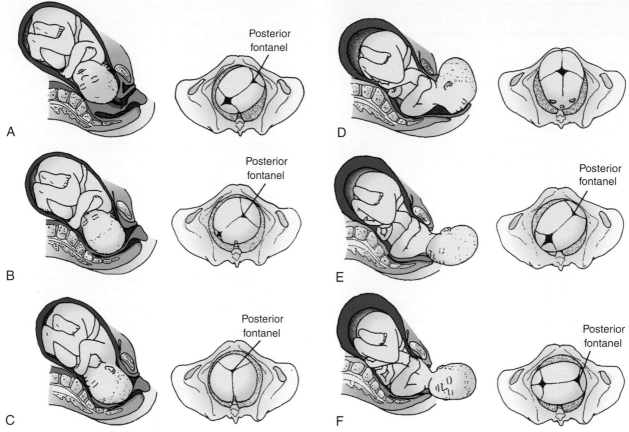

Fig. 6.17 Cardinal Movements of the Mechanism of Labor Left Occipitoanterior (LOA) Position. Pelvic figures show the position of the fetal head as seen by the birth attendant. (A) Engagement and descent. (B) Flexion. (C) Internal rotation to occipitoanterior position (OA). (D) Extension. (E) External rotation beginning (restitution). (F) External rotation. (From Lowdermilk, D. L., Perry, S. E., Cashion, M., & Alden, K. [2012]. *Maternity and women's health care* [10th ed.]. St. Louis, MO: Mosby.)

5. Observe for blood loss and ask obstetric provider for estimate of blood loss (EBL).
6. Dry and suction infant, perform Apgar assessment at 1 and 5 minutes after birth.
7. Encourage skin-to-skin contact with mother after delivery if possible. Facilitate attachment with mother and support person by encouraging touching of newborn and breastfeeding if desired.
8. Gently cleanse perineal area with warm water; apply a perineal pad or ice pack to perineum (Table 6.14).

Fourth Stage of Labor

Description: Begins after delivery of the placenta and includes at least the first 2 hours after delivery of placenta until the woman is stable.

Clinical Judgment Measures

A. Review antepartum and L&D records for possible complications.
   1. PPH
   2. Uterine hyperstimulation
   3. Uterine overdistention

   4. Dystocia
   5. Antepartum hemorrhage
   6. Magnesium sulfate therapy
   7. Bladder distention

B. Routine postpartum physical assessment
   1. Assess maternal BP, pulse, and respirations every 15 minutes for the first 2 hours. Temperature is assessed at the beginning of recovery and then every 4 hours for the first 8 hours after birth.
   2. Assess fundal firmness and height, bladder, lochia, and perineum every 15 minutes for one hour, then as ordered.
      a. Fundus: Firm, midline, at or below the umbilicus. Massage if soft or boggy to contract uterus and expel any clots prior to measuring. Suspect full bladder if above umbilicus and to the right side of abdomen. If the nurse finds the fundus soft, boggy, and displaced above and to the right of the umbilicus, the nurse should perform fundal massage, then have the client empty her bladder. Encourage frequent voiding (Fig. 6.18).
      b. Lochia: Rubra (red), moderate, and clots less than 2 to 3 cm. Amount similar to a heavy menstrual period.

TABLE 6.14 Clinical Judgment Measures: Third Stage of Labor (Placental Expulsion)

Clinical Judgment Measure	Assessment Characteristics
Recognize Cues (after delivery of the fetus	Vaginal bleeding Abdominal cramping Umbilical cord length Consistency of uterus
Analyze Cues	Determine where cramping is located and verify constitution of pain (cramping is typically the return of moderate to strong uterine contractions to facilitate placental expulsion) Determine the amount of vaginal bleeding present (trickle, gushing) Verify any lengthening of the umbilical cord (the portion of umbilical cord noted outside of the vagina) Verify consistency of uterus, i.e., firm and contracting or boggy
Prioritize Cues	Determine risk factors for retained placenta Determine if it has been longer than 15 min since delivery of the fetus Verify normalcy of third-stage bleeding pattern; significant estimated blood loss, concern for immediate postpartum hemorrhage Verify apparent lengthening of umbilical cord as placenta descends to introitus Assess for any change in vital signs
Solutions	Teach clients about expectations for delivery of the placenta Be prepared for potential complications of retained placenta, immediate postpartum hemorrhage Assess vital signs every 15 min to observe for maternal stability Assess for early signs of placental separation Assist mother to push to facilitate expulsion of the placenta when appropriate
Actions	Monitor blood loss Provide uterine fundal massage as soon as the placenta is expelled Administer oxytocic medication as ordered to assist with uterine contraction and prevent hemorrhage Keep mother and partner informed of progress of third stage and answer any questions After placental expulsion, obtain blood sample from umbilical cord as ordered (used to determine baby's blood type, Rh status)

HESI HINT A first-degree perineal laceration extends through skin and structures superficial to muscles. A second-degree laceration extends through muscles of perineal body. A third-degree laceration continues through external anal sphincter muscle. A fourth-degree laceration extends completely through anal sphincter and rectal mucosa. Tears cause pain and swelling and may impact voiding or bowel movements. Avoid rectal manipulations.

C. Monitor infusion of IV oxytocin (Pitocin) as ordered.
D. Administer analgesics as prescribed.
E. Report any abnormal vital signs, uterus not becoming firm with massage, second perineal pad soaked in 15 minutes, signs of hypovolemic shock: pale, clammy, tachycardic, lightheaded, hypotensive.
F. Support parental emotional needs and promote bonding with infant.
   1. Allow extended family time post-birth so family can hold and examine the newborn if status of mother and newborn allows. Encourage skin-to-skin contact.
   2. Encourage initiation of breastfeeding within 1 to 2 hours of birth if desired. In some cultures mothers may choose to delay initiation of breastfeeding.
   3. Provide a warm, darkened environment.
   4. Perform newborn admission and routine procedures in room with parents when possible (Table 6.15).

LABOR AND BIRTH COMPLICATIONS

Preterm Labor

Description: Regular contractions accompanied by a change in cervical status that occurs between 20 and 36 6/7 weeks' gestation. Predisposing factors include medical conditions (diabetes, cardiac disease, preeclampsia, and placenta previa), infections (UTI, STIs), overdistention of uterus (multifetal gestation, hydramnios), substance abuse, high levels of personal stress.
A. Symptoms
   1. Frequent contractions with cervical changes occurring
   2. Menstrual-like cramps; low, dull backache; and pelvic pressure
   3. Urinary frequency
   4. Increase or change in vaginal discharge
   5. ROM
B. Labs
   1. Fetal fibronectin test obtained from a cervical swab indicates the client is at higher risk for preterm labor.
   2. CBC, urinalysis, and cervical cultures may be ordered
C. Diagnostics
   1. US may be ordered to check cervical length or as part of a BPP/NST to check on fetal well-being.
D. Clinical Judgment Measures
   1. Teach symptoms of preterm labor early in prenatal care.
   2. Educate on self-management of symptoms and when to notify obstetric provider.

Suspect undetected laceration if fundus is firm and bright-red blood continues to trickle. Always check perineal pad *and* under buttocks.
   c. Perineum: Observe in good lighting. Should be intact or assess lacerations/episiotomy for redness, edema, ecchymosis, drainage, and approximation (REEDA). Suspect hematomas if very tender or discolored or if pain is disproportionate to vaginal delivery.

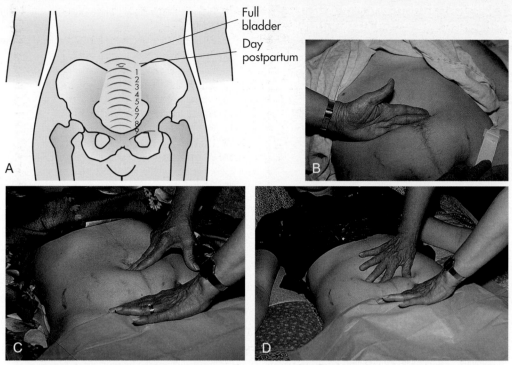

Fig. 6.18 Assessment of Involution of Uterus After Birth. (A) Normal progress, days 1 to 9. (B) Size and position of uterus 2 hours after birth. (C) Two days after birth. (D) Four days after birth. Note linea nigra and striae gravidarum ("stretch marks") in B–D. ([B–D] Courtesy Marjorie Pyle, RNC, Lifecircle, Costa Mesa, CA.) (From Lowdermilk, D. L., Perry, S. E., Cashion, K., Alden, K., & Olshansky, E. [2020]. *Maternity and women's health care* [12th ed., 10]. St. Louis, MO: Elsevier.)

3. Select women may be managed at home with activity restriction, pelvic rest (avoidance of sexual activity), oral medications, adequate hydration.
   a. Teach about side effects and warning signs of medications.
4. Many women will be admitted for observation, bed rest, and management with tocolytics (i.e., indomethacin, nifedipine, magnesium sulfate, terbutaline) to arrest labor after uterine contractions and cervical change has occurred.
   a. Follow protocols for continuous uterine and FHR monitoring, assessment of maternal vital signs.
5. Glucocorticoids (betamethasone) may be administered to women between 24 and 34 weeks' gestation to accelerate fetal lung maturity (stimulates fetal surfactant production). Typically two IM injections are given to the mother, 24 hours a part.
6. If labor continues to progress despite interventions, the obstetric provider should be notified immediately, and the nurse should prepare for emergent delivery of a preterm infant. Personnel who are skilled at neonatal resuscitation should be present at the birth (Table 6.16).

Dystocia

Description: A lack of progress in labor for any reason. May result from any one or all of the 5 P's: **P**owers (primary uterine contractions and secondary abdominal bearing-down efforts), **P**assage (maternal pelvis, uterus, cervix, vagina, perineum), **P**assenger (fetus and placenta), **P**syche (response to labor by woman), and **P**osition (position of the laboring woman).

A. Symptoms

Dystocia is suspected when there is a
1. Lack of progress in cervical dilatation
2. Lack of fetal descent, or
3. Uterine contractions become ineffective (hypertonic, hypotonic).
4. Abnormal labor patterns

B. Clinical Judgment Measures
1. Continuous uterine and fetal monitoring; notify obstetric provider if abnormal labor patterns occur.
   a. Assist with placement of intrauterine pressure catheter, fetal scalp electrode.
2. Assist with diagnostic procedures (ultrasound, pelvimetry, vaginal examination) to rule out CPD.
3. Assist with amniotomy. Artificial rupture of membranes (AROM) may enhance labor forces.
   a. Explain procedure.
   b. Assess FHR.
   c. Assess fluid for color, odor, and consistency (blood, meconium, or vernix particles).
4. Administer oxytocin infusion for induction (initiation) or augmentation (stimulation) of labor as ordered (Box 6.3).

TABLE 6.15 Clinical Judgment Measures: Fourth Stage of Labor (Parental Attachment After Vaginal Birth)

Clinical Judgment Measure	Assessment Characteristics
Recognize Cues	Mother and support person are holding infant, making eye contact
	Mother is examining infant and verbalizing physical likeness to parents, counting fingers, toes, and commenting on hair, calling newborn by name
	Monitor attempts to feed infant, note mother's choice of feeding method
Analyze Cues	Recognize any circumstances that prohibit mother-infant contact, i.e., unstable infant needing neonatal intensive care unit admission, mother is experiencing acute postpartum hemorrhage, VS are unstable
	If mother and infant are stable, note any skin-to-skin contact
	Note any verbal expression of exhaustion by mother, physical inability to hold infant
	Note engagement of support partner, other parent
	Note ability to comfort a crying infant
	Note any cultural considerations (some cultural practices may not be congruent with standard practices associated with the Anglo-American culture)
Prioritize Cues	Determine need to manage unstable maternal VS, control unusual vaginal bleeding, address maternal pain
	Determine if newborn is in need of additional interventions (suctioning, swaddling)
	Note any physical concerns that would prohibit early attachment (IVs in place, blood pressure cuff)
	Determine need to model early attachment behaviors (holding, eye contact, talking to infant)
Solutions	Assess mother and parents' comfort level in caring for a newborn (is this the first child for the family?)
	Encourage skin-to-skin contact and assist with establishing this contact
	Teach clients about early newborn behavior
	Demonstrate newborn cares (diapering, umbilical cord care, bathing)
	Discuss and demonstrate newborn comfort techniques (swaddling, talking, rocking)
	Assist with feeding (positioning, burping, latch if breastfeeding) and discuss normal newborn feeding behaviors
	Discuss rooming-in options

❓ REVIEW OF INTRAPARTUM NURSING CARE

1. List five prodromal signs of labor the nurse might teach the client.
2. How is true labor discriminated from false labor?
3. State two ways to determine whether the membranes have truly ruptured.
4. Hyperventilation often occurs in the laboring client. What results from hyperventilation, and what actions should the nurse take to relieve the condition?
5. Describe the maternal changes that characterize the transition phase of labor.
6. When should a laboring client be examined vaginally?
7. Define cervical effacement.
8. Where is the fetal heart rate (FHR) best heard?
9. Normal FHR during labor is _____.
10. Normal maternal BP during labor is _____.
11. Normal maternal pulse during labor is _____.
12. Normal maternal temperature during labor is _____.
13. List three signs of placental separation.
14. When should the postpartum dosage of oxytocin be administered? Why is it administered?
15. What is the danger associated with regional blocks?
16. Why are PO medications avoided in labor?
17. When is it dangerous to administer an agonist/antagonist narcotic to a woman in labor?
18. Hypotension commonly occurs after the laboring client receives a regional block. What is one of the first signs the nurse might observe?
19. State three actions the nurse should take when hypotension occurs in a laboring client.
20. How is the fourth stage of labor defined?
21. What actions can the nurse take to assist in preventing postpartum hemorrhage?
22. What nursing interventions are used to enhance maternal–infant bonding during the fourth stage of labor?
23. List the symptoms of a full bladder that might occur in the fourth stage of labor.
24. What action should the nurse take first when a soft, boggy uterus is palpated?
25. What are the symptoms of hypovolemic shock?
26. How often should the nurse check the fundus during the fourth stage of labor?

See Answer Key at the end of this text for suggested responses.

Normal Puerperium (Postpartum)

Description: The interval between birth and return of reproductive organs to normal nonpregnant state. It is sometimes called the fourth trimester. This has traditionally been considered to last 6 weeks, however physiological and emotional recovery varies for every woman and the entire first year after delivery is considered to be the postpartum period.
A. Care during this period is focused on recovery and wellness.
B. Teaching must be initiated early to cover the physical self-care needs and the emotional needs of the mother, infant, and family.

Normal Puerperium Physiologic Changes
A. Maternal Adaptations
   1. Vital Signs
      a. Temperature: slight risk in first 24 hours, then afebrile
      b. Pulse: Slightly elevated in first 24 hours, then decreases over 48 hours; puerperal bradycardia (40 to 50 beats/min) can temporarily occur.
      c. Respirations: should be within normal
      d. Blood pressure: transient increase over first few days after birth but should return to normal within a few

days. Orthostatic hypotension can develop in first 48 hours

1) Increases greater than 140/90, measured on 2 occasions at least 4 hours apart, can indicate gestational HTN or preeclampsia.

2) About half of women may experience "shivering" during first hour after birth; exact cause unknown.

2. Uterus

a. Uterine contractions occur for several days after delivery. During the first 2 hours postdelivery they

---

TABLE 6.16 Tocolytic Therapy for Preterm Labor

Medication and Action	Dosage and Route	Adverse Effects	Nursing Considerations
Magnesium Sulfate			
CNS depressant; relaxes smooth muscle, including uterus	IV fluid should contain 40 g in 1000 mL, piggyback to primary infusion, and administer using controller pump: Loading dose: 4–6 g over 20–30 min Maintenance dose: 1–4 g/h Use for stabilization only Discontinue within 24–48 h at the maintenance dose or if intolerable adverse effects occur	**Maternal:** • Hot flushes, sweating, burning at the IV insertion site, nausea and vomiting, dry mouth, drowsiness, blurred vision, diplopia, headache, ileus, generalized muscle weakness, lethargy, dizziness • Hypocalcemia • Dyspnea • Transient hypotension • Some reactions may subside when loading dose is completed **Intolerable:** • Respiratory rate fewer than 12 breaths/min • Pulmonary edema • Absent DTRs • Chest pain • Severe hypotension • Altered level of consciousness • Extreme muscle weakness • Urine output <25–30 mL/h or <100 mL/4 h • Serum magnesium level of 10 mEq/L (9 mg/dL) or greater **Fetal (uncommon):** • Decreased breathing movement • Reduced FHR variability • Nonreactive NST	Assess woman and fetus to obtain baseline before beginning therapy and then before and after each incremental change; follow frequency of agency protocol. Drug is almost always given IV but can also be administered IM. Monitor serum magnesium levels with higher doses; therapeutic range is 4–7.5 mEq/L or 5–8 mg/dL. Discontinue infusion and notify health care provider if intolerable adverse effects occur. Ensure that calcium gluconate is available for emergency administration to reverse magnesium sulfate toxicity. Do not give to women with myasthenia gravis. Total IV intake should be limited to 125 mL/h.
β-Adrenergic Agonist (β-Mimetic)			
Terbutaline (Brethine) relaxes smooth muscle, inhibiting uterine activity and causing bronchodilation	Subcutaneous injection of 0.25 mg every 4 h Treatment should last no longer than 24 h Discontinue use if intolerable adverse effects occur	**Maternal (most are mild and of limited duration):** • Tachycardia, chest discomfort, palpitations, arrhythmias • Tremors, dizziness, nervousness • Headache • Nasal congestion • Nausea and vomiting • Hypokalemia • Hyperglycemia • Hypotension **Intolerable:** • Tachycardia >130 beats/min • BP <90/60 • Chest pain • Cardiac arrhythmias • Myocardial infarction • Pulmonary edema	Should not be used in women with known or suspected heart disease, pregestational or gestational diabetes, preeclampsia with severe features or eclampsia, hyperthyroidism, or with significant hemorrhage or possible chorioamnionitis. Myocardial infarction leading to death has been reported after use.

Continued

TABLE 6.16 Tocolytic Therapy for Preterm Labor—cont'd

Medication and Action	Dosage and Route	Adverse Effects	Nursing Considerations
β-Adrenergic Agonist (β-Mimetic)—cont'd		**Fetal:** • Tachycardia • Hyperinsulinemia • Hyperglycemia	Assess woman and fetus according to agency protocol, being alert for adverse effects. Assess maternal glucose and potassium levels before treatment is initiated and periodically during treatment. Significant hyperglycemia (>180 mg/dL) and hypokalemia (<2.5 mEq/L) may occur. Notify health care provider if the following are noted: Maternal heart rate >130 beats/min; arrhythmias, chest pain BP <90/60 mm Hg Signs of pulmonary edema (e.g., dyspnea, crackles, decreased SaO₂). Fetal heart rate >180 beats/min. Hyperglycemia occurs more frequently in women who are being treated simultaneously with corticosteroids. Ensure that propranolol (Inderal) is available to reverse adverse effects related to cardiovascular function.
Prostaglandin Synthetase Inhibitors (NSAIDs)			
Indomethacin (Indocin) relaxes uterine smooth muscle by inhibiting prostaglandins	Loading dose: 50 mg orally, then 25–50 mg orally every 6 h for 48 h	**Maternal (common):** • Nausea and vomiting • Heartburn (Less common but more serious): b. GI bleeding c. Prolonged bleeding time d. Thrombocytopenia e. Asthma in aspirin-sensitive clients **Fetal:** b. Constriction of ductus arteriosus c. Oligohydramnios, caused by reduced fetal urine production d. Neonatal pulmonary hypertension	b. The long-acting formulations decrease the incidence of adverse effects. c. Used only if gestational age is <32 weeks. d. Administer for 48 h or less. e. Do not use in women with renal or hepatic disease, active peptic ulcer disease, poorly controlled hypertension, asthma, or coagulation disorders. f. Can mask maternal fever. g. Assess woman and fetus according to agency policy, being alert for adverse effects. h. Determine amniotic fluid volume and function of fetal ductus arteriosus before initiating therapy and within 48 h of discontinuing therapy; assessment is critical if therapy continues for more than 48 h. i. Administer with food to decrease GI distress. j. Monitor for signs of postpartum hemorrhage.
Calcium Channel Blockers			
Nifedipine (Adalat, Procardia) relaxes smooth muscle including the uterus by blocking calcium entry	Initial dose: 10–20 mg, orally, every 3–6 h until contractions are rare, followed by long-acting formulations of 30 or 60 mg every 8–12 h for 48 h while corticosteroids are being given (however, the ideal dose has not been established)	**Maternal (most effects are mild):** • Hypotension • Headache • Flushing • Dizziness • Nausea **Fetal:** • Hypotension (questionable)	Avoid concurrent use with magnesium sulfate because skeletal muscle blockade can result. Should not be given simultaneously with or immediately after terbutaline because of effects on heart rate and blood pressure. Assess woman and fetus according to agency protocol, being alert for adverse effects. Do not use sublingual route of administration.

NOTE: There are variations in recommended administration protocols; always consult agency protocol, which should be evidence based.
BP, Blood pressure; *CNS,* central nervous system; *DTRs,* deep tendon reflexes; *FHR,* fetal heart rate; *GI,* gastrointestinal; *IM,* intramuscular; *IV,* intravenous; *NSAIDs,* nonsteroidal antiinflammatory drugs; *NST,* nonstress test; *SaO₂,* arterial oxygen saturation; *SOB,* shortness of breath.
Adapted from Lowdermilk, D. L., Perry, S. E., Cashion, K., Alden, K., & Olshansky, E. (2020). *Maternity and women's health care* (12th ed.). St. Louis, MO: Elsevier.

BOX 6.3 Medication Guide: Oxytocin

Medication	Action	Adverse Reactions	Nursing Implications
Oxytocin (Pitocin)	Used for labor induction and augmentation, also used to control postpartum bleeding	Uterine tachysystole Placental abruption Uterine rupture Water intoxication, severe hyponatremia Abnormal fetal heart rate pattern, fetal hypoxia Unplanned cesarean birth secondary to adverse effects	This is a high-alert medication Assess maternal and fetal vital signs prior to administration and frequently during administration A primary IV infusion line is started first and oxytocin is administered through a secondary line Assess I&O Monitor contraction pattern and uterine tone frequently and per institutional protocol Discontinue oxytocin if uterine tachysystole occurs

Adapted from Lowdermilk, D. L., Perry, S. E., Cashion, K., Alden, K., & Olshansky, E. (2020). *Maternity and women's health care* (12th ed., 10). St. Louis, MO: Elsevier. (Medication Guide: Oxytocin, p 703.) Data from American College of Obstetricians and Gynecologists. (2009, reaffirmed 2019). Practice bulletin no. 107: Induction of labor. *Obstetrics & Gynecology, 114*(2, pt 1), 386–397; Clark, S., Simpson, K., Knox, G., & Garite, T. J. (2009). Oxytocin: New perspectives on an old drug. *American Journal of Obstetrics and Gynecology, 200*(1), 35.e1–35.e6; Hill, W., & Harvey, C. (2013). Induction of labor. In N. Troiano, C. Harvey, & B. Chez (Eds.), *AWHONN's high risk and critical care obstetrics* (3rd ed.). Philadelphia: Wolters Kluwer/Lippincott Williams & Wilkins; Mahlmeister, L. (2008). Best practices in perinatal care: Evidence-based management of oxytocin induction and augmentation of labor. *Journal of Perinatal and Neonatal Nursing, 22*(4), 259–263; Simpson, K. R., & O'Brien-Abel, N. (2014). Labor and birth. In K. R. Simpson & P. Creehan (Eds.), *AWHONN's perinatal nursing* (4th ed.). Philadelphia: Lippincott; and Simpson, K., & Knox, G. (2009). Oxytocin as a high-alert medication: Implications for perinatal patient safety. *American Journal of Maternal/Child Nursing, 34*(1), 8–15.

may decrease in intensity and become uncoordinated. Therefore, exogenous oxytocin is usually administered IV or IM immediately after delivery of the placenta to help the uterus remain firm and well contracted. Endogenous oxytocin also helps strengthen and coordinate uterine contractions. Breastfeeding increases the release of endogenous oxytocin. Primiparous women may perceive only minimal contractions but afterpains are more common in subsequent pregnancies and may be experienced for 3 to 7 days after birth.

  b. Involution (return of uterus to nonpregnant state). Occurs (1 to 2 cm/day).

    1) End of third stage: Uterus is midline, about 2 cm below level of umbilicus

    2) Within 12 hours, fundus can rise to about 1 cm above umbilicus.

    3) Over the next few days, the fundus descends 1 to 2 cm every 24 hours.

    4) By 2 weeks postpartum, the uterus should not be palpable abdominally.

  c. Uterine placenta site contracts and heals without scarring secondary to endometrial growth and sloughing of necrotic tissue. Endometrial regeneration begins within 3 days after birth and regeneration of placental site is complete by week 6.

  d. Lochia (post-birth uterine discharge, vaginal bleeding)

    1) Lochia rubra: Blood-tinged discharge, including shreds of tissue and decidua; lochia rubra lasts 1 to 3 days postpartum.

    2) Lochia serosa: Pale pinkish to brownish discharge lasting up to 10 days postpartum

    3) Lochia alba: Thicker, whitish-yellowish discharge with leukocytes and degenerated cells; lochia alba can last up to 6 weeks postpartum

3. Cervix

  a. Bruised and edematous immediately after birth. By 3 days postpartum, shortens, becomes firm and regains form. The cervical os closes gradually and is about 1 cm dilated by 1 week post birth. External os never regains prepregnancy appearance and appears as a transverse slit. Typically healed within 6 weeks

4. Vagina

  a. Rugae (folds) reappear within 3 weeks but are more flattened. Walls are atrophic and can have localized dryness until ovarian function and menstruation resumes. Mucosa may remain atrophic during lactation and vaginal dryness is common in breastfeeding mothers.

  b. Introitus is edematous and erythematous after birth. Episiotomy and laceration repairs may be present. Initial healing of repairs occurs within 2 to 3 weeks but full healing may take 4 to 6 months.

5. Breasts

  Both breastfeeding and non-breastfeeding women should be educated about symptoms of engorgement (breasts are distended, firm, tender to touch secondary to milk production, temporary venous congestions, lymphatic circulation for 24 to 48 hours) and encouraged to observe for erythema, cracked nipples, indications of mastitis (infection in milk duct with accompanying fever, erythema, flu-like symptoms).

  a. Non-breastfeeding

    1) Nodules may be palpable, bilateral, and diffuse.

    2) Colostrum is present. Engorgement may occur 3 to 5 days postpartum but will spontaneously

resolve without milk expression. Lactation will typically cease within about 1 week. Ice bags and supportive bra may help with discomfort.
   b. Breastfeeding
      1) Milk sinuses (lumps) are palpable.
      2) Colostrum (yellowish fluid) is present. Thick yellow fluid. Breasts gradually become fuller, tender, may feel warm. Colostrum color transitions to whiter appearance eventually becoming mature milk that is bluish-white.
      3) Encourage frequent breastfeeding to help establish milk supply.
6. Cardiovascular system
   a. At delivery maternal blood volume can decrease secondary to blood loss during delivery. Average blood loss for vaginal birth: 300 to 500 mL (10% blood volume). Average blood loss for cesarean birth: 500 to 1000 mL (15% to 30% blood volume)
   b. Over the first 72 hours, cardiac output increases slightly over first hours after birth by 60% to 80% over pre-labor values; returns to prepregnant levels in 2 to 3 weeks.
7. Hematologic system
   a. Hct level drops moderately for 3 to 4 days after birth, then increases to nonpregnant levels by 8 weeks postpartum.
   b. WBC count is elevated (up to 30,000 mm^3).
   c. Blood-clotting factors remain elevated immediately postpartum; increases risk for thromboembolism.
8. Urinary system
   a. Diuresis of tissue fluid accumulated during pregnancy occurs within 12 hours after birth; woman excretes up to 3000 mL/day of urine during first 2 to 3 days after birth. Diaphoresis also frequently occurs and can be especially heavy at night.
   b. Bladder distention and incomplete emptying are common and may occur due to birth trauma, increased bladder capacity after birth, effects of anesthesia. With adequate emptying, tone is generally restored within 1 week.
   c. Dilation of ureter and renal pelvis return to nonpregnant state in 6 to 8 weeks; persistent dilation of urinary tract for 3 months or longer can increase risk for UTI.
9. Gastrointestinal system
   a. Excess analgesia and anesthesia may decrease peristalsis. Mothers often feel very hungry after full recovery from analgesia, anesthesia.
   b. Bowel movements can be delayed for 2 to 3 days.
10. Integumentary system
   a. Melasma (Chloasma or "mask of pregnancy") and hyperpigmentation areas (linea nigra, areolae) regress; some areas may remain permanently darker in about 30% of women.
   b. Striae gravidarum (stretch marks) may fade but usually do not fully disappear.
   c. Palmar erythema declines quickly.

   d. Spider nevi fade; some in legs may remain.
   e. Hair loss may occur over first 3 months postpartum.
11. Musculoskeletal system
   a. Pelvic muscles regain tone in 3 to 6 weeks.
   b. Abdominal muscles regain tone in 6 weeks. Persistence of diastasis recti (separation of rectus abdominis muscles) can occur but becomes less apparent over time.
   c. Relaxation and subsequent hypermobility of joints as well as change in maternal center of gravity that occurred during pregnancy generally resolve in a few weeks to months after birth.
12. Neurologic system
   a. Postpartum headaches can be common but must be evaluated for postpartum onset of preeclampsia, stress, leaking of cerebrospinal fluid into extradural space with epidural or spinal anesthesia.
13. Psychosocial system
   a. A variety of emotions secondary to hormonal changes, fatigue, and transition to parenthood are common.
   b. Postpartum blues can occur in the first 10 to 14 days postpartum and include symptoms of decreased appetite, sleep interference, emotional lability.

HESI HINT Client and family teaching is a common subject of NCLEX-RN questions. Remember that, when teaching, the first step is to assess the clients' (parents') level of knowledge and to identify their readiness to learn. Client teaching regarding lochia changes, perineal care, breastfeeding, and sore nipples are subjects that are commonly tested.

B. Clinical Judgment Measures
1. Review prenatal, antepartum, L&D, and early postpartum records for status, laboratory data, and possible complications.
2. Review newborn's record for Apgar scores, sex, possible complications, and relevant psychosocial information (adoption, single parent, etc.).
3. Assess maternal postpartum status
   a. Vital signs. Monitor blood pressure and pulse every 15 minutes for the first 2 hours after birth. Assess temperature every 4 hours for the first 8 hours after birth and then at least every 8 hours.
   b. Fundal height. Check fundal height and firmness. Massage the fundus if it is soft or boggy by stabilizing the bottom of the uterus before applying pressure. Teach about the normalcy of afterpains.
   c. Lochia. Frequently assess and document lochia saturation on perineal pad; check under buttocks.
      1) Scant: (<2.5 cm)
      2) Light: (<10 cm)
      3) Moderate: (>10cm)
      4) Heavy: Saturated pad within 2 hours

5) A perineal pad saturated in 15 minutes or less and pooling under buttocks requires immediate intervention; notify obstetric provider

6) Clots

7) Odor: Fleshy, not foul

d. Perineum. Assess perineum and episiotomy site.

1) Place woman in lateral position, wear gloves, and use flashlight to increase accuracy of visualization.

2) Check for redness, edema, intactness, and presence of hematomas; teach self-inspection with mirror.

3) Teach hygiene and comfort and healing measures.

 a) Instruct to change pad as needed and with every voiding and defecation.

 b) Instruct to wipe perineum front to back.

 c) Instruct to use good handwashing technique.

 d) Teach about use of ice packs, sitz baths, using a squeeze bottle for perineal lavage, and topical application of anesthetic spray and pads.

e. Breasts.

1) Assess nipples for cracks, fissures, redness, and tenderness.

2) Palpate breasts for lumps and nodules.

3) Determine mother's desired feeding method: breastfeeding or bottle feeding.

 a) For breastfeeding mothers

  (1) Assess breasts for engorgement.

  (2) Teach mothers how to prevent engorgement.

  (3) Assist mother and infant with breastfeeding.

 b) If not breastfeeding, teach woman nonpharmacologic measures of milk suppression: supportive bra or soft binder, ice packs, and avoiding breast stimulation.

4) Teach breast self-examination.

f. Bladder and urine output.

1) Palpate for spongy, full feeling over symphysis.

2) Check urge to void when bladder is palpated.

3) Assist client to ambulate for first void (orthostatic hypotension may occur); measure if possible.

 a) Client should void within 4 hours of delivery.

 b) Monitor client closely for urine retention. Suspect retention if voiding is frequent and less than 100 mL per voiding.

 c) Run warm water over perineum or place spirit of peppermint in bedpan to relax urethra if necessary.

 d) Catheterize only if necessary.

 e) Teach symptoms of UTI: dysuria, frequency, and urgency.

 f) Bowel and anal area:

  (1) Inspect for hemorrhoids; describe size, and number.

  (2) Auscultate bowel sounds; check abdominal distention.

  (3) Document flatus and bowel movement.

  (4) Encourage early ambulation.

  (5) Encourage increased fluids and use of roughage and bulk in diet.

  (6) Administer stool softeners as prescribed. Rectal suppositories and enemas should not be administered to women with 3rd- or 4th-degree perineal lacerations and repairs as they can cause hemorrhage or damage to sutures and predispose women to infection.

4. Assess maternal–infant bonding and identify teaching needs of mother and family.

a. Assess mother–infant bonding behaviors:

1) Eye contact between mother and neonate

2) Exploration of infant from head to toe

3) Stroking, kissing, and fondling the neonate

4) Smiling, talking, singing to the neonate

5) Absence of negative statements, such as, "She just doesn't like me."

b. Promote bonding opportunities

1) Ensure mother is comfortable; provide pain relief, hygiene, adequate rest.

2) If possible, have baby room-in; include family in teaching; praise and reinforce positive parenting behaviors.

3) Teach about neonatal behavioral traits.

4) Teach responses to cues from the baby.

5. Maintain safety.

a. Women may feel lightheaded or have a syncopal (fainting) episode on the first ambulation after delivery (usually related to vasomotor changes, orthostatic hypotension).

6. Prevent venous thromboembolism (VTE).

a. Encourage early ambulation.

b. Encourage flexion and extension of feet and legs. Rotate ankles in circular motion.

c. Examine legs of postpartum client frequently for pain, warmth, and tenderness or a swollen vein that is tender to the touch.

7. Prevent Rh isoimmunization

a. Determine the need for Rh immune globulin within 72 hours after birth for Rh-negative clients who have newborns who are Rh-positive (RhoGAM).

b. Determine the need for vaccinations

1) Rubella vaccination for women who are serologically nonimmune, Rubella titer of ≤1.10 or enzyme immunoassay (EIA) of ≤0.10. Vaccine should be administered prior to discharge. Caution to avoid pregnancy for at least 28 days after receiving vaccination.

2) Varicella vaccination for postpartum women who have no immunity. Should be administered prior to discharge. A second dose will be given at 4 to 8 weeks postpartum. Caution to avoid pregnancy for at least 28 days after receiving each varicella vaccination.

3) Tetanus-diphtheria-acellular pertussis vaccination (Tdap) is recommended for clients who have not previously had this vaccine or did not receive this vaccine

during pregnancy (ideally between 27 and 36 weeks of pregnancy). Breastfeeding is not contraindicated. Advise that other adults and children who will be around the newborn should be vaccinated with Tdap if they have previously not received the vaccine.

8. Assess maternal psychological adaptation.
   a. Review effects of birth experience.
   b. Assess for signs of potential psychosocial concerns (see Box 6.4).
   c. Consider family structure, cultural beliefs, and practices.
   d. Encourage verbalization of feelings; offer support in nonjudgmental manner.

> **HESI HINT** Informed consent should be obtained for vaccinations in the postpartum period and include information about possible side effects. Women should understand that they should not become pregnant for 28 days after rubella and varicella vaccinations.

C. Discharge teaching

1. Instruct client to notify obstetric provider promptly of
   a. Heavy vaginal bleeding with clots
   b. Temperature of 38°C or higher lasting 24 hours or longer
   c. A red, warm lump in breast
   d. Pain on urination
   e. Tenderness in calf
   f. Symptoms of preeclampsia
2. Teach self-care.
   a. Instruct to continue perineal care and regular pad changes.
   b. Encourage balanced diet and fluid intake.
   c. Encourage client to rest or nap when newborn does.

> **BOX 6.4 Signs of Potential Complications: Postpartum Psychosocial Concerns**
>
> The following signs suggest potentially serious complications and should be reported to the health care provider or clinic (these may be noticed by the partner or other family members):
> - Unable or unwilling to discuss labor and birth experience
> - Refers to self as ugly and useless
> - Excessively preoccupied with self (body image)
> - Markedly depressed
> - Lacks a support system
> - Partner or other family members react negatively to the baby
> - Refuses to interact with or care for baby; for example, does not name baby, does not want to hold or feed baby, is upset by vomiting and wet or soiled diapers (cultural appropriateness of actions must be considered)
> - Expresses disappointment over baby's sex
> - Sees baby as messy or unattractive
> - Baby reminds mother of family member or friend she does not like
> - Has difficulty sleeping
> - Experiences loss of appetite

d. Educate about signs of baby blues and postpartum depression (Box 6.5).

3. Discuss sexual activity and contraception.
   a. Encourage to abstain from sexual intercourse until bleeding has stopped and perineum is healed. Most couples can resume sexual intercourse by 4 to 6 weeks after birth unless directed otherwise but this will vary for every couple.
   b. Inform that first sexual experience may be uncomfortable because of vaginal dryness, perineal repairs, fear of pain with intercourse.
   c. Discuss contraceptive options before discharge. Include partner in discussion if client desires. Discuss use, risks, side effects, and available options postpartum and with breastfeeding (see Tables 6.17 and 6.18).

Nonhormonal Methods of Contraception

There are several options for nonhormonal contraception. All require commitment to use with each act of sexual intercourse if preventing pregnancy is the goal. These options do not have systemic adverse effects. Nonhormonal methods may fit within many cultural beliefs (see Table 6.17).

Hormonal Methods of Contraception

There are several hormonal options of contraception available to the woman. They may contain both progestin and estrogen (combined) or progestin only. The primary mechanism of

---

> **BOX 6.5 Signs of Postpartum Blues, Depression, and Psychosis**
>
> - Signs of baby blues (these should go away in a few days or a week):
>   - Sad, anxious, or overwhelmed feelings
>   - Crying spells
>   - Loss of appetite
>   - Difficulty sleeping
> - Signs of postpartum depression (can begin any time in the first year):
>   - Same signs as baby blues, but they last longer and are more severe
>   - Thoughts of harming yourself or your baby
>   - Not having any interest in the baby
> - Signs of postpartum psychosis:
>   - Seeing or hearing things that are not there
>   - Feelings of confusion
>   - Rapid mood swings
>   - Trying to hurt yourself or your baby
> - When to call your health care provider:
>   - The baby blues continue for more than 2 weeks
>   - Symptoms of depression get worse
>   - Difficulty performing tasks at home or at work
>   - Inability to care for yourself or your baby
>   - Thoughts of harming yourself or your baby

From Lowdermilk, D. L., Perry, S. E., Cashion, K., Alden, K., & Olshansky, E. (2020). *Maternity and women's health care* (12th ed.). St. Louis, MO: Elsevier. Data from US Department of Health and Human Services Office of Women's Health. (2018). *Depression during and after pregnancy fact sheet*. Retrieved from http://www.womenshealth.gov/publications/our-publications/fact-sheet/depression-pregnancy.html.

TABLE 6.17 Nonhormonal Methods of Contraception

Method	Considerations
Barrier Methods • Diaphragm • Cervical caps • Condoms (male and internal) • Contraceptive sponge	• All barrier methods must be applied near the time of sexual intercourse • Barrier methods are less effective than hormonal methods • Diaphragms and cervical caps should be used with spermicide; some condoms are lubricated with a spermicide • Diaphragms, cervical caps must be fitted by a health care provider; not recommended for use immediately postpartum (cervix should be healed) and woman's weight should be stabilized (diaphragm must be refitted if excessive weight gain or loss occurs) • Condoms and sponges are single use only • Ideally, diaphragms, cervical caps, and sponges should not be left in the vagina for more than 24 h • Only condoms protect against sexually transmitted infections
Fertility Awareness-Based Methods (FABM) • Determines when a woman is most fertile during each month and uses abstinence or barrier contraception during that time to prevent pregnancy • Calendar methods, basal body temperature charting • CycleBeads • Postovulation method, cervical mucus assessment	• Most women will benefit from detailed education about FABM • It can be more difficult for women to identify their fertile window if ovulation is impacted by the postpartum recovery period (irregular menses) or by breastfeeding (absence of menses)
Lactational Amenorrhea Method • The act of infant suckling during breastfeeding increases maternal prolactin levels which inhibits ovulation	• Three conditions should be present to increase the effectiveness of this method: (a) amenorrhea (no vaginal bleeding after 56 days postpartum), (b) exclusive or near-exclusive breastfeeding, and (c) infant younger than 6 months
• Permanent Contraception (Sterilization) • May be chosen when the woman and /or the couple decides they no longer want children • Tubal Occlusion • Vasectomy	• Tubal occlusion may be done in the hospital after delivery and prior to discharge; should be discussed with provider prior to the birth • Both methods are highly effective in preventing pregnancy

Adapted from Current NCLEX-RN Examination (2021) Philadelphia: Elsevier and Schuiling, K., & Likis, F. (2022). *Gynecologic health care* (4th ed.). Burlington, MA: Jones & Bartlett Learning.

TABLE 6.18 Hormonal Contraception

Composition	Route of Administration	Duration of Effect
Combination estrogen and progestin (synthetic estrogens and progestins in varying doses and formulations)	Oral Transdermal Vaginal ring insertion	24 h; extended cycle 12 weeks 7 days 3 weeks
Progestin only Norethindrone, norgestrel Medroxyprogesterone acetate Progestin, etonogestrel Levonorgestrel	Oral Intramuscular injection; subcutaneous injection Subdermal implant Intrauterine device	24 h 3 months Up to 3 years Up to 5 years

From Lowdermilk, D. L., Perry, S. E., Cashion, K., Alden, K., & Olshansky, E. (2020). *Maternity and women's health care* (12th ed.). St. Louis, MO: Elsevier.

action is to prevent ovulation, however progestin-only products can also thicken cervical mucus and alter the endometrium. Long-acting reversible contraception (LARC) methods like intrauterine contraception (Copper IUD or Progestin IUDs containing levonorgestrel) and emergency contraceptive options are also available.

Hormonal contraceptives are very effective in preventing pregnancy but may have adverse side effects like headache, nausea, breast pain, mood changes, and metabolic effects. Increased risk of VTE is primarily a concern with combined

methods. Initiation of combined hormonal methods are contraindicated until 21 days postpartum and preferably delayed until after 42 days postpartum (elevated risk for VTE). Most progestin-only methods can be initiated within the first month postpartum.

Women who are breastfeeding should also be aware that estrogen-containing products may affect milk supply. Combined methods are typically delayed until breastfeeding is well established. Some women may choose to initiate combined methods when they wean from breastfeeding. Progestin-only methods may typically be initiated within the first month postpartum without known adverse effects on breastfeeding (see Table 6.18).

    4. Review Schedule of Postpartum Care

       a. All women should have contact with obstetric care provider within first 3 weeks after delivery. This may vary for women with chronic medical conditions, hypertensive disorders, high risk of mood or anxiety disorders, or breastfeeding mothers with lactation concerns.

       b. Breastfeeding newborns should be seen by a pediatric provider within 3 to 5 days after birth or 48 to 72 hours after hospital discharge to assess feeding adequacy and weight loss.

       c. Encourage client to contact obstetric provider sooner if complications arise or she has questions or concerns.

       d. A comprehensive well woman visit and exam should occur no later than 12 weeks after delivery.

    5. Offer information and referral information for community resources.

❓ REVIEW OF NORMAL PUERPERIUM (POSTPARTUM)

1. A nurse discovers a postpartum client with a boggy uterus that is displaced above and to the right of the umbilicus. What nursing action is indicated?
2. Which women experience afterpains more than others?
3. Upon admission to the postpartum room, 3 hours after delivery, a client has a temperature of 37.5°C. What nursing actions are indicated?
4. A client feels faint on the way to the bathroom. What nursing assessments should be made?
5. What factor places the postpartum client at risk for thromboembolism?
6. A breastfeeding mother complains of very tender nipples. What nursing actions should be taken?
7. Three days postpartum, a lactating mother has full, warm, taut, tender breasts. What nursing actions should be taken?
8. What information should be given to a client regarding resumption of sexual intercourse after delivery?
9. A woman asks why she is urinating so much in the postpartum period. The nurse bases the response on what information?
10. A woman's WBC count is 17,000 mm³; she is afebrile and has no symptoms of infection. What nursing action is indicated?
12. What is the most common cause of uterine atony in the first 24 hours postpartum?
12. What is the purpose of giving docusate sodium to the postpartum client?
13. What should the fundal height be at 3 days postpartum for a woman who has had a vaginal delivery?
14. List three signs of positive bonding between parents and newborn.

See Answer Key at the end of this text for suggested responses.

POSTPARTUM COMPLICATIONS

Postpartum Infections

Description: Any clinical infection that occurs within 28 days of delivery, after spontaneous or induced abortion. The presence of a fever (38°C or higher) on two successive days of the first 10 days postpartum. Typical sites of infection include the vagina, perineum, uterus, bladder, or breasts. Risk factors include prolonged ROM, any lacerations, or operative incisions (forceps, episiotomy, or cesarean section), hemorrhage, intrauterine manipulation, manual removal of placenta, retained placental fragments, anemia.

A. Symptoms

    1. Wound (abdomen, perineum)

       a. Fever

       b. Red, swollen, very tender

       c. Purulent and/or foul-smelling drainage, induration

    2. Endometritis (infection of lining of uterus)

       a. Fever

       b. Chills

       c. Increased pulse

       d. Malaise, anorexia

       e. Excess fundal tenderness long after it is expected, pelvic pain

       f. Uterine subinvolution

       g. Lochia returning to rubra from serosa

       h. Foul-smelling lochia

    3. UTI (can progress to pyelonephritis if not identified and treated)

       a. Slight or no fever

       b. May have chills

       c. Dysuria, frequency, urgency, suprapubic tenderness

       d. Hematuria, bacteriuria

       e. Cloudy urine

       f. Development of flank pain or costovertebral-angle tenderness, nausea or vomiting may indicate progression to pyelonephritis.

    4. Mastitis (secondary to breast engorgement, blocked ducts, trauma, improper latch with breastfeeding, infrequent breastfeeding)

       a. Nipple fissures

       b. Fatigue

       c. Flulike symptoms: malaise, chills, and fever

       d. Red, warm, hard lump in breast (typically unilateral)

B. Clinical Judgment Measures

    Implement general care pertinent to any client with a diagnosed infection.

    1. Use and teach good hygiene techniques, aseptic technique with wound care.

    2. Frequently assess and record vital signs, including pain

    3. Manage fever by increasing fluids, providing comfort measures. Administer fever-reducing medications as ordered.

    4. Analgesics as ordered.

    5. Emphasize adherence to medication regimen

       a. Broad-spectrum antibiotics. Administer IV as directed if client is hospitalized.

       b. Educate about proper antibiotic use, need to complete entire course, side effects, directions for home use (Table 6.19).

    6. Site specific interventions:

TABLE 6.19 Antibiotics

Drugs	Indications	Adverse Reactions	Nursing Implications
Clindamycin	Broad-spectrum antibiotic used to treat postpartum endometritis	• Nausea, vomiting • GI irritation • Diarrhea	• Must be used in combination with gentamicin
Ampicillin-sulbactam	Broad-spectrum antibiotic used to treat postpartum endometritis	• Rash, dermatitis • Nausea, vomiting • GI irritation	• Do not administer to clients with penicillin sensitivity. • Alternative to clindamycin and gentamicin combination
Gentamicin sulfate	Aminoglycoside antibiotic used for serious puerperal infections	• GI irritation • Nephrotoxicity • Ototoxicity • Neurotoxicity • Possible hypersensitivity	• Do not mix with any other drug. • Observe for ototoxicity: ataxia, tinnitus, headache. • Observe for nephrotoxicity: elevated blood urea nitrogen (BUN) and creatinine levels. • Observe for neurotoxicity: paresthesia, muscle weakness. • Monitor I&O closely.
Cephalexin	Broad-spectrum antibiotic used to treat lactational mastitis	• Rash, dermatitis • Nausea, vomiting	• Do not administer to clients with penicillin allergy.

a. Perineal: Assist with sitz bath, cool compresses, encourage meticulous perineal care.
b. Endometritis: Assess lochia, obtain vaginal cultures if ordered
c. Mastitis: Encourage frequent breastfeeding, educate on breastfeeding technique, well-fitting bra (no underwire), use of breast pads (frequent changing, cleanliness), monitor for abscess formation or worsening symptoms, educate on when to contact obstetric provider.

C. Labs
1. Collect specimens for cultures as indicated.
2. CBC if applicable

HESI HINT Remember, the risk for postpartum infections is higher in clients who experienced problems during pregnancy (e.g., anemia, diabetes) and who experienced trauma during L&D (Table 6.20).

Postpartum Hemorrhage

Description: Obstetric emergency. It is a leading cause of maternal mortality that demands prompt recognition and intervention. The definition of acute PPH, also known as early or primary PPH, is a cumulative blood loss of greater than or equal to 1000 mL or bleeding associated with signs/symptoms of hypovolemia within 24 hours of birth, regardless of type of birth. Contributing factors for hemorrhage include uterine atony (overdistention of the uterus: polyhydramnios, multiple gestation, large neonate), lacerations of the genital tract, hematomas, placental complications (retained fragments, placenta accrete syndrome, abruption, previa), high parity, dystocia, prolonged labor, operative delivery (cesarean or forceps delivery, intrauterine manipulation), and previous history. Late, or secondary, PPH is possible but less common. The

definition of a late PPH is a hemorrhage that occurs more than 24 hours but less than 6 weeks after the birth.

A. Symptoms
1. Increase in lochia
   a. Perineal pad is soaked within 15 minutes
   b. Bleeding may be a continuous trickle or spurts
2. Large blood clots may be present (larger than a quarter in size)
3. Hypotonic (boggy) uterus
   a. Fundus that does not firm up with massage
4. Change in vital signs: hypotension, increased pulse
5. Pallor, cool, clammy skin

B. Clinical Judgment Measures

Acute Postpartum Hemorrhage

1. Review chart for predisposing factors.
2. Monitor vital signs, fundus, lochia frequently, and according to institution's policy.
a. Count pads saturated and time required to saturate.
3. Monitor level of consciousness.
4. Keep the bladder empty.
5. Contact obstetric provider if atony or bleeding continues despite massage.
6. Anticipate administering uterine stimulant medication as ordered (Table 6.21).
7. Monitor I&O (at least 30 mL/h output); maintain fluid replacement.

Late Postpartum Hemorrhage

Anticipate hospitalization, pelvic examination/labs/diagnostics to determine cause of bleeding and subsequent treatment. Subinvolution (uterus remains enlarged, often from placental fragments or pelvic infection) is a common cause of late PPH.

TABLE 6.20 Clinical Judgment Measures: Mastitis in a Breastfeeding Mother

Clinical Judgment Measure	Assessment Characteristics
Recognize Cues	Choice of newborn feeding method (breastfeeding or non-breastfeeding mother)
	Number of days postpartum (most cases of mastitis occur 2—4 weeks postpartum, but can occur at any time)
	Breast pain, areas of redness, warmth
	Sudden onset of influenza-like symptoms (fever, chills, malaise, body aches, headache, nausea, vomiting)
Analyze Cues	Determine where breast pain is located (mastitis typically presents unilaterally in the upper outer quadrant of the breast)
	Assess vital signs (especially temperature)
	Assess for signs of engorgement
	Assess for axillary lymphadenopathy
	Assess for cracked, sore, reddened nipples
	Observe integrity of breast tissue for signs of abscess or open areas, areas of warmth, redness
	Determine frequency of breastfeeding episodes daily, i.e., feeding every 2—3 h vs. feeding every 6 h; any pumping
	Determine if mother is still able to breastfeed (since onset of symptoms), is pumping only, or has stopped breastfeeding completely
Prioritize Cues	Determine need for any surgical intervention (abscess requiring I&D, aspiration)
	Determine if newborn is receiving adequate, uninterrupted nutrition
Solutions	Teach clients about symptoms of mastitis before discharge from birthing facility and when to notify health care provider
	Encourage prevention measures: frequent breastfeeding on both breasts, adequate rest and nutrition for mother, appropriate breast hygiene, and hand washing
	Advise to avoid use of underwire bras
Actions	Warm compresses for discomfort
	Take antibiotics (complete entire course) and analgesics as ordered
	Teach mother to contact provider if symptoms are not relieved with antibiotic therapy or worsen
	Review proper breastfeeding technique, latch
	Refer to lactation consultant for assistance as appropriate Educate on safety of continued breastfeeding, safety of breastmilk when mastitis is present; safety of breastfeeding with antibiotic therapy
	Educate about mastitis and answer any questions

Lochia persists and may have irregular patterns or become excessive with brisk periods of lochia rubra. A dilation and curettage (D&C) may be necessary.

1. Frequent vital signs
2. Initiate IV access.
3. Type and crossmatch for possible blood transfusion.
4. Obtain cultures if ordered.

5. Administer antibiotics as prescribed.
6. Keep the client warm and be alert for symptoms of shock.
7. Prepare client for possible surgical repair of laceration, evacuation of hematomas, or curettage for removal of placental fragments.

C. Labs
1. CBC
2. Blood type and cross match
3. Coagulation studies

D. Diagnostics
1. US may be ordered.

HESI HINT During medical emergencies such as bleeding episodes, clients need calm, direct explanations, and assurance that everything possible is being done to care for the woman. If possible, allow support person at bedside.

Cesarean Birth

Description: The birth of the fetus or fetuses through a transabdominal uterine incision. This may be scheduled or unplanned and may be the choice of birth when maternal and/or fetal complications arise. A woman may have a vaginal birth after cesarean (VBAC) if she has no contraindications, is at low risk for uterine rupture, and she desires to do this after consultation with her obstetric provider. A trial of labor (TOL) to observe the mother and fetus for a reasonable period of spontaneous labor may be required before proceeding with a VBAC. Preparations must be in place for any emergent needs like an immediate cesarean birth.

A. Symptoms
1. Planned
2. Maternal or fetal complications requiring immediate operative delivery

B. Clinical Judgment Measures
1. Obtain informed consent; explain procedure.
2. Provide emotional support.
3. Monitor vital signs.
4. Assess fetal well-being (FHR).
5. Establish IV access, initiate IV fluids as ordered.
6. Assist with anesthesia.
7. Administer preoperative medications if prescribed.
8. Maintain safety.
9. Intraoperative care: Place client in supine position with wedge under one hip to displace uterus laterally and prevent compression of vena cava; monitor vital signs, I&O, IV fluids, FHR, assist per institutional protocol.
10. Post-surgical care: Review complete surgery report, conduct standard postpartum assessments for vital signs, I&O, fundal height, lochia, signs of infection, excessive bleeding. Administer pain medications as prescribed.
11. Encourage early ambulation.
12. Encourage participation in infant care as soon as possible, including initiation of breastfeeding.

TABLE 6.21 Uterotonic Drugs to Manage Postpartum Hemorrhage

Drug	Side Effects	Contraindications	Nursing Considerations
Oxytocin (Pitocin)	Infrequent: water intoxication, nausea and vomiting	None for PPH	Continue to monitor vaginal bleeding and uterine tone.
Misoprostol (Cytotec)	Headache, nausea, vomiting, diarrhea, fever, chills	None	Continue to monitor vaginal bleeding and uterine tone.
Methylergonovine (Methergine)	Hypertension, hypotension, nausea, vomiting, headache	Hypertension, preeclampsia, cardiac disease	Check blood pressure before giving, and do not give if >140/90 mm Hg; continue monitoring vaginal bleeding and uterine tone.
15-Methylprostaglandin $F_2\alpha$ (Prostin/15 m; Carboprost, Hemabate)	Headache, nausea and vomiting, fever, chills, tachycardia, hypertension, diarrhea	Avoid with asthma or hypertension	Continue to monitor vaginal bleeding and uterine tone.
Dinoprostone (Prostin E_2)	Headache, nausea and vomiting, fever, chills, diarrhea	Use with caution with history of asthma, hypertension, or hypotension	Continue to monitor vaginal bleeding and uterine tone.

IM, Intramuscular; *IV,* intravenous; *PO,* by mouth; *PPH,* postpartum hemorrhage. Adapted from Lowdermilk, D. L., Perry, S. E., Cashion, K., Alden, K., & Olshansky, E. (2020). *Maternity and women's health care* (12th ed.). St. Louis, MO: Elsevier. Data from Francois, K. E., & Foley, M. R. (2017). Antepartum and postpartum hemorrhage. In S. G. Gabbe, J. R. Niebyl, J. L. Simpson, et al. (Eds.), *Obstetrics: Normal and problem pregnancies* (7th ed.). Philadelphia: Elsevier; and Lyndon, A., Lagrew, D., Shields, L., et al. (Eds.). (2015). *California maternal quality care collaborative toolkit to transform maternity care: Improving health care response to obstetric hemorrhage version 2.0.* Stanford, CA: California Maternal Quality Care Collaborative (CMQCC). Retrieved from https://www.cmqcc.org/ob_hemorrhage.

C. Labs
1. Blood type, Rh and crossmatch
2. CBC, may be repeated post-op
3. Chemistry panel

D. Discharge
1. Provide discharge instructions and follow-up care as ordered.
   a. Information about PPH, preeclampsia, infection, pulmonary embolism, deep vein thrombosis, thrombophlebitis, postpartum depression

❓ REVIEW OF POSTPARTUM COMPLICATIONS

1. May women with a positive HIV antibody try to breastfeed?
2. What are the common side effects of antibiotics used to treat puerperal infection?
3. How does the nurse differentiate the symptomatology of cystitis from that of pyelonephritis?
4. What are the signs of endometritis?
5. State four risk factors for or predisposing factors to postpartum infection.
6. State four risk factors for or predisposing factors to postpartum hemorrhage.
7. What immediate nursing actions should be taken when a postpartum hemorrhage is detected?
8. Must women diagnosed with mastitis stop breastfeeding?

See Answer Key at the end of this text for suggested responses.

THE NORMAL NEWBORN

Description: During the immediate transitional period (first 6 to 8 hours of life) and the early newborn period (first few days of life), the nurse assesses, plans, and provides nursing interventions based on the outcomes of the individual newborn's examination.

Newborn Transition to Extrauterine Life

The newborn should be carefully observed during the initial 6 to 8 hours after birth for adaptation of key systems to extrauterine life.

A. Respiratory
1. Establishment of respirations after umbilical cord is clamped and cut (clamping causes a rise in BP which increases circulation and lung perfusion)
2. Initiation of respirations occurs because of chemical, mechanical, thermal, and sensory factors.

B. Cardiovascular
1. Cord clamping and cutting causes changes in pressures of cardiovascular system triggering functional closure of the foramen ovale, ductus arteriosus, and ductus venosus.
2. BP range: 60 to 80 mm Hg systolic/40 to 50 mm Hg diastolic

C. Thermogenic
1. Heat regulation is critical to survival.
2. Newborns have only a thin layer of subcutaneous fat, blood vessels are close to the skin's surface, and they have a larger body surface-to-body weight (mass) ratio.
3. Thermoregulation is the balance between heat loss and heat production. Hypothermia (heat loss) leads to depletion of glucose and, therefore, to the use of brown fat (special fat deposits fetus develops in last trimester; they are important to thermoregulation) for energy (Table 6.22).

TABLE 6.22	**Newborn Vital Sign Norms**	
Vital sign	**Normal**	**Nursing Implications**

Respirations	Rate: 30—60 breaths/min	• Remember the ABCs (airway, breathing, circulation).
		• Count 1 full minute by observing abdomen or auscultating breath sounds.
		• Note five symptoms of respiratory distress
		  • Tachypnea
		  • Cyanosis
		  • Flaring nares
		  • Expiratory grunt
		  • Retractions

Heart rate	110—160 beats/min; may decrease as low as 100 during sleep; may increase as high as 180 during crying	• Auscultate for 1 full minute at the PMI (point of maximal impulse): third to fourth intercostal space.
Temperature	Range: 36.5°C—37.5°C	• Rectal approach may perforate rectum; if taken rectally, insert only ¼ to ½ inch for 5 min and hold legs firmly to prevent trauma.
Blood pressure	Average 80/50 mm Hg	• Not usually measured unless problems in circulation have been assessed.

Immediate Care of Newborn After Delivery

Description: Nursing care provided to the newborn immediately after birth that includes a brief, initial assessment of systems and identification of any abnormalities requiring emergency interventions. If possible, the assessment should be completed while skin-to-skin contact is maintained with the mother.

A. Brief initial exam

1. Observe for life-threatening abnormalities (poor muscle tone, not crying, not breathing or respiratory distress), need for resuscitation, birth injuries.
2. Immediately dry infant, place cap on head, and establish skin-to-skin contact with mother by laying infant on mother's chest or abdomen. Infant may alternatively be placed on radiant warmer.
3. Nasal and oral secretions should be wiped away; suction mouth and nose with bulb syringe if needed; keep head slightly lower than body; and assess airway status.
4. Place identity bands on neonate and mother.

> **HESI HINT** Suction the mouth first and then the nose. Stimulating the nares can initiate inspiration, which could cause aspiration of mucus in oral pharynx.

B. Apar Score

1. Obtain Apgar score at 1 and 5 minutes (Table 6.23).

C. Physical Assessment

1. General physical assessment should be completed as soon as possible after birth. Check for gross anomalies, including no back lesions and a patent anus.
2. Encourage parent's presence during exam.
3. Assess vital signs, including body length, weight, and head circumference (Table 6.24).
4. Collect cord blood and capillary stick for lab analysis as ordered.
   a. Blood type and Rh status
   b. CBC

TABLE 6.23	**Apgar Assessment**
Performed at exactly 1 and 5 min after birth. Cannot just eyeball; must have hands-on examination. Score: • 7—10: Good • 4—6: Needs moderate resuscitative efforts • 0—3: Severe need for resuscitation	
Heart rate	Absent = 0; <100 = 1; ≥100 = 2
Respiratory effort	No cry = 0; weak cry = 1; vigorous cry = 2
Muscle tone	Flaccid = 0; some flexion = 1; total flexion = 2
Reflex irritability	No response to foot tap = 0; slight response to foot tap (grimace) = 1; quick foot removal = 2
Color	Dusky, cyanotic = 0; acrocyanotic = 1; totally pink = 2

   c. Glucose
   d. Bilirubin
5. Examine cord clamp for closure, absence of blood oozing from cord; check for presence of three vessels (Table 6.25).

Ongoing Newborn Assessment

A. History

1. Review L&D report of neonatal history to determine risks during newborn transition caused by medical and obstetric complications.
   a. Cesarean delivery
   b. Prematurity or postmaturity
   c. Medical conditions of the mother (GDM, HTN)
   d. Prolonged ROM greater than 24 hours: sepsis workup
   e. Rh+ isoimmunization (positive direct Coombs test)
   f. Traumatic (forceps or vacuum suction) delivery
2. Review L&D report of neonatal history to determine risks during newborn transition caused by analgesia and anesthesia during L&D.
   a. Magnesium sulfate during labor: Hypermagnesemia in neonate causes depressed respirations, hypocalcemia, and hypotonia.

TABLE 6.24 Physical Measurements

Assessment	Normal	Nursing Implications
Weight	• Majority weigh between 2700 and 4000 g (6—9 lb)	• Weigh at birth and daily, with neonate completely naked. • Normally lose 5%—15% (average 10%) of birth weight in first week of life; weight should be documented carefully.
Length	• Average range: 46—52.5 cm	• Measured from crown to rump and rump to heel, or from crown to heel at birth
Head circumference	• Average range: 33—35 cm (normally, 2 cm larger than chest circumference)	• Tape measure placed above eyebrows and stretched around fullest part of occiput, at posterior fontanel (frontal-occipital circumference [FOC])
Chest circumference	• Average range: 31—33 cm	• Tape measure is stretched around scapulae and over nipple line.

   b. Late administration of narcotic analgesics; causes decreased respirations and hypotonia.
   c. Epidural or spinal anesthesia
   d. General anesthesia
3. Review L&D report of neonatal history to determine risks during newborn transition caused by degree of birth asphyxia.
   a. Potential asphyxia events during labor: documented late decelerations, decreased variability, severe variable decelerations
4. Review significant maternal social history: partner and support system, infections (TORCH, STDs), cultural influences (language, preferences for newborn care), maternal substance use.

B. Clinical Judgment Measures

The nurse is responsible for monitoring the newborn whether the infant is rooming-in or in the nursery. Parent—infant attachment and bonding should be encouraged.
1. Maintain oxygen supply
2. Maintain body temperature.
   a. Keep newborn warm and dry.
   b. If newborn's temperature falls below 36.4°C, place in radiant warmer and apply skin temperature probe to regulate isolette temperature. May also double-wrap or put skin to skin (kangaroo) with mother.
3. Assess for neonatal pain.
   a. Every neonate should have an initial pain assessment and pain management plan.
      1) Physiologic pain responses may be noted by a change in vital signs, decreased oxygenation, skin pallor or sweating, increased muscle tone, or dilated pupils.
      2) Behavioral pain responses may be noted by crying, whimpering, grimace, furrowed brows, chin quivering, thrashing, rigidity or flaccidity, fist clenching, irritability.
4. Document the infant's elimination pattern daily.
   a. Stool progression: Meconium (black, tarry, sticky) stool within the first 24 hours to transitional (yellowish-green) to milk stool (yellow). Report if no stool within 24 hours.
   b. Infant should void within 4 to 6 hours of birth; then should use one diaper for each day of life, minimum, until day 6. On day 6 and beyond infant should use a minimum of six to eight diapers per day. Report if there is no urination within 24 hours. There may be brick-red "dust" in the first voidings (uric acid crystals).
   c. To evaluate exact urine output, weigh dry diaper before applying. Weigh the wet diaper after infant has voided. Calculate and record each gram of added weight as 1 mL urine.
5. Document nutrition intake and calculate nutrition needs.
   a. Demand feeding (bottle or breast) is preferred.
   b. Most bottle-fed newborns eat every 3 to 4 hours; breastfed infants eat every 1 to 3 hours (the breast milk is digested more quickly).
   c. After the initial weight loss period, the infant should gain approximately 1 oz (30 g) per day.
   d. An infant needs about 50 calories/lb or 108 calories/kg of body weight for the first 6 months.

C. Medications

1. Eye prophylaxis
   a. Recommended to prevent ophthalmia neonatorum
   b. Erythromycin ophthalmic ointment 0.5% is recommended.
   c. Administer within first hour of birth. If parents desire an open-eye bonding period, may delay eye prophylaxis for up to 2 hours.
2. Vitamin K Prophylaxis
   a. Neonates have low vitamin K levels at birth.
   b. Recommended to prevent vitamin K-dependent hemorrhagic disease of the newborn.
   c. Administer phytonadione 0.5 to 1 mg IM soon after birth.
   d. May be delayed until after first breastfeeding.
3. Hepatitis B vaccination
   a. Recommended for all newborns before discharge
   b. If mother is positive for Hepatitis B, infant should receive HepB vaccine and HepB immune globulin (HBIG) within 12 hours of birth.

D. Gestational assessment

Description: Assessment of the gestational age of the infant examines six physical and six neuromuscular signs. A frequently used method is the New Ballard Score. The initial examination should be performed in the first 48 hours of life (Fig. 6.19, pp. XXX and Tables 6.26 and 6.27, pp. XXX).

TABLE 6.25 Physical Examination of Newborn

Normal	Abnormal	Rationale
General Appearance		
• Awake	• Little subcutaneous fat	• Intrauterine growth problems
• Flexed extremities		• Fetal stress
• Moves all extremities	• Frog position	• Prematurity
• Strong, lusty cry	• Flaccid	• Asphyxia
• Obvious presence of subcutaneous fat		• Prematurity
• No obvious anomalies	• Hard to arouse	• Sepsis
		• CNS problems
		• Asphyxia
	• High-pitched cry	• CNS damage or anomalies
		• Hypoglycemia
		• Drug withdrawal
Integument		
• Smooth, elastic turgor and subcutaneous fat, superficial peeling after 24 h; veins rarely visible	• Extreme desquamation	• Postmaturity
	• Many visible veins	• Prematurity
• Milia, vernix increases	• Meconium staining	• Fetal distress
• Lanugo, mottling	• Cyanosis	• Heart disease
• Harlequin sign (pink-red skin on one side of body)		• Asphyxia
• Erythema toxicum (pink papular rash is normal)	• Jaundice (within 24 h)	• Blood incompatibilities
		• Sepsis
• Mongolian spots		• Drug reactions
• Telangiectatic nevi (stork bites)	• Vesicle	• Herpes, syphilis
	• Café-au-lait spots	• Neurofibromatosis
Head		
• Round or slightly molded	• Bulging fontanel	• Increased intracranial pressure (ICP)
• Caput succedaneum (edema over occiput)	• Crosses suture line, present at birth	
• Open, flat anterior and posterior fontanels, sutures slightly separated or overlapping due to molding	• Sunken fontanel	• Dehydration
	• Widely separated sutures	• Hydrocephalus
	• Premature suture closure	• Genetic disorders
	• Cephalohematoma	• Blood under periosteum due to trauma; can cause hyperbilirubinemia
Eyes		
• Symmetrically placed	• Purulent discharge	• Gonorrhea or chlamydia
• Pseudostrabismus	• Brushfield spots in iris	• Down syndrome
• Chemical conjunctivitis (from eye prophylaxis)	• Absence of red reflex	• Congenital cataracts
• Clear cornea	• Epicanthal folds	• Down syndrome
• White-blue sclera	• Setting-sun sign	• CNS disorders
• Subconjunctival hemorrhage from pressure	• Absent glabellar reflex (blink)	• CNS or neuromuscular problem
• Absence of tears		
• Doll's eye movement (slight nystagmus)		
Ears		
• Pinna at or above level of line drawn from outer canthus of eye	• Low set	• Down syndrome
	• Unformed, soft	• Prematurity
• Well-formed and firm with instant recoil if folded against head	• Preauricular sinus	• Possible renal anomaly
Nose		
• In midline	• Short, upturned, small philtrum (creases under nose)	• Fetal alcohol syndrome
• Appears flattened		
• Is being used for breathing	• Nasal flaring	• Respiratory distress
• Occasional sneezing	• Grunting	• Respiratory distress
		• Choanal atresia (obstruction between nares and pharynx)
	• Snuffles	• Syphilis
	• Excessive sneezing	• Drug withdrawal

Continued

Mouth and Chin

- Symmetrical movement
- Intact lip and palate
- Epstein pearls
- Mobile tongue
- Sucking pads in cheeks
- Presence of rooting, sucking, swallowing, and gagging reflexes

- Asymmetry
- Cleft lip
- White plaques on cheeks, tongue
- Absence of protective reflexes

- Excessive drooling

- Facial nerve injury (Bell palsy)
- Genetic disorder
- Monilia infection/thrush
- Prematurity
- CNS disorders
- Esophageal atresia

Neck

- Short
- Range of motion
- Nonpalpable thyroid
- Ability to lift head momentarily

- Limited range of motion
- Nuchal rigidity
- Enlarged thyroid
- Crepitus over clavicle

- Torticollis (wry neck)
- Meningitis
- Hyperthyroidism
- Fractured clavicle

Chest

- Symmetrical excursion
- Breath sounds clear and equal
- Transient rales at birth
- Round
- Breast engorgement (hormonal)
- Transient murmurs

- Persistent murmur
- Visible activity over precordium

- Retractions
- Asymmetrical chest

- Patent ductus arteriosus
- Congenital heart anomaly
- Heart failure
- Respiratory distress
- Pneumothorax

Back, Hips, Buttocks, and Anus

- Spine intact
- Symmetrical gluteal folds
- Equal limb lengths
- Patent anus

- Pilonidal dimple or sinus (at base of sacrum)
- Hip click
- Unequal limb lengths
- Asymmetrical gluteal folds
- Absence of stools after 24 h

- CNS anomaly
- Covert spina bifida
- Congenital hip dislocation

- Imperforate anus
- GI obstruction

Abdomen

- Full, rounded, soft
- Present bowel sounds
- Palpable liver 1–2 cm below right costal margin
- Two arteries, one vein in cord; white cord with Wharton jelly

- Scaphoid
- Distention

- Hepatosplenomegaly
- Purulent discharge at base of cord, foul odor
- One artery
- Omphalocele
- Gastroschisis

- Diaphragmatic hernia
- Meconium ileus
- GI obstruction
- Hirschsprung disease
- Sepsis
- Omphalitis (cord infection)

- Renal or heart anomalies
- Abdominal contents in umbilicus (anomaly)
- Abdominal contents outside of abdomen (anomaly)

Genitals
Female

- Slightly edematous labia covering clitoris and labia minora
- Pseudomenstruation
- Visible hymenal tag

- Labia minora and clitoris visible

- Prematurity

Male

- Penis with foreskin intact
- Meatus in middle at tip of penis
- Descended testes
- Slight edema of scrotum
- Rugae on scrotum

- Undescended testes
- Meatus on dorsal surface penis
- Meatus on ventral surface penis
- Fluid in testes
- Intestine in inguinal canal

- Prematurity
- Epispadias
- Hypospadias
- Hydrocele
- Inguinal hernia

Continued

TABLE 6.25 Physical Examination of Newborn—cont'd

Normal	Abnormal	Rationale
Extremities • Arms, hands, fingers, legs, feet, toes • Flexion • Symmetrical movement • Palpable brachial and radial pulses • Palmar and plantar grasp reflex present • Strong grasp reflex • Multiple palmar and plantar creases • Slightly bowed legs • Femoral pulses present • Positive Babinski reflex	• Incurving little finger • Simian crease • Flapping tremors • Polydactyly • Syndactyly • Difference in pulses between upper and lower extremities • Absence of plantar creases • Rigid fixation of ankle • Absent Babinski reflex	• Down syndrome • Drug withdrawal • Extra digit (family trait) • Webbed digit (family trait) • Coarctation of aorta • Prematurity • Club feet (talipes) • CNS injury

CNS, Central nervous system; *GI,* gastrointestinal.

NEUROMUSCULAR MATURITY

	−1	0	1	2	3	4	5
Posture							
Square Window (wrist)	> 90°	90°	60°	45°	30°	0°	
Arm Recoil		180°	140°–180°	110°–140°	90°–110°	< 90°	
Popliteal Angle	180°	160°	140°	120°	100°	90°	< 90°
Scarf Sign							
Heel to Ear							

PHYSICAL MATURITY

Skin	sticky friable transparent	gelatinous red, translucent	smooth pink, visible veins	superficial peeling or rash, few veins	cracking pale areas rare veins	parchment deep cracking no vessels	leathery cracked wrinkled
Lanugo	none	sparse	abundant	thinning	bald areas	mostly bald	
Plantar Surface	heel-toe 40–50 mm: −1 <40 mm: −2	>50 mm no crease	faint red marks	anterior transverse crease only	creases ant. 2/3	creases over entire sole	
Breast	imperceptible	barely perceptible	flat areola no bud	stippled areola 1–2 mm bud	raised areola 3–4 mm bud	full areola 5–10 mm bud	
Eye/Ear	lids fused loosely: −1 tightly: −2	lids open pinna flat stays folded	sl. curved pinna; soft; slow recoil	well-curved pinna; soft but ready recoil	formed & firm instant recoil	thick cartilage ear stiff	
Genitals (male)	scrotum flat, smooth	scrotum empty faint rugae	testes in upper canal rare rugae	testes descending few rugae	testes down good rugae	testes pendulous deep rugae	
Genitals (female)	clitoris prominent labia flat	prominent clitoris small labia minora	prominent clitoris enlarging minora	majora & minora equally prominent	majora large minora small	majora cover clitoris & minora	

MATURITY RATING

score	weeks
−10	20
−5	22
0	24
5	26
10	28
15	30
20	32
25	34
30	36
35	38
40	40
45	42
50	44

Fig. 6.19 Estimation of Gestational Age. New Ballard scale for newborn maturity rating. Expanded scale includes extremely premature infants and has been refined to improve accuracy in more mature infants. (From Ballard, J. L., Khoury, J. C., Wedig, K., Wang, L., Eilers-Walsman, B. L., & Lipp, R. [1991]. New Ballard score, expanded to include extremely premature infants. *The Journal of Pediatrics, 119*[3], 4177.)

TABLE 6.26   Neuromuscular Assessment

Reflex	Normal Response	Lasts Until
Rooting	Baby turns toward stimulus when cheek or corner of lip is touched.	3–4 months (possibly 1 year)
Moro	When startled, baby symmetrically extends and abducts all extremities. Forefingers form a C shape.	3–4 months
Tonic neck	When neck is turned to side, baby assumes fencing posture.	3–4 months
Babinski	When sole of foot is stroked from heel to ball, toes hyperextend and fan apart from big toe.	1 year–18 months
Palmar grasp	When examiner's finger is placed in the infant's palm, the newborn will curl his or her fingers around the examiner's finger.	Lessens by 3–4 months
Plantar	A finger at base of toes causes them to curl downward.	8 months
Stepping	When infant is held in upright position with feet touching a hard surface, walking motions are made.	3–4 months

TABLE 6.27   Gestational Age Assessment

By Date	By Weight
Preterm: 20–37 weeks gestation	Small for gestational age (SGA): Weight below the tenth percentile for estimated weeks of gestation
Term: 38–42 weeks gestation	Average for gestational age (AGA): Weight between the tenth and ninetieth percentiles for estimated weeks of gestation
Postterm: >42 weeks gestation	Large for gestational age (LGA): Weight above the ninetieth percentile for estimated weeks of gestation

E. Labs and Diagnostic Tests

1. Universal newborn screening (usually completed in the first 24 hours of life). Screens for core disorders (hemoglobinopathies, inborn errors of metabolism [PKU, galactosemia]) and secondary disorders. State laws differ regarding informed consent newborn screening.
2. Hearing screening. Early detection of hearing loss allows for early intervention and treatment.
3. Critical congenital heart disease (CCHD) screening. Uses pulse oximetry testing at 24 and 48 hours of age to detect critical congenital heart defects that present with hypoxemia.
4. Monitor laboratory values (Table 6.28).

F. Assessment of Physiologic Problems

G. Hypoglycemia

Description: Blood glucose level inadequate to support the newborn. At-risk infants include those born preterm or late preterm, small-for-gestational-age (SGA), large-for-gestational-age (LGA), low birth weight, infants born to mothers with diabetes, infants who experienced respiratory, asphyxia, or cold stress.

1. Perform a heelstick blood glucose assessment on all SGA or LGA babies, on infants of diabetic mothers (IDMs), on jittery babies, and on babies with high-pitched cries (Box 6.6).
2. Report any blood glucose levels under 40 mg/dL. Normal serum glucose is 40 to 80 mg/dL. Administer glucose gel if ordered and per institution protocol.
3. Feed the baby early (breast milk or formula) if a low glucose level is detected. In addition, review orders and institution protocol to apply glucose gel for infants with a blood glucose level under 40 mg/dL. Notify provider.
4. Prevent cold stress, which leads to hypoglycemia.

H. Hyperbilirubinemia

1. **Description:** Elevation of serum bilirubin. Most newborns will experience some level of jaundice. Physiologic jaundice is caused by increased levels of unconjugated bilirubin, is usually self-limiting, and often requires no treatment. Evaluate for Rh isoimmunization (Rh+ newborn, Rh− mother; maternal Rh+ antibodies are passed to the fetus and cause RBC hemolysis) and for ABO incompatibility (mother blood type O, newborn blood type A or B; maternal anti-A or anti-B antibodies are passed to newborn and cause less severe hemolysis).
2. Promote stooling by early feedings of milk (bilirubin, a byproduct of RBC destruction, binds to protein for excretion or metabolism).
3. Assess at birth and at least every 8 to 12 hours for presence of jaundice.
   a. Visual assessment to look for yellowish skin color, sclera, and mucous membranes; jaundice tends to proceed cephalocaudally (relationship between the head and the base of the spine).
      1) Assess skin for jaundice: apply pressure with thumb over bony prominences to blanch skin. After the thumb is removed, the area will look yellow before normal skin color reappears.
      2) The best areas for assessment are the nose, forehead, and sternum. In dark-skinned infants, observe conjunctival sac and oral mucosa.
      3) Visual assessment alone does not provide an accurate assessment. Also follow POC transcutaneous bilirubin level (TcB) protocols.
   b. Measurements for total serum bilirubin level (TSB) or (TcB) should be conducted as ordered. Repeat testing is based on risk level, age of neonate, and progression of jaundice.
4. Assist with phototherapy if ordered (Table 6.29).

TABLE 6.28 Standard Laboratory Values in a Term Neonate

Hematology	Values
Hemoglobin (g/dL)	15—24
Hematocrit (%)	44—70
Red blood cells (RBCs)/μL	4.8×10^6 to 7.1×10^6
Reticulocytes (%)	1.8—4.6
Fetal hemoglobin (% of total)	50—70
Platelet count/mm³	
≤1 week	84,000—478,000
>1 week	150,000—300,000
White blood cells (WBCs)/μL	9000—30,000
Bilirubin, total (mg/dL)[a]	
24 h	2—6
48 h	6—7
3— days	4—6
Serum glucose (mg/dL)	
<1 day	40—60
>1 day	50—90
Arterial blood gases	
pH	7.35—7.45
P_{CO_2}	35—45 mm Hg
P_{O_2}	60—80 mm Hg
HCO_3	18—26 mEq/L
Base excess	(−5) to (+5)
O_2 saturation	92%—94%

[a]Bilirubin levels should be interpreted according to the hour-specific nomogram (AAP Subcommittee on Hyperbilirubinemia, 2004).

dL, Deciliter; *μL*, microliter; *P_{CO_2}*, partial pressure of carbon dioxide; *P_{O_2}*, partial pressure of oxygen.

Data from American Academy of Pediatrics [AAP] Subcommittee on Hyperbilirubinemia. (2004). Clinical practice guideline: Management of hyperbilirubinemia in the newborn infant 35 or more weeks of gestation. *Pediatrics, 114*(1), 297—316; Blackburn, S. T. (2018). *Maternal, fetal, and neonatal physiology* (5th ed.). St. Louis, MO: Elsevier; Kliegman, R. M., Stanton, B. F., St. Geme III, et al. (Eds.). (2016). *Nelson textbook of pediatrics* (20th ed.). Philadelphia: Elsevier; Pagana, K. D., & Pagana, T. J. (2014). *Mosby's manual of diagnostic and laboratory tests* (5th ed.). St. Louis, MO: Elsevier; Barry, J. S., Deacon, J., Hernández, C., et al. (2016). Acid-base homeostasis and oxygenation. In: S. L. Gardner, B. S. Carter, M. Enzman-Hines, et al., (Eds.), *Merenstein & Gardner's handbook of neonatal intensive care* (8th ed.). St. Louis, MO: Elsevier.

HESI HINT Physiologic jaundice, which occurs after 24 h of age, peaks at about 3—5 days in term infants, and resolves after 1—2 weeks. It is due to the immature liver's normal inability to keep up with RBC destruction and to bind bilirubin. Remember that unconjugated bilirubin is the culprit.

HESI HINT When phototherapy is used, the infant's eyes must be protected by a special opaque mask designed to prevent retinal damage and no ointments, creams, or lotions should be applied to the newborn's skin to prevent burns.

I. Newborn Discharge Teaching
1. Provide parent and family with teaching plan for newborn care.

BOX 6.6 Heelstick Procedure for Newborns
- Wash hands and put on gloves.
- Clean heel with alcohol and dry with a gauze pad.
- Choose a site for puncture that avoids the plantar artery in the middle of the heel.
- Use only the lateral surfaces of the heel.
- Puncture deep enough to trigger a free flow of blood. Wipe away first drop with sterile gauze pad.
- Collect blood in appropriate tube, on card, or on glucose "stick."

---

a. Bathing. Teach *not* to submerge infant in water until cord falls off (10 to 14 days); continue cord care and keep diaper off cord.

b. Diapering. Teach to use warm water to clean infant after voiding; use mild soap and water with stools. (Remember, cleanse female perineum front to back); dry completely before applying next diaper.

c. Crying. Teach that all infants cry. Instruct on strategies to calm a crying or fussy baby. Encourage picking the baby up.

d. Comfort. Encourage parents to implement swaddling, back massage, rhythmic movement such as rocking to help with calming infant.

2. Teach to recognize signs and symptoms of a sick newborn who needs medical attention.

a. Lethargy or difficulty waking

b. Temperature above 37.8°C

c. Vomiting (large emesis, not spitting up)

d. Green, liquid stools

e. Refusal of two feedings in a row

f. Presence of fever

3. Review follow-up care. Most infants will have an appointment with a health care provider within 48 to 72 hours of discharge. This is especially important for breastfed infants to monitor weight and hydration status.

HESI HINT Teach parents to take infant's temperature, both axillary and rectal. Axillary is recommended, but some pediatricians request a rectal (core) temperature.

❓ REVIEW OF THE NORMAL NEWBORN

1. The newborn transitional period consists of the first _____ of life.
2. The nurse anticipates which newborns will be at greater risk for problems in the transitional period. State three factors that predispose to respiratory depression in the newborn.
3. What is the danger to the newborn of heat loss in the first few hours of life?
4. Normal newborn temperature is _____. Normal newborn heart rate is _____. Normal newborn respiratory rate is ___. Normal newborn BP is ____.
5. The nurse records a temperature below 36.1°C on admission of the newborn. What nursing actions should be taken?

TABLE 6.29 Clinical Judgment Measures: Pathologic Jaundice in Newborn

Clinical Judgment Measure	Assessment Characteristics
Recognize Cues	Jaundice appearing before 24 h of age usually indicates a pathologic condition
	TSB levels increase by more than 0.2 mg/dL/h; TSB is >95th percentile for age in hours
	Direct serum bilirubin levels exceed 1.5–2 mg/dL
Analyze Cues	Review maternal history and labor/birth record for potential risk factors
	a. Rh incompatibility; ABO incompatibility; other hemolytic disease (G6PD deficiency)
	b. Prematurity
	c. Sepsis
	d. Maternal diabetes, intrauterine infections
	e. Native American or Asian race
	f. Birth trauma (including vacuum or forceps assisted delivery); cephalohematoma
	g. Previous sibling who received phototherapy
	Monitor serum bilirubin levels closely; repeat testing as ordered
	Review other labs as ordered (direct Coombs test, reticulocyte count, Hgb, Hct)
	Monitor urine and stools
	Document visual assessment of jaundice (in addition to serum levels);
	Observe and document changes in infant behavior
Prioritize Cues	The time of onset of jaundice is a key factor in evaluating its cause and determining needed treatment; increasing levels of unconjugated bilirubin that are left untreated can quickly result in
	a. Acute bilirubin encephalopathy with symptoms of lethargy, hypotonia, irritability, seizures, coma, death
	b. Kernicterus (irreversible, long-term consequences of bilirubin toxicity (hypotonia, delayed motor skills, hearing loss, cerebral palsy)
Solutions	Encourage frequent and adequate feedings
	Assess for risk factors prior to delivery
	Closely observe infant in the first 24 h of life for signs of jaundice
	Teach parents about the differences between physiologic and pathologic jaundice; answer questions
Actions	Treatment will depend on TSB levels, infant's gestational age, presence of risk factors; goal is to reduce the newborn's serum levels of unconjugated bilirubin
	Phototherapy or exchange infusion may be needed to reduce unconjugated bilirubin levels
	Teach parents the importance of follow-up care and clearly review discharge instructions
Evaluate Outcomes	The overall status of the newborn will be determined by decreasing TSB levels, behavior, and reduction in visible jaundice
	Early identification and treatment will prevent acute bilirubin encephalopathy and kernicterus

Hct, Hematocrit; *Hgb,* hemoglobin; *TSB,* total serum bilirubin level.

6. True or false: The newborn's head is usually smaller than the chest.
7. During the physical examination of the newborn, the nurse notes the cry is shrill, high-pitched, and weak. What are the possible causes?
8. The nurse notes a swelling over the back part of the newborn's head. Is this a normal newborn variation?
9. Should the normal newborn have a positive or negative Babinski reflex?
10. When suctioning the newborn with a bulb syringe, which should be suctioned first, the mouth or the nose?
11. A new mother asks the nurse whether circumcision is medically indicated in the newborn. How should the nurse respond?
12. Normal blood glucose in the term neonate is _____.
13. Why does the newborn need vitamin K in the first hour after birth?
14. Physiologic jaundice in the newborn occurs _____. It is caused by _____.
15. When is the screening test for PKU done?
16. A term newborn needs to take in _____ calories per pound per day. After the initial weight loss is sustained, the newborn should gain _____ per day.
17. List five signs and symptoms new parents should be taught to report immediately to a health care provider or clinic.

See Answer Key at the end of this text for suggested responses.

NEWBORN COMPLICATIONS

Neonatal Sepsis

Description: One of most significant causes of neonatal mortality and morbidity. Classified into either early-onset sepsis (within first 7 days of life) or late-onset (occurring 7 to 30 days of age). Neonatal infections may be bacterial, viral, or fungal.

A. General Symptoms (may vary with causative agent)
  1. Earliest symptoms are often nonspecific and include lethargy, poor feeding, and temperature instability.
  2. Subtle color changes: mottling, duskiness
  3. Subtle changes in behavior
  4. Respiratory distress, apnea

Example: Group B Streptococcus

Description: GBS lives in human GI and genitourinary tracts. It is a leading cause of perinatal infections. In the newborn it can cause focal or systemic disease. Women who are GBS positive during pregnancy can pass the infection on to the newborn; however, the practice of providing prophylactic intrapartum antibiotics to women with GBS has greatly reduced the incidence in newborns. GBS disease in the newborn can be early-onset (within the first 7 days of birth, usually form vertical transmission during birth) or late-onset (from 7 days of life to 3 months of age).

Risk factors include preterm birth, ROM greater than 18 hours before birth, intrapartum maternal fever, maternal GBS bacteriuria during current pregnancy.

A. GBS Symptoms
1. Early-onset typically presents with severe respiratory distress (rapid breathing, grunting, apnea), being fussy, lethargic, change in blood pressure.
2. Late-onset disease associated with meningitis, osteomyelitis, musculoskeletal pain, or decreased movement

B. Clinical Judgment Measures for neonates with sepsis
1. Prevent infection in the newborn
   a. Meticulous handwashing
   b. Maintain sterile technique during procedures.
   c. Universal precautions. Wear gloves; clean environment and equipment, change linens.
2. Review maternal chart for risk factors.
3. Monitor vital signs.
4. Monitor daily weights.
5. Monitor I&O, fluid status.
6. Maintain adequate nutrition: Calculate calorie, protein, and fluid needs according to weight.
7. Administer antibiotics, antivirals, antifungals as prescribed.
   a. Dosage is typically based on the neonate's weight in kilograms.

C. Labs
1. Blood, urine, CSF cultures
2. CBC with differential
3. C-reactive protein/Procalcitonin
4. Chemistry panel

D. Discharge Instructions
1. Provide emotional support to parents.
2. Provide instructions for medication use, follow-up care.

HESI HINT Sepsis can be indicated by both a temperature increase and a temperature decrease.

Preterm Newborn

Description: Infants born after 20 weeks gestation and before the completion of 37 weeks gestation. Additional classifications include late preterm infants, born from 34 (0/7) weeks' through 36 (6/7) weeks' gestation; and early term infants, born from 37 (0/7) weeks' through 38 (6/7) weeks' gestation. Supportive care for the neonate born at less than 38 weeks' gestation is based on the level of immaturity identified by gestational age and physical assessment.

A. Symptoms will vary according to system response to prematurity
1. Respiratory system. Signs of distress (apnea, tachypnea, flaring nares, retractions, seesaw breathing, grunting, abnormal blood gases) due to
   a. Lung immaturity
   b. Deficient surfactant levels
   c. Immaturity of respiratory center in brain causing apnea and bradycardia
2. Cardiovascular system. Signs of distress include abnormal rate and rhythm, persistent murmurs, differentials in pulse, dusky skin color, circumoral cyanosis.
3. Thermoregulation. Temperature instability related to
   a. Insufficient subcutaneous fat
   b. Larger ratio of body surface area to body weight
   c. Extended, open body position
   d. Immature hypothalamus
4. CNS System. Function is dependent on gestational age. Clinical signs may include
   a. Lethargy
   b. High-pitched cry or weak cry
   c. Hyperirritability, seizure activity
   d. Increased intracranial pressure
   e. Hypotonia
5. Nutrition problems related to intake and metabolism.
   a. Weak or absent suck, swallow, gag reflexes
   b. Difficulty coordinating suck and swallow
   c. Small stomach capacity
   d. Immature digestion process: lacks some gastric and pancreatic enzymes, decreased gastric emptying time
6. Immunity
   a. Shortage of stored maternal immunoglobulins
   b. Impaired ability to make antibodies
   c. increased risk for thin skin barrier

B. Clinical Judgment Measures
1. Conduct initial, rapid assessment at birth, perform resuscitation measures if needed, and transfer infant to neonatal intensive care unit (NICU) for advanced care.
2. Promote growth and development through an extrauterine environment that approximates that of the fetus.
3. Continual assessment of physiologic status of each system
4. Monitor vital signs.
5. Provide and monitor O_2 therapy.
6. Monitor thermoregulation.
   a. Place infant under radiant warmer.
   b. Infants may be placed in polyethylene bag to reduce heat and insensible water loss as applicable.
   c. Warm all things that touch newborn: hands, equipment, O_2, and surfaces.
7. Monitor fluid and electrolytes. Observe for signs of
   a. Hypoglycemia: Jitteriness, tremors, lethargy, hypotonia, apnea, weak or high-pitched cry, eye rolling, and seizures

b. Over hydration: Edema, tachycardia, bulging fontanels, crackles in lungs, increased weight gain

c. Dehydration: Sunken fontanels, poor skin turgor, and dry mucous membranes, weight loss, decreased urine output

d. Maintain urine output of 1 mL/kg/h and specific gravity of 1.005 to 1.012.

8. Maintain nutrition: Human milk is the best source of nutrition.

a. Administer nutrition (parental or enteral) as prescribed; infant may need IV or gavage feedings (see Box 6.7 and Fig. 6.20)

b. Once infant is able to tolerate oral nipple feedings, observe for coordinated suck-swallow ability and gag reflex as well as signs of fatigue or tachycardia.

c. Provide options for non-nutritive sucking as applicable; i.e., pacifier.

9. Support family and parental adjustment.

a. Initiate early visitation and accompany parents on visits to the NICU.

b. Provide information to parents daily.

c. Teach caregiving skills.

d. Continue to enhance parent–infant bonding. Physical contact is important to establish bonding.

e. Expect that some parents may experience anticipatory grief over potential loss of a preterm infant or the loss of the delivery of a healthy, full-term infant. Provide ongoing support.

10. Plan for discharge using multidisciplinary approach.

Respiratory Distress Syndrome

Description: Lung disorder that is caused by a lack of pulmonary surfactant. Complications include progressive atelectasis, respiratory acidosis, infection, intraventricular hemorrhage (IVH). The incidence and severity of respiratory distress syndrome (RDS) increase as gestational age decreases. Risk factors include prematurity, perinatal asphyxia (meconium aspiration, nuchal cord or cord prolapse), maternal diabetes, familial predisposition, cesarean birth without labor.

A. **Symptoms**

1. Usually appear immediately after or within 6 hours of birth but clinical course is variable
2. Lung sounds: crackles, poor air exchange
3. Pallor; cyanosis
4. Use of accessory muscles (retractions)
5. Nasal flaring, grunting
6. Apnea

B. **Clinical Judgment Measures**

1. Immediate initial assessment of respiratory status at birth and frequently thereafter
   a. Prepare for newborn resuscitation measures if needed.
2. Supportive measures
   a. Establish and maintain ventilation, oxygenation (may include positive-pressure ventilation, nasal CPAP, oxygen therapy).

b. Monitor pulse oximetry and arterial blood gases (ABGs).

3. Administer exogenous surfactant as ordered.
4. Monitor thermoregulation.
5. Maintain nutrition, fluids, electrolytes.
6. Monitor I&O.
7. Provide emotional support to parents and educate about ongoing interventions.

C. **Labs**

1. ABGs/CBC
2. CBC with differential; cultures (blood and urine) if sepsis suspected
3. Lumbar puncture may be considered.

BOX 6.7 Procedure for Inserting a Gavage Feeding Tube

Equipment

- Infant feeding tube
  - For infants less than 1 kg (2.2 lb), size 4 Fr
  - For infants more than 1 kg (2.2 lb), size 5—6 Fr
- Stethoscope
- Sterile water (lubricant)
- Syringe: 5—10 mL
- Tape, optional transparent dressing
- Gloves

Procedure

- Measure the length of the gavage tube from the tip of the nose to the earlobe to the midpoint between the xiphoid process and the umbilicus. Mark the tube with indelible ink or a piece of tape.
- Lubricate the tip of the tube with sterile water and insert gently through the nose or mouth until the predetermined mark is reached. Placement of the tube in the trachea will cause the infant to gag, cough, or become cyanotic.
- Check correct placement of the tube by:
  a. Pulling back on the plunger to aspirate stomach contents. Lack of stomach aspirate or fluid is not necessarily evidence of improper placement. Aspiration of respiratory secretions can be mistaken for stomach contents; however, the pH of the stomach contents is much lower (more acidic) than the pH of respiratory secretions.
  b. Injecting a small amount of air (1—3 mL) into the tube while listening for gurgling by using a stethoscope placed over the stomach. Ensure that the tube is inserted to the mark; air entering the stomach can be heard even if the tube is positioned above the gastroesophageal (cardiac) sphincter.
  c. Abdominal or chest radiography. This is the only definitive way to verify tube placement.
- Using tape or a transparent dressing, secure the tube in place and tape it to the cheek to prevent accidental dislodgment and incorrect positioning
  a. Assess the infant's skin integrity before taping the tube.
  b. Edematous or very preterm infants should have a pectin barrier placed under the tape to prevent abrasions, or a hydrocolloid adhesive should be used to prevent epidermal stripping.
- Tube placement *must* be assessed before each feeding.

From Lowdermilk, D. L., Perry, S. E., Cashion, K., Alden, K., & Olshansky, E. (2020). *Maternity and women's health care* (12th ed.). St. Louis, MO: Elsevier.

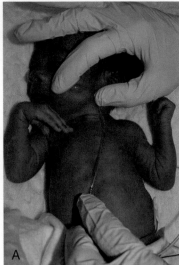

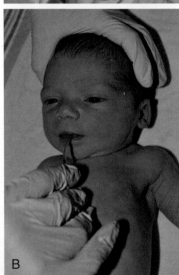

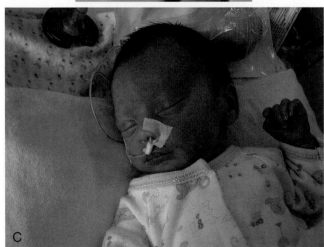

Fig. 6.20 Gavage Feeding. (A) Measurement of gavage feeding tube from tip of nose to earlobe and to midpoint between end of xiphoid process and umbilicus. Tape may be used to mark correct length on tube. For accurate measure the infant should be facing up. (B) Insertion of gavage tube using orogastric route. (C) Indwelling gavage tube, nasogastric route. After feeding by orogastric or nasogastric tube, infant is propped on right side or placed prone (preterm infant) for 1 hour to facilitate emptying of stomach into small intestine. (From Lowdermilk,

D. **Diagnostics**
   1. Chest x-ray
E. **Discharge**
   1. Educate on signs of respiratory distress.
   2. Teach parents importance of follow-up care.

Effects of Substance Abuse on the Neonate

Description: Maternal substance use and abuse can greatly impact the developing fetus. Polysubstance use is common and includes alcohol, tobacco, illicit drugs, and prescription drugs. In recent years, the opioid crisis has brought more attention to prescription opioid misuse and opioid use disorders. The effects of individual drugs as well as collective use may vary according to dose, route of administration, genotype of the mother or fetus, and timing of the drug exposure.

The newborn can experience withdrawal symptoms at birth or several hours or even days after birth. Neonatal abstinence syndrome (NAS) refers to the clinical signs that can be associated with withdrawal from any substance (Box 6.8). Neonatal opioid withdrawal syndrome (NOWS) refers to the clinical signs associated specifically with withdrawal from opioids.

A. **Symptoms of NAS**
B. **Consequences of maternal substance misuse and abuse**
   1. Many drugs have vasoconstrictive effects which cause hypoxemia and contribute to fetal growth delays (small size, IUGR) and fetal distress.
   2. Increased risk for spontaneous abortion, preterm labor and birth, placental abruption.
   3. Cognitive and developmental delays; often not fully recognized until childhood.
   4. Alcohol is specifically causative for an umbrella of fetal alcohol spectrum disorders (FASDs) that include fetal alcohol syndrome (FAS), partial FAS, alcohol-related neurodevelopmental disorder (ARND), alcohol-related birth defects (ARBDs), and neurobehavioral disorder associated with prenatal alcohol exposure.
      a. FAS is the most severe FASD and criteria for diagnosis include specific dysmorphic facial features, growth deficiency, and CNS abnormalities (Fig. 6.21).
C. **Clinical Judgment Measures**
   1. Review maternal prenatal record and history noting documentation of any substance use.
   2. Conduct a thorough assessment of the newborn, including gestational age, maturity, and behavior.
      a. Nurses typically document an additional, ongoing neonatal abstinence scoring system assessment to monitor changes in withdrawal symptoms and guide nonpharmacologic and pharmacologic treatment regimens. Two of the most common systems in use are the Finnegan Neonatal Abstinence Scoring System and the Eat, Sleep, Console (ESC) approach.

D. L., Perry, S. E., Cashion, K., Alden, K., & Olshansky, E. [2020]. *Maternity and women's health care* [12th ed., 10]. St. Louis, MO: Elsevier. A and B, Courtesy Cheryl Briggs, RNC, Annapolis, MD. C, Courtesy Randi and Jacob Wills, Clayton, NC.)

BOX 6.8   Signs of Neonatal Abstinence Syndrome

Acute Signs and Symptoms That May Persist for Several Weeks

Restlessness

Tremors (disturbed at first to undisturbed)

High-pitched cry

Increased muscle tone

Irritability and inconsolability

Increased deep tendon reflexes

Exaggerated Moro reflex

Seizures in approximately 1%—2% of heroin-exposed neonates and approximately 7% of methadone-exposed neonates

Subacute Signs and Symptoms That May Persist for 4—6 months

- Irritability
- Sleep pattern disturbance
- Hyperactivity
- Feeding problems
- Hypertonia

From Lowdermilk, D. L., Perry, S. E., Cashion, K., Alden, K., & Olshansky, E. (2020). *Maternity and women's health care* (12th ed.). St. Louis, MO: Elsevier. Data from Weiner, S. M., & Finnegan, L. P. (2016). Drug withdrawal in the neonate. In S. L. Gardner, B. S. Carter, M. Enzman-Hines, & J. A. Hernandez (Eds.), *Merenstein & Gardner's handbook of neonatal intensive care* (8th ed.). St. Louis, MO: Mosby.

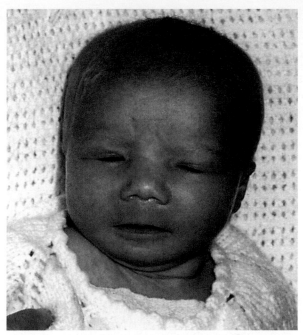

Fig. 6.21 Infant With Fetal Alcohol Syndrome. (From Markiewicz, M., & Abrahamson, E. [1999]. *Diagnosis in color: Neonatology*. St. Louis, MO: Mosby. From Lowdermilk, D. L., Perry, S. E., Cashion, K., Alden, K., & Olshansky, E. [2020]. *Maternity and women's health care* [12th ed., p. 777, 10]. St. Louis, MO: Elsevier.)

3. Monitor vital signs.

4. Monitor fluids and electrolytes.

5. Nonpharmacologic interventions include swaddling, gentle handling, decreasing environmental stimuli, providing nonnutritive suckling with a pacifier.

6. Administer pharmacologic agents as ordered. Pharmacotherapy is usually based on severity of withdrawal symptoms.

7. Provide education and support to parents.

D. **Labs**

1. Drug screen of urine, meconium, or umbilical cord testing may be ordered.

2. Possible labs:

   a. CBC

   b. Chemistry panel

E. **Discharge**

1. Teach parents about importance of ongoing follow-up care.

2. Provide community resources for referrals for addiction services, social services as indicated and desired.

💡 REVIEW OF NEWBORN COMPLICATIONS

1. List the major central nervous system danger signals that occur in the neonate.

2. A baby is delivered blue, limp, has a heart rate less than 100, and is gasping. The nurse dries the infant, suctions the oropharynx, and gently stimulates the infant while blowing O_2 over the face. The infant still does not respond. What is the next nursing action?

3. What conditions make oxygenation of the newborn more difficult?

4. What are the cardinal symptoms of sepsis in a newborn?

5. A premature baby is born and develops hypothermia. State the major nursing interventions to treat hypothermia.

6. What factors does a nurse look for in determining a newborn's ability to take in nourishment by nipple and mouth?

7. List four nursing interventions to enhance family and parent adjustment to a high-risk newborn.

8. List the risk factors for hyperbilirubinemia.

9. List the symptoms of hyperbilirubinemia in the neonate.

10. List three nursing interventions for the neonate undergoing phototherapy.

11. List the symptoms of neonatal abstinence syndrome.

12. Neonates with complications may receive too much stimulation in the form of invasive procedures and handling and too little developmentally appropriate stimulation and affection. How might such an infant respond?

13. How should a nurse determine the length of a tube needed for the oral gavage feeding of a newborn?

14. What are the two best ways to test for correct placement of the gavage tube in the infant's stomach?

15. What characteristics would the nurse expect to see in a neonate with fetal alcohol syndrome?

See Answer Key at the end of this text for suggested responses.

For more review, go to http://evolve.elsevier.com/HESI/RN for HESI's online study examinations.

NEXT-GENERATION NCLEX® EXAMINATION-STYLE QUESTIONS

| Health History | Nurses' Notes | Vital Signs | Lab Results |

Ms. Betty is a 34-year-old Caucasian woman (G5T3P1A0L4). She entered into prenatal care at 32 weeks' gestation. Obstetric history was significant for opioid use disorder currently being treated with methadone, and intimate partner violence. Ms. Betty reported contractions at 36 4/7 weeks' gestation and was directed to the ER for further evaluation.

Labor and Delivery Record

Ms. Betty presented to the ER in active labor and had a precipitous birth at 36 4/7 weeks' gestation. She was admitted to the postpartum floor and the infant boy was admitted to the NICU for observation.

Orders

Begin assessment using Neonatal Abstinence Scoring System, Vital signs, monitor lab values, IV fluids, I&O.

Instructions

Complete the diagram by selecting from the choices below to specify which potential condition the client is most likely experiencing, 2 actions to take, and 2 parameters the nurse would monitor to assess the client's progress.

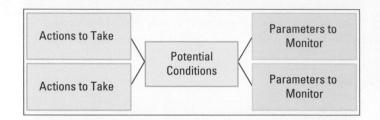

Nursing Actions	Potential Conditions	Parameters to Monitor
Gestational Assessment	Seizures	Observe skin color
Use of bright lights to enhance physical assessment skills	Excessive sleep patterns	Temperature
Serum glucose testing	Large for gestional age	Eye Contact
Swaddle infant with legs flexed	Neonatal hyperglycemia	Output
Provide extra feedings		Mother baby bonding

REFERENCES AND BIBLIOGRAPHY

American College of Obstetricians and Gynecologists (ACOG). (2019). ACOG Practice bulletin no. 202: Gestational hypertension and preeclampsia. *Obstetrics & Gynecology, 133*(1), e1–e25.

American College of Obstetricians and Gynecologists (ACOG). (2020). *Nutrition during pregnancy.* Retrieved from https://www.acog.org/womens-health/faqs/nutrition-during-pregnancy.

King, T., Brucker, M., Osborne, K., & Jevitt, C. (2019). *Varney's midwifery* (6th ed.). Burlington, MA: Jones & Bartlett Learning.

Lowdermilk, D. L., Perry, S. E., Cashion, K., Alden, K., & Olshansky, E. (2020). *Maternity and women's health care* (12th ed.). St. Louis, MO: Elsevier.

Schuiling, K., & Likis, F. (2022). *Gynecologic health care* (4th ed.). Burlington, MA: Jones & Bartlett Learning.

Psychiatric Nursing

The United States is amid a national mental health dilemma. More than 50% of all Americans experience some form of mental illness in their lifetime (NAMI, 2021), and over 20% of adults experience a mental illness each year (NAMI, 2021). Of those, only about 50% receive treatment. Nonetheless, many opportunities exist for nurses to intervene to improve outcomes of patients who seek mental health service. Psychiatric-mental health (PMH) nurses are ideally suited for identification and management of mental illness (Rice, 2019).

Psychiatric registered and practical nurses (PNs) focus their attention primarily on individuals with chronic or major mental illnesses and have assumed case management roles with multidisciplinary teams. Developments of psychopharmacology have changed treatment for mental illness. Consequently, the use of psychotropic medications to treat mental illness and manage symptoms and behaviors through psychopharmacology has led to a decrease in overall hospitalization and institutionalization, earlier discharges, and return of patients to community-dwelling status. This change has led to a major shift away from less-invasive forms of therapy, such as counseling, as the main psychiatric treatment to treatment with medications (Whitaker, 2011). Although many nurses are trained to use psychosocial interventions, the potential for nurses to deliver cognitive-behavioral therapy to those with common mental disorders has not been fully realized (Gournay, K., Kelly Winstanley, et al., 2018), yet the need for cognitive-behavioral therapies has not declined. The phenomenon of briefer inpatient stays, and fewer patient-nurse interactions has led to an ever-growing need for nurses to provide short patient-nurse encounters. Both registered and PNss conduct brief meetings providing short-term interventions that screen, identify, and prioritize individual care along the health care continuum from inpatient to community-based settings. Such interventions focus on safe and secure therapeutic environments of care, psychotropic psychoeducational administration, and management, and promote self-care and self-management for individuals with mental health conditions.

PNs perform necessary roles in caring for individuals who need psychiatric care and in supporting patients in managing their mental health and well-being (Delaney et al., 2017). Several nursing roles include providing patients with *safe*, therapeutic, and recovery-oriented treatment by means of *structure, support, and self-management*, which provides the framework for the clinical judgment measures for psychiatric nursing (Shattell & Delaney, 2015).

SAFETY

At the most basic level, inpatient treatment environments must be safe. A fundamental nursing responsibility is to ensure that staff and patients are free from harm (Delaney & Johnson, 2012). Safety is connected to reducing aggression, violence, and avoiding coercive interventions such as seclusion and restraints. Principles of safety also includes the techniques that nurses and other health care workers employ to avoid such confrontations or events, and to offer patients' choices in difficult situations. With an increased emphasis on and initiating measures to engage, anticipate risk, and intervene early prior for an escalating situation, safety has taken a broader meaning beyond preventing physical aggression, violence, or harm to include maintaining both the physical *and* trauma-informed care approach of psychological safety (Bryson et al., 2017). This requires nurses to promote positive interactions in patient settings and maintain supportive environments that promote healing and recovery (Delaney & Johnson, 2012).

Fundamentally, safety demands creating a physical environment that is free of any object that could be used for self-harm or that could easily harm others. Nurses and other staff members must consistently follow policies and protocols surrounding sharp objects (sharps) and other potentially dangerous items. Safety plans should include unit safety checks for contraband and for tracking incidents of safety breaches. Units must also have a system of precautions for monitoring aggression or suicide risks that determines the frequency of monitoring commensurate with the risk (Delaney et al., 2018).

Nurses must be aware of less obvious measures that assure safety, such as adequate staffing and ensuring that nurses and staff are appropriately trained. Training needs to be consistent with inpatient psychiatric assessment, early intervention, restraint reduction techniques, and noncoercive interventions and less restrictive measures (Scanlan, 2009). Nurses should evaluate their interventions by using debriefing techniques and reviewing data that improves patient outcomes and improve their practice (Azeem et al., 2011).

STRUCTURE

Structure encompasses a unit's rules and expectations. Many episodes of aggression occur following interactions where staff impose unit rules when dealing with a specific patient request (Bowers, 2014). In maintaining structure, staff constantly balance the need for consistency while avoiding infringements on the individual's sense of personal control (Voogt et al., 2013). To achieve this, balance demands that structure depend on nurses and other staff members' assessment skills, clinical judgment measures, and critical thinking.

These moment-to-moment decisions around rules and subsequent responses to an individual's behaviors also set the culture of the unit. A unit culture can easily slip into a rule-driven mindset, and the staff's role becomes enforcing expectations. Alternately, a unit can adopt a flexible interpretation of rules/norms prioritizing how to use structure to meet individual needs. The later approach helps to develop coping skills and begin to see caregivers as helpful to remain organized and in control.

SUPPORT

An important nursing role is to promote a culture of caring. Providing support also demands that nurses and staff interact with patients and engage with the individual (Polacek et al., 2015). Engagement that operates at the interpersonal level involves empathy, adjustment to the individual's experience, and understanding what is meaningful to them (Salamone-Violi et al., 2015) while maintaining boundaries (Ward, 2014). Nurses attempt to engage with patients by interacting at the interpersonal level, directing attention to establishing a presence, and tailoring responses based on the patients' individual experiences (Delaney et al., 2017). Patients may lack insight into connecting events to behaviors and emotions or they may be unable to articulate emotions and distress in a manner of behavior that is appropriate (Foster & Smedley, 2016). For example, patients on inpatient units struggle with maintaining control of their behaviors or managing emotions such as anger and frustration (Delaney, 2018). Nurses must recognize expressions of distress through behaviors and emotions and then interpret the underlying meaning of the behaviors (Geanellos, 2002).

SELF-MANAGEMENT

The final important aspect of engagement is related to activities that foster self-management among patients. This includes educating patients on health and/or management of symptoms associated with an illness (Delaney et al., 2000). Typically, nurses should employ a collaborative problem-solving approach (Bobier et al., 2009; Pollastri et al., 2013) when developing strategies to manage psychiatric patients.

Self-management strategies should be geared to the population of clients being treated on the unit. For instance, for children hospitalized secondary to suicidal ideations, interventions should be geared toward teaching coping behaviors but delivered in the context of a supportive, collaborative approach (Montreuil et al., 2015). For adolescents, specific strategies to address suicidal thoughts may include family interventions and individual skills training around emotional regulation and problem solving (Glenn et al., 2014).

THERAPEUTIC MODALITIES

PNs should make themselves aware of the current treatment modalities that they or their patients may encounter in mental health and psychiatric treatment. These may include a range of options such as electroconvulsive therapy (ECT) or individual and group therapy. Most of these options strive to assist individuals with the promotion of mental health for individuals, and social and family functioning.

Electroconvulsive therapy (ECT). ECT involves using electrically induced seizures for psychiatric purposes. It is used for the severely depressed clients who do not respond to antidepressant medications and therapy. PNs assist with ECT because of their close involvement with patients before and after the procedure. Although ECT has been found to be one of the most robust and rapid treatments for severe depression, it is widely underused partly because of negative perceptions and inaccurate knowledge about the treatment (Tsai et al., 2021). PNs must apprise themselves of the knowledge and attitude of the nursing staff working in ECT rooms, which can have a direct impact on the quality of their nursing practice.

1. Client care prior to ECT
   a. Prepare client by teaching about ECT.
   b. Avoid using the word "shock."
   c. Assist the RN with administration of medication before and after the procedure.
   d. Provide an emergency cart, suction equipment, and oxygen available in the room.
2. Client care post ECT
   a. Maintain patent airway; the client is unconscious immediately after ECT.
   b. Check vital signs frequently according to institutional policy.
   c. Reorient client after ECT.
   d. Common complaints that often occur after anesthesia is administered may include modest headache, mild muscle soreness, moderate nausea, and retrograde pain.

> **HESI HINT** Vomiting by an unconscious post electroconvulsive therapy client can lead to aspiration. Remember to maintain a patent airway in these clients.

? REVIEW OF THERAPEUTIC COMMUNICATION AND TREATMENT MODALITIES

1. A nurse plans to teach a patient about a new diagnosis of bipolar disorder so that the patient can be more aware of fluctuating moods over time. This would be best be described as:
   a. Self-management
   b. Safety
   c. Structure
   d. Therapy
2. On an inpatient psychiatric unit, clients are expected to get up at a certain time, attend breakfast at a certain time, and come for their medication at the correct time. What form of therapy is incorporated into this unit?
3. The 10-year-old boy, his sister, his mother, and his mother's live-in boyfriend are asked to attend a therapy meeting. Who is the "client" that will be treated during this session?
4. Describe the nursing interventions used to care for a client during and after electroconvulsive therapy.

See Answer Key at the end of this text for suggested responses.

COMMON MENTAL HEALTH TREATMENTS AND INTERVENTIONS

Although nurses do not typically participate or conduct therapy, they should be aware that individuals they encounter or care for may be participating in therapy. Nurses who understand the basic goals and structures of therapies can help patients by showing empathy for the challenges that patients' face. Nurses can identify patient problems and concerns or make recommendations to health providers for referral or treatment. Moreover, nurses are expected to provide brief clinical interventions when interacting with individuals in their care. Knowledge of the intervention types available can help nurses to remain consistent with the patients' therapy and assist in the delivery of nurse-driven brief clinical interventions.

Group Therapy

Group therapy is a form of treatment that is reserved for individuals with various issues and may include addiction, anger management, depression, and anxiety. An important aspect of group therapy is that it brings people together and creates a dynamic of support and inclusion. Because each participant is present for a similar purpose, participants can feel comfortable about sharing problems and struggles with the group. In addition to togetherness and support, group therapy provides an excellent opportunity for its participants to learn and listen. Hearing about others' challenges can be insightful and help the participant to gain alternative perspectives. The benefits and flexibility that comes along with group therapy are one of the many reasons why group therapy is commonly used. Groups may be closed (a predetermined group) or open (members may join and leave) and focus on psychoeducation, providing support, psychotherapy, or self-help. The advantages associated with groups include developing socializing techniques, providing opportunities for feedback, and promoting a feeling of universality (not being alone in experiencing problems).

Interpersonal Therapy

Interpersonal therapy is a brief, attachment-focused form of therapy that aims to help patients address challenges in managing relationships and ultimately to improve the symptoms of mood disorders, such as depression (Van Hees et al., 2013). This type of therapy is commonly used because healthy relationships with other people is extremely conducive to an individual's success and opportunities in life. Someone who struggles to get along with other people will experience difficulties in the workplace and other critical aspects of life.

Interpersonal therapy largely focuses on relationship stressors and the root cause of the issues that impact the patient's ability to maintain healthy relationships with those around them. The underlying cause can vary depending on a series of factors; however, once the root cause of the problem is identified and addressed, the patient can begin to heal and learn appropriate methods for developing healthy, positive relationships.

Family Therapy

While family therapy is common, it does share a separate distinction from other types of individual psychological treatment. Family therapy can help members of a family to define or explain problems in relational networks (Colapinto, 2019) or terms of family structures, boundaries, hierarchies, roles, rules, and patterns of interaction and coalitions (Tadros & Finney, 2018). One important goal of family therapy is to strengthen family interactions and to improve behavioral outcomes (Collyer & Eisler, 2020).

Brief Interventions

Brief interventions are typically face-to-face sessions, with or without the addition of written materials such as self-help manuals, workbooks, or self-monitoring diaries with the purpose of addressing specific problems (Heather, 1995, p. 287). The primary goal of brief interventions is to raise awareness of problems such as (alcohol and substance use) and then to recommend a specific change or activity or motivate the client to change (Miller & Munoz, 1982; Rollnick & Miller, 1991). The brevity and lower delivery costs of these brief approaches make them ideal mechanisms for use in settings where cost and time constraints are a consideration. The person delivering the brief intervention is usually trained to be empathic, warm, and encouraging and nonconfrontational. Brief interventions ranged from relatively unstructured counseling and feedback to more formal structured therapy (Miller & Hester, 1986). Treatment staff or other professionals may deliver brief interventions, and do not require extensive training, making it suitable for nurses at various levels of experience and education. A PN may identify a problem and ask how much the problems interfere with daily functioning and then make suggestions for further treatment, self-help, or to continue to focus on the problem as opportunities arise on the unit.

> **HESI HINT** A practical nurse may use any private interaction with a patient as an opportunity for a properly executed brief intervention.

A PN may identify clients who may benefit from types of therapies. The PN can arrange for therapy, schedule an appropriately trained therapist, and encourage and provide support for attendance.

? REVIEW OF COMMON MENTAL HEALTH TREATMENTS AND INTERVENTIONS

Practical nurses (PNs) may have assessed clients on a unit and viewed each as an individual that would benefit from tailored interventions that address personal, emotional, mental health, and family needs. This contrasts with a "fits-all" approach.

1. A client arrives to a busy emergency department smelling of alcohol after an altercation with his significant other. The client states this has happened before while drinking. The PN asks "How often is alcohol a factor in arguments?" This is an example of?
2. Describe the PN's role in preparing a client for electroconvulsive therapy.

Continued

❓ REVIEW OF COMMON MENTAL HEALTH TREATMENTS AND INTERVENTIONS—cont'd

3. A client has received an individualized plan in the morning describing scheduled therapies for the entire day. What is the proposed purpose of such an intervention?

4. A 55-year-old client arrives to an inpatient unit angry and verbally abusive to staff. How should a PN approach and manage this situation?

5. A 24-year-old was admitted after a suicide attempt. The client expresses lots of problems getting along with friends. What types of therapies might be appropriate for this client and why?

6. A 61-year-old client with schizophrenia states, "I never could trust anyone in my life, including you." Describe how a nurse may explore for distortions in thinking.

See Answer Key at the end of this text for suggested responses.

PSYCHIATRIC ASSESSMENT STRATEGIES FOR INPATIENTS: RESOURCES WITH A PURPOSE

Adults with psychiatric conditions who are admitted as inpatients need to be assessed carefully to ensure they receive the best possible care. Although PNs do not diagnose, a PN's observations can help providers in the formulation of diagnoses and a treatment plan. PNs should observe and record pertinent information based on patient's statement, behaviors, family history, chief complaint, and other information such a circumstance surrounding admission. The RN, who is familiar with psychiatric diagnoses, their presentation, and psychopathology, completes the clinical assessment.

Schizophrenia and Schizoaffective Disorder

Clinicians consider five domains when assessing patients for schizophrenia or schizoaffective disorder—delusions, hallucinations, disorganized thinking, and speech, grossly disorganized or abnormal motor behavior (including catatonia), and negative symptoms.

> **HESI HINT** Catatonia occurs across several categories of disorders and can be present in depressive, bipolar, and psychotic disorders.

Delusions are fixed beliefs not amenable to change even considering conflicting evidence (excluding religious beliefs commonly held in the community).

Examples include:
- delusions of persecution ("someone is out to get me")
- nihilistic delusions ("something bad is going to happen")
- somatic delusions ("something is terribly wrong with me")
- control delusions ("someone is making me do something")
- thought-withdrawal delusions ("aliens are stealing my thoughts")
- thought-insertion delusions ("aliens are putting thoughts into my head")
- thought-broadcasting delusions ("everyone can hear my thoughts")
- referential delusions ("people are talking about me")
- delusions of grandeur (for instance, a patient thinks she's royalty and should be treated as such)
- erotomania (a false belief that others are in love with the patient).

Hallucinations are perception-like experiences that occur without an external stimulus. In schizophrenics, auditory hallucinations (AHs) are more common than visual or other hallucinations. Visual hallucinations (VHs) may be illusions (misinterpretation of visual stimuli; for instance, a shadow becomes a menacing black dog). VHs can occur with other medical conditions, such as alcohol withdrawal, or may manifest as an aura with a seizure or brain injury. AHs and VHs rarely occur at the same time.

Disorganized thinking and speech may include:
- circumstantiality (verbalization of concrete details that's slow in getting to the point)
- concrete thinking (making literal rather than figurative interpretations; for instance, the patient answers "I took the bus" when asked how he or she ended up in the hospital)
- clang associations (rhyming words and not completing sentences)
- loose associations (sentences or phrases not logically connected to those coming before or after)
- tangentiality (going from topic to topic without making a point)
- neologisms (making up words that have meaning only to the patient)
- "word salad" (a stream of unconnected words).

Grossly disorganized and abnormal motor behavior may manifest as:
- unpredictable behavior that interferes with task completion or causes agitation
- failure to follow instructions to move
- holding a fixed bizarre position
- lack of verbal or physical response
- purposeless or repetitive movements
- staring at staff
- catatonic stupor not caused by a physical problem.
- negative symptoms refer to lack of something, including:
  - lack of emotional expressions
  - avolition (lack of motivation for goal-oriented tasks)
- alogia (decreased speech)
- anhedonia (lack of pleasure from activities previously enjoyed)
- a sociality (lack of interest in others).

A schizophrenic patient with negative symptoms seems to lack personality.

Clinical signs and symptoms of schizoaffective disorder include:
- a major mood episode of either major depression or mania for at least 1 month
- at least 2 weeks of delusions or hallucinations that don't occur at the same time as a major mood episode.

Clinical Assessment Tips

If your patient seems to be hearing voices, observe him or her to determine the following:

- Is the patient talking to a wall or an empty space?
- Is he or she mumbling or yelling? If so, can you make out words or themes?
- Are the patient's eyes darting, staring, or frightened?
- Does the patient seem to be lost in thought?
- Is the patient thought-blocking (stopped talking abruptly)?
- What is the patient's affect (nonverbal expression of feelings, including posture, facial expression, and tone of voice)?

Try to determine if the patient seems internally preoccupied or is behaving in a way that's consistent with AHs. Once you've formed general impressions, ask the patient questions such as the following:

- Are the voices frightening?
- What are they saying?
- Are they telling you to do something?
- Are they loud?
- Do you believe the voices?
- How often do you hear them?

Keep in mind that paranoid patients may not admit to hearing voices until they have developed trust in you or until antipsychotic medications start to take effect. Try to identify a theme to what the voices are saying; for example, are they worried something bad will happen? Unfortunately, voices rarely go away completely even when the patient is well-managed on medications (Table 7.1).

Bipolar I Disorder

Bipolar I disorder involves manic episodes that last at least 1 week or manic symptoms severe enough to require immediate hospital care. Mixed episodes (mania and depression at the same time) may occur as well. Some patients also experience episodes of hypomania (similar to mania but less intense). The episodes do not stem from a medical condition or substance use.

Clinical signs and symptoms of bipolar I disorder include:
- persistent elevated mood, including high energy output, expansiveness, persistence, task, and goal orientation, or marked irritability
- significant behavior changes, such as grandiose behavior, constantly moving without purpose, participating in high-risk activities, such as sex with strangers, or incessant rapid speech.

In many cases, patients with bipolar disorder require hospitalization to protect themselves from their own behavior.

TABLE 7.1 Clinical Judgment Measures: Spectrum of Schizophrenia

Clinical Judgment Measure	Assessment Characteristics
Recognize Cues	• Delusions • Hallucinations • Disorganized speech • Disorganized behavior
Analyze Cues	• Assess disturbance in perceptions • Assess affect • Assess interpersonal relationships
Prioritize Cues	• Establish trust • Help with physical hygiene and Activities of daily living (ADL) • Use clear, simple concrete terms when talking to client • Set limits on behavior • Avoid stressful situations
Solutions	• Encourage client to identify positive characteristics related to self • Praise socially acceptable behavior
Actions	• Provide safe environment • Establish trust
Evaluate Outcomes	• Determine ability to return to ADL • Communication is linear, organized, rational, and logical.

Clinical Assessment Tips

When assessing the patient, ask yourself these questions:
- What is the patient's mood? (Document this in the patient's own words.)
- What is the patient's affect? (How does the patient appear to be feeling?)
- What is the quality and content of the patient's behavior and speech?

Documentation Tips

Describe specific risks of the patient's manic behavior, including taking sexual risks, antagonizing others, making intrusive phone calls, making life-defining decisions, or losing weight because the patient can't sit long enough to eat a meal. Keep in mind that a patient with bipolar I disorder may be in the depressed phase of the condition, so be sure to assess for depression, suicide risk, and marked shifts in mood or affect. When documenting the quality and content of the patient's behavior and speech, be as specific as possible.

Major Depressive Disorder

Major depressive disorder causes severe symptoms that affect how the patient thinks and feels. It also may affect such activities as sleeping, eating, and working. The patient must have signs or symptoms for at least 2 weeks. In 2014, an estimated 15.7 million adults aged 18 or older in the United States had at least one major depressive episode in the past year, making it one of the most common mental health disorders.

Essential information to communicate during care transitions includes:

- pain management history
- pain assessment tools and scales used
- complementary and pharmacologic interventions tried and shown to be either effective or ineffective
- patient goals for pain outcomes.

Clinical decision-making tools, such as alerts in the electronic health record regarding inappropriate or high-alert medications, flag alerts for frail elders, and embedded standard communication and pain assessment tools, may promote effective communication and documentation.

Clinical Signs and Symptoms

Patients with a major depressive disorder have a depressed mood or loss of pleasure or interest in activities that usually provide pleasure. Other signs and symptoms include:

- unintentional weight loss or gain (5% or more in 1 month)
- insomnia or hypersomnia
- psychomotor agitation
- fatigue
- feelings of worthlessness or excessive guilt
- decreased ability to concentrate
- suicidal thoughts or a suicide attempt.

Be aware that depression differs from dementia and delirium. Dementia is a gradual neurocognitive decline involving decreased logic and memory; for instance, patients try to answer questions but give the wrong answer. Delirium is marked by sudden onset of rapid fluctuations in behavior and level of consciousness; it stems from medication, substance use, or a medical condition. Delirium usually is a medical emergency.

Clinical Assessment Tips

When assessing patients with a suspected major depressive disorder, start by evaluating their risk for suicidal ideation or behavior (Table 7.2). Ask the patient how he or she is feeling and document the answer in the patient's own words; for instance, "Patient states that mood is happy." Also ask the patient to rate his or her mood on a scale of 1 to 10, with 10 indicating the most severe feelings of depression. Note the patient's affect (how he or she appears to be feeling) and determine if it matches the stated mood. Next, assess the amount and pattern of the patient's sleep, fluid and food intake, recent weight changes, activity and behavior level, and self-care (noting how much prompting or assistance the patient needs). Keep in mind that depressed patients typically give brief answers or may say they don't care or don't know the answer. Also, patients with depression who have an unknown history of manic or hypomanic episodes may be tipped into a manic phase when they begin antidepressants without also taking mood-stabilizing medication.

Clinical Judgment Measures

A. Maintain client's physical health. Provide nutrition, rest, and hygiene.
B. Provide a safe environment.
C. Decrease environmental stimulation.
D. Implement suicide precautions.
E. Use consistent approach to minimize manipulative behavior.
F. Use frequent, brief contacts to decrease anxiety.
G. Implement constructive limit setting.
H. Avoid giving attention to bizarre behavior.
I. Try to meet needs as soon as possible to keep client from becoming aggressive.
J. Provide small frequent feedings of food.
K. Engage in simple, active, noncompetitive activities.
L. Avoid distracting or stimulating activities in the evening to help promote sleep and rest.
M. Praise self-control, acceptable behavior.
N. Promote family involvement in therapy, teaching, and medication compliance.
O. Assist the RN with the administration of sedatives and antipsychotics as prescribed (Table 7.3).

TABLE 7.2 **Columbia-Suicide Severity Rating Scale**		
	Past 1 Month	
1) Have you wished you were dead or wished you could go to sleep and not wake up?		
2) Have you had any thoughts about killing yourself?		
If **YES** to 2, answer questions 3, 4, 5, and 6. If **NO** to 2, go directly to question 6.		
3) Have you thought about how you might do this?		
4) Have you had any intention of acting on these thoughts of killing yourself, as opposed to you having the thoughts but you definitely would not act on them?	High Risk	
5) Have you started to work out or worked out the details of how to kill yourself? Did you intend to carry out this plan?	High Risk	
Always Ask Question 6	**Life-time**	**Past 3 Months**
6) Have you done anything, started to do anything, or prepared to do anything to end your life?		High Risk
Examples: Collected pills, obtained a gun, gave away valuables, wrote a will or suicide note, held a gun but changed your mind, cut yourself, tried to hang yourself, etc.		

From Posner, K., Brown, G. K., Stanley, B., Brent, D. A., Yershova, K. V., & Oquendo, M. A., et al. (2011). The Columbia-Suicide Severity Rating Scale: Initial validity and internal consistency findings from three multisite studies with adolescents and adults. *American Journal of Psychiatry, 168*(12), 1266–1277.

TABLE 7.3 Antipsychotic Drugs

Traditional Drugs	Indications	Adverse Reactions	Nursing Implications
Phenothiazines • Chlorpromazine HCl (Thorazine) • Trifluoperazine HCl (Stelazine) • Thioridazine HCl (Mellaril) • Perphenazine (Trilafon) • Triflupromazine (Vesprin) • Loxapine (Loxitane)	• To control psychotic behavior: hallucinations, delusions, and bizarre behavior	• Drowsiness • Orthostatic hypotension • Weight gain • Anticholinergic effects • Extrapyramidal effects • Pseudoparkinsonism • Akathisia • Dystonia • Tardive dyskinesia • Photosensitivity • Blood dyscrasias: granulocytosis, leukopenia • Neuroleptic malignant syndrome	• Extrapyramidal effects are *major* concern • Monitor elderly clients closely • Takes 2–3 weeks to achieve therapeutic effect. • Keep client supine for 1 h after administration and advise to change positions slowly because of effects of orthostatic hypotension. • Teach client to avoid: • Alcohol. • Sedatives (potentiate effect of central nervous system (CNS) depressants). • Antacids (reduce absorption of drug).
• Fluphenazine HCl (Prolixin)	• To control psychotic behavior • Useful in treatment of psychomotor agitation associated with thought disorders	• Same as other phenothiazines	• Absorbed slowly. • Used with noncompliant clients because it can be administered IM once every 14 days.
Nonphenothiazines • Haloperidol (Haldol) • Thiothixene HCl (Navane) • Pimozide (Orap)	• To control psychotic behavior • Less sedative than phenothiazines	• Severe extrapyramidal reactions • Leukocytosis • Blurred vision • Dry mouth • Urinary retention	• Teach client to avoid alcohol. • Orap is used only for Tourette's syndrome.
Long Acting • Fluphenazine decanoate (Prolixin Decanoate) • Haloperidol decanoate (Haldol Decanoate)	• Clients who require supervision with medication regimens	• Similar to Prolixin and Haldol	• Similar to Haldol and Prolixin. • Prolixin Decanoate can be given every 7–28 days. • Haldol Decanoate can be given every 4 weeks. • Requires several months to reach steady-state drug levels.
Atypical Antipsychotic Drugs • Risperidone (Risperdal) • Olanzapine (Zyprexa) • Quetiapine (Seroquel) • Aripiprazole (Abilify) • Ziprasidone (Geodon) • Clozapine (Clozaril)	• Treat positive and negative symptoms of schizophrenia without significant extrapyramidal syndrome (EPS) • Clients who have not responded well to typical antipsychotics or who have side effects with typical antipsychotics • Fewer side effects • Clozapine has superior efficacy in clients who have been treatment resistant	• Risperdal: neuroleptic malignant syndrome (NMS), EPS, dizziness, GI symptoms (nausea, constipation), anxiety • Zyprexa: drowsiness, dizziness, EPS, agitation • Seroquel: drowsiness, dizziness, headache, EPS, weight gain, anticholinergic effects • Clozaril: agranulocytosis, drowsiness, dizziness, gastrointestinal (GI) symptoms, neuroleptic malignant syndrome	• Monitor white blood cells (WBC) weekly for first 6 months, then biweekly. • Baseline vital signs (VS) and ECG; report abnormal VS. • Monitor for symptoms of NMS and EPS. • Teach to change positions slowly. • Abilify is a new class of antipsychotic drugs, dopamine system stabilizers (DSSs) for schizophrenia, and acute bipolar mania. • Seroquel: monitor lipids, especially for obese, diabetic, or hypertensive clients.

P. Redirect negative behavior or verbal abuse in a calm, firm, nonjudgmental nondefense manner.
  1. Suggest a walk or another physical activity.
  2. Set limits on intrusive behavior.
  3. If a client becomes totally out of control, RN should administer medication or use seclusion if the client is a danger to self or others.

HESI HINT Clients who are experiencing mania can be very caustic toward authority figures. Be prepared for personal putdowns. Avoid arguing or becoming defensive.

❓ REVIEW OF MOOD DISORDERS

1. Identify the physiologic changes that commonly occur with depression.
2. A client who has been withdrawn and tearful comes to breakfast one morning smiling and interacting with her peers. Before breakfast, she gave her roommate her favorite necklace. What actions should the nurse take and why?
3. Name the components of a suicide assessment.
4. A client on your unit refuses to go to group therapy. What is the most appropriate nursing intervention?
5. A client is standing on a table loudly singing "The Star-Spangled Banner" and is encircled by sheets, which have been set afire. In order of priority, describe appropriate nursing actions.

See Answer Key at the end of this text for suggested responses.

ALCOHOL WITHDRAWAL SYNDROME

Alcohol withdrawal syndrome occurs when a person reduces or stops consuming alcohol, especially after a period of heavy or prolonged drinking. Severe withdrawal symptoms require medical attention and possibly hospitalization for detoxification.

Clinical Signs and Symptoms

- Autonomic hyperactivity (diaphoresis, increased pulse)
- Tremor (usually of the hands)
- Insomnia
- Nausea and vomiting
- Hallucinations or illusions, which typically start as sensitivity (for instance, the patient complains that lights are too bright, or sounds are too loud) and then develop into hallucinations (usually tactile or visual). Other signs and symptoms include anxiety, general tonic-clonic seizures, inability to sit still, and constant purposeless movement or fidgeting (Table 7.4).

Clinical Judgment Measures

- Maintain safety, nutrition, hygiene, and rest.
- Obtain a blood alcohol level on admission or when the client appears intoxicated.

- Monitor vital signs
- I&O
- Observe for DTs.
- Prevent aspiration: implement seizure precautions.
- Reduce environment stimuli.
- RN to medicate with antianxiety medication (Table 7.5).
- Provide high-protein diet and adequate fluid intake.
- Provide vitamin supplements (B1 and B complex).
- Provide emotional support.
- Provide care during withdrawal:
  - Use a direct, nonjudgmental attitude.
  - Confront denial and rationalization (main coping styles used by alcoholics).
  - Confront any manipulation.
  - Set short-term realistic goals.
  - Help increase self-esteem.
  - Explore ways to increase frustration tolerance without alcohol.
  - Identify ways to decrease loneliness.
  - Identify support groups (AA).
  - Identify friendships not related to drinking.
  - Provide group and family therapy (family AA groups).

Assist the RN with patient and family teaching regarding the side effects of disulfiram (Anabuse) (Table 7.6).

Encourage an outpatient day center or AA when the patient is discharged.

OPIOID WITHDRAWAL

Opioids include heroin, methadone, oxycodone, hydrocodone, and certain other substances. Heavy opioid use over several weeks changes brain chemistry. Opioid withdrawal occurs when the person stops using opioids.

Clinical Signs and Symptoms

Patients with opioid withdrawal may have insomnia or a sad or depressed mood. Physiologic signs and symptoms may include:
- nausea and vomiting
- muscle ache
- lacrimation (tearing eyes)
- rhinorrhea (running nose)
- pupil dilation
- piloerection
- diaphoresis
- diarrhea
- yawning
- fever.

Clinical Judgment Measures

A. Assess level of consciousness and vital signs. (Rapid withdrawal can be fatal for persons addicted to barbiturates and antianxiety medications and hypnotics.)
B. Monitor I&O and electrolytes.
C. Implement suicide precautions if assessment indicates risk.
D. Provide adequate nutrition, hydration, and rest.

TABLE 7.4 Drug Withdrawal and Overdose Symptoms

Drugs	Withdrawal	Overdose	Effect
Opiates • Heroin • Morphine • Codeine • Opium • Methadone	• Watery eyes, runny nose, dilated pupils • Anxiety • Diaphoresis, fever • Nausea, vomiting, and diarrhea • Achiness • Abdominal cramps • Insomnia • Tachycardia	• Respiratory depression leading to respiratory arrest • Circulatory depression leading to cardiac arrest • Unconsciousness leading to coma • Death	• General physical and mental deterioration • Rapid tolerance • Impaired judgment
• Cocaine	• Depression • Fatigue • Disturbed sleep • Anxiety • Psychomotor agitation	• Tachycardia • Pupillary dilation • Increased BP • Cardiac dysrhythmias • Perspiration, chills • Nausea, vomiting	• Psychological dependence • Tolerance within hours or days
• Amphetamines	• Depression • Fatigue • Disturbed sleep	• Restlessness • Tremors • Rapid respiration • Confusion • Assaultive behavior • Hallucinations • Panic	• Paranoid delusions
• Hallucinogenics	• No withdrawal	• Panic • Psychosis	• Flashbacks • Impaired judgment

Antianxiety Drugs
• Benzodiazepines:
  • diazepam (Valium)
  • oxazepam (Serax)
  • lorazepam (Ativan)
	• Tremors
	• Agitation
	• Anxiety
	• Abdominal cramps
	• Grand mal seizures
		• Drowsiness
		• Confusion
		• Hypotension
		• Coma
		• Death
			• Withdrawal occurs if there is abrupt cessation
			• Temporary psychosis

TABLE 7.5 Antianxiety Drugs

Drugs	Indications	Reactions	Nursing Implications
Benzodiazepines • Chlordiazepoxide HCl (Librium) • Diazepam (Valium) • Alprazolam (Xanax) • Clorazepate dipotassium (Tranxene) • Lorazepam (Ativan)	• Reduce anxiety • Induce sedation, relax muscles, inhibit convulsions • Treat alcohol and drug withdrawal symptoms • Safer than sedative-hypnotics	• Sedation • Drowsiness • Ataxia • Dizziness • Irritability • Blood dyscrasias • Habituation and increased tolerance	• Administer at bedtime to alleviate daytime sedation. • Greatest harm occurs when combined with alcohol or other CNS depressants. • Instruct to avoid driving or working around equipment. • Gradually taper drug therapy due to withdrawal effects; do not stop suddenly. • Used only as short-term drug and as supplement to other medications.
Nonbenzodiazepines • Buspirone (BuSpar)	• Reduces anxiety • Helps to control symptoms such as insomnia, sweating, and palpitations associated with anxiety	• Dizziness	• Takes several weeks for antianxiety effects to become apparent. • Intended for short-term use.
• Zolpidem (Ambien) • Ramelteon (Rozerem)	• Used for short-term treatment of insomnia • Approved for long-term treatment of insomnia • Selectively binds to melatonin receptors	• Daytime drowsiness • Dizziness	• Give with food 1–1½ h before bedtime. • Appropriate for clients with delayed sleep onset.

TABLE 7.6   Alcohol Deterrents

Drugs	Indications	Adverse Reactions	Nursing Implications
• Disulfiram (Antabuse)	• Treatment of alcoholism; aversion therapy • Interferes with breakdown of alcohol causing an accumulation of acetaldehyde (a byproduct of alcohol in the body)	• Severe side effects occur if alcohol is consumed • Nausea and vomiting • Hypotension, headaches • Rapid pulse and respirations • Flushed face and bloodshot eyes • Confusion • Chest pain • Weakness, dizziness	• Teach client what to expect if alcohol is consumed while taking the drug. • Be aware that some alcoholic clients use the side effects as a means of "punishing" themselves or as a form of masochism, and if a client repeatedly consumes alcohol while taking the drug, the health care provider should be notified. • Persons with serious heart disease, diabetes, epilepsy, liver impairment, or mental illness should not take Antabuse. • Use in motivated clients who have shown the ability to stay sober.
• Acamprosate (Campral)	• Treatment of alcohol dependence by reducing anxiety and unpleasant effects that trigger resuming drinking • Balances Gamma-aminobutyric acid (GABA) and glutamate neurotransmitters	• Headache • Nausea and diarrhea	• Helps reduce cravings • Does not reduce or eliminate withdrawal symptoms

E. Assist RN in the administration of medications according to detoxification protocol of medical unit.

F. Phenothiazines, benzodiazepines, beta-blockers, clonidine, and anticonvulsants may be used to decrease the discomfort of withdrawal.

G. Confront denial
   1. Focus on the substance abuse problem.
   2. Confront the placing of blame on external problems.

H. Reinforce reality in simple, concrete terms.

I. Encourage verbal expressions of anger and depression.

Stimulant Withdrawal

Stimulants include amphetamine, methylphenidate (Ritalin), amphetamine with dextroamphetamine (Adderall), cocaine, and certain other substances. They cause changes in brain chemistry after short periods of use and have a short half-life. Withdrawal occurs after the person stops using stimulants.

Clinical Signs and Symptoms

Patients with stimulant withdrawal may have a dysphoric mood along with:

- vivid and scary dreams
- insomnia or hypersomnia
- increased appetite
- psychomotor retardation
- inability to sit still
- constant, purposeless movement or fidgeting

Key Points to Remember

When assessing patients for mental illness or substance withdrawal, always assess the risk for suicidal and aggressive behavior, regardless of the patient's specific diagnosis. Also, be aware that a patient may not admit to experiencing certain symptoms until he or she trusts you. Finally, be sure to fully document your observations in the health record so psychiatric physicians and nurse practitioners can more easily diagnose the patient's specific problem using the *Diagnostic and Statistical Manual of Mental Disorders*, 5th Edition (DSM-5).

❓ REVIEW OF SUBSTANCE ABUSE DISORDERS

1. A client was admitted 3 days ago to the medical unit for a gastrointestinal bleed. His BP and pulse rate gradually increased, and he developed a low-grade fever. What assessment data should the nurse obtain?

2. What physical signs might indicate that a client is abusing intravenous medications?

3. What behaviors would indicate to a nurse that an employee has a possible substance abuse problem? To whom would the nurse report these concerns?

4. A client becomes extremely agitated, abusive, and very suspicious. He is currently undergoing detoxification from alcohol with chlordiazepoxide (Librium) 50 mg every 6 h. What nursing actions are indicated?

5. A client in the third week of a cocaine rehabilitation program returns from an unsupervised pass. The nurse notices that he is euphoric and is socializing with the other clients more than he has in the past. What nursing actions are indicated?

See Answer Key at the end of this text for suggested responses.

NEXT-GENERATION NCLEX EXAMINATION-STYLE QUESTIONS

Orders

Admit to Psy. Ward. Monitor I&O, daily weights, suicide precautions, administer lithium, sedatives, and antipsychotics, obtain routine bloodwork, provide safe environment

Health History	Nurses' Notes	Vital Signs	Lab Results

Carrie Smith, a 29-year woman, is admitted to the emergency room with feelings of being on a high. She has had grandiose feelings for 2 weeks and today she was brought in by her son because she was talking constantly and had a bizarre and severe dress that did not match her other clothes. She was screaming in pain stating that her doctor told her to come to the E.R. Additionally, Ms. Smith was extremely talkative and kept fidgeting with her hair.

Instructions

Complete the diagram by selecting from the choices below to specify which potential condition the client is most likely experiencing, 2 actions to take, and 2 parameters the nurse would monitor to assess the client's progress.

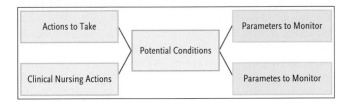

Clinical Nursing Actions	Potential Conditions	Parameters to Monitor
Praise self-control, acceptable behavior	Attention-Deficit Disorder	Increase conversations with client to establish more attention
Restrain individual for own safety	Bipolar disorder or manic-depressive illness	Provide small, frequent, feedings, record I&O
Provide frequent stimulation such as playing physical games	Delirium	Monitor physical activity/overstimulation
Monitor I&O	Overuse of amphetamines	Use a variety of approaches to maximize manipulative behavior.
Obtain an order for pain medication.		Provide additional stimulation for client.

REFERENCES AND BIBLIOGRAPHY

Azeem, M. W., Aujla, A., Rammerth, M., Binsfeld, G., & Jones, R. B. (2011). Effectiveness of six core strategies based on trauma informed care in reducing; seclusions and restraints at a child and adolescent psychiatric hospital. *Journal of Child and Adolescent Psychiatric Nursing, 24*(1), 11–15.

Bobier, C., Dowell, J., & Swadi, H. (2009). An examination of frequent nursing interventions and outcomes in an adolescent psychiatric inpatient unit. *International Journal of Mental Health Nursing, 18*(5), 301–309.

Bowers, L. (2014). Safewards: A new model of conflict and containment on psychiatric wards. *Journal of Psychiatric and Mental Health Nursing, 21*(6), 499–508.

Bryson, S. A., Gauvin, E., Jamieson, A. et. al. (2017). What are effective strategies for implementing trauma-informed care in youth inpatient psychiatric and residential treatment settings? *A realist systematic review.* May 11;11:36. https://doi.org/10.1186/s13033-017-0137-3.eCollection.

Colapinto, J. (2019). Structural family therapy. In: Fiese, B. H., Celano, M., Deater-Deckard, K., Jouriles, E. N., & Whisman, M. A. (Eds.), *APA handbook of contemporary family psychology: Family therapy and training* (pp. 107–121). American Psychological Association. https://doi.org/10.1037/0000101-007.

Collyer, H., Eisler, I., & Woolgar, M. (2020). Systematic literature review and meta-analysis of the relationship between adherence, competence and outcome in psychotherapy for children and adolescents. *European Child & Adolescent Psychiatry, 29*(4), 417–431. PMID: 30604132 https://doi.org/10.1007/s00787-018-1265-2. PMCID: PMC7103576.

Delaney, C., Barrere, C., Robertson, S., Zahourek, R., Diaz, D., & Lachapelle, L. (2016). Pilot Testing of the NURSE stress management intervention. *J Holist Nurs, 34*(4), 369–389. https://doi.org/10.1177/0898010115622295. Epub 2015 Dec 30. PMID: 26721516.

Delaney, K. R., Pitula, C. R., & Perraud, S. (2000). Psychiatric hospitalization and process description: what will nursing add? *Journal of Psychosocial Nursing and Mental Health Services, 38*(3), 7–13. PMID: 10779939 https://doi.org/10.3928/0279-3695-20000301-08.

Delaney, K. R., Naegle, M. A., Valentine, N. M., Antai-Otong, D., Groh, C. J., & Brennaman, L. (2018). The effective use of psychiatric mental health nurses in integrated care: Policy implications for increasing quality and access to care. *The Journal of Behavioral Health Services & Research, 45*(2), 300–309. PMID: 28484943 https://doi.org/10.1007/s11414-017-9555-x.

Delaney, K. R., Shattell, M., & Johnson, M. E. (2017). Capturing the interpersonal process of psychiatric nurses: A model for engagement. *Archives of Psychiatric Nursing, 31*(6), 634–640.

Foster, C., & Smedley, K. (2019). Understanding the nature of mental health nursing within CAMHS PICU:Identifying nursing interventions that contribute to the recovery journey of young people. *Journal of Psychiatric Intensive Care, 15*(2), 87–102. https://doi/org/10.20299/jpi.2010.012.

Geanellos, R. (2002). Exploring the therapeutic potential of friendliness and friendship in nurse-client relationships. *Contemporary Nurse, 12*(3), 235–245.

Glenn, C. R., Franklin, J. C., & Nock, M. K. (2014). Evidence-based psychosocial treatments for self-injurious thoughts and behaviors in youth. *Journal of Clinical Child and Adolescent Psychology, 44*(1), 1–29.

Gournay, K., Kelly Winstanley, Ashley Mancey-Johnson, Noel Tracey (2018). *British Journal of Mental Health Nursing*, pp. 161–166. https://doi.org/10.12968/bjmh.2019.0034

Heather, N. (1995). Treatment approaches to alcohol problems. *WHO Reg Publ Eur Ser, 65*, 1–201.

Miller, W. R., & Hester, R. K. (1986). The effectiveness of alcoholism treatment. In *Treating addictive behaviors* (pp. 121–174).

Miller, W. R., & Hester, R. K. (1986). Inpatient alcoholism treatment. Who benefits? *American Psychologist, 41*(7), 794–805. https://doi.org/10.1037//0003-066x.41.7.794.

Miller, W. R., & Muñoz, R. F. (1982). *How to control your drinking* (pp. 150–169). University of New Mexico Press.

Montreuil, M., Butler, K. J. D., Stachura, M., & Pugnaire Gros, C. (2015). Exploring helpful nursing care in pediatric mental health settings: The perceptions of children with suicide risk factors and their parents. *Issues in Mental Health Nursing, 36*(11), 849–859.

NAMI: National Alliance on Mental Illness. (2021). *Americans' Stigma Against Depression May Finally Be Fading: Study*. Posted on Dec 22 2021. https://www.nami.org/Press-Media/In-The-News/2021

Polacek, M. J., Allen, D. E., Damin-Moss, R. S., Schwartz, A. J. A., Sharp, D., Shattell, M., et al. (2015). Engagement as an element of safe inpatient psychiatric environments. *Journal of the American Psychiatric Nurses Association, 21*(3), 181–190.

Pollastri, A. R., Epstein, L. D., Heath, G. H., & Ablon, J. S. (2013). The collaborative problem solving approach: Outcomes across settings. *Harvard Review of Psychiatry, 21*(4), 188–199.

Rice, M. J., Stalling, J., & Monastero, A. (2019). Psychiatric-mental health nursing: Data-driven policy platform for a psychiatric mental healthcare workforce. *Journal of the American Psychiatric Nurses Association, 25*(1), 27–37. https://doi.org/10.1177/1078390318808368.

Rollnick, S., & Miller, W. R. (1991). *Motivational interviewing : preparing people to change addictive behavior* (pp. 114–155). United Kingdom: Guilford Publications.

Salamone-Violi, G. M. L., Chur-Hansen, A., & Winefield, H. R. (2015). I don't want to be here, but I feel safe": Referral and admission to a child and adolescent psychiatric inpatient unit: The young person's perspective. *International Journal of Mental Health Nursing, 24*(6), 569–576.

Scanlan, J. N. (2009). Interventions to reduce the use of seclusion and restraint in inpatient psychiatric settings: what we know so far a review of the literature. *Int J Soc Psychiatry, 56*(4), 412–423. Epub Jul 17. PMID: 19617275 https://doi.org/10.1177/0020764009106630.

Tadros, E., & Finney, N. (2019). Exploring the utilization of structural and medical family therapy with an incarcerated mother living with HIV. *International Journal of Offender Therapy and Comparative Criminology, 63*(4), 624–640.

Tsai, J., et al. (2021). Twenty-year trends in use of electroconvulsive therapy among homeless and domiciled veterans with mental illness. *CNS Spectrums, 1-7*. https://doi.org/10.1017/S1092852921001061.

van Hees, M. L., Rotter, T., Ellermann, T., & Evers, S. M. (2013). The effectiveness of individual interpersonal psychotherapy as a treatment for major depressive disorder in adult outpatients: a systematic review. *BMC Psychiatry, 13*, 22. PMID: 23312024 https://doi.org/10.1186/1471-244X-13-22. PMCID: PMC3558333.

Voogt, L. A., Goossens, P. J. J., Nugter, A., & van Achterberg, T. (2013). An observational study of providing structure as a psychiatric nursing intervention. *Perspectives in Psychiatric Care, 50*(1), 7–18.

Ward, L. (2014). Record-keeping and documentation. *Nurs Stand, 29*(15), 61. PMID: 25492793 https://doi.org/10.7748/ns.29.15.61.s49.

Whitaker, R. (2011). *Anatomy of an epidemic: Magic bullets, psychiatric drugs, and the astonishing rise of mental illness in America*. New York, NY: Broadway Books.

Gerontologic Nursing

AGING AND THE OLDER ADULT

A. Overview of aging and the older adult

1. The number of people aged 60 years and older was 1 billion in 2019 and will increase to 1.4 billion by 2030 and 2.1 billion by 2050 (Aging and Health, 2019).
2. Aging has been defined as young-old (65 to 74), middle-old (75 to 84), old-old (over 85), elite-old (over 90), centenarian (100+), and super-centenarian (110+).
3. Healthy aging is now an achievable goal for many.
4. Aging and disease are separate entities.

B. Theories of aging

1. Psychosocial theories
   a. Disengagement theory: Progressive social disengagement occurs naturally with aging and is accepted by the older adult.
   b. Activity theory: Successful aging requires a high level of activity and involvement to maintain life satisfaction and positive self-esteem.
2. Biologic theories
   a. Pacemaker theory: A programmed decline or cessation of many components occurs in the nervous and endocrine systems.
   b. Immunity theory: A programmed accumulation of damage and decline of the immune system's function (immunosenescence) takes place due to oxidative stress.
   c. Wear-and-tear theory: After repeated use, damaged cells in the body structures wear out from the harmful effects of internal and external stressors, now known as *free radicals.*
3. Developmental theories
   a. Erik Erikson's theory: Theory identifies eight stages of developmental tasks throughout the life span; the eighth stage is integrity versus despair.
   b. Maslow's theory: Maslow's hierarchy of needs ranks an individual's needs from the most basic to the most complex. Maslow uses the terms *physiologic, safety and security, belonging, self-esteem,* and *self-actualization* needs to describe the process that generally motivates individuals to move through life.

> **HESI HINT** The concept of aging is shifting from viewing older adults as frail and dependent to being able to engage in healthy living. Your clinical judgment abilities differentiates the health and well-being of individuals depending on their age range. The majority of those aged 65 and older regard their health as good or excellent. The clinical judgment measure to differentiate the ability of an older person to perform activities of daily living (ADLs) is a more accurate measure of an older person's age than chronological age.

C. Physiologic changes

1. Aging affects every cell in every organ of the body, but not at the same rate.
2. Three physiologic changes are clinically significant in making older adults vulnerable to injury and disease.
   a. Loss in compensatory reserve
   b. Progressive loss in efficiency of the body to repair damaged tissue
   c. Decreased functioning of the immune system processes
3. Diseases in older adults do not always present with classic signs and symptoms.
4. Physiologic changes increase more rapidly with increasing age.
5. Aging changes are influenced by genetic makeup and environment.

> **HESI HINT The NGN-NCLEX-PN will measure your clinical judgment ability.** Clinical judgment measures may include the development of preventive care such as exercise, teaching about good nutrition and rehabilitation programs for the older adult. Keep in mind that the type of prevention programs should be tailored to the age of the person as well as diagnosis of the chronic disease.

COMMUNICATION

Communicating With Older Adults

Communication is the beginning of understanding. Older adults often have difficulty in hearing or speech. As a result, the role of the nurse is to not only to observe verbal and nonverbal behaviors, but to be able to listen, interpret, and provide effective communication skills during an initial assessment of a patient.

A. Address client with respect: "Good morning, Mrs. Jones."
B. Orient the client to time, place, and purpose of conversation.
C. Give the older adult time to respond because verbal response slows with age.
D. Choose words based on the client's sociocultural background and formal education
E. Keep questions short and to the point.

F. Give nonverbal cues and responses such as nodding and direct eye contact; avoid patting or stroking the client.

G. Active listening validates the older person. Reminiscence is an excellent way to obtain data about the client's current health problems and support system.

H. To help cognitive losses due to alcohol consumption, smoking, and breathing polluted air, the nurse should teach older clients to shop during less crowded times in stores that are familiar to them, slow down well in advance of traffic signals, stay in the slower lane of the freeway, avoid freeways during rush hours, and leave for appointments well ahead of time.

I. Discuss the problems family members have in dealing with clients with Alzheimer disease in relation to the following disease manifestations:
   1. Depression
   2. Night wandering
   3. Aggressiveness or passiveness
   4. Inability to recognize family members

CLINICAL JUDGMENT MEASURES

Clinical Judgement Measures (CJM) refers to a systematic method of reflecting on a clinical issue. It consists of six levels of critical thinking: recognizing cues, analyzing cues, prioritization, solutions, actions, and evaluation of outcomes. For each of the psychosocial and physiologic changes that occur during aging, it is important to systematically review the CJM associated with each of these systems. For example, each system that will be presented will provide a table that will list the identified clinical measure and the assessment characteristics associated with each. The essential content will be systematically presented to facilitate a comprehensive review about the essential content needed to understand the overall concept. This will facilitate an understanding as to how to prioritize the practical nursing care associated with the older adult. It is essential to be able to accurately use CJM when providing the nursing care needs of the older adult.

Other issues that that will be reviewed include content associated with the health and preventive care for older adults, healthcare maintenance and interventions associated with end-of-life care. The overall nursing care needs of the older adult not only includes their psychological and physiological needs but includes their ability about healthy aging and safe environments.

AGING AND ITS EFFECT ON BODY SYSTEMS

Integumentary System Changes

A. Overview of integumentary system changes
   1. Changes in the skin, hair, and nails can cause problems concerning discomfort and self-esteem.

B. Causes of integumentary system changes
   1. Thin skin provides a less effective barrier to trauma due to
      a. A loss of subcutaneous tissue.
      b. Increased risk for dehydration due to decline in lean mass and loss of body water
      c. Decreased ability of the skin to detect and regulate temperature
      d. Dry skin resulting from a decrease in endocrine secretion
      e. Loss of elastin and increased vascular fragility
   2. Keratinocytes become smaller and regeneration slows; wound healing is slower.
   3. Hair loss occurs; women have increased facial hair.
   4. Vascular hyperplasia causes more varicosities (brown or blue discolorations).
   5. Increased appearance of "age spots" and/or "liver spots" and raised lesions (seborrheic keratosis).
   6. Nails become brittle and thick.

C. Risk factors
   1. Age
   2. Nutrition
   3. Immobility
   4. Obesity
   5. Poor tissue perfusion

Table 8.1 provides an example of a clinical judgment checklist applicable to the Integumentary System.

Musculoskeletal System

A. Overview of musculoskeletal system changes
   1. Age-related changes in the musculoskeletal system are gradual but have a significant impact on levels of mobility, which puts older adults at risk for falls and fractures.
   2. The musculoskeletal system is composed of bones, joints, tendons, ligaments, and muscles.
   3. Age-related changes are not life threatening but can affect function and quality of life.
   4. Bone loss begins around age 40 and is more common in women than in men; thus, osteoporosis occurs more often in women.
   5. There is a shortening of the trunk due to thinning of vertebral disks.

B. Loss of bone calcium, atrophic cartilage, and muscle occurs.

C. Complications of musculoskeletal system changes
   1. Bone mineral density (BMD) decreases, resulting in osteopenia and osteoporosis.
   2. Range of motion (ROM) of joints decreases.
   3. Progressive loss of cartilage occurs, resulting in osteoarthritis.
   4. Muscle cells are lost and not replaced.
   5. Lean body mass decreases with increased body fat.
   6. Impaired mobility, impaired skin integrity, decreased peripheral circulation, and a lack of physical activity places older adults at risk for developing ulcers.
   7. Pain

Table 8.2 provides an example of a clinical judgment checklist applicable to the Musculoskeletal System.

TABLE 8.1 Clinical Judgment Measures: Integumentary System

Clinical Judgment Measure	Assessment Characteristics
Recognize cues	• Skin dryness and tears • Nails for changes in shape, color, and brittleness • Lesions to differentiate normal from abnormal • Bony prominences for signs of pressure ulcers
Analyze cues	• Determine types of skin (open wound, infection) • Potential skin integrity issues that impact on assessment
Prioritize cues	• Determine if problem is emergent • Determine wound scale measurement score (Braden's scale 9—23, lower score = higher risk) • Determine impact of problem on Patient's overall health status
Solutions	• Encourage the use of oils or lubricants on the skin at least twice a day • Discourage the use of powder, which can be drying • Teach to avoid overexposure to sunlight • Encourage balanced nutrition and increased fluid intake • Teach to maintain adequate humidity in the environment • Teach to avoid temperature extremes • Teach good foot care • Observe bony prominences for signs of pressure • Teach that poor peripheral circulation may slow the healing of foot and hand lesions
Actions	• Apply topical moisturizing non-allergic lubricant to skin every morning and evening • Measure humidity in the room so that it is in normal limits (below 30%—60%, Wolkoff, 2018) • Perform foot care and have patient demonstrate understanding back to you
Evaluate Outcomes	• The overall status of the patient's skin has improved from the first to the second visit (improved skin turgor, no signs or symptoms of skin tears or wounds) • Height and weight is normal for age

---

> **HESI HINT** Clinical judgment includes an understanding of fractures such as hip replacements in older persons. When fractured hips are replaced, it is important to teach about the proper way to sit and rise after hip replacement so that the hip is not adducted and not flexed more than 90 degrees. They should not lean forward while sitting (can cause dislocation of the prosthesis).

Cardiovascular System

A. Overview of cardiovascular system changes
   1. Age-related changes in the cardiovascular system predispose the older person to the development of dysrhythmias and other cardiac problems.

B. Causes of cardiovascular system changes
   1. Cardiac output decreases because of a decrease in heart rate and stroke volume (heart rate slows with age resting heart rate remains unchanged).
   2. Cardiac output decreases because vessels lose elasticity. The heart's contractility decreases in response to increased demands.

C. Risk factors for cardiovascular system changes
   1. Age
   2. Nutrition
   3. Rest
   4. Obesity
   5. Sedentary lifestyle

D. Complications of cardiovascular system changes
   1. Diastolic murmurs are present in more than one-half of older adults because the mitral and aortic valves become thick and rigid.
   2. Dysrhythmias (bradycardia, tachycardia, atrial fibrillation, and heart block) become more common as one ages, in part because of higher systolic blood pressure (BP) and increased size of the atria.
   3. Significant increases in systolic BP occur because of altered distribution of blood flow and increased peripheral resistance.
   4. Arteriosclerosis increases with age and can cause cardiovascular problems.
       a. Peripheral vascular disease
       b. Edema
       c. Coronary artery disease: acute coronary insufficiency, myocardial infarction, dysrhythmias, heart failure (HF)

> **HESI HINT** Clinical judgment parameters for both systolic and diastolic BPs tend to increase with normal aging, but the elevation of the systolic BP is greater. The physiology of BP is expressed as a ratio of systolic to diastolic BP. Systolic refers to the level of BP during the contraction phase, whereas diastolic refers to the stage when the chambers of the heart are filling with blood (relaxation phase). The healthy older heart can sustain adequate function for everyday live.

TABLE 8.2 Clinical Judgment Measures: Musculoskeletal System

Clinical Judgment Measure	Assessment Characteristics
Recognize Cues	• Dietary intake of calcium and vitamin D • Weight; underweight or overweight • Height • Lifestyle habits; inappropriate nutrition, smoking, and inadequate exercise • History of fractures • Range of motion (ROM) • Pain and chronic pain management strategies
Analyze Cues	• Determine type of diet for adequate intake • Verify lifestyle habits (smoking, exercise) • Ascertain ability to functionally move (ROM, walk without limp or pain)
Prioritize Cues	• Determine risk factors for fractures (emergent versus non-emergent) • Clarify nutritional factors • Establish weight parameters
Solutions	• Teach that adequate calcium intake may help lessen osteoporotic changes • Establish muscle-strengthening program (small weights, aquatic therapy) • Prevent accidents by ensuring a clutter-free, safe environment • Provide adequate lighting day and night to prevent falls • Teach clients not to back up but to turn around to move in the direction they wish to go • Teach clients to walk looking straight ahead instead of looking down at their feet to optimize balance • Encourage regular exercise inclusive of balance, weight-bearing, and low-resistance training • Teach to avoid excessive joint strain • Teach that medications (diuretics and sedatives) may contribute to falls • The following are ways to help prevent or decrease the occurrence of falls: • Install adequate lighting • Install grab bars in bathtubs • Wear proper footwear that supports the foot and contributes to balance; shoes should be made of non-slippery materials • Place a bell on any resident cats; cats move quickly and can get underfoot • Paint the edges of stairs a bright color • Discourage excessive alcohol intake and encourage smoking cessation • Encourage older people to change positions slowly to prevent orthostatic hypotension
Actions	• Provide patient with nutritionist appointment • Communicate which exercise programs are available • Enroll patient into fall prevention class • Educate patient about healthy lifestyle (cessation of smoking, overeating, immobility)
Evaluate Outcomes	• The overall status of the patient's musculoskeletal system has improved from the first to the second visit (improved balance, walking without cane, no signs or symptoms of joint injuries) • Weight is improved (loss or added)

Table 8.3 provides an example of a clinical judgment checklist applicable for the Cardiovascular System.

HESI HINT Clinical judgment parameters such as dysrhythmias in older adults are particularly serious because they cannot tolerate decreased cardiac output, which can result in syncope, falls, and transient ischemic attacks. The pulse may be rapid, slow, or irregular. Angina symptoms may be absent in older adults or may be confused with gastrointestinal (GI) symptoms such as esophagitis or musculoskeletal disorders. Your ability to differentiate among all these symptoms is dependent on the questions you ask the patient and your physical assessment skills.

Respiratory System

A. Overview of respiratory system changes

1. Older adults have increased demands for oxygen. The life span of an older adult increases the chance for exposure to toxic or infectious agents. Due to the aging process, multiple exposures over time can be damaging to the lungs and even life threatening.
B. Causes of respiratory system changes
   1. Breathing mechanics: Lungs lose elasticity; muscles become rigid and lose muscle mass and strength. Declining muscle strength may impair cough efficiency. This fact makes older people more susceptible to chronic bronchitis, emphysema, and pneumonia.
   2. Oxygenation: Increased ventilation and perfusion are imbalanced; increased dead space in the lungs and a decrease of alveolar surface area
   3. Ventilation control: Decreased reaction of peripheral and central chemoreceptors to hypoxia and hypercapnia

TABLE 8.3 Clinical Judgment Measures: Cardiovascular System

Clinical Judgment Measure	Assessment Characteristics

Recognize Cues	• Blood pressure (BP) and vital signs
	• History of dizziness or blackouts with sudden position change (orthostatic hypotension)
	• Diuresis after lying down
	• Feelings of heart palpitations
	• Angina
	    1. Angina symptoms may be absent in older adults
	    2. They can also be confused with gastrointestinal (GI) symptoms
	• Swelling in hands and feet (rings and shoes have become tight)
	• Weight gain without changes in eating pattern
	• Difficulty breathing at night (without elevation of the head of the bed). Confusion and personality changes can result from oxygen deficit

Analyze Cues	• BP and vital signs are consistent with age & diagnosis of patient • Neuro status is stable (no dizziness, movement) • Breathing patterns are regular for age & diagnosis of patient • Mini-mental exam reliable for patient status
Prioritize Cues	• Keep in mind any emergent issue related to: airway, breathing, or circulation (A, B, Cs) • Mentation intact measured by mini-mental exam (confusion, speech, responses)
Solutions	• Monitor BP in lying, sitting, and standing positions • Encourage frequent rest periods to avoid fatigue • Encourage regular, low-impact exercise • Teach to change positions slowly to avoid falls and injuries • Take apical and radial pulse; note deficits or rhythm abnormalities • Teach to avoid extreme hot and cold because of decreased peripheral sensation • Teach to avoid sitting with feet in a dependent position • Assess edema: Weigh daily if indicated • Encourage strict adherence to medication regimen • Teach not to stop medications without prior approval from health care provider
Actions	• Check vital signs for normalcy of patient's age • List up-coming doctor appointments • Evaluate patient's understanding of current cardiac medications • Examine patient's ability to understand changes in cardiac status (when to call 911, when to contact doctor) • Reassess patient's overall ability to ambulate and do routine activities of daily living (ADLs)
Evaluate Outcomes	• The patient's overall cardiac status is stable for health condition • Patient or caregiver demonstrates an understanding of cardiac medications and follow up health visits • Patient's functional status is intact (ADL)

4. Immune response: Decrease of cilia; decreased ability to clear mucus secretions, decreased ability to cough and deep breathe, and a decreased immune response
5. Exercise capability: Decrease of strength and muscle mass in the body
6. Breathing ability: Decreased reaction to hypoxemia and hypercapnia

C. Risk factors for respiratory changes
 1. Age; Nutrition; Rest; Obesity; Sedentary lifestyle

D. Complications of respiratory system changes
 1. Infection
 2. Poor tissue perfusion
 3. Confusion
 4. Weakness, increased risk for falls and injury
 5. Respiratory arrest
 6. Cardiac arrest
 7. Death

Table 8.4 provides an example of a clinical judgment checklist applicable to the Respiratory System.

Gastrointestinal System

A. Overview of GI System changes
 1. Age-related changes are bothersome and can affect comfort, function, and quality of life, but are rarely a direct cause of death.
 2. The production of pepsin and hydrochloric acid decreases

B. Causes of GI system changes
 1. Decreased saliva and dry mouth (xerostomia) are common.
 2. Dental caries (tooth decay) and loss of teeth increase, resulting in decreased ability to chew food.
 3. Diminished taste sensation due to loss of taste buds.

C. Risk factors for GI system changes
 1. Age
 2. Tobacco use
 3. Medications
 4. Nutrition
 5. Injury/trauma

TABLE 8.4 Clinical Judgment Measures: Respiratory System

Clinical Judgment Measure	Assessment Characteristics
Recognize Cues	• Confusion (may be the first sign of respiratory infection) • Vital signs for elevated temperature, blood pressure (BP) or elevated/decreased respiratory rate • Lungs for congestion or atelectasis Vital capacity • Dyspnea and fatigue • Cough reflex and sputum production
Analyze Cues	• Breathing patterns are consistent with age of patient without (SOB, confusion, orthopnea) • Respiratory rate, BP, and other vital signs are consistent with age and diagnosis of patient • Productive/non-productive cough
Prioritize Cues	• Keep in mind any emergent issue related to: airway, breathing, or circulation (A, B, C) • Mentation is what is expected for age and diagnosis without confusion in speech, or wrong responses to questions) • Change in skin color (pale, cyanosis)
Solutions	• Encourage clients to receive an influenza vaccine yearly • Encourage clients to receive the pneumonia vaccine after age 65 (a second dose may be given one additional time after about 5 years) • Remember that hypoxia can manifest as confusion • If the client is a smoker, encourage him or her to stop. (Regardless of age, cardiovascular and respiratory status improves with smoking cessation and exercise.) • For older postoperative clients, turning, deep breathing, and use of incentive spirometer are imperative to prevent complications • Encourage deep breathing • Teach breathing techniques such as pursed lip breathing to facilitate respirations
Actions	• Test mental status (date, time, place) • Check vital signs for normalcy of patient's age • Note that respiratory rate is within normal limits • Review medications for respiratory system (have patient recite medication, dosage and routine) • Auscultate lungs for consolidation • Reassess patient's overall ability to ambulate and do routine activities of daily living (ADLs)
Evaluate Outcomes	• Respiratory status has improved (respiratory rate normal, color good, use of oxygen properly if ordered for age and patient's diagnosis) • Mentation within normal limits (recites date, time, mini-mental exam) • Respiratory rate consistent with activity (walking, ADL) • Patient is able to recite list of respiratory medications and dosage

D. Complications of GI system changes
1. Decreased ability to chew food
2. Decreased hunger sensations
3. Relaxation of the lower esophageal sphincter or a sliding hiatal hernia.
4. Delayed gastric emptying makes digestion of large amounts of food difficult.
5. Decreased peristalsis and decreased absorption in the small intestine. Protein, fats, minerals (calcium), vitamins B$_1$ and B$_2$, and carbohydrates contribute to constipation problems. Decreased muscle tone of the colon also causes constipation.
6. Decreased enzyme production in the liver affects drug metabolism and detoxification processes.
7. Weight changes, especially weight loss, can be early indicators of health problems.

Table 8.5 provides an example of a clinical judgment checklist applicable to the Respiratory System.

HESI HINT The following changes occur with aging that contribute to chronic constipation:
• The number of enzymes in the small intestine is reduced and simple sugars are absorbed more slowly, resulting in decreased efficiency of the digestive process.
• Smooth muscle content and muscle tone of the wall of the colon decrease.
• Anatomic changes in the large intestine result in decreased intestinal motility.
• Psychological factors, as well as abuse of over-the-counter laxatives, can contribute to constipation.
• Decreases in fluid intake and mobility contribute to constipation.

HESI HINT Poor or inadequate nutrition and malnutrition are significant concerns in the older adult. Some reasons for poor nutrition include chronic illnesses that suppress appetite, hospitalizations and surgery, difficulty chewing, alcohol use, cognitive changes, depression, grief, loneliness, social isolation, and problems with food procurement. An early sign of nutritional problems may be changes inn weight.

TABLE 8.5 Clinical Judgment Measures: Gastrointestinal System

Clinical Judgment Measure	Assessment Characteristics
Recognize Cues	• Brittle teeth due to thinning enamel • Receding gums resulting from periodontal disease (the major cause of tooth loss after the age of 30) • Decrease in taste sensation and appetite • Dry mouth due to a decrease in saliva production • Elimination pattern for evidence of constipation or diarrhea • Use of pain medications that may cause constipation • Poor tolerance of high-fat meals and poor absorption of fat-soluble vitamins • Decreased glucose tolerance • Fluid intake • Weight change
Analyze Cues	• Condition of teeth consistent with age (repairs, dentures, gums) • Taste, appetite and eating patterns suitable for age • Bowel habits acceptable for age • Food tolerance (regular, soft, portion size) consistent with age
Prioritize Cues	• Nutritional status (gain or loss of weight) proper for age • Fluid intake of 7–8 (8 oz./day) Picetti et al. (2017). Vitamin intake consistent with recommendations for people over 51: (https://www.nia.nih.gov/health/vitamins-and-minerals-older-adults)

Solutions	• Encourage good oral hygiene (the use of a soft tooth, dental floss, and regular dental visits)
	• Assess dentures for proper fit
	• Educate older clients about hidden sodium (canned soups, antacids, over-the-counter medications)
	• Promote adequate bowel functioning
	• Determine what is normal gastrointestinal (GI) functioning for each individual.
	   1. Encourage client to increase fiber and bulk in the diet
	   2. Provide adequate hydration
	   3. Encourage regular exercise
	   4. Encourage eating small, frequent meals
	   5. Discourage the use of laxatives and enemas
	   6. Document bowel movements: frequency and consistency

Actions	• Verify nutritional status (nutrition for age and weight). Provide vitamins for any deficiency • Check height and weight • Provide list of community services for seniors (food banks, meals on wheels, community lunches)
Evaluate Outcomes	• Patient maintains healthy weight for age • Annual or semi-annual dental visits • Patient is engaged in senior lunch programs

Genitourinary System

A. Overview of the genitourinary system changes
1. There are functional and structural changes, as well as psychosocial changes, in the older adult pertaining to the urinary system.
2. Older persons have a higher risk of developing renal failure because normal age-related changes result in compromised renal functioning. The nurse should pay careful attention to urinary output in older clients because it is the first sign of loss of renal integrity.

B. Causes of genitourinary system changes
1. Size and weight of the kidney decrease due to reduced renal tissue growth.
2. Glomerular filtration rate decreases due to a decrease in renal blood flow resulting from lower cardiac output. Decreased renal clearance of drugs is the result.
3. Tubular function diminishes.
4. Increased risk for reflux of urine into the ureters.
5. Chronic diseases such as atherosclerosis and hypertension also decrease renal functioning in older adults.

C. Risk factors for genitourinary system changes
1. Age
2. Nutrition
3. Tobacco use
4. Alcohol use
5. Hygiene
6. Medications

D. Complications of genitourinary system changes
1. Electrolyte imbalance
2. Fluid imbalance
3. Infection
4. Sexual dysfunction
5. The capacity of the bladder decreases by one-half, resulting in urinary frequency and nocturia.
6. Emptying the bladder may become difficult because of a weakening of the bladder and perineal muscles, and because of a decrease in sensation of urge to void. (This sets up a propensity for urinary tract infections [UTIs] due to residual urine in the bladder.)
7. Increased frequency and dribbling may occur in men because of a weakened bladder and enlarged prostate.

8. Prostatic enlargement may also cause urinary retention and bladder infection in men.

9. Women may experience stress incontinence.

HESI HINT The total number of functioning glomeruli decreases with age until renal function has been reduced by nearly 50%. Medications such as penicillin, tetracycline, and digoxin are primarily cleared from the bloodstream by the kidneys and remain active longer in an older person's system. Drug levels may be more potent, indicating a need to adjust/reduce the dose and frequency of administration.

Table 8.6 provides an example of a clinical judgment checklist applicable to the Genitourinary System.

TABLE 8.6 Clinical Judgment Measures: Genitourinary System

Clinical Judgment Measure	Assessment Characteristics
Recognize Cues *Kidney* *Bladder*	Signs of dehydration or electrolyte imbalance • Decreased skin turgor (tenting) • Intake/output • Confusion • Concentrated urine • Medications such as diuretics Laboratory values • Proteinuria • Increased blood urea nitrogen and creatinine • Presence of blood in urine Signs of urinary tract infection (UTI) • Urinary elimination patterns: normal voiding patterns and symptoms such as burning, urgency, and frequency • Mental status (knowledge of name, date, time, place)
Analyze Cues *Kidney* *Bladder*	• Laboratory values assessed for the development of acute kidney insufficiency (an elevated blood urea nitrogen (BUN) level, an elevation in serum creatinine, and a decrease in creatinine clearance accompanied by a decrease in urine output) • Urinary output consistent for age (urinary output measured 800—2400 mL/day (Corder et al., 2020)
Prioritize Cues *Kidney* *Bladder*	• Keep in mind acute renal failure issues (blood pressure changes, laboratory value changes) for age and diagnosis • Changes in heart rate (heart failure) • Impaired cognition (disorientation) • Immune function (infection/sepsis) Monitor symptoms: • Lower UTI: dysuria, urgency, frequency, and hematuria • Upper UTI: chills, fever, flank pain, mentation changes (septicemia)

Solutions
Kidney
Bladder
	• Encourage an intake of at least 2—3 L of fluid daily, if not contraindicated
	• Instruct client about signs and symptoms of dehydration and to contact health care provider immediately
	• Instruct client about the importance of completing antibiotics until the entire prescription is gone, even if symptoms go away
	• Write out antibiotic schedule, including any special instructions. Print in large letters
	• Initiate a bladder-training program if indicated
	• Encourage older women to void at first urge when possible
	• Initiate a skin-care program if incontinence is present
	• Provide methods of dealing with incontinence. Kegel exercises can help
	• Kegel exercises consist of tightening and relaxing the vaginal and urinary meatus muscles
	  • Teach to avoid sleeping pills and sedation, which may cause nocturnal incontinence
	  • Teach to avoid caffeine because it promotes diuresis
	  • Caffeine inhibits the production of antidiuretic hormone (ADH)

Actions *Kidney* *Bladder*	• Monitor vital signs • Monitor fluid intake and urinary output • Monitor laboratory values • Determine suitable mentation for age and diagnosis • Monitor fluid intake and urinary output • Monitor vital signs • Provide mini-mental health score • Monitor sleep patterns (waking up to urinate, frequency, odor)
Evaluate Outcomes *Kidney* *Bladder*	• Quality of life report is good for age and patient's condition • Renal function is stable (levels of BUN, creatinine, hematocrit, fluid and electrolytes are normal for age) • Vital signs, functional status, activities of daily living for age and health condition is fitting

HESI HINT CJM include psychosocial effects since older adults may be embarrassed because they have become incontinent. They may seek isolation or become depressed, thereby predisposing themselves to loneliness.

Reproductive System

A. Overview of reproductive system changes
1. Many older adults are sexually active and maintain an interest in sexual activities. A sexual assessment should be obtained among older men and women in the acute care, community, and long-term care settings.
2. Age-related changes are related to hormonal and nervous system control for both men and women.
B. Causes of reproductive system changes
1. Age-related changes affect women more than men
   a. Women's ovarian function decreases; breast tissue involutes.
   b. Ovaries and the uterus slowly atrophy, and neither may be palpable.
   c. Perineal muscle weakness and atrophy of the vulva occur with age.
   d. Vaginal mucous membrane becomes dry, elasticity of tissue decreases, surface becomes smooth, and secretions become reduced and more alkaline. May lead to dyspareunia (painful intercourse).
   e. Risk of vaginal yeast infection increases.
   f. Libido may or may not decline
   g. Lower estrogen levels due to menopause may cause cardiovascular changes, reduce cholesterol, or increase risk of osteoporosis.
C. Age-related changes in men include:
1. Testes atrophy, lose weight, and soften.
2. Erectile dysfunction (less frequent erections, inability to have an erection).
3. Erection changes occur:
   a. An erection that is less firm
   b. Shorter duration of erection
   c. Diminished force of ejaculation
4. Prostate enlargement due to changes in testosterone levels
5. Testosterone production decreases and libido can decline.
Table 8.7 provides an example of a clinical judgment checklist applicable to the Reproductive System in Women and Men.

HESI HINT Sexually active older adults are at risk for sexually transmitted diseases if they seek sexual relations with different partners. An important CJM is to ascertain number of sexual partners and knowledge of HIV infection among older adults (Heidari, 2016).

TABLE 8.7 Clinical Judgment Measures: Reproductive System Women and Men

Clinical Judgment Measure	Assessment Characteristics
Recognize Cues	• Vital signs (temperature), discharge, or labial or vulvar redness and pruritus for possible infections (vaginitis)
Women	• Complaints of hot flashes, mood swings, or night sweat
Men	• Dyspareunia (painful intercourse)
	• Complaints of urinary problems (dribbling, incontinence, frequent waking up at night to urinate), prostate enlargement
	• Testosterone hormone levels
Analyze Cues	• All vital signs are consistent for age of patient
Women	• Loss of pubic muscle tone may cause bladder to fall (prolapse) of uterus
Men	• Benign prostatic hyperplasia (BPH) can cause slowed urine or ejaculation
	• Medication (antihypertensives) use may decrease libido
Prioritize Cues	• Monitor changes in vital signs (increased temperature)
Women	• Changes in discharge (infection, vaginitis)
Men	• Monitor vital signs (increase in temperature)
	• Prostatitis risk (greater in men over 50)
Solutions	• Teach client signs of vaginitis; report and treat if present
Women	• Promote perineal care as needed
Men	• Prescription creams can help with vaginal dryness
	• Encourage client to obtain mammogram per guidelines
	• Encourage annual digital examination for early identification of prostate cancer
Actions	• Monitor vital signs for normalcy for age
Women	• List signs and symptoms of vaginitis
Men	• Promote creams that help with vaginal dryness
	• Encourage wellness plan: annual mammogram and annual physical
	• Monitor vital signs for normalcy for age
	• Encourage annual physical exam following prostate guidelines
Evaluate Outcomes	• Stable vital signs during annual physical exam
Women	• No pain during sexual encounters
Men	• Stable vital signs during annual physical exam
	• Signs and symptoms of prostatitis is negative

Neurologic System

A. Overview of neurologic system changes
1. Neurocognitive disorders (DSM-5) are the major cause of disability in older adults. Dementia (Box 8.1), cerebrovascular disorders, and movement disorders (e.g., Parkinson disease) are the major disorders in this category.
2. The nervous system is the most complex of all systems and functions alone and in conjunction with many systems.
3. There is a decrease of neurons and neurotransmitters in the brain, which do not regenerate.
4. The neurologic system consists of two main components: the central nervous system (CNS) and the peripheral nervous system (PNS): decrease in both CNS and PNS functioning with age.
5. Intelligence remains constant in the healthy older adult.
6. Central processing decreases; performance of tasks is slower.

B. Causes of neurologic system changes
1. Older adults experience a decrease of neurons and neurotransmitters in the brain, which do not regenerate

C. Risk factors for neurologic system changes
1. Decreased cerebral tissue diffusion
2. Disease process
3. Medications
4. Substance abuse

D. Complications of neurologic system changes
1. Significantly lower or nonexistent vibratory senses in the lower extremities
2. Decrease of tactile sensitivity
3. Loss of connection in nerve endings in the skin
4. Loss of proprioception, affecting balance
   a. Sleep disturbances

HESI HINT Alzheimer disease is the most common irreversible dementia of old age. It is characterized by deficits in attention, learning, memory, and language skills. Discuss the problems family members have in dealing with patients with Alzheimer disease in relation to the following disease manifestations:
- Depression, night wandering: aggressiveness or passiveness; failure to recognize family members; living in the past

Table 8.8 provides an example of a clinical judgment checklist applicable to the Neurologic System.

HESI HINT The most common neurological disorders in the older adult include cognitive disorders, behavioral changes and alterations in physical abilities. CJM are most crucial to differentiate the signs and symptoms that the older adult may exhibit during the assessment phase.

Endocrine System

A. Overview of endocrine system changes
1. In the older adult, glands atrophy and decrease the rate of secretion. The impact is unclear, except it is more prevalent in women than in men due to the decline of estrogen, which causes menopause.
2. The endocrine system consists of the thyroid, parathyroid, pituitary, adrenal, and pineal glands; the thymus; and the endocrine pancreas
3. Thyroid activity decreases with age. Symptoms are commonly undiagnosed in the older adult because they are attributed to being "normal for age."

B. Causes of endocrine system changes
1. Metabolic rate slows.
2. Estrogen production ceases with menopause; ovaries, uterus, and vaginal tissue atrophy.
3. Gonadal secretion of progesterone and testosterone decreases.
4. Insulin production decreases or insulin resistance increases.
5. Thyroxine (T_4) and triiodothyronine (T_3) secreted by the thyroid gland levels decrease and appear to be age-related. Production of parathyroid hormone decreases, which is made evident by osteoporosis.

BOX 8.1 Delirium and Dementia

Delirium	Dementia
Description: An acute process that, if treated, is usually reversible. It is recognized by its *sudden* onset.	**Description:** Cognitive impairment characterized by gradual, progressive onset; it is irreversible. Judgment, memory, abstract thinking, and social behavior are affected.
A. Occurs in response to a specific stressor such as:	A. Most frequently seen in:
1. Infection	1. Alzheimer disease (Table 8.9)
2. Drug reaction	2. Multi-infarctions (brain)
3. Substance intoxication or withdrawal	B. Also occurs in:
4. Electrolyte imbalance	1. Huntington chorea
5. Head trauma	2. Parkinson disease
6. Sleep deprivation	3. Multiple sclerosis and brain tumors
B. Treatment of choice is the correction of the causative disorder	4. Wernicke–Korsakoff syndrome (chronic alcoholism)

TABLE 8.8   Clinical Judgment Measures: Neurologic System

Clinical Judgment Measure	Assessment Characteristics
Recognize Cues	• Comprehensive functional assessment; weaknesses, tremors, and gait disturbances • History of falls • Pain, headaches, range of motion (ROM), and neuropathies in extremities • Sudden changes in vision, cognition, and muscle weakness • Depression • Sleep patterns
Analyze Cues	• Sleep disorders (sleep-wake cycle) consistent for age • Answers related to old and new information dependable for age, memory reliable • Hearing, smell, vibratory sensations, taste consistent for age • Balance steady for age • Mini cog—screens for cognitive impairment, consistent for age • Mental status assessment: attention, memory, orientation, etc. intact for age and diagnosis • Neurologic assessment: cranial nerves, gait, balance, distal deep tendon reflexes, plantar responses, primary sensory modalities in lower extremities, and cerebrovascular integrity intact for age • Functional assessment: Dementia Severity Rating Scale (DSRS) normal score 4 or less (increases with age), consistent for age • Mini cog—screens for cognitive impairment, consistent for age • Screen for age associated issues: The three Ds: depression, delirium, and dementia: consistent for age
Prioritize Cues	• Keep in mind acute changes with patient: changes in vital signs, stroke assessment (headaches, vomiting, seizures, mental status changes (including coma), fevers, and electrocardiogram (ECG) changes mentation, slurred speech, ABCs • Cognitive changes, outbursts, disorientation, emotional or sensory overload, confusion, agitation
Solutions	• Perform a complete mental status examination • Screen for depression • Screen for cognitive impairment • Monitor for conditions caused by lack of sleep • Fatigue, confusion, disorientation • Monitor blood pressure and hydration status • Request physical and occupational service evaluations, if indicated • Provide assistive devices as needed for ambulation • Encourage walking, ROM, and balance exercises • Teach individual relaxation techniques, stress management, and adaptive self-care management • Minimize potential sources of injury in the environment • Educate family and caregivers about support groups and other resources (agencies)
Actions	• Vital signs assess and normal for age • Mini-mental status exam intact • Functional status exam stable for age • Judgment, home activities, personal care, speech and language recognition, feeding, incontinence, and mobility or walking consistent for age • Physical activities consistent for age (ROM, balance, gait) and appraised by care provider
Evaluate Outcomes	• Check vital signs for normalcy for age • Behavioral changes (mood, sleep patterns, fatigue, confusion, orientation) consistent for age and diagnosis of patient as reported by care provider and/or patient • No gait or balance issues, no falls in home environment • Effectiveness of health teaching evident in patient's ability to effectively balance when walking and report by care giver about community senior support groups

TABLE 8.9   Alzheimer's Medications

Drugs	Adverse Reactions	Nursing Implications
Acetyl Cholinesterase Inhibitors		
• Tacrine hydrochloride • Donepezil HCl • Rivastigmine • Galantamine	• Overall: nausea and diarrhea • Cognex: considerable gastrointestinal (GI) distress, elevated liver enzymes	• For early to moderate stage • Reinforce teaching to clients that they should take no anticholinergic medication • Medications should not be used in cases of severe liver impairment • Take with meals to avoid GI upset • Do not discontinue abruptly • Implement the established plan of care • Report significant changes to the registered nurse
N-Methyl D-Aspartate (NMDA) Antagonist		
• Aduhelm • Memantine	• Headaches, ARIA-H microhemorrhage • Headaches, dizziness, and constipation	• Used to treat Alzheimer disease • Add to acetyl cholinesterase inhibitors in moderate to severe Alzheimer disease

TABLE 8.10 Clinical Judgment Measures: Endocrine System

Clinical Judgment Measure	Assessment Characteristics
Recognize Cues	• Signs and symptoms of diabetes in older adults; dehydration and confusion • History of recurrent infections, fatigue, and nausea; delayed wound healing; paresthesia • Weight loss or gain without change in eating pattern • Laboratory values; hemoglobin A1c, aldosterone, and cortisol levels • Bone density testing • Sleeping pattern • Depression
Analyze Cues	• Vital signs are consistent for age of patient • Laboratory values are normal (hemoglobin A1c in normal limits) • No sleepiness, no changes in mentation
Prioritize Cues	• Concentrate on vital signs, changes in mental status (mini-mental test) • Keep in mind changes in blood sugar (sleepiness, cognitive responses, slurred speech)
Solutions	• Encourage thyroid testing for older clients who seem depressed. Hypothyroidism is often dismissed as depression • Refer to "Hypothyroidism (Hashimoto Disease, Myxedema)" in Chapter 4: Medical-Surgical Nursing • Older clients may have difficulty with lifelong medication regimens. Develop memory cues for medications and caution against abrupt withdrawal • See "Diabetes Mellitus (DM) in Chapter 4: Medical-Surgical Nursing • Encourage annual physical examination with routine laboratory tests • Encourage annual eye examinations • Teach daily foot care and monthly toenail care
Actions	• Vital signs assessed for normalcy for age • Mini-mental status exam intact • Functional status exam stable for age • Judgment intact for activities of daily living
Evaluate Outcomes	• Check vital signs for normalcy for age • Functional status exam normal for age as reported by caregiver • Behavioral changes not evident (sleep patterns, no fatigue or confusion)

6. Adrenal changes may affect circadian patterns of adrenocorticotropic hormone (ACTH).

C. Risk factors for endocrine system changes
   1. Age
   2. Medications
   3. Nutrition
   4. Substance abuse

D. Complications of endocrine system changes
   1. Electrolyte imbalance
   2. Impaired nutrition
   3. Disturbed sleep
   4. Blood glucose imbalance

Table 8.10 provides an example of a clinical judgment checklist applicable to the Neurologic System.

HESI HINT CJM that differentiate between thyroid dysfunction and type 2 diabetes is important since both disorders are common endocrine syndromes of the older adult.

Sensory System

A. Overview of sensory system changes
   1. The sensory system consists of vision, hearing, taste, touch, and smell. Changes in the sensory system, including balance, occur gradually and are often unnoticed.

B. Causes of sensory system changes
   1. A loss of cells in the olfactory bulb of the brain and a decrease in sensory cells in the nasal lining occur.
   2. Taste perception decreases due to loss of taste buds on the tongue.

C. Risk factors for sensory system changes
   1. Aging
   2. Tobacco use
   3. Substance abuse
   4. Disease process
   5. Medications

D. Complications of sensory system changes
   1. Sensitivity to smell declines
   2. Tear production decreases.
   3. Abnormal, progressive clouding or opacity of the lens in the eyes occurs (cataracts).
   4. A partial or complete white ring encircles the periphery of the cornea (arcus senilis).
   5. Increased intraocular pressure (IOP), usually bilaterally, leads to optic nerve damage (glaucoma).
   6. Hearing of high pitches diminishes first; the ability to discriminate tones is lost (presbycusis).

HESI HINT Lower the tone of your voice when speaking to an older person with hearing impairment. High-pitched tones (i.e., Women's voices are the first heating to go: therefore, lowering the pitch of your voice increases the likelihood that an older person with a hearing loss will be able to hear you speak.

HESI HINT CJM associated with changes in the sensory system are important to determine the overall functional status of older adults.

Psychosocial Changes

A. Overview of loss
1. Loss includes loss of functional ability, decreased self-image, and death of significant others (family members, friends, or pets).
2. Loss is a universal, incontestable event of the human experience.

Injury

Table 8.11 provides an example of a clinical judgment checklist applicable to the Sensory System.

TABLE 8.11 Clinical Judgment Measures: Sensory System

Clinical Judgment Measure	Assessment Characteristics
Recognize Cues	• Monitor visual and hearing acuity, as well as glasses and/or hearing aids used • Eyes for cloudiness or opacity • Ears for wax and hearing loss • Evaluate dietary intake for unplanned weight loss and salt and sugar intake
Analyze Cues	• Vital signs are consistent for age of patient • Able to clearly read (patient reads simple list, assess for accuracy) • Understands simple directions (responds to healthcare provider without increasing voice) • Weight consistent for age
Prioritize Cues	• Concentrate on vital signs, mentation changes (acute disorientation) • Acute pain in eyes, ears, nose or mouth

Solutions	• Provide interventions to supplement loss of sensory input
	• Encourage social interaction
	• Make the client's environment as safe as possible to increase orientation and decrease confusion
	• Maximize visual and nonvisual aids, such as bright colors, large print for written material, recorded books, lighted mirror, and glasses, if applicable
	• Encourage the use of hearing aids with frequent battery changes, if applicable
	• The nurse should use a lower tone of voice when talking to an older person who is hearing impaired
	• High-pitched tones (e.g., women's voices) are the first to become difficult to hear
	• Encourage the use of glasses and frequent cleaning, if applicable
	• Diminished eyesight results in the following:
	   A loss of independence (driving and the ability to perform activities of daily living [ADLs])
	   A lack of stimulation
	   The inability to read (recommend audiotapes)
	   The fear of blindness
	   Decreased independence due to fear of not
	   being able to clearly see
	• Encourage the use of artificial tears; teach to avoid rubbing and touching of the eyes (increases risk for infection)
	• Encourage regular eye examinations
	• Directly face hearing-impaired clients so they may read lips and view facial expressions
	• Adapt ethnic favorites to dietary and taste limitations
	• Use frequent touch to compensate for visual and auditory sensory loss and decrease the sense of isolation
	• The nurse should make the older adult aware that he or she is going to touch and should therefore ask permission before touching the client. The nurse should be cognizant of cultural differences with direct eye contact, touch, and taste
	• The nurse should teach the caregiver or patient to carefully use sharp kitchen utensils since the patient may unintentionally injure themselves
	• Educate the client's support system about interventions to maintain a safe and comfortable environment

Actions	• Vital signs normal for age • Mini-mental status exam intact • Functional exam for vision, hearing and taste stable for age (use of glasses, hearing aids, diet recall) • Judgment intact for ADLs
Evaluate Outcomes	• Check vital signs for consistency for age • Functional status exam normal for age related to vision (screen with SNELLEN exam), screen for hearing • ADLs as reported by caregiver (able to eat and feed self, smell intact)

3. Regardless of the loss, each event has the potential to cause grief and the process called *bereavement* or *mourning*.
4. Grief is an individual response and is different depending on social and cultural norms.

B. Causes of loss
   1. Illness
   2. Injury
   3. Death
C. Risk factors for loss
   1. Age
   2. Illness
   3. Infection
   4. Inadequate nutrition
   5. Substance abuse
D. Complications of loss
   1. Losses may be compounded (e.g., relocation, loss of support network, economic changes, and/or role changes), causing bereavement overload.
   2. Suicide

> **HESI HINT** Older people undergo a great many changes, which are usually associated with loss (loss of spouse, friends, career, home, health, etc.). Therefore, older people are extremely vulnerable to emotional and mental stress, depression, and substance abuse.

Table 8.12 provides an example of a clinical judgment checklist applicable to Psychosocial changes: Loss.

> **HESI HINT** *Integrity versus despair* is Erikson's final stage of growth and development. Reminiscing is a means of setting one's life in order (accepting life and self, which is the task of this stage of Erikson's developmental theory. The goal of this stage is to feel a sense of meaning in one's life rather than feel despair or bitterness that life was wasted. The major task of old age is to redefine self in relation to a "changed role." Those persons who had been in charge of situations most of their lives may now find themselves in dependent positions. Role adjustment is a major task of old age.

Dementia

A. Overview of dementia
   1. There are many conditions that can imitate dementia in older adults. A key role for the nurse is to be observe and to rule out other possible causes of particular behavior, for example, acute infections (UTI), dehydration (electrolyte imbalance, medication, pain and metabolic disorders.
   2. Dementia is the permanent, progressive impairment in cognitive functioning manifested by memory loss (both long term and short term) and accompanied by impairment in judgment, abstract thinking, and social behavior.
   3. Dementia is characterized by the following:
      a. Personality changes: confusion, disorientation
      b. Deterioration of intellectual functioning, loss of memory
      c. Decline of appropriate judgment and ADLs
      d. Difficulty performing familiar tasks
      e. Misplacing things
      f. Problems with abstract thinking

TABLE 8.12   Clinical Judgment Measures: Psychosocial Changes: Loss

Clinical Judgment Measure	Assessment Characteristics
Recognize Cues	• Any loss or losses • The older adult's day-to-day functioning (e.g., eating and sleeping and work or social patterns) • Level of depression and suicide risk • The support system in place to assist with loss • Ability to express emotions related to the loss or losses • Any feelings of uselessness and nonparticipation in social events • Any loss of income that affects health care needs and quality of life • New or increased alcohol consumption on a daily or weekly basis • Past coping styles used with past losses
Analyze Cues	• Scores on the Geriatric Depression Scale (GDS) are within normal limits (no indication of symptoms related to loss, self-image, or late-life depression • Activities of daily living (ADLs) within normal limits (no change in sleeping or eating patterns)
Prioritize Cues	• Vital signs normal for age • Keep in mind symptoms associated with loss (recent spouse, child) feelings of uselessness, loneliness • Changes in income status (retirement, social security)
Solutions	• If needed, offer or refer to grief counseling or a support group • Encourage activities that allow the individual to use past coping strategies that will promote a feeling of self-worth and increased self-esteem • Encourage the individual to share his or her feelings • Encourage socialization with family peers and reminiscing about significant life experiences
Actions	• Vital signs normal for age • Oral responses consistent without evidence of depression, loneliness during examination • Evidence of social support by family members and friends
Evaluate Outcomes	• Vital signs normal for age • GDS scores normal (no evidence of depression) • ADLs normal for age (no evidence of changes in eating or sleep patterns

g. Changes in mood or behavior

h. The four A's of cognitive impairment are agnosia, amnesia, apraxia, and aphasia.

B. Causes of dementia

1. Alzheimer disease: the brains of individuals with Alzheimer disease have an abundance of beta amyloid plaques, neurofibrillary tangles, and atrophic brain cells and tissue. Alzheimer disease is the most common brain disorder and is one of the leading causes of death in the older adult.

2. Vascular or multifocal dementia: ischemic brain lesions develop as a result of a history of hyperlipidemia, hypertension, smoking, or obesity.

3. Dementia with Lewy bodies (DLB): microscopic deposits develop in the brain that damage nerve cells.

4. Frontotemporal dementia (Pick disease): the frontal and temporal lobes of the brain degenerate.

C. Risk factors of dementia

1. Cardiovascular disease

2. Depression

3. Diabetes

4. Midlife obesity

5. Sleep impairment

D. Complications of Dementia

1. Chronic confusion

2. self-neglect

3. Injury

4. Malnutrition

Table 8.13 provides an example of a clinical judgment checklist applicable to the Neurocognitive Disorder (NCD): Dementia.

> **HESI HINT** The major task of old age, according to Erikson, is to transition and redefine one's self in relation to a changed role. CJM associated with the understanding of dependent and independent situations present differently for older individuals thus awareness of the sense of control is important when providing goals associated with ADLs.

Health Promotion of Older Adults

A. Overview of health promotion of older adults

1. Diseases and conditions that affect older adults are the same as those that affect younger adults. However, in older adults, the signs and symptoms of pathology may be subtle, slow to develop, and very different from those seen in younger people (Table 8.14).

B. CJM for health promotion in the older adult

1. Encourage periodic health appraisal and counseling to prevent illness.

2. Electrocardiogram to detect subtle heart abnormalities

3. Chest radiograph to detect tuberculosis or lung cancer

4. Pulmonary function tests to detect chronic bronchitis and emphysema

5. Tonometer test to measure IOP as a test for glaucoma

6. Blood glucose to detect diabetes mellitus

7. Pap smear to detect cancer of the cervix; digital rectal examination to detect cancer of the prostate

8. Hearing and vision testing to detect sensory deprivation

9. Breast self-examination and mammogram, if indicated

10. Serum cholesterol as indicated by health status

11. Screen at-risk older adults for bone density, thyroid functioning, and abdominal aneurysm (in males).

12. Screen for depression and cognitive impairment.

13. Screen for BP as indicated by health status.

14. Screen for obesity.

15. Screen for substance abuse.

16. Screen for physical or emotional abuse.

C. Promote accident prevention.

1. Educate about safety measures to take to prevent falls.

2. Encourage physical and mental activities to promote mobility and confidence.

3. Encourage regular muscle-strengthening and balance-training exercises.

4. Encourage the use of assistive devices when needed (e.g., cane, walker, glasses, hearing aids).

5. Monitor driving skills; encourage American Association of Retired Persons (AARP) driving evaluation and training.

D. Protect against infectious diseases.

1. Encourage handwashing.

2. Educate older adults to avoid individuals who are ill.

3. Encourage immunization for influenza, pneumonia, Td/Tdap COVID-19.

4. Recommend herpes zoster (shingles); hepatitis A and B; and measles, mumps, rubella, and varicella immunizations if risk factors are present.

E. Avoid temperature extremes; prevent hypothermia.

F. Encourage the older person to stop smoking and discourage excessive alcohol intake.

G. Educate clients about proper foot care.

H. Encourage proper nutrition and weight control.

J. Encourage social interaction and use of support services (e.g., Meals on Wheels) and support groups (e.g., church).

K. Discourage the use of over-the-counter medications.

L. Review all medications yearly and encourage the client to throw away outdated drugs and prescriptions.

M. Diseases and conditions that affect older adults are the same as those that affect younger adults. However, in older adults, the signs and symptoms of pathology may be subtle, slow to develop, and quite different from those seen in younger people (see Table 8.14).

Elder Abuse

A. Overview of elder abuse

1. Interpersonal violence among older adults is defined as intentional acts of abuse and neglect that cause harm to create serious risk of harm to vulnerable older adults perpetrated by a caregiver or other person who is engaged in a trusting relationship with the older adult.

2. Abuse and neglect include the caregiver's failure to meet the older adult's basic physical needs, failure to protect the older adult from harm, or exploitation of their finance. The practical nurse (PN) is legally and

TABLE 8.13   Clinical Judgment Measures: Neurocognitive Disorder: Dementia

Clinical Judgment Measure	Assessment Characteristics

Recognize Cues	• Memory complaints: short term/long term; recognition of family, friends, or environment
	• Impaired physical functioning: shuffling, difficulty swallowing, and inability to perform activities of daily living (ADLs)
	• Conditions that mimic dementia
	• Unrecognized medical conditions
	  • Acute infection (urinary tract infection), dehydration (electrolyte imbalance), medication, pain, and metabolic disorder
	  • Medications, adverse reactions & nursing implications (Table 8.1)

Analyze Cues	• Vital signs are normal for age • Mini-mental score is normal (cognitive assessment score is not elevated, able to complete a clock drawing test with number spacing that is correct) • Laboratory values normal (WBC count normal) • No nausea or vomiting associated with medications
Prioritize Cues	• Vital signs normal for age • Acute cognitive changes (delirium, no recognition of family or caregiver) • Headache, dizziness or gastrointestinal (GI) distress
Solutions	• Administer screening tools for depression and cognitive impairment • Keep the client functioning and actively involved in social and family activities for as long as possible • Maintain an orderly, almost ritualistic, schedule to promote a sense of security • Maintain a regularly scheduled reality orientation on a daily basis • Keep the client oriented as to time, place, and person (repeatedly) • Keep a calendar and clock within sight at all times • Display a calendar and clock that can be read by the older person (i.e., a clock with large numbers and a calendar that can be read by those with deteriorating vision) • Be sure the date and time are accurate (i.e., keep the calendar current and the clock in working order) • Keep familiar objects, such as family pictures, in the older adult's environment to promote a sense of continuity and security • Administer prescribed drugs to reduce emotional lability, agitation, and irritability or prescribed antidepressant, as indicated • Speak in a slow, calm voice; avoid excitement • Redirect the client who exhibits combative behavior • Educate family and caregivers on safe home environment • Provide support and education to family and long-term caregivers • Encourage end-of-life planning, including a will, do not resuscitate status, power of attorney, and funeral arrangements
Actions	• Vital signs normal for age • Oriented to place, time, environment • Mini-mental status exam intact • ADLs intact (teach family/caregiver changes in ability to complete daily activities: eating, bathing) • Medication regime adequate for diagnosis • Teach family/caregiver to take medications with meals to avoid GI upset
Evaluate Outcomes	• Check vital signs for consistency for age • Mini-mental status exam intact for age • ADLs as reported by caregiver (able to eat, feed self, and bathe self) • Medication compliance adherence as reported by family or caregiver

ethically responsible for reporting elder abuse to the appropriate agency. Most of the abuse is committed by spouses and children, but other caregivers can also be perpetrators.

3. In the United States, legislatures in each state have passed elder abuse prevention laws.

B. Causes of elder abuse
  1. Elder abuse may be defined as intentional acts.
     a. Physical abuse—inflicting physical pain or injury to an older adult (e.g., slapping, hitting, bruising, or physical restraint)
     b. Sexual abuse—sexual contact, of any kind, without consent
     c. Neglect—failure by the responsible individuals to provide food, shelter, or health care
     d. Exploitation—misuse, concealment, or illegal taking of funds, property, or assets of an elder for someone else's use
     e. Emotional abuse—using verbal or nonverbal actions to inflict distress or mental pain on an older adult (e.g., intimidation, humiliation, or threats)
     f. Desertion—the leaving alone of a vulnerable older adult by someone who has assumed responsibility for the care of the older adult

C. Risks of elder abuse
  1. Cognitive impairment

TABLE 8.14 Diseases and Conditions in the Older Adults

Disease or Condition	Description in Terms of the Older Adult	Nursing Implications
Delirium	• Acute confused state with rapid onset, usually the result of systemic illness or medication • Decreased level of consciousness • Client is often disoriented and/or incoherent with severe memory disturbances • Hallucinations and delusions may be present	• Establish a meaningful environment • Help maintain body awareness • Help client cope with confusion, delusions, and illusions • Is usually transient • Usually occurs secondary to another medical condition substance abuse (withdrawal), medication, or toxic exposures
Dementia	• Slow onset of symptoms • Level of consciousness may be intact	• Dementia is a major neurocognitive disorder • Characterized by multiple cognitive deficits • 80% of dementias are irreversible • See nursing interventions for dementia
Cardiac Dysrhythmias	• Incidence increases with age • More serious in older adults because of lower tolerance of decreased cardiac output (can result in syncope, falls, transient ischemic attacks, and confusion) • Symptoms result from compromised circulation and O_2 deficit	• Monitor, prevent, and manage dysrhythmias • Advise smoking cessation • Encourage exercise and weight control
Cataracts	• Often a result of normal aging changes • Most common pathologic problem affecting the eyesight of older adults • Treatment is surgical removal	• Teach instillation of eye drops • Reduce glare in environment • Assistance is required postoperatively because affected eye is covered and disorientation may occur
Glaucoma	• Risk of acquiring increases with age	• Loss of sensory input can result in confusion • Prevention: yearly intraocular pressure examinations
Macular Degeneration	• Principal cause of blindness	• Loss of sensory input can result in confusion • Prevention: yearly examinations
Cerebrovascular Accident	• Interruption of cerebral circulation, caused by occlusion or hemorrhage in the brain • Risk increases with age	• Prevent deterioration of client's condition • Maximize functional abilities (occupational therapy) • Assist client in accepting physical deficits • Check gag reflex before client receives food or fluids • Prevent injuries to paralyzed limbs
Pressure Ulcer	• Immobility puts older adults at risk for the development of pressure ulcers	• Reposition frequently • Provide adequate nutrition
Hypothyroidism	• Usually occurs after age 50 • Symptoms are often similar to normal aging changes and have an insidious onset, making it difficult to detect in older adults • Older adults are at greater risk for development of myxedema coma, which is life threatening	• Often diagnosed as depression; with treatment, signs of depression disappear • Caution against abruptly discontinuing medication
Thyrotoxicosis (Graves Disease)	• Symptoms may be absent or attributed to other, more common diseases in older adults • Weight loss and heart failure may be predominant symptoms	• It is precipitated by stressful events such as trauma, surgery, or infection. Be alert for signs and symptoms • Can be fatal if untreated
Chronic obstructive pulmonary disease	• A major cause of respiratory disability in older adults • Most older people exhibit both chronic bronchitis and chronic emphysema • Fatigue is a common result because of the increased work required to breathe (dyspnea)	• Encourage client to stop smoking • Keep in mind older person's state of confusion when teaching about treatment regimen • Plan rest periods to allow client to maintain oxygen levels
Urinary Tract Infections (UTIs)	• Incidence increases with age • Older people are often asymptomatic or exhibit vague, ill-defined symptoms • With infections, older people often become confused	• Suspect UTI when client's voiding habits change

2. Physical impairment
3. Dependency
4. Caregiver stress
5. Family conflict
6. Isolation
7. Addiction

D. Complications of elder abuse

1. Injury
2. Infections
3. Death
4. Impaired self-esteem

E. Nursing assessment (data collection) of elder abuse
  1. Bruises on the upper arms (bilaterally, from being shaken)
  2. Broken bones from falls (resulting from being pushed)

3. Dehydration or malnourishment
4. Overmedication
5. Poor physical hygiene: improper medical care
6. Withdrawn behavior, feelings of hopelessness, helplessness
7. May be demanding, belligerent, and aggressive
8. Repeated visits to health care agency for injuries/falls
9. Injuries that do not correlate with state cause
10. Misuse of money by children or legal guardians

F. Clinical judgment plans and interventions for elder abuse
1. PNs are legally required to report all the cases of suspected elder abuse to the appropriate local and state agencies
2. Follow the policy and procedures of the institution. Report the observed data to the registered nurse (RN).
3. Establish trust; use nonjudgmental approach.
4. Meet physical needs: treat wounds or injuries.
5. Document factual, objective statements of client's physical condition, injuries, and interaction with significant other and family.
6. Collaborate with the RN to arrange community resources to provide "respite care" for the caregiver.
7. Collaborate with the RN to arrange visiting nurses, nutritional services, or adult day care if possible.

> **HESI HINT** It is difficult for an older adult to admit abuse for fear of being placed in a nursing home or being abandoned. Therefore, it is imperative to establish a trusting relationship with the older adult client.

End-of-Life Care

A. Overview of end-of life care
1. End-of-life care shifts care from invasive interventions aimed at prolonging life to supportive interventions that focus on control of symptoms.
2. Insurance and hospice entities view the end-of-life stage as 6 months before death. However, a major problem with this definition is the difficulty in predicting the period of client survival. Health care providers may overestimate or underestimate survival time.

B. Clinical Nursing Judgment interventions for end-of-life care includes the following:
1. Pain management is a priority in end-of-life care because untreated or undertreated pain consumes energy; interferes with function; affects quality of life and social interactions; and contributes to sleep disturbances, hopelessness, and loss of control.
2. Alleviating dyspnea can contribute to the client's comfort and decrease the family's anxiety. Dyspnea (distressing shortness of breath) may be related to pulmonary, cardiac, neuromuscular, or metabolic disorders; obesity; anxiety; and spiritual distress. Families need support, in particular when the gurgling sound ("death rattle") occurs close to the end of life.
3. Listening, reassuring, and reinforcing nonpharmacologic interventions to help manage anxiety (a mild to severe subjective feeling of apprehension, tension, insecurity, and uneasiness) may need to be followed by pharmacologic agents.
4. Managing GI symptoms of nausea, vomiting, gastritis, constipation, and diarrhea ensures comfort and quality of life.
5. Assessing for psychiatric symptoms of depression and delirium common at the end of life and providing care as needed. If unrecognized, they can rob clients of quality of life and quality of care.
6. Recognizing the spiritual needs of older adults can help them come to terms with their illness and the end of their lives. *Spirituality* is a broad concept that encompasses the search for meaning in life experiences, relationships with others, and a sense of connectedness to a personal deity. Recognition of spiritual distress is important to help the dying client come to terms with the end of life.
7. Supporting family caregivers is important because family caregivers may do everything for the client, from assisting with ADLs to giving medications and managing medical equipment and treatments. Often, they are the ones who serve as go-betweens for the client and health care providers. Although caregivers may find great satisfaction in their role, they often experience stress and diminished physical health.
8. Family bereavement support is essential because survivors are at an increased risk for illness or death. Normal responses to grief can be physical, psychological, cognitive, and/or spiritual. Uncomplicated grief is a dynamic, pervasive, and highly individualized process. Individuals who are overwhelmed or remain interminably in the state of grief without progression through the mourning process to completion may be experiencing complicated grief. When the nurse identifies complicated grief, it should be reported so that a referral for help can be made to the correct provider, such as a bereavement counselor.

💡 REVIEW OF GERONTOLOGIC NURSING

1. What are the normal memory changes that occur as one ages?
2. What three physiologic changes are clinically significant in older adults?
3. Why can the BP of older adults be expected to increase?
4. What is the major cause of respiratory disability in older adults?
5. List five nursing interventions to promote adequate bowel functioning for older people.
6. What lifestyle factors negatively affect nearly every system in the older adult's body?
7. What visual problem most commonly occurs in older adults?
8. What are the three most common disorders that result from changes in the neurologic system?
9. What is the difference between delirium and NCD?
10. Falls are the result of what physiologic changes?
11. What are two factors that cause a decrease in the excretion of drugs by the kidneys?
12. What areas are important for end-of-life care?

See Answer Key at the end of this text for suggested responses.
For more review, go to http://evolve.elsevier.com/HESI/RN for HESI's online study examinations.

NEXT-GENERATION NCLEX® EXAMINATION-STYLE QUESTIONS

Orders

stat 12-lead EKG, chest X-ray, CBC, SMA-12, safety parameters, vital signs q.4 h.

| Health History | Nurses' Notes | Vital Signs | Lab Results |

Mrs. Smith, an 84-year-old female, has been brought to the emergency room for chest pain. She has been living with her sister Cecelia for the last 5 years and states that her sister helps her with bathing and ADLs. When the PN enters the room, Mrs. Smith states that her chest hurts. The PN helps her into a hospital gown and notices that she is bruised on her chest and back. Additionally, she had bruises on the front and back of her arms with open cuts to her upper thighs. Mrs. Smith states that she fell several times at home and the open cuts were from her accidentally cutting herself when cutting vegetables. The PN tends to her bruises by putting ice on her chest for pain relief, and cleans and bandages her wounds on her thighs. As the PN gets ready to leave the room she notices that Mrs. Smith is crying.

Instructions

Complete the diagram by selecting from the choices below to specify which potential condition the client is most likely experiencing, 2 actions to take, and 2 parameters the nurse would monitor to assess the client's progress.

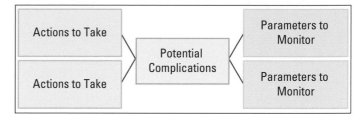

Nursing Actions	Potential Conditions	Parameters to Monitor
Report the observed data to the registered nurse (RN)	Myocardial infarction (MI)	Chest pain level
Obtain MRI	Elderly abuse/physical	Complications associated with bruising and open wounds
Document factual, objective data related to the patient's physical condition and injuries.	Cardiovascular ischemia	Pulse oximetry
Administer oxygen 2 L/min NC	Situational depression	I & O
Call dermatology for consult		Complete Glascow scale every 4 hr

---

REFERENCES AND BIBLIOGRAPHY

Corder, C. J., Rathi, B. M., Sharif, S., & Leslie, S. W. (2020). 24-hour urine collection. In *StatPearls* [Internet]. Treasure Island, FL: StatPearls Publishing. Retrieved from: https://www.ncbi.nlm.nih.gov/books/NBK482482/.

Dumic, I., Nordin, T., Jecmenica, M., Stojkovic Lalosevic, M., Milosavljevic, T., & Milovanovic, T. (2019). Gastrointestinal tract disorders in older age. *Canadian Journal of Gastroenterology & Hepatology.* https://doi.org/10.1155/2019/6757524, 2019, 6757524 https://www.ncbi.nlm.nih.gov/pmc/articles/PMC6354172/.

Gamache, J., & Hoo, G. W. S. (2018). What is the mortality rate of aspiration pneumonia? In *Aspiration pneumonitis and pneumonia.* Retrieved from https://www.medscape.com/answers/296198-38080/what-is-the-mortality-rate-of-aspiration-pneumonia (accessed on February 13, 2021).

Gridley, K., Aspinal, F., Parker, G., Weatherly, H., Faria, R., Longo, F., et al. (2019). *Specialist nursing support for unpaid carers of people with dementia: A mixed-methods feasibility study.* Bethesda, Maryland. NIHR Journals Library. Health Services and Delivery Research, No. 7.12. Bookshelf ID: NBK539055.

Heidari, S. (2016). Sexuality and older people: A neglected issue. *Reproductive Health Matters, 24*(48), 1—5. https://doi.org/10.1016/j.rhm.2016.11.011.

National Institute on Aging. *Healthy Eating. Vitamins and Minerals for Older Adults.* www.nia.nih.gov/health/vitamins-and-minerals-older-adults (accessed on February 12, 2021).

Picetti, D., Foster, S., Pangle, A. K., Schrader, A., George, M., Wei, J. Y., et al. (2017). Hydration health literacy in the elderly. *Nutrition and Healthy Aging, 4*(3), 227—237. https://doi.org/10.3233/NHA-170026.

Varghese, M., & Dahale, A. B. (2018). The geropsychiatric interview—assessment and diagnosis. *Indian Journal of Psychiatry, 60*(Suppl. 3),

S301—S311. https://doi.org/10.4103/0019-5545.224471. https://www.ncbi.nlm.nih.gov/pubmed/29535466.

Weil, A., Fulmer, T., Stuart, B., Konetzka, R. T., Ornstein, K. A., Leff, B., et al. (2019, September 24). *Event. Aging and health: Improving care for older adults. HealthAffairs.* National Press Club. https://doi.org/10.1377/he20190829.971169.

Wolkoff, P. (2018). Indoor air humidity, air quality, and health—an overview. *International Journal of Hygiene and Environmental Health,* *221*(3), 376—390. https://doi.org/10.1016/j.ijheh.2018.01.015. https://s100.copyright.com/AppDispatchServlet?publisherName=ELS&contentID=S1438463917306946&orderBeanReset=true.

World Health Organization. (2018). *Aging and health.* Retrieved from https://www.who.int/news-room/fact-sheets/detail/ageing-and-health (accessed on February 14, 2021).

Normal Values

Test	Adult	Child	Infant/Newborn	Elder	Nursing Implications
Hematologic					
Hgb Hemoglobin: g/dL	Male: 14—18 Female: 12—16 Pregnant: >11	1—6 years: 9.5—14 6—18 years: 10—15.5	0—28 days: 14—24 1—2 months: 12—20 2—6 months: 10—17 6 months—1 year: 9.5—14	Values slightly decreased	High-altitude living increases values Drug therapy can alter values Slight Hgb decreases normally occur during pregnancy
Hct Hematocrit: %	Male: 42—52 Female: 37—47 Pregnant: >33	6—12 years: 31—38 12—18 years: 31—41	Newborn: 37—47 15—30 days: 41—43 Male Female 34—42 61—180 days: 31—38 6 months—2 years: 31—36	Values slightly decreased	Prolonged stasis from vaso-constriction secondary to the tourniquet can alter values Abnormalities in RBC size may alter Hct values
RBC Red blood cell count:1012/L (mm3)	Male: 4.7—6.1 Female: 4.2—5.4	1—6 years: 4.0—5.5 1—18 years: 4.5—5	Newborn: 4.8—7.1 2—8 weeks: 4—6 2—6 months: 3.5—5.5 6 mo—1 year: 3.5—5.2	Same as adult	Never draw specimen from an arm with an infusing IV Exercise and high altitudes can cause an increase in values Pregnancy values are usually lower Drug therapy can alter values
WBC White blood cell count: 109/L (mm3)	Both genders: 5—10	≤ 2 years: 6.2—17 ≥ 2 years: 5—10	Newborn, term: 9—30	Same as adult	Anesthetics, stress, exercise, and convulsions can cause increased values Drug therapy can decrease values 24—48 h postpartum: normal count may be as high as 25
Platelet count: 109/L (mm3)	Both genders: 5—10	150—400	Premature infant: 100—300 Newborn: 150—300 Infant: 200—475	Same as adult	Values may increase at high altitudes, with strenuous ex-ercise, or taking oral contraceptives Values may decrease because of hemorrhage, DIC, reduced production of platelets, in-fections, prosthetic heart valves, and drugs (acetamin-ophen, aspirin, chemo-therapy, H_2-blockers, INH, Levaquin, streptomycin, sul-fonamides, thiazide diuretics)

The laboratory values that are most important to know for the NCLEX-PN exam are Hgb, Hct, WBCs, Na, K, BUN (Blood urea nitrogen), blood glucose, ABGs (blood gases), bilirubin for newborns, and therapeutic range for PT/INR and PTT.

Continued

Test	Adult	Child	Infant/Newborn	Elder	Nursing Implications
SED rate, ESR Erythrocyte sedimentation rate: mm/hr	Male: up to 15 Female: up to 20 Pregnant (all trimesters); up to 10 Both genders 11—12.5	Same as adult	Newborn: 0—2	Same as adult	Rate is elevated during 2nd and 3rd trimester of pregnancy
PT Prothrombin time: seconds	Both genders: 11—12.5 Pregnant: Slight ↓	Same as adult	Same as adult	Same as adult	Used in regulating warfarin (Coumadin) dosages Therapeutic range is 1.5 to 2 times normal or control
INR International Normalized Ratio	Both genders: 0.8—1.1	Same as adult	Same as adult	Same as adult	Used to monitor anticoagulation therapy. INR must be individualized Certain clients with: (1) Atrial fibrillation and deep vein thrombosis: between 2.0—3.0 (2) Mechanical heart valves: between 3.0—4.0
PTT Partial thromboplastin time: seconds (see APTT)	Both genders: 60—70 Pregnant: Slight ↓	Same as adult	Same as adult	Same as adult	It is used in regulating heparin therapy Therapeutic range is 1.5 to 2.5 times normal or control
APTT Activated partial thromboplastin time: seconds	Both genders: 30—40	Same as adult	Same as adult	Same as adult	It is used to partially regulate heparin dosages Therapeutic range is 1.5 to 2.5 times normal or control
Blood Chemistry					
Alkaline phosphatase: U/L	Both genders: 30—120	1—3 years: 185—383 4—6 years: 191—450 7—9 years: 218—499 10—11 years: Male 174—624 12—13 years: Male 245—584 Female 144—499 14—15 years: Male 168—618 Female 103—283 16—19 years: Male 97—317 Female 82—169	No information listed	Slightly higher than adults	Hemolysis of specimen can cause falsely elevated values.
Albumin: g/dL	Both genders: 3.5 to 5 Pregnant: slight ↑	4.5—9	Premature infant: 3—4.2 Newborn: 3.5—5.4 Infant 4.4—5.4	Same as adult	No special preparation is needed
Bilirubin total: mg/dL	Total: 0.3—1 Indirect: 0.2—0.8 Direct: 0.1—0.3	Same as adult	Newborn: 1—12	Same as adult	Client is to be NPO (NPO means "nothing by mouth," from the Latin nil per os) except for water for 8—12 hours before testing Prevent hemolysis of blood during venipuncture Do *not* shake tube; it can cause inaccurate values Protect blood sample from bright light
Calcium total: mg/dL	Both genders: 9—10.5	8.8—10.8	<10 days: 7.6—10.4 Cord: 9—11.5 10 days—2 years: 9—10.6	Values tend to decrease	No special preparation is needed Use of thiazide diuretics may increase calcium values.

Continued

Test	Adult	Child	Infant/Newborn	Elder	Nursing Implications
Chloride: mEq/l	Both genders: 98—106	90—110	Newborn: 96—106 Premature infant: 95—110	Same as adult	Do not collect from an arm with an infusing IV solution
Cholesterol: mg/dL	Both genders: <200	10—11 years: Male 120—228 Female: 122—242	7—12 months: Male 83—205 Female 68—216 Newborn (0—1 mo) Male 348—174 Female 56—195	Same as adult	Do not collect from an arm with an infusing IV solution.
High-density lipoprotein [HDL] (alpha lipoproteins)	Both genders: 30—70 mg/dL	1 to 9 years: 53—56 10 to 14 years: 52—55 15 to 19 years: 46—52	Newborn: 35	Same as adult	
Low-density lipoprotein (LDL) (beta lipoproteins)	Both genders: <130 mg/dL	1 to 9 years: 93—100 10 to 14 years: 97 15 to 19 years: 94—96	Newborn: 29	Same as adult	Target LDL is <70 for client with high risk for CHD.
CPK Creatine phosphokinase: IU/l	Male: 55—170 Female: 30—135	Same as adult	Newborn: 65—580	Same as adult	Specimen must not be stored before running test
Creatinine: mg/dL	Male: 0.6—1.2 Female: 0.5—1.1	Child/Adolescent 1 —18 years: 0.2—0.7	Newborn 0—1 week: 0.6—1.1 Infant 7 days —12 months: 0.2—0.4	Decrease in muscle mass may cause decreased values	It is preferred but not necessary to be NPO 8 hours before testing A ratio of 20:1, BUN to creatine, indicates adequate kidney functioning
Glucose: mg/dL	Both genders: 70—100	≤2 years: 60—100 >2 years: 70—110	Cord: 45—96 Premature infant: 20—60 Newborn: 30—60 Infant: 40—90	Increase in normal range after age 50	Client to be NPO except for water 8 hours before testing Caffeine can cause increased values Stress, infection, and caffeine can cause increased values.
Glycosylated hemoglobin (%)	Nondiabetic: 4—5.9 Diabetic Good control <7	Same	Same	Same	Used to monitor diabetic treatment Amount depends on glucose available over RBC's life span
HCO3: mEq/l	Both genders: 21—28	Same as adult	Infant: 20—28 Newborn: 13—22	Same as adult	None
Iron: mcg/dL	Male: 80—180 Female: 60—160	Child 4—10 years: Male: 15—128 Female: 28—122	Newborn: Male: 72—203 Female: 75—235	Same as adult	It is preferred but not necessary to be NPO 8 hours before testing
TIBC Total iron binding capacity: mcg/dL	Both genders: 250—460	Same as adult	Newborn: 94—232	Same as adult	None
LDH Lactic dehydrogenase: IU/l	Both genders: 100—190	60—170	Infant: 100—250 Newborn: 160—450	Same as adult	No IM injections are to be given 8 to 12 hours before testing Hemolysis of blood will cause false positive
Potassium: mEq/l	Both genders: 3.5—5	3.4—4.7	Infant: 4.1—5.3 Newborn: 3—5.9	Same as adult	Hemolysis of specimen can result in falsely elevated values Exercise of the forearm with tourniquet in place may cause increased potassium levels
Protein total: g/dL	Both genders 6.4—8.3	6.2—8	Premature infant: 4.2—7.6 Newborn: 4.6—7.4 Infant: 6—6.7	Same as adult	It is preferred but not necessary to be NPO 8 hours before testing

Continued

Test	Adult	Child	Infant/Newborn	Elder	Nursing Implications
AST/SGOT Aspartate amino-transferase: IU/l	0—35 Female slightly lower than adult males	3—6 years: 15—50 6—12 years: 10—50 12—18 years: 10—40	0—5 days: 35—140 <3 years: 15—60	Slightly higher than adult	Hemolysis of specimen can result in falsely elevated values Exercise may cause an increased value
ALT/SGPT Alanine aminotrans-ferase: IU/mL	Both genders: 4—36	Similar to adult	Infant may be twice as high as an adult	Slightly higher than adult	Hemolysis of specimen can result in falsely elevated values Exercise may cause an increased value
Sodium: mEq/l	Both genders: 136—145	136—145	Infant: 134—150 Newborn: 134—144	Same as adult	Do not collect from an arm with an infusing IV solution
Triglycerides: mg/dL	Male: 40—160 Female: 35—135	4—6 years: 32—116 7—9 years: 28—129 10—11 years: Male: 24—137 Female: 39—140 12—13 years: Male: 24—145 Female: 37—130 14—15 years: Male: 34—165 Female: 38—135 16—19 years: Male: 34—140 Female: 37—140	Male: 0—3 years: 27—125 Female: 32—99	Same as adult	Client is to be NPO 12 hours before testing No alcohol for 24 hours before test
Urea nitrogen: mg/dL	Both genders: 10—20	5—18	Infant: 5—18 Newborn: 3—12 Cord: 21—40	Slightly higher	None
Thyroid- Stimulating Hormone (TSH, Thyrotropin) μ/mL	Both genders: 2—10	Same as adult	Newborn: 3—18 Cord: 3—12	Same as adult	The TSH test is used to differentiate primary and secondary hypothyroidism
Triiodothyronine (T3) ng/dL	Both genders: 70—205	1—5 years: 105—270 6—10 years: 95—240 ng/dL 11—15 years: 80—215 ng/dL 16—20 years: 80—210 ng/dL	Newborn: 100—740 Infant: 105—245	>50 years: 40—180	Primarily to diagnose hyperthyroidism
Total thyroxine (T4) mcg/dL	Male: 4—12 Female: 5—12	1—5 years: 7—15 5—10 years: 6—13 10—15 years: 5—12	Newborn: 1—3 days: 11—22 1—2 weeks: 10—16 Infant: 8—16	> 60 years: 5—11	Newborns are screened to detect hypothyroidism so mental retardation can be prevented with early diagnosis. A heel stick is used to collect the blood
Arterial Blood Chemistry pH	Both genders: 7.35—7.45	Child >2 years: Same as adult	2 months—2 years: 7.34—7.46 Newborn: 7.32—7.49	Same as adult	Specimen must be heparinized Specimen must be iced for transport All air bubbles must be expelled from sample Direct pressure to puncture site must be maintained

Continued

Test	Adult	Child	Infant/Newborn	Elder	Nursing Implications
Pco2: mmHg	Both genders: 35—45	Same as adult	<2 years: 26—41	Same as adult	Specimen must be heparinized Specimen must be iced for transport All air bubbles must be expelled from sample Direct pressure to puncture site must be maintained
Po2: mmHg	Both genders: 80—100	Same as adult	Newborn/Infant: 16—24	Same as adult	Specimen must be heparinized Specimen must be iced for transport All air bubbles must be expelled from sample Direct pressure to puncture site must be maintained
HCO3: mEq/l	Both genders: 21—28	Same as adult	Infant/Newborn: 16—24	Same as adult	Specimen must be heparinized Specimen must be iced for transport All air bubbles must be expelled from sample Direct pressure to puncture site must be maintained
O2 saturation: %	Both genders: 95—100	Same as adult	Newborn: 40—90	95	Specimen must be heparinized Specimen must be iced for transport All air bubbles must be expelled from sample Direct pressure to puncture site must be maintained

Urinalysis (UA)

Characteristic	Normal	Nursing Implications
Appearance	Clear	May be a midstream, clean-catch specimen Cloudy urine may be caused by the presence of pus (necrotic WBCs), RBCs, or bacteria, or ingestion of certain foods Urine that has been refrigerated for longer than 1 hour can become cloudy
Color	Yellow to amber	Pale yellow to amber color because of the pigment urochrome (product of bilirubin metabolism) The color indicates the concentration of the urine (dilute urine: straw colored; concentrated urine: deep amber and varies with specific gravity) Color can change with ingestion of certain foods or medications Urine darkens with prolonged standing
Odor	Aromatic	Diabetic ketoacidosis has the strong, sweet smell of acetone UTI, the urine may have a foul odor
pH	4.6—8.0 (average, 6.0)	Bacteria, UTI, or a diet high in citrus fruits or vegetables may cause increased urine pH
Protein	0—8 mg/dL 50—80 mg/24 h (at rest) <250 mg/24 h (during exercise)	Proteinuria is an indicator of renal disease Test urine of all pregnant women for proteinuria, an indicator of preeclampsia. If significant protein is noted at urinalysis, a 24-hour urine specimen should be collected so that the quantity of protein can be measured A first-voided specimen is best to test for protein

Continued

Characteristic	Normal	Nursing Implications
Specific gravity	Adult: 1.005—1.030 (usually, 1.010—1.025) Older adults: values decrease with age Newborn: 1.001—1.020	Renal disease tends to diminish concentrating capability Specific gravity is also a measurement of hydration status: overhydration of urine is more dilute, dehydration of urine is more concentrated
Ketones	None	Ketonuria is associated with poorly controlled diabetes Ketonuria may occur with acute febrile illnesses, especially in infants and children Special diets (carbohydrate-free, high-protein, high-fat) and some drugs may cause ketonuria
Red blood cells (RBCs)	≤2	Hematuria can be microscopic or gross Bladder, ureteral, and urethral diseases are the most common causes of RBCs in the urine
Volume		24-hour specimen is required If a 24-hour urine collection is needed, refrigerate urine during the collection period
Glucose	In fresh specimen: none 24—hour specimen: 50—300 mg/24 h	Glucose is not excreted by the kidney unless blood levels exceed approximately 180 mg/dL so can reflect the degree of glucose elevation in the blood Collect a fresh double-voided specimen In pregnancy glycosuria is common, but persistent and significantly high levels may indicate gestational diabetes or other obstetric illness
White blood cells (WBCs)	0—4 per low-power field	The presence of five or more WBCs in the urine indicates a UTI involving the bladder or kidneys, or both. A clean-catch urine culture should be done for further evaluation Vaginal discharge may contaminate the urine specimen and factitiously cause WBCs in the urine

APTT, Activated partial thromboplastin time; *Hct,* Hematocrit; *Hgb,* Hemoglobin; *INR,* International Normalized Ratio; *LDL,* Low-density lipoprotein; *PT,* Prothrombin time; *PTT,* Partial thromboplastin time; *RBC,* Red blood cell; *TSH,* Thyroid- stimulating hormone; *WBC,* White blood cell.
Source: Pagana KD & Pagana TJ. (2013): *Mosby's diagnostic and laboratory test reference,* (11th ed), St. Louis, Mosby.

Answers to Review Questions

CHAPTER 1

No review questions in this chapter.

CHAPTER 2

Review of Leadership and Management

1. Aspects of supervision:
   A. Checks on the staff after making assignments.
   B. Carefully explains details of an assignment.
   C. Suggests an improvement in a technique to UAP after completing a task.
2. Right task, right person, right situation, right communication, and right supervision.
3. Which of these tasks can be delegated to a UAP?
   a. Should not be delegated because it is a sterile procedure.
   b. Can be delegated because it is an intervention that is part of the implementation phase of the nursing process.
   c. Requires nursing knowledge and skills and thus cannot be delegated.
   d. Must be performed by a nurse and cannot be delegated.
4. Nursing process.
5. Which assignment should be appropriate for the PN to delegate to a UAP? Select all that apply (correct answer is highlighted).
   A. Explain the side effects of chemotherapy to the client.
   B. Feed a client who is 2 days postop.
   C. Calculate the intake and output (I&O) on the client who is on TPN.
   D. Hang intravenous piggyback (IVPB) antibiotics.
   E. Assist a client who is 2 days postop to the bathroom.

Review of Legal Aspects of Nursing

1. Has the PN received sufficient education, training, and experience? Refer to the job description, policies, and procedures of the health care facility; be consistent with the state's Nurse Practice Act.
2. Is the action something that a rational, responsible, and prudent nurse would do in a similar situation?
3. *Duty:* nurse was responsible for delivering care; *breach of duty:* failure to perform according to established standards; *causation:* failure to follow the standard resulted in client injury or damage; and *damages:* client suffers a physical, mental, or financial loss.
4. *Assault:* threats or acts that cause fear; *battery:* unauthorized physical contact; *defamation:* using false information to harm another's reputation; *false imprisonment:* unauthorized interference with someone's personal freedom; *fraud:* providing false information with the potential to cause harm; and *invasion of privacy:* failure to protect bodily and confidential property.
5. A person's ability to make responsible decisions; client must be alert, coherent, emancipated, or have a parent or legal guardian. A person declared incompetent cannot vote, make contracts or wills, drive a car, sue or be sued, or hold a professional license.
6. Client is declared a threat to self, or others, as certified by a licensed health care provider (one or two required). Client must receive a legal hearing shortly after admission; confinement is usually limited to 90 days and may possibly be extended to a 1-year commitment.
7. Must be written, voluntary, informed, witnessed, and signed by a competent adult, emancipated minor, or parent or legal guardian.
8. When the client is fully informed, the client voluntarily agrees to the procedure, verbal consent is obtained, and is necessary to save "life or limb."
9. The Good Samaritan Law. The person rendering aid is not held liable for civil acts for emergency care rendered "in good faith." The care delivered must be reasonable and prudent.
10. The PN should inform the health care provider, record that the health care provider was informed, and record the health care provider's response to such information. The PN should inform the nursing supervisor and decline to perform the order.
11. Apply restraints according to the manufacturer's instructions and institutional policy; check restraints regularly and frequently; prevent injury from the restraint; record all monitoring; remove restraints as soon as possible; and demonstrate and record repeated efforts to avoid restraint use.
12. Client must give written consent before health care providers can use or disclose personal health information; health care providers must give clients notice about provider responsibilities regarding client confidentiality; clients must have access to their medical records; providers who restrict access must explain why and must offer clients a description of the complaint process; clients have the right to request that changes be made in their medical records to correct inaccuracies; health care providers must follow specific tracking procedures or any disclosures made that ensure accountability for the maintenance of client confidentiality; and clients have the right to request that health care providers restrict use and disclosure of

their personal health information, although the provider may decline to do so.

Review of Disaster Nursing

1. Disaster preparedness, disaster response, and disaster recovery.
2. *Primary:* assist with development of plan, training/education plan, train/educate personnel and public; *secondary:* triage, treatment shelter supervision; *tertiary:* follow-up, recovery assistance, prevention of future disasters.
3. To sort or categorize.
4. Anthrax, pneumonic plague, botulism, smallpox, inhalation tularemia, viral hemorrhagic fever, ricin, sarin, radiation.

NEXT-GENERATION PN-NCLEX® EXAMINATION-STYLE QUESTION

Actions to Take	Potential Conditions	Parameters to Monitor
Take a temperature	Eczema-related inflammation	Fall precautions
Obtain MRI for suspected head injury	Suspect child abuse	Monitor oximeter
Report suspicion of child abuse to RN and social worker	Lesions due to falls	Observe interaction between mom and child (report to RN as needed)
Provide toys for the child	Cardiac distress	Restrain child for safety
Complete an assessment of the child's friends		Check I & O

CHAPTER 3

Review of Respiratory Failure

1. Less than 60 mm Hg.
2. P_{CO_2} greater than 5o mm Hg.
3. Hypoxemia.
4. Dyspnea/tachypnea, intercostal retractions, cyanosis.
5. Congenital heart disease, infection or sepsis, respiratory distress syndrome, aspiration, fluid overload, or dehydration.
6. 100%.

Review of Shock and DIC

1. Widespread, serious reduction of tissue perfusion, which leads to generalized impairment of cellular function.
2. Hypovolemia.
3. Release of endotoxins from bacteria that act on nerves in vascular space in the periphery, causing vascular pooling,

reduced venous return, and decreased cardiac output, resulting in poor systemic perfusion.
4. Quick restoration of cardiac output and tissue perfusion.
5. Warm rapid infusion of volume-expanding fluids.
6. History of MI with left ventricular failure or possible cardiomyopathy, with symptoms of pulmonary edema.
7. Pulmonary edema; administer cardiotonic drugs such as digitalis preparations.
8. 30 mL/h.
9. BP mean of 80 to 90 mm Hg; P_{O_2} more than 50 mm Hg; CVP greater than 6 cm of H_2O; urine output at least 30 mL/h.
10. A coagulation disorder in which there is paradoxical thrombosis and hemorrhage.
11. Prothrombin time—prolonged; partial thromboplastin time—prolonged; platelets—decreased.
12. Heparin.
13. Gently provide oral care with mouth swabs. Minimize needle sticks and use the smallest-gauge needle possible when injections are necessary. Eliminate pressure by turning the client frequently. Minimize the number of BPs taken by cuff. Use gentle suction to prevent trauma to the mucosa. Apply pressure to any oozing site.

Review of Resuscitation

1. Call 9-1-1 (or send someone to do that) and begin CPR by pushing hard and fast on the center of the chest.
2. Necrosis of the heart muscle because of poor perfusion of the heart.
3. Palpate for at least but no more than 10 seconds, recognizing that dysrhythmias or bradycardia could be occurring.
4. Thirty compressions and two breaths.
5. Adults 30:2; use chest compression rate of ~100 to 120/min for infants and children; single rescuer compression to ventilation rate of 30:2, two rescuers 15:2.
6. Watch for chest excursion and auscultate bilaterally for breath sounds.
7. When the person points to his or her throat and can no longer cough, talk, or make sounds.
8. This may result in the object possibly being pushed farther down into the throat.

Review of Fluid and Electrolyte Balance

1. GI causes: vomiting, diarrhea, GI suctioning; decrease in fluid intake; increase in fluid output, such as sweating; massive edema, ascites.
2. Heart failure (HF); renal failure; cirrhosis; excess ingestion of table salt; or overhydration with sodium-containing fluids.
3. Ringer's lactate; normal saline.
4. Lungs; kidneys; chemical buffers.
5. Normal levels include:
   a. 7.35 to 7.45 pH.
   b. 35 to 45 mm Hg P_{CO_2}.
   c. 21 to 28 mEq/L HCO_3.

Review of Electrocardiogram (ECG)

1. P wave, QRS complex, T wave, ST segment, PR interval.
2. Represented by the P wave.
3. QRS complex.
4. The time required for the impulse to travel from the atria through the AV node.
5. Hypokalemia.
6. Count the number of RR intervals in the 30 large squares and multiply by 10 to determine the heart rate for 1 minute.
7. Ability of the client to tolerate the dysrhythmia.
8. Any atrial or ventricle dysrhythmia that becomes unstable—that is, atrial fib, atrial flutter, ventricle fib, ventricle flutter, third-degree AV block.

Review of Perioperative Care

1. Age: very young and very old; obesity and malnutrition; preoperative dehydration/hypovolemia; preoperative infection; use of anticoagulants preoperative (aspirin).
2. Impairs ability to detoxify medications used during surgery. Impairs ability to produce prothrombin to reduce hemorrhage.
3. Respiratory activities: coughing and breathing, use of a spirometer. Exercises: range of motion exercises, leg exercises, turning. Pain management: medications, splinting. Dietary restrictions: NPO to progressive diet. Dressings and drains. Orientation to the recovery room environment.
4. Contact lenses, glasses, dentures, partial plates, wigs, jewelry, prostheses, makeup, and nail polish.
5. Usually on the side or with head to side to prevent aspiration of any emesis.
6. Splint incision when coughing, encourage coughing/deep breathing in the *early* postoperative period when sutures are *strong*. Monitor for signs of infection, malnutrition, and dehydration. Encourage a high-protein diet.
7. Avoid postoperative catheterization. Increase oral fluid intake. Empty bladder every 4 to 6 hours, early ambulation; teach patient how to brace site with a pillow when coughing, note any stain on the incision site, report any strain on the incision site to the health care provider and the RN.
8. Early ambulation. Limit use of narcotic analgesics. NG tube decompression.
9. Perform in-bed leg exercises. Early ambulation. Apply antiembolus stockings. Avoid positions/pressure that obstruct venous flow.
10. Ascertain correct sponge, needle, and instrument count. Position patient to avoid injury. Apply ground during electrocautery use. Strict use of surgical asepsis.
11. SBAR (Situation-Background-Assessment-Recommendation) technique provides a framework for communication between members of the health care team about a patient's condition: S = situation (a concise statement of the problem), B = background (pertinent and brief information related to the situation), A = assessment (analysis and considerations of options — what you found/think), and R = recommendation (action requested/recommendation)

Review of HIV Infection

1. Transmitted through blood and body fluids—for example, unprotected sexual contact with an infected person, sharing needles among drug-abusing persons, infected blood products (rare), maternal-to-fetus transmission through maternal placental circulation, breaks in universal precautions (needle sticks or similar occurrences).
2. Vertical transmission occurs less than 2% of the time in the U.S. due to ability to test early in pregnancy.
3. Protection from blood and body fluids is the goal of standard precautions. Standard precautions: initiate barrier protection between caregiver and patient through handwashing, use of gloves, use of gown and mask, eye protection as indicated, depending on activity of care and the likelihood of exposure. Prevent needle sticks by not recapping needles.
4. CD4+ T-cell count describes the number of infection-fighting lymphocytes that are available per person.
5. CD4+ T-cell count drops because the virus destroys CD4 T-cells as it invades them and replicates.
6. Through infected blood products, sexual abuse, and/or breast milk.

Review of Pain

1. Massage, heat and cold, acupuncture, TENS.
2. Knowledge about what relieves the pain, based on the individual's experience with pain.
3. Acupuncture, administration of placebos, TENS.
4. Location, intensity, comfort measures, quality, chronology, and subjective view of pain.
5. NSAIDs act by a peripheral mechanism at the level of damaged tissue by inhibiting prostaglandin synthesis and other chemical mediators involved in pain transmission.
6. Initiation of withdrawal symptoms.
7. Nausea/vomiting, constipation, CNS depression, respiratory depression.
8. Naloxone (Narcan).
9. Decreased duration of drug effectiveness.
10. Intravenous push or bolus.
11. Heat and cold applications, TENS, massage, distraction, relaxation techniques, biofeedback techniques.

Review of Death and Grief

1. Denial, anger, bargaining, depression, acceptance.
2. Denial.
3. Gently point out both the positive and negative aspects of her relationship with her father. Try to minimize the idealization of the deceased.
4. This is a normal expression of anger and guilt that occurs. Try to minimize the rumination of these thoughts.
5. This is a dysfunctional grief reaction. Mrs. Green has never moved out of the denial stage of her grief work.

NEXT-GENERATION PN-NCLEX® EXAMINATION-STYLE QUESTION

Actions to Take	Potential Conditions	Parameters to Monitor
Start the I.V. and monitor the amount of fluids	Anxiety	Heart rate and cuff blood pressure
Obtain CT scan	Pulmonary embolism	Monitor for internal bleeding
Assess level of chest pain and report to RN	Myocardial Infarction (MI)	Assess the skin for any bruises or petechiae
Monitor ECG and contact RN if immediate change occurs	Gastrointestinal discomfort or GERD	Chest discomfort/pain
Do bedside sonogram		Monitor antibiotic use

CHAPTER 4

Review of Respiratory System

1. Tachypnea, fever with chills, productive cough, bronchial breath sounds.
2. Deep breathing, fluid intake increased to 3 L/day, use humidity to loosen secretions, suction airway to stimulate coughing.
3. Confusion, lethargy, anorexia, rapid respiratory rate.
4. The flow rate should be 1 to 2 L per nasal cannula; too much O_2 may eliminate the COPD patient's stimulus to breathe. A COPD patient has a hypoxic drive to breathe.
5. Deliver 100% oxygen (hyperinflating) before and after each endotracheal suctioning.
6. Monitor the patient's respiratory status and secure connections, establish a communication mechanism with the patient, keep airway clear by coughing/suctioning.
7. Barrel chest, dry or productive cough, decreased breath sounds, dyspnea, crackles in lung fields.
8. Smoking.
9. Involve family/patient in manipulation of tracheostomy equipment before surgery, plan acceptable communication method, refer to a speech pathologist, discuss rehabilitation program.
10. Maintain a dry occlusive dressing on the chest tube site at all times. Keep all tubing connections tight and taped and monitor the patient's clinical status. Encourage the patient to breathe deeply periodically. Monitor the fluid drainage and mark the time of measurement and fluid level.
11. Place the end of the tube in a sterile water container at a 2-cm level. Immediately reestablish the water-seal system and attach a new drainage system as soon as possible. Apply a dry, sterile dressing and notify the health care provider *STAT.*
12. Do *not* wash off lines; wear soft cotton garments; avoid use of powders/creams on radiation site.
13. Mask for anyone entering room; private room; client *must* wear mask if leaving room.
14. Cough into tissues and dispose immediately into special bags. Long-term need for daily medication. Good handwashing technique. Report symptoms of deterioration, such as blood in secretions.

Review of Renal System

1. Acute kidney injury: often reversible, abrupt deterioration of kidney function. Chronic kidney failure: irreversible, slow deterioration of kidney function characterized by increasing BUN and creatinine. Eventually, dialysis is required.
2. Toxic metabolites that accumulate in the blood (urea, creatinine) are derived mainly from protein catabolism.
3. Do not take BP or perform venipunctures on the arm with the A-V shunt, fistula, or graft. Assess access site for thrill and bruit.
4. Risk of imbalanced fluid volume.
5. Calcium and aluminum antacids bind phosphates and help to keep phosphates from being absorbed into the bloodstream, thereby preventing rising phosphate levels. These antacids must be taken with meals.
6. Fluid intake 3 L/day; good handwashing; void every 2 to 3 hours during waking hours; take all prescribed medications; wear cotton undergarments.
7. Straining all urine is the most important intervention. Other interventions include accurate intake and output documentation and administering analgesics as needed.
8. Maintain a high fluid intake of 3 to 4 L/day. Follow-up care (stones tend to recur). Follow the prescribed diet based on the calculi content. Avoid supine position.
9. Fourth day.
10. Continued strict I&O. Continued observations for hematuria. Inform client that burning and frequency may last for a week.
11. Respiratory status (breathing is guarded because of pain); circulatory status (the kidney is very vascular, and excessive bleeding can occur); pain assessment; urinary assessment (most importantly, assessment of urinary output).

Review of Cardiovascular System

1. Described as squeezing, heavy, burning, radiates to the left arm or shoulder. It may transient or prolonged.
2. Take at first sign of anginal pain. Take no more than three, 5 minutes apart. Call for emergency attention if no relief within 10 minutes.
3. Greater than 140/90.
4. Essential has no known cause, whereas secondary hypertension develops in response to an identifiable mechanism.
5. Explain how and when to take medication; state the reason for medication, necessity of compliance, need for follow-up visits while on medication, need for certain laboratory tests, vital sign parameters while initiating therapy.
6. Pain related to peripheral vascular disease occurring with exercise and disappearing with rest.

7. Keep extremities elevated when sitting, rest at the first sign of pain, keep extremities warm (but do *not* use heating pad), change position often, avoid crossing legs, wear unrestrictive clothing.
8. Atherosclerosis.
9. PTT, PT, Hgb, Hct, and platelets.
10. When they begin to occur more often than once in every 10 beats, occur in 2 s or 3 s, land near the T wave, or take on multiple configurations.
11. Left-sided failure results in pulmonary congestion due to backup of circulation in the left ventricle. Right-sided failure results in peripheral congestion due to backup of circulation in the right ventricle.
12. Dysrhythmias, headache, nausea, and vomiting.
13. When the client is hypokalemic (which is more common when diuretics and digitalis preparations are given together).
14. Cease cigarette smoking if applicable, control weight, exercise regularly, and maintain a low-fat/low-cholesterol diet.
15. Place the client on immediate strict bed rest to lower oxygen demands on the heart; administer oxygen by nasal cannula at 2 to 5 L/min; and take measures to alleviate pain and anxiety (administer PRN pain medications and antianxiety medications).
16. Dry mouth and thirst, drowsiness and lethargy, muscle weakness and aches, and tachycardia.
17. 60 beats/min; 100 beats/min.
18. Take prophylactic antibiotics.

Review of Gastrointestinal System

1. Sit up while eating and for 1 hour after eating. Eat small, frequent meals. Eliminate foods that are problematic.
2. Antacids, histamine-2 receptor-blockers, mucosal healing agents, PPIs.
3. Upper GI: melena, hematemesis, tarry stools. Lower GI: bloody stools, tarry stools. Similar: tarry stools.
4. Early mechanical obstruction: high-pitched sounds; late mechanical obstruction: diminished or absent bowel sounds.
5. Irrigate daily at the same time; use warm water for irrigations; wash around the stoma with mild soap and water after each ostomy bag change; the pouch opening should extend at least 1/8 inch around the stoma.
6. Icteric sclerae or scleral icterus (yellow sclera), dark urine, chalky or clay-colored stools.
7. Fried, spicy, and/or fatty foods.
8. Rectal bleeding, change in bowel habits, sense of incomplete evacuation, abdominal pain with nausea, weight loss.
9. Avoid injections, use small-bore needles for IV insertion, maintain pressure for 5 minutes on all venipuncture sites, use an electric razor, use a soft-bristle toothbrush for mouth care, check stools and emesis for occult blood.
10. Diarrhea.
11. Homosexual males, IV drug users, those with recent piercing or tattooing, and health care workers.
12. Give with meals or snacks. Powder forms should be mixed with fruit juices.

Review of Endocrine System

1. T$_3$, T$_4$.
2. Hypothyroidism, requiring thyroid replacement.
3. Hyperthyroidism: weight loss, heat intolerance, diarrhea. Hypothyroidism: fatigue, cold intolerance, weight gain.
4. Continue medication until weaning plan is begun by physician; monitor serum potassium, glucose, and sodium frequently; weigh daily and report gain of more than 5 lb/wk; monitor BP and pulse closely; teach symptoms of Cushing syndrome.
5. Moon face, obesity in trunk, buffalo hump in back, muscle atrophy, and thin skin.
6. Type 1, insulin-dependent diabetes mellitus.
7. Type 2, non—insulin-dependent diabetes mellitus.
8. Polydipsia, polyuria, polyphagia, weakness, weight loss.
9. Hunger, lethargy, confusion, tremors or shakes, sweating.
10. The underlying pathophysiology of the disease, its management/treatment regimen, meal planning, exercise program, insulin administration, sick-day management, symptoms of hyperglycemia (not enough insulin), symptoms of hypoglycemia (too much insulin, too much exercise, not enough food).
11. All but the current bottle in use should be kept in the refrigerator.
12. Rapid-acting regular insulin: 1 to 4 hours. Intermediate-acting insulin: 6 to 12 hours. Long-acting insulin: peakless.
13. Stress and stress hormones usually increase glucose production and increase insulin need; exercise can increase the chance for an insulin reaction; therefore the client should always have a sugar snack available when exercising (to treat hypoglycemia); a bedtime snack can prevent insulin reactions.
14. Hypoglycemia/insulin reaction.
15. Check feet daily and report any breaks, sores, or blisters to the health care provider; wear well-fitting shoes; never go barefoot or wear sandals; never personally remove corns or calluses; cut or file nails straight across; wash feet daily with mild soap and warm water.

Review of Musculoskeletal System

1. Rheumatoid arthritis occurs bilaterally. Degenerative joint disease occurs asymmetrically.
2. NSAIDs (nonsteroidal antiinflammatory drugs), of which salicylates are the cornerstone of treatment, and corticosteroids (used when arthritic symptoms are severe).
3. Warm, moist heat (compresses, baths, showers), diversionary activities (imaging, distraction, self-hypnosis, biofeedback), and medications.
4. Estrogen replacement after menopause for some women, high calcium and vitamin D intake beginning in early adulthood, calcium supplements after menopause, and weight-bearing exercise.

5. GI irritation, tinnitus, thrombocytopenia, mild liver enzyme elevation.
6. Administer or reinforce client teaching about taking drugs with food or milk.
7. Hip, knee, finger.
8. Elevate residual limb (stump) first 24 hours. Do not elevate the residual limb (stump) after 48 hours. Keep the residual limb (stump) in an extended position and turn prone three times a day to prevent flexion contracture.
9. Be aware that phantom pain is real and will eventually disappear. Administer pain medication; phantom pain responds to medication.
10. Fat embolism, which is characterized by hypoxemia, respiratory distress, irritability, restlessness, fever, and petechiae.
11. Notify health care provider STAT, draw blood gases, administer oxygen according to blood gas results, assist with endotracheal intubation and treatment of respiratory failure.
12. Venous thrombosis, urinary calculi, skin integrity problems.
13. Passive range of motion exercises, elastic stockings, and elevation of foot of bed 25 degrees to increase venous return.

Review of Neurosensory/Neurologic Systems

1. Parasympathomimetics for pupillary constriction, beta-adrenergic receptor-blocking agents to inhibit the formation of aqueous humor, carbonic anhydrase inhibitors to reduce aqueous humor production, and prostaglandin agonists to increase aqueous humor outflow.
2. Conductive (transmission of sound to inner ear is blocked) and sensorineural (damage to eighth cranial nerve).
3. *Care of the blind client:* announce presence clearly, call by name, orient carefully to surroundings, guide by walking in front of client with his or her hand on your elbow. *Care of the deaf client:* reduce distraction before beginning conversation, look at and listen to client, give client full attention if he or she is a lip reader, face client directly.
4. An objective assessment of the level of consciousness based on a score of 3 to 15, with scores of 7 or less indicative of coma.
5. Ineffective breathing pattern, ineffective airway clearance, impaired gas exchange, and decreased cardiac output.
6. Position for maximum ventilation (prone or semiprone and slightly to one side), insert airway if tongue is obstructing; suction airway efficiently; monitor arterial Po_2 and Pco_2; and hyperventilate with 100% oxygen before suctioning.
7. Persons with a history of hypertension, previous transient ischemic attacks, cardiac disease (atrial flutter/fibrillation), diabetes, oral contraceptive use, and older adults.
8. Frequent range-of-motion exercises, frequent (every 2 hours) position changes, and avoidance of positions that decrease venous return.
9. Anoxia, distended bladder, covert bleeding, or a return to consciousness.

10. Irrigation of eyes as needed with sterile prescribed solution, application of ophthalmic ointment (every 8 hours), and close assessment for corneal ulceration drying.
11. When peristalsis resumes, as evidenced by active bowel sounds, passage of flatus or bowel movement.
12. Establishment of regularity.
13. A disruption of blood supply to a part of the brain, which results in a sudden loss of brain function.
14. Left.
15. Hypotension, bladder and bowel distention, total paralysis, and lack of sensation below the lesion.
16. Hypertension, bladder and bowel distention, exaggerated autonomic responses, headache, sweating, goosebumps, and bradycardia.
17. A change in the level of responsiveness.
18. Increased BP, widening pulse pressure, increased or decreased pulse, respiratory irregularities, and temperature increase.
19. Call his health care provider now and inform him or her of the fall. Symptoms needing medical attention would include vertigo, confusion, or any subtle behavioral change; headache; vomiting; ataxia (imbalance); or seizure.
20. Change in bed position, extreme hip flexion, endotracheal suctioning, compression of jugular veins, coughing, vomiting, or straining of any kind.
21. Dehydrate the brain and reduce cerebral edema by holding water in the renal tubules to prevent reabsorption and by drawing fluid from the extravascular spaces into the plasma.
22. Narcotics mask the level of responsiveness as well as pupillary response.
23. Headache that is more severe upon awakening and vomiting not associated with nausea are symptoms of a brain tumor. Supratentorial—elevated; infratentorial—flat. All o.k.
24. Supratentorial–
25. Yes.
26. No.
27. Anticholinesterase drugs, which inhibit the action of cholinesterase at the nerve endings to promote the accumulation of acetylcholine at receptor sites; should improve neuronal transmission to muscles.

Review of Hematology/Oncology

1. Diet lacking in iron, folate, and/or vitamin B_{12}; use of salicylates, thiazides, diuretics; exposure to toxic agents such as lead or insecticides.
2. Activity intolerance and ineffective tissue perfusion.
3. Normal saline.
4. Turn off transfusion. Take temperature. Send blood being transfused to laboratory. Obtain urine sample. Keep vein patent with normal saline.
5. Use a soft toothbrush; avoid salicylates; do not use suppositories.
6. Oral cavity and genital area.
7. Glandular meats (liver), milk, green leafy vegetables.
8. Double-check order with another nurse. Check for blood return before administration to ensure that medication

does not go into tissue. Use a new IV site daily for peripheral chemotherapy. Wear gloves when handling the drugs, and dispose of waste in special containers to avoid contact with toxic substances.

9. *Collection of trough*: draw blood 30 minutes before administration of antibiotic. *Collection of peak*: draw blood 30 minutes after administration of antibiotic.

10. Protect from infection. Observe for anemia. Encourage high-nutrient foods. Provide emotional support to client and family.

11. Handwashing technique. Avoid infected persons. Avoid crowds. Maintain daily hygiene to prevent the spread of microorganisms.

Review of Reproductive System

1. Severe menorrhagia leading to anemia, severe dysmenorrhea requiring narcotic analgesics, severe uterine enlargement causing pressure on other organs, and severe low back and pelvic pain.

2. Symptoms include incontinence/stress incontinence, urinary retention, and recurrent bladder infections. Conditions associated with cystocele include multiparity, trauma in childbirth, and aging.

3. Avoid rectal temps and/or rectal manipulation; manage pain; and encourage early ambulation.

4. Do not permit pregnant visitors or pregnant caretakers in the room. Discourage visits by small children. Confine client to room. Nurse must wear radiation badge. Nurse limits time in room. Keep supplies and equipment within client's reach.

5. Pap smear. Women aged 30 to 65 years should have Pap smears every 3 years. Screened for HPV.

6. Altered body image related to uterine removal. Pain related to postoperative incision.

7. Breast self-examination monthly; annual mammograms for women ages 45 to 54; physical examination by a health professional skilled in examination of the breast.

8. Position arm on operative side on pillow. Avoid BP measurements, injections, or venipunctures in operative arm. Encourage hand activity and use.

9. Arrange for Reach-to-Recovery visit. Discuss the grief process with the client. Have health care provider discuss with client the reconstruction options.

10. Chlamydia trachomatis.

11. *Treponema pallidum* (spirochete bacteria).

12. *Trichomonas vaginalis.*

13. Herpes simplex type II.

14. Signs and symptoms of STI. Mode of transmission. Avoid sex while infected. Provide concise written instructions regarding treatment and request a return verbalization to ensure the client understands. Collaborate with the RN to develop and implement a teaching plan about "safer sex" practices.

Review of Burns

1. Thermal, radiation, chemical, and electrical.

2. Superficial partial-thickness: first degree = pink to red skin (i.e., sunburn), slight edema, and pain relieved by cooling. Deep partial-thickness: second degree = destruction of epidermis and upper layers of dermis; white or red, very edematous, sensitive to touch and cold air, hair does not pull out easily. Full-thickness: third degree = total destruction of dermis and epidermis; reddened areas do not blanch with pressure, not painful, inelastic, waxy, white skin to brown, leathery eschar.

3. Stage I (Emergent Phase): Replacement of fluids is titrated to urine output. Stage II (Acute Phase): Maintain patent infusion site in case supplemental IV fluids are needed; saline lock is helpful; may use colloids. Stage III (Rehabilitation Phase): No extra fluids are needed, but high-protein drinks are recommended.

4. Administer pain medication, especially before dressing the wound. Reinforce distraction/relaxation techniques and the use of guided imagery.

5. Provide a patent airway as intubation may be necessary. Determine baseline data. Initiate fluid and electrolyte therapy. Administer pain medication. Determine depth and extent of burn. Administer tetanus toxoid. Insert NG tube.

6. High-calorie, high-protein, high-carbohydrate diet. Medications with juice or milk; *no* "free" water. Tube feeding at night. Maintain accurate, daily calorie counts. Weigh client daily.

7. Thermal: remove clothing, immerse in tepid water. Chemical: flush with water or saline. Electrical: separate client from electrical source.

8. Singed nasal hairs, circumoral burns; sooty or bloody sputum, hoarseness, and pulmonary signs including asymmetry of respirations, rales, or wheezing.

9. Water may interfere with electrolyte balance. Client needs to ingest food products with highest biologic value.

10. Use of client's own skin for grafting.

NEXT-GENERATION NCLEX® EXAMINATION-STYLE QUESTION

Action to Take	Potential Conditions	Parameters to Monitor
Administer Acetaminophen 650 mg q 6 hours PRN for Fever	Appendicitis	Electrocardiogram (EKG)
Obtain a urine sample for culture	Influenza	Neurologic status
Call laboratory for blood culture draw	Diabetic ketoacidosis	Monitor pulses
Provide K+ as indicated	Food Poisoning	Fall precautions
Reorient client as needed		Blood glucose level

CHAPTER 5

Review of CHILD Health Promotion

1. Immunocompromised child or a child in a household with an immunocompromised individual.
2. Different techniques to assess pain in children include observation of nonverbal signs of pain: grimacing, irritability, restlessness, and difficulty sleeping. May use pain indicators such as FACES that provides a scale of how bad the pain may be.
3. Nonaccidental trauma (NAT) signs and symptoms include: child is frightened, and injuries include soft tissue such as bruising in unusual places, burns, bald patches, or hx. of fractures.
4. Anemia, pale conjunctiva, pale skin color, atrophy of papillae on tongue, brittle/ridged/spoon-shaped nails, and thyroid edema.
5. Present nutritional status is measured by weight, skinfold thickness, and arm circumference.
6. Poor skin turgor, absence of tears, dry mucous membranes, weight loss, depressed fontanel, and decreased urinary output.
7. Lab findings for dehydrated children include: Loss of bicarbonate (serum pH, 7.33; bicarbonate level less than 18 mEq/L; elevated hematocrit and elevated urea nitrogen.
8. Use the Lund-Browder chart, which takes into account the changing proportions of the child's body.
9. Fluid replacement in children will result in increased skin turgor, increased urinary output, and increased activity.
10. Lock all cabinets, safely store all toxic household items in locked cabinets, and examine the house from the child's point of view.
11. Observe and report to RN the child's respiratory, cardiac, and neurologic statuses.
12. Early CNS signs of lead poisoning include hyperactivity, aggression, impulsiveness, decreased interest in play, and irritability.

Review of Respiratory Disorders

1. Reverse bronchospasm and open airways.
2. Expiratory wheezing, rales, tight cough, and signs of altered blood gases.
3. Pancreatic enzyme replacement, fat-soluble vitamins, and a moderate- to low-carbohydrate, high-protein, moderate-fat diet.
4. The disease is autosomal recessive in its genetic pattern.
5. Restlessness, tachycardia, tachypnea, diaphoresis, flaring nostrils, retractions, and grunting.
6. Upright, sitting, with chin out and tongue protruding ("tripod" position).
7. The child is at risk for dehydration and acid–base imbalance.
8. Hearing loss. (otitis media)
9. Hemorrhage; frequent swallowing, vomiting fresh blood, and clearing throat. (tonsillectomy)

Review of Cardiovascular Disorders

1. A left-to-right shunt moves oxygenated blood back through the pulmonary circulation. A right-to-left shunt bypasses the lungs and delivers unoxygenated blood to the systemic circulation, causing cyanosis.
2. VSD, overriding aorta, pulmonary stenosis, and right ventricular hypertrophy.
3. Poor feeding, poor weight gain, respiratory distress/infections, edema, and cyanosis.
4. Reduce the workload of the heart and increase cardiac output.
5. Small, frequent feedings or gavage feedings. Plan frequent rest periods. Maintain a neutral thermal environment. Organize activities to disturb child only as indicated.
6. Aortic valve stenosis and mitral valve stenosis
7. Penicillin, erythromycin, and aspirin

Review of Neuromuscular Disorders

1. Simian creases of palms, hypotonia, protruding tongue, and upward/outward slant of eyes.
2. A common characteristic of spastic cerebral palsy in infants. The legs are extended and crossed over each other; feet are plantarflexed.
3. Prevention of infection of the sac and monitoring for hydrocephalus (measure head circumference; check fontanel; assess neurologic functioning).
4. Irritability, change in LOC, motor dysfunction, headache, vomiting, unequal pupil response, and seizures.
5. Signs of infection and increased ICP (see Signs of Increased ICP and Meningitis; shunt should not be pumped. Child will need revisions because of growth. Provide guidance for growth and development.
6. Maintain patent airway, protect from injury, and observe carefully.
7. Gingival hyperplasia of the gums, dermatitis, ataxia, gastrointestinal distress.
8. Fever, irritability, vomiting, neck stiffness, opisthotonus, positive Kernig sign, positive Brudzinski sign. Infant does not show all classic signs but is very ill.
9. Ampicillin, ceftriaxone, and/or chloramphenicol.
10. Suctioning and positioning/turning.
11. Duchenne muscular dystrophy is inherited as an X-linked recessive trait.
12. Gowers' sign is an indicator of muscular dystrophy. The child has to "walk" up legs using their hands to stand.

Review of Renal Disorders

1. AGN: gross hematuria, recent streptococcus infection, hypertension, and mild edema. Nephrosis: severe edema, massive proteinuria, frothy-appearing urine, and anorexia.
2. Beta-hemolytic streptococcus infection.
3. AGN: low-sodium diet with no added salt. Nephrosis: high-protein, low-salt diet.
4. Hypoproteinemia occurs because the glomeruli are permeable to serum proteins.

5. Long-term prednisone should be given every other day. Signs of edema, mood changes, and gastrointestinal distress should be noted and reported. The drug should be tapered, not discontinued suddenly.

6. Avoid bubble baths; void frequently; drink adequate fluids, especially acidic fluids such as apple or cranberry juice; and clean the genital area from front to back.

7. A malfunction of the valves at the end of the ureters, allowing urine to reflux out of the bladder into the ureters and possibly the kidneys.

8. Protect the child from injury to the encapsulated tumor. Prepare the family/child for surgery.

9. Preschoolers fear castration, are achieving sexual identity, and are acquiring independent toileting skills.

Review of Gastrointestinal Disorders

1. Lamb's nipple or prosthesis. Feed child upright with frequent burping.

2. Choking, coughing, cyanosis, and excess salivation.

3. NPO immediately and suction secretions.

4. Maintain IV hydration. Provide small, frequent oral feedings of glucose and/or electrolyte solutions within 4 to 6 hours. Gradually increase to full-strength formula. Position on right side in semi-Fowler position after feeding.

5. Check vital signs and take axillary temperatures. Provide bowel-cleansing program and teach about colostomy. Observe for bowel perforation; measure abdominal girth.

6. Family needs education about skin care and appliances. Referral to an enterostomal therapist is appropriate.

7. A newborn who does not pass meconium within 24 hours, meconium appearing from a fistula or in the urine, or an unusual-appearing anal dimple.

8. Maintain fluid balance (I&O, NG suction, monitor electrolytes), monitor vital signs, care of drains if present, assess bowel function, prevent infection of incisional area and other postoperative complications, and support child/family with appropriate teaching.

Review of Hematologic Disorders

1. Give oral iron on an empty stomach and with vitamin C. Use straws to avoid discoloring teeth. Tarry stools are normal. Increase dietary sources of iron.

2. Meat, green leafy vegetables, fish, liver, whole grains, legumes.

3. Genetic transmission of hemophilia is X-linked recessive chromosome (mother is the carrier).

4. The sequence of events in a vasoocclusive crisis in SCD is fever, pain (abdomina), hand-foot syndrome (edema) and arthralgia.

5. Hydration promotes hemodilution and circulation of the red cells through the blood vessels.

6. Keep child well hydrated. Avoid known sources of infections. Avoid high altitudes. Avoid strenuous exercise.

7. Anemia (decreased erythrocytes). Infection (neutropenia). Bleeding thrombocytopenia (decreased platelets).

Review of Metabolic and Endocrine Disorders

1. Newborn screening revealing a low T4 and high TSH.

2. Large, protruding tongue; coarse hair; lethargy; sleepiness; and constipation.

3. Cognitive impairment and growth failure.

4. CNS damage, cognitive impairment, and decreased melanin.

omit

5. Meat, milk, dairy products, and eggs.

6. Polydipsia, polyphagia, and polyuria.

7. Hypoglycemia: tremors, sweating, headache, hunger, nausea, lethargy, confusion, slurred speech, anxiety, tingling around mouth, nightmares. Hyperglycemia: polydipsia, polyuria, polyphagia, blurred vision, weakness, weight loss, and syncope.

8. Provide care for an unconscious child, monitor blood gas values, and maintain strict I&O.

9. Need to be like peers. Assuming responsibility for own care. Modification of diet, snacks, and exercise in school.

10. During exercise, insulin uptake is increased and the risk of hypoglycemia occurs.

Review of Skeletal Disorders

1. Warm extremity, brisk capillary refill, free movement, normal sensation of the affected extremity, and equal pulses.

2. Damage to nerves and vasculature of an extremity due to compression.

3. Abnormal neurovascular assessment: severe pain, cold extremity, inability to move the extremity, and poor capillary refill.

4. Fractures of the epiphyseal plate (growth plate) may affect the growth of the limb.

5. Skeletal traction is maintained by pins or wires applied to the distal fragment of the fracture.

6. Check circulation. Keep cast dry. Do not stick anything under cast. Prevent cast soilage during toileting or diapering. Do not turn with abductor bar.

7. Unequal skin folds of the buttocks, Ortolani sign (performed by HCP), limited abduction of the affected hip, and unequal leg lengths.

8. Ask the child to bend forward from the hips with arms hanging free. Examine the child for a curve of the spine, rib hump, and hip asymmetry.

9. Wear the brace 23 hours per day. Wear T-shirt under brace. Check skin for irritation. Perform back and abdominal exercises. Modify clothing. Encourage the child to maintain normal activities as able.

10. Prescribed exercise to maintain mobility, splinting of affected joints, and teaching medication management and side effects of drugs.

NEXT-GENERATION NCLEX® EXAMINATION-STYLE QUESTION

Actions to Take	Potential Conditions	Parameters to Monitor
Obtain post-op orders	Fracture to left ribs and thoracic cage	60 cc h. up to 1000 cc per IV fluid per day
Contact social services for child abuse assessment	Exacerbated respiratory syndrome	Monitor ecg and heart rate
Initiate physical therapy treatment	First and second-degree burns	Oriented to time, person and place
Monitor I & O	Acute skin abrasions secondary to fall	Assess pain level
separate the mom from her daughter		have the doctor order a MRI

CHAPTER 6

Review of Anatomy and Physiology of Reproduction and Antepartum Nursing Care

1. Abundant, thin, and clear cervical mucus; Spinnbarkeit (egg-white stretchiness) of cervical mucus; open cervical os; slight drop in basal body temperature and then 0.5 degree to 1 degree F rise; ferning under the microscope.
2. 14 days.
3. 10 lunar months; 9 calendar months consisting of three trimesters of 3 months each; 40 weeks; 280 days.
4. Nausea and vomiting: crackers before rising; fatigue: rest periods and naps; and 7 to 8 hours of sleep at night.
5. At the umbilicus;
6. Total gain should average 11,340 and 15,876 g (25 to 35 lb). Gain should be consistent throughout pregnancy. An average of 1 lb/week should be gained in the second and third trimesters.
7. 10 to 12.
8. Once every 4 weeks until 28 weeks; once every 2 weeks from 28 to 36 weeks; then once a week until delivery.

Review of Fetal and Maternal Assessment Techniques

1. Diagnosis of preeclampsia, diabetes mellitus, or cardiac disease; less than 3 months between pregnancies; maternal age (under 17 or over 34 years of age); parity (over 5).
2. Fetal well-being.
3. Have client fill bladder. Do not allow client to void. Position client supine with a uterine wedge.
4. Can be done between 8 and 12 weeks' gestation, with results returned within 1 week, which allows for decision about termination while still in first trimester.
5. To determine AFP levels: elevated AFP may indicate the presence of neural tube defects; or low AFP levels may indicate trisomy 21.
6. L/S ratio (lung maturity, lung surfactant development).
7. FHR acceleration of 15 bpm for 15 seconds in response to fetal movement.
8. The inability to control oxytocin "dosage" and the chance of tachysystole.

Review of Antepartum Complications

1. Maintain strict bed rest for 24 to 48 hours. Avoid sexual intercourse for 2 weeks.
2. Weigh daily; check urine ketones three times daily; give progressive diet; check FHR every 8 hours; monitor for electrolyte imbalances.
3. Prevent pregnancy for 1 year. Return to clinic or healthcare provider for monthly hCG levels for 1 year. Postoperative D & C instructions: Call if bright-red vaginal bleeding or foul-smelling vaginal discharge occurs or temperature spikes over 38°C.
4. Ectopic pregnancy.
5. Abruptio placentae: fetal distress; rigid board-like abdomen; pain; dark-red or absent bleeding. Previa: pain-free; bright-red vaginal bleeding; normal FHR; soft uterus.
6. More than five contractions per hour; cramps; low, dull backache; pelvic pressure; change in vaginal discharge.
7. Urinary tract infection; overdistention of uterus; diabetes; preeclampsia; cardiac disease; placenta previa, psychosocial factors such as stress.
8. Answers are as follows:
   A. To prevent seizures by decreasing CNS irritability.
   B. CNS depression (seizure prevention).
   C. Calcium gluconate.
   D. Reduced urinary output, reduced respiratory rate, and decreased reflexes.
9. Systolic blood pressure of 160 mm Hg or more, or diastolic blood pressure of 110 mm Hg or more on two occasions at least 4 hours apart (unless antihypertensive therapy is initiated before this time).
10. No. Oral tolbutamide is suspected to be teratogenic to the fetus. Insulin will be used.
11. Maternal: hypoglycemia, hyperglycemia, ketoacidosis. Fetal: macrosomia, hypoglycemia at birth, fetal anomalies.
12. Monitor for signs of blood loss. Continue to assess BP and DTRs every 4 hours. Monitor for uterine atony.
13. Late in the third trimester and in the postpartum period when insulin needs drop sharply (the diabetogenic effects of pregnancy drop precipitously).
14. It is short acting, predictable, can be infused intravenously, and can be discontinued quickly if necessary.
15. Preeclampsia, hydramnios, infection.

Review of Intrapartum Nursing Care

1. Lightening, Braxton Hicks contractions, increased bloody show, loss of mucous plug, burst of energy, and nesting behaviors.
2. True labor: regular, rhythmic contractions that intensify with ambulation, pain in the abdomen sweeping around

from the back, and cervical changes. False labor: irregular rhythm, abdominal pain (not in back) that decreases with ambulation, and no cervical change.

3. Nitrazine testing: Paper turns dark blue or black. Demonstration of fluid ferning under microscope.

4. Respiratory alkalosis occurs; it is caused by blowing off CO_2 and is relieved by breathing into a paper bag or cupped hands.

5. Irritability and unwillingness to be touched but does not want to be left alone; nausea, vomiting, and hiccupping.

6. Vaginal examinations should be done before analgesia and anesthesia to rule out cord prolapse, to determine labor progress if it is questioned, and to determine when pushing can begin.

7. The taking up of the lower cervical segment into the upper segment; the shortening of the cervix expressed in percentages from 0% to 100%, or complete effacement.

8. Through the fetal back in vertex, OA positions.

9. 110 to 160 bpm.

10. <140/90.

11. <100 bpm.

12. 38°C.

13. Gush of blood, lengthening of cord, and globular shape of uterus.

14. Give immediately after placenta is delivered to prevent postpartum hemorrhage and atony.

15. Hypotension resulting from vasodilatation below the block, which pools blood in the periphery, reducing venous return.

16. Gastric activity slows or stops in labor, decreasing absorption from PO route; it may cause vomiting.

17. When the client has an undiagnosed substance use disorder of narcotics, it can cause immediate withdrawal symptoms.

18. Nausea.

19. Turn client to left side. Administer O_2 by mask at 10 L/min. Increase speed of intravenous infusion (if it does not contain medication).

20. The first 1 to 4 hours after delivery of placenta.

21. Massage the fundus (gently) and keep the bladder emptied.

22. Withhold eye prophylaxis for up to 1 hour. Perform newborn admission and routine procedures in room with parents. Encourage early initiation of breastfeeding. Darken room to encourage newborn to open eyes.

23. Fundus above umbilicus, dextroverted (to the right side of abdomen), increased bleeding (uterine atony).

24. Perform fundal massage.

25. Pallor, clammy skin, tachycardia, lightheadedness, and hypotension.

26. Every 15 minutes for 1 hour; every 30 minutes for 2 hours if normal.

Review of Normal Puerperium (Postpartum)

1. Perform immediate fundal massage. Ambulate to the bathroom or use bedpan to empty bladder because cardinal signs of bladder distention are present.

2. Breastfeeding women, multiparas, and women who experienced overdistention of the uterus.

3. Temperature is probably elevated due to dehydration and work of labor; force fluids and retake temperature in an hour; notify healthcare provider if above 38°C.

4. Assess BP sitting and lying; assess Hgb and Hct for anemia.

5. Increased clotting factors.

6. Have her demonstrate infant position on breast (incorrect positioning often causes tenderness). Leave bra open to air-dry nipples for 15 minutes three times daily. Express colostrum and rub on nipples.

7. She is engorged; have the newborn suckle frequently; take measures to increase milk flow: warm water, breast massage, and supportive bra.

8. Avoid until postpartum examination. Use water-soluble jelly. Expect slight discomfort due to vaginal changes.

9. Up to 3000 mL per day can be voided because of the reduction in the 40% plasma volume increase during pregnancy.

10. Continue routine assessments; normal leukocytosis occurs during postpartal period because of placental site healing.

11. A full bladder.

12. To soften the stool in mothers with third- or fourth-degree tears or episiotomies, hemorrhoids, or cesarean section delivery.

13. Three fingerbreadths/cm below the umbilicus.

14. Calling infant by name, exploring newborn head to toe, eye contact between parent and neonate.

Review of Pospartum Complications

1. No. HIV has been found in breastmilk.

2. GI adverse reactions: nausea, vomiting, diarrhea, and cramping. Hypersensitivity reactions: rashes, urticaria, and hives.

3. Pyelonephritis has the same symptoms as cystitis (dysuria, frequency, and urgency) with the addition of flank pain, fever, and pain at costovertebral angle.

4. Subinvolution (boggy, high uterus); lochia returning to rubra with possible foul smell; temperature 38.0°C or higher; unusual fundal tenderness.

5. Operative delivery, intrauterine manipulation, anemia or poor physical health, traumatic delivery, and hemorrhage.

6. Dystocia or prolonged labor, overdistention of the uterus, abruptio placentae, and infection.

7. Fundal massage. Notify healthcare provider if massage does not firm fundus. Count pads to estimate blood loss. Assess and record vital signs. Increase IV fluids and administer oxytocin infusion as prescribed.

8. No. Women who stop breastfeeding abruptly may make the situation worse by increasing congestion and engorgement and providing further media for bacterial growth. Client may have to discontinue breastfeeding if pus is present or if antibiotics are contraindicated for neonate.

Review of the Normal Newborn

1. 6 to 8 hours
2. Cesarean section delivery; magnesium sulfate given to mother in labor; asphyxia or fetal distress during labor.
3. It leads to depletion of glucose (there is very little glycogen storage in immature liver); body begins to use brown fat for energy, producing ketones, and causing subsequent ketoacidosis and shock.
4. 36.5°C to 37.4°C; 110 to 160 bpm; 30 to 60; 80/50.
5. Place newborn in isolette or under radiant warmer, and attach a temperature skin probe to regulate temperature in isolette or radiant warmer. Double-wrap newborn if no isolette or warmer is available, and put cap on head. Watch for signs of hypothermia and hypoglycemia.
6. False: The head is usually 2 cm larger, unless severe molding occurred.
7. CNS anomalies, brain damage, hypoglycemia, drug withdrawal.
8. It depends on the finding. If it crosses suture lines and is a caput (edema), it is normal. If it does not cross suture lines, it is a cephalohematoma with bleeding between the skull and periosteum. This could cause hyperbilirubinemia. This is an abnormal variation.
9. Positive; the transient reflex is present until 12 to 18 months of age.
10. The mouth; stimulating the nares can initiate inspiration, which could cause aspiration of mucus in the oral pharynx.
11. There is controversy concerning this issue, but we do know it causes pain and trauma to the newborn, and the medical indications (prevention of penile and cervical cancer) may be unfounded.
12. 40 to 80 mg/dL.
13. The sterile gut at delivery lacks intestinal bacteria necessary for the synthesis of vitamin K; vitamin K is needed in the clotting cascade to prevent hemorrhagic disorders.
14. Jaundice occurs at 2 to 3 days of life and is caused by immature liver's inability to keep up with the bilirubin production resulting from normal RBC destruction.
15. At 2 to 3 days of life, or after enough breast milk or formula, usually after 24 hours, is ingested to allow for determination of body's ability to metabolize amino acid phenylalanine.
16. 50; 1 oz, or 30 g.
17. Lethargy, temperature greater than 37.7°C, vomiting, green stools, refusal of two feeds in a row.

Review of Newborn Complications

1. Lethargy, high-pitched cry, jitteriness, seizures, and bulging fontanels.
2. Begin oxygenation by bag and mask at 30 to 50 breaths per minute. If heart rate is less than 60, start cardiac massage at 120 events per minute (30 breaths and 90 compressions). Assist health care provider in setting up for intubation procedure.
3. RDS: alveolar prematurity and lack of surfactant; anemia; and polycythemia.
4. Lethargy, temperature instability, difficulty feeding, subtle color changes, subtle behavioral changes, and hyperbilirubinemia.
5. Place under radiant warmer or in incubator with temperature skink probe over liver. Warm all items touching newborn. Place plastic wrap over neonate.
6. Infant has good suck, has coordinated suck-swallow, takes less than 20 minutes to feed, gains 20 to 30 g/day.
7. Initiate early visitation at ICU. Provide daily information to family. Encourage participation in support groups for parents. Encourage all attempts at caregiving (enhances bonding).
8. Rh incompatibility, ABO incompatibility, prematurity, sepsis, perinatal asphyxia.
9. Bilirubin levels rising 5 mg/day, jaundice, dark urine, anemia, high reticulocyte (RBC) cunt, and dark stools.
10. Apply opaque mask over eyes. Leave diaper loose so stools and urine can be monitored but cover genitalia. Turn every 2 hours. Watch for dehydration.
11. Irritability, hyperactivity, high-pitched cry, frantic sucking, tremors, and poor feeding.
12. Failure to thrive, absence of crying.
13. Measure from the bridge of the nose to the earlobe and then to a point halfway between the xiphoid and the umbilicus.
14. Aspiration of stomach contents and pH testing; auscultation of an air bubble injected into the stomach.
15. Microcephaly, growth retardation, short palpebral fissures, thin upper lip, smooth filtrum.

NEXT-GENERATION NCLEX® EXAMINATION-STYLE QUESTIONS

Actions to Take	Potential Conditions	Parameters to Monitor
Gestational Assessment	Seizures	Observe skin color
Use of bright lights to enhance physical assessment skills	Excessive sleep patterns	Temperature
Serum glucose testing	Large for gestional age	Eye Contact
Swaddle infant with legs flexed	Neonatal hyperglycemia	Output
Provide extra feedings		Mother baby bonding

CHAPTER 7

Review of Therapeutic Communication and Treatment Modalities

1. Safety
2. Milieu
3. The entire family.
4. Maintain patent airway. Check vital signs every 15 minutes until client is alert. Remain with the client after treatment until client is conscious. Reorient if client is confused. Insert into key from p. 4 of Chapter 7

Review of Common Mental Health Treatments and Interventions

1. Obtaining assessment data related to substance abuse and frequency of use of alcohol.
2. PN's role in ECT is dictated by the PN's scope of practice and by the agency's policies and procedures.
3. This is an example of milieu therapy that focuses on the here and now and assists the patient to deal with realities of today rather than focusing on situations and behaviors of the past. It involves the patient in making decisions about his or her own care.
4. Establish trust; use calm approach and direct, simple questions. Provide a safe environment. Draw the patient's attention away from situation. Reinforce and encourage positive thoughts.
5. Identify the method chosen; the more lethal the method, the higher the probability that an attempt is imminent. Assess need for depression; use antidepressants.
6. Quietly approach the client and note the behavior. Assess verbal and nonverbal cues for escalating behavior. Avoid "why" questions and redirect feelings to a safe alternative.

Review of Mood Disorders

1. Report the following information to the RN: weight change (loss or gain), constipation, fatigue, lack of sexual interest, somatic complaints, and sleep disturbances.
2. In collaboration with the RN and the interprofessional team: assess for suicidal ideation, plan, and means of carrying out plan. Place on precautions as indicated. A sudden change in mood and giving away possessions are two possible signs that a suicide plan has been developed.
3. Notify RN of existence of a plan, existence of a method, availability of method chosen, lethality of method chosen, identified support system, and history of previous attempts.
4. Accompany client to the group; do not give client option. Client needs to be mobilized.
5. Remove client and other persons in the vicinity to a safe area and have someone activate the hospital fire plan.

When area is safe, place client in quiet environment with low stimulation and medicate as indicated.

Review of Substance Abuse Disorders

1. Obtain a drug and alcohol consumption assessment, including type, frequency, and time of last dose or drink. Notify the RN and report findings. Anticipate withdrawal and DTs. Provide a quiet, safe environment. Place on seizure precautions. Anticipate giving a medication such as chlordiazepoxide (Librium). Call the health care provider and report findings.
2. Needle track marks; cellulitis at puncture site; poor nutritional status.
3. Change in work performance, withdrawal, increase in absences (especially Mondays and Fridays), increase in number of times tardy, long breaks, lateness returning from lunch.
4. Notify the RN and the health care provider immediately and anticipate an increase in dose or frequency of Librium to 100 mg. Provide a quiet, safe environment. Approach the client in a quiet, calm manner. Avoid touching the client.
5. Notify the RN and health care provider of observed behavior change. Get a urine drug screen as prescribed. Confront client with observed behavior change.

NEXT-GENERATION NCLEX® EXAMINATION-STYLE QUESTIONS

Actions to Take	Potential Conditions	Parameters to Monitor
Praise self-control, acceptable behavior.	Attention-Deficit Disorder	Increase conversations with client to establish more attention.
Restrain individual for own safety.	Bipolar disorder or manic-depressive illness.	Provide small, frequent feedings, record I & O.
Provide frequent stimulation such as playing physical games.	Delirium	Monitor physical activity/over-stimulation.
Monitor I & O.	Over-use of amphetamines.	Use a variety of approaches to maximize manipulative behavior.
Obtain an order for pain medication.		Provide additional stimulation for client.

CHAPTER 8

Review of Gerontologic Nursing

1. Short-term memory declines, whereas long-term memory stays the same.
2. Loss in compensatory reserve, progressive loss in efficiency of the body to repair damaged tissue, and decreased functioning of the immune system processes.
3. The heart's work increases in response to increased peripheral resistance.
4. Chronic obstructive pulmonary disease.
5. Determine what is "normal" GI functioning for each individual, increase fiber and bulk in the diet, provide adequate hydration, encourage regular exercise, and encourage eating small meals frequently.
6. Smoking, excessive alcohol intake, sedentary lifestyle (inactivity), and excessive dietary intake versus energy output.
7. Cataracts
8. Dementia disorders, cerebrovascular disorders, and movement disorders (e.g., Parkinson disease).
9. Delirium has a sudden onset and is reversible; dementia is a slowly progressive and irreversible disease.
10. Falls are the result of cardiovascular, musculoskeletal, and neurological system changes.
11. Decreased glomerular filtration and slowed organ functioning.
12. Relief of pain, anxiety, gastrointestinal symptoms, psychiatric symptoms, spirituality, support for family members and support during bereavement period are important for end-of-life care.

NEXT-GENERATION NCLEX® EXAMINATION-STYLE QUESTIONS

Actions to Take	Potential Conditions	Parameters to Monitor
Report the observed data to the registered nurse (RN)	Myocardial Infarction (MI)	Chest Pain Level
Obtain MRI	Elderly Abuse/physical	Complications associated with bruising and open wounds
Document factual, objective data related to the patient's physical condition and injuries.	Cardiovascular Ischemia	Pulse oximetry
Administer oxygen 2 L/min NC.	Situational Depression	I & O
Call dermatology for consult.		Complete Glascow scale every 4 hr.

Note: Page numbers followed by "f " indicate figures, "t" indicate tables, and "b" indicate boxes.

A

AAA. *See* Abdominal aortic aneurysm
Abciximab (Reopro), 94t—95t
Abdomen, newborn, 262t—264t
Abdominal aortic aneurysm (AAA), 91, 91b
  nursing assessment for, 91
  nursing plans and interventions for, 91—92
Abortions, 216
  spontaneous, 220—221
Abruptio placentae, 222
  causes of, 223t
  Clinical Judgment Measures, 224t
  symptoms of, 223t
Absence seizure, 186
Acamprosate (Campral), 282t
Acarbose (Precose), 114t
Acceleration-deceleration injury, 129f
Acetazolamide (Diamox), 123t
Acetyl cholinesterase inhibitors, 295t
Acid-base balance, 41
Acid-base disorders, 42
Acid-base imbalance
  in ARDS, 21, 23t
  clinical manifestations of, 22f, 24t
Acquired immunodeficiency syndrome (AIDS), 48b, 50t, 228
ACTH. *See* Adrenocorticotropic hormone
Activity theory, of aging, 285
Acupressure, 64
Acute glomerulonephritis (AGN), 190
Acute HIV infection, 48b, 50t
Acute kidney injury (AKI), 77—78, 77b
  nursing assessment for, 77
  nursing plans and interventions for, 77—78
  types of, 77t
Acute lymphocytic leukemia (ALL), 139, 199—200, 200b
Acute myelogenous leukemia (AML), 139
Acute pain, 56
Acute pancreatitis
  nursing assessment for, 106
  nursing plans and interventions for, 106—107
Acute postpartum hemorrhage, 257
Acute respiratory distress syndrome (ARDS), 21
  Clinical Judgment Measures, 25t
Acyanotic heart defects, pediatric nursing, 173—176, 174t, 178b
Acyclovir sodium (Zovirax), 52t
Addison crisis, 110b—111b
Addison disease, 110—111, 110b

Adenectomy, 109
Adenosine (Adenocard), 94t—95t
ADH. *See* Antidiuretic hormone
ADHD. *See* Attention-deficit/hyperactivity disorder
Adjuvant therapy, 141
Adolescent
  growth and development of, 158—159, 159b
  pain assessment and management in, 159
Adrenal glands, electrolyte balance and, 37
Adrenergics, 72t, 170t
Adrenocorticotropic hormone (ACTH), 110
Aduhelm, 295t
Adults
  foreign body airway obstruction in, 31
  human immunodeficiency virus (HIV) infection in, 49—50
Aging, 285b
  definition of, 285
  effect on body systems, 286—302
  and older adult, 285
  physiologic changes of, 285
  theories of, 285
AGN. *See* Acute glomerulonephritis
Agraphia, 137b
AIDS. *See* Acquired immunodeficiency syndrome
Albuterol (Proventil), 72t
Alcohol
  newborn affected by maternal use of, 270
  withdrawal syndrome, 280
Alcohol deterrents, 282t
Alexia, 137b
ALL. *See* Acute lymphocytic leukemia
α-adrenergic agonist, 249t—250t
Alpha-adrenergic blockers, 88t—89t
Alpha agonists, 123t
Alpha beta-blockers, combined, 88t—89t
Alpha-glucosidase inhibitors, 114t
Alprazolam (Xanax), 281t
Altered state of consciousness, 126—128
  nursing assessment for, 126—127
  nursing plans and interventions for, 127—128
Aluminum hydroxide/magnesium hydroxide (Maalox, Mylanta, Riopan, Gelusil II), 100t
Alzheimer disease
  dementia associated with, 294b, 299
  medications for, 295t
Amantadine HCL (Symmetrel), 135t
Amikacin sulfate, 66t—68t
Amiloride (Midamor), 87t

Aminoglycosides, 66t—68t
Aminophylline, 72t
Amiodarone HCL (Cordarone), 94t—95t
AML. *See* Acute myelogenous leukemia
Amlodipine (Norvasc), 88t—89t
Ammonia, cirrhosis and, 104b
Ammonia detoxicant/stimulant laxative, 105t
Amniocentesis, 219
Amphetamines, withdrawal and overdose symptoms, 281t
Amphotericin B (Fungizone), 52t
Ampicillin, 66t—68t
Ampicillin-sulbactam, 257t
Ampicillin + sulbactam (Unasyn), 66t—68t
Amprenavir (Agenerase), 52t
Amputation, 121—122
Analgesia, labor with, 241—243
Analgesics, 242t
  routes of administration for, 57t
Anaphylactic shock, 26
Anemia, 137—138
  iron deficiency, 197—198, 197b
  nursing assessment for, 137—138
  nursing plans and interventions for, 138
  during pregnancy, 227
  sickle cell, 198
Anesthesia
  labor with, 241—243
  local, 242
  regional block, 242—243
Angina
  nursing assessment for, 83
  nursing plans and interventions for, 83—84
Angiotensin-converting enzyme (ACE) inhibitors, 88t—89t
Angiotensin II receptor antagonists, 88t—89t
Anidulafungin (Eraxis), 52t
Anorectal malformations, 196—197
Antacids, 100t
Antepartum, 223—224
Antepartum complications, 220—222
  abruptio placentae and placenta previa, 222
  causes of, 223t
  Clinical Judgment Measures, 224t
  symptoms of, 223t
  ectopic pregnancy, 222, 222b
  hyperemesis gravidarum, 221
  molar pregnancy (hydatidiform mole), 221—222
  review of, 230b
  spontaneous abortion, 220—221

Antepartum fetal and maternal assessments, 218—220
  amniocentesis, 219
  biophysical profile, 220
  chorionic villi sampling, 219
  contraction stress test/oxytocin challenge test, 220
  nonstress test, 219—220
  review of, 220b
  ultrasonography, 218—219
Antepartum nursing care, 216—218
  first prenatal visit, 216—217
  prenatal nutrition, 217—218
  review of, 218b
  subsequent antepartum visits, 217
Antianemic drug, 79t
Antianginals, 84t
Antianxiety drugs, 281t
Antibiotics, 257t
Anticholinergics, 72t
Anticoagulants, 90t, 92b
Anticonvulsants, 183t
Antidiuretic hormone (ADH), 37
Antidysrhythmics, 94t—95t
Antifungal drugs, 52t
Antigen/antibody test, 49
Antihypertensives, 88t—89t
Anti-infectives, 66t—68t, 179t
Antilipemics, 85t
Antimicrobial agents, topical, 151t
Antiparkinsonian drugs, 135t
Antiplatelet agent, 90t
Antiprotozoal drugs, 52t
Antipseudomonal penicillins, 66t—68t
Antipsychotic drugs, 279t
Antiretroviral therapy (ART), 47—48
Antiulcer drugs, 100t
Antiviral drugs, 52t
Anus, newborn, 262t—264t
Aorta, coarctation of, 175, 176f
Aortic stenosis, 176, 176f
Apgar scoring system, 260t
Aphasia, 137b
Appendicitis, 197
Apraclonidine (Iopidine), 123t
Apraxia, 137b
ARDS. See Acute respiratory distress syndrome
Aripiprazole (Abilify), 279t
AROM. See Artificial rupture of membranes
Aromatherapy, 64
Arterial blood gas (ABG)
  comparisons, 41t
  values, 23t
Arteriolar vasodilator, 225t
Arteriosclerosis, 287
Arthrectomy, 83
Arthritis
  juvenile/juvenile idiopathic, 206—207
  rheumatoid, 116—117, 116b—117b

Artificial rupture of membranes (AROM), 247
Ascites, cirrhosis and, 104b
Aspart (NovoLog), 115t
Assault and battery, 11—12
Asthma, 68, 69t
  pediatric nursing, 169—170, 171f
Atazanavir (Reyataz), 52t
Atelectasis, postoperative, 46t
Atenolol (Tenormin), 84t, 88t—89t, 94t—95t
Atonic seizure, 186
Atorvastatin (Lipitor), 85t
Atovaquone (Mepron), 52t
Atrial fibrillation, 93, 93f
Atrial flutter, 93, 93f
Atrial septal defect (ASD), 175, 175f
Atrioventricular canal (AVC), 175
Atropine sulfate (Atropisol), 94t—95t, 135t
Attention-deficit/hyperactivity disorder (ADHD), 183—184
  types of, 183—184
Atypical antipsychotic drugs, 279t
Auditory hallucinations (AHs), 276
AVC. See Atrioventricular canal (AVC)
Azilsartan (Edarbi), 88t—89t
Azithromycin (Zithromax), 66t—68t
Aztreonam (Azactam), 66t—68t

B
Babinski reflex, 265t
Baby blues, 254b
Bachelor's buttons. See Feverfew
Back, newborn, 262t—264t
Bacterial meningitis, 187—188, 188b
Bacterial vaginosis, 228—230
Barlow test, 204, 205f
Barrel chest, 70b
Basic life support (BLS), 29b
  pediatric, 32f—33f
Battery, definition of, 11
Becker muscular dystrophy (BMD), 189
Beclomethasone dipropionate (Vanceril), 72t
Benazepril (Lotensin), 88t—89t
Benign prostatic hyperplasia (BPH), 81—82, 82b
Benzathine penicillin (Bicillin L-A), 66t—68t
Benzodiazepines, 281t
Benztropine mesylate (Cogentin), 135t
Beta-adrenergic receptor-blocking agents, 123t
β-adrenergic agonist, 249t—250t
Beta-blockers, 88t—89t
Betamethasone, 246—247
Betaxolol (Betoptic S), 123t
Bicarbonate-carbonic acid buffer, 41
Biguanides, 114t
Bimatoprost (Lumigan), 123t
Biologic theories, of aging, 285
Biophysical profile (BPP), 218, 220

Bioterrorism, 16
Bipolar I disorder, 277
Bisoprolol (Zebeta), 88t—89t
Bleeding, gastrointestinal, 100b
Blood glucose, 116b
  self-monitoring of, 116b
Blood lead level (BLL) test, 168
Blood pressure (BP)
  age-related changes in, 211, 254b
  newborn, 259, 260t
  physiology of, 287b
Blood urea nitrogen (BUN), elevated, 37t
Blood/urine testing, for pregnancy, 211
BMD. See Becker muscular dystrophy (BMD)
Body temperature, newborn, 259, 260t
Bowel obstructions, 102b
BPH. See Benign prostatic hyperplasia
Bradycardia, 236—238
Bradypnea, 23
Brain tumor, 132, 132b, 188—189, 188b
  causes of, 188
  clinical assessment of, 188
  clinical interventions for, 188—189
  complications of, 188
Breach of duty, definition of, 11
Breast
  postpartum changes in, 251—252
  self-examination, 253
Breast cancer, 143—144
  nursing assessment for, 144
  nursing plans and interventions for, 144
Brief interventions, 275—276
Brimonidine (Alphagan P), 123t
Brinzolamide (Azopt), 123t
Bromocriptine mesylate (Parlodel), 135t
Bronchiolitis, pediatric nursing, 172
Bronchitis, 68, 69t
Bronchodilators, 72t
Bryant traction, 203
Buck extension traction, 203
Budesonide (Pulmicort), 72t
Budesonide + formoterol (Symbicort), 72t
Bumetanide (Bumex), 87t
BUN. See Blood urea nitrogen
Burn care, stages of, 149
Burns, 148—152
  categories of, 148
  depth of, 148—149, 148f
  estimation of, 149f
  nursing assessment for, 149
  nursing plans and interventions for, 149—152
  pediatric nursing, 165—166, 165f, 166b
  review of, 152b
Buspirone (BuSpar), 281t
Buttocks, newborn, 262t—264t

C
CAL. See Chronic airflow limitation
Calcium channel blockers, 88t—89t
  for preterm labor, 249t—250t

Calcium disodium EDTA, 168
Calcium, serum, 109b
Cancer, 140
  breast, 143–144
  colon, 102–104
  of larynx, 72–73
  lung, 74–77
  ovarian, 143, 143b
  prostate, 145
  testicular, 144–145
  warning signs of, 141
Candesartan (Atacand), 88t–89t
Candida albicans, 146t–147t
Candidiasis, 48, 146t–147t, 230
  of oral cavity and esophagus, 49t
Cane, 120
Capreomycin (Capastat), 75t
Captopril (Capoten), 88t–89t
Caput succedaneum, 262t–264t
Carbamazepine, 183t
Carbapenems, 66t–68t
Carbonic anhydrase inhibitors, 123t
Carcinoma, 140
Cardiac arrest algorithm, pediatric, 34f
Cardiac dysrhythmias, 301t
Cardiogenic shock, 26
  signs of, 85b
Cardiopulmonary arrest, 29
  clinical assessment (in-hospital care),
    29–30
  clinical judgment interventions, 30
Cardiovascular disorders, pediatric nursing,
    173–181
  acyanotic heart defects, 173–176
  Clinical Judgment Measures, 180t
  congenital heart disorders, 173, 174t
  heart failure, 178, 178t, 178b
  Kawasaki disease, 180–181
  review of, 181b
  rheumatic fever, 178–180
  truncus arteriosus, 176–177, 177f
Cardiovascular system, 83–98
  abdominal aortic aneurysm, 91
  age-related changes in, 287–288
  angina, 83–84
  Clinical Judgment Measures, 289t
  dysrhythmias, 92–94
  heart failure, 94–96
  hypertension, 86–89
  inflammatory and infectious heart disease,
    96–97
  myocardial infarction, 84–86
  peripheral vascular disease, 89–91
  postpartum changes in, 252
  review of, 98b
  thrombophlebitis, 91–92
  valvular heart disease, 97–98
Cardioversion, 93b
Caring, 63, 63b
Carteolol (Ocupress), 123t
Carvedilol (Coreg), 88t–89t
Caspofungin (Cancidas), 52t

CAT. See Computer adaptive testing
    (CAT)
Cataract, 124, 124b
  in older adults, 301t
Catatonia, 276b
Catechol-O-methyl transferase (COMT)
    inhibitor, 135t
CCR5 inhibitors, 52t
CDC. See Centers for Disease Control and
    Prevention
Cefaclor (Ceclor), 66t–68t
Cefamandole (Mandol), 66t–68t
Cefazolin (Kefzol), 66t–68t
Cefdinir (Omnicef), 66t–68t
Cefepime (Maxipime), 66t–68t
Cefixime (Suprax), 66t–68t
Cefotaxime (Claforan), 66t–68t
Cefotetan (Cefotan), 66t–68t
Cefoxitin (Mefoxin), 66t–68t
Cefpodoxime (Vantin), 66t–68t
Cefprozil (Cefzil), 66t–68t
Ceftazidime (Fortaz), 66t–68t
Ceftibuten (Cedax), 66t–68t
Ceftriaxone (Rocephin), 66t–68t
Cefuroxime (Ceftin-PO), 66t–68t
Centers for Disease Control and Preven-
    tion (CDC), AIDS defined by, 47
Central-acting inhibitors, 88t–89t
Cephalexin (Keflex), 66t–68t, 257t
Cephalosporins, 66t–68t
Cerebral palsy, 182–183, 183b
  causes of, 182
  clinical assessment of, 182
  clinical interventions for, 182–183
  complications of, 182
  risk factors, 182
Cerebral vascular accident (CVA),
    136–137, 136b. See also Stroke
  diagnosis of, 136
  location of disruption in, 136t
  nursing assessment for, 137
  nursing plans and interventions for, 137
  in older adults, 301t
  risk for, 136
Cerebrospinal fluid (CSF) leakage, 129,
    129b
Cervical assessment, during labor, 233
Cervical cap, contraception with, 255t
Cervix
  cancer of, 142–143
  postpartum changes in, 251
Cesarean birth, 258–259
Chadwick's sign, 211
Chemical buffer system, 41–42
Chemotherapy
  for acute lymphocytic leukemia, 200
  for brain tumor, 132
  for Hodgkin disease, 140
  for lung cancer, 76
Chest circumference, newborn, 261t
Chest, newborn, 262t–264t
Chest tubes, 74–75, 75b, 76f

Child abuse, assessment for, 167f
Children
  with cognitive developmental delays, 160
  with communicable disease, 163t
    clinical care for, 160, 160b
  with congenital heart disease, 177–178
  foreign body airway obstruction in, 31
  respiratory failure in, 23–24
Chin, newborn, 262t–264t
Chlamydia, 145b, 146t–147t, 228t
Chlamydia trachomatis, 146t–147t
Chlordiazepoxide HCl (Librium), 281t
Chlorpromazine HCl (Thorazine), 279t
Chlorpropamide (Diabinese), 114t
Chlorthalidone (Hygroton), 87t
Cholecystectomy, 107
Cholecystitis, 107, 107b
Cholelithiasis, 107
Cholinergic crisis, 134t
Chorionic villi sampling (CVS), 219
Chronic airflow limitation (CAL), 68–72,
    69t
  nursing assessment for, 69–70
  nursing plans and interventions for,
    70–72, 71f, 71t
Chronic HIV infection, 48b, 50t
Chronic kidney disease, 78–80
  nursing assessment for, 78
  nursing plans and interventions for,
    79–80
Chronic lymphocytic leukemia, 139
Chronic myelogenous leukemia, 139
Chronic obstructive pulmonary disease
    (COPD), 68
  in older adults, 301t
Chronic pain, 56
Chronic pancreatitis
  nursing assessment for, 106
  nursing plans and interventions for, 107
Cimetidine (Tagamet), 100t
Ciprofloxacin (Cipro), 66t–68t
Circumstantiality, 276
Cirrhosis, 104–105
  nursing assessment for, 104
  nursing plans and interventions for,
    104–105
Civil procedures, 12
Clang associations, 276
Clarithromycin (Biaxin), 66t–68t
Cleft lip/palate, 193–194, 194f, 194b
Clindamycin, 257t
Clindamycin HCl (Cleocin HCl), 66t–68t
Clinical concepts, advanced, 21–61
Clinical Judgment Measurement Model,
    1–2, 2f
Clinical Judgment Measures (CJM)
  for ARDS, 25t
  cardiovascular system, 289t
  for death, 59–60
  definition of, 286
  dementia, 300t
  dystocia, 247

Clinical Judgment Measures (CJM) (Continued)
endocrine system, 296t
gastrointestinal system, 291t
with general anesthesia, 243
genitourinary system, 292t
integumentary system, 287t
labor
first stage of, 244t
fourth stage of, 245–246, 248t
second stage of, 244
third stage of, 244–245, 246t
musculoskeletal system, 288t
for nerve block analgesia and anesthesia, 243
neurologic system, 295t
newborn, 261
for pain, 57–58
postpartum period, 252–254
for pregnancy
first trimester, 211–213, 213t
second trimester, 213–214
third trimester, 215, 215t
preterm labor, 246–247
psychosocial changes, 298t
reproductive system, 293t
respiratory system, 290t
Clinical nursing judgment measures
for disaster nursing and crisis intervention, 16–17
for disseminated intravascular coagulation, 29
for shock, 27–28
CLL. See Chronic lymphocytic leukemia
Clofibrate (Claripex), 85t
Clonazepam, 183t
Clonidine (Catapres), 88t–89t
Clopidogrel (Plavix), 90t
Clorazepate dipotassium (Tranxene), 281t
Closed fracture, 119
Closed head injury, 128
Cloxacillin sodium, 66t–68t
Clozapine (Clozaril), 279t
CML. See Chronic myelogenous leukemia
Coagulation, disseminated intravascular, 28–29
Coarctation, of aorta, 175, 176f
Cocaine, withdrawal and overdose symptoms, 281t
Codeine, 58t
withdrawal and overdose symptoms, 281t
Cognitive development, 155
Colesevelam (Welchol), 85t
Colestipol HCL (Colestid), 85t
Colon cancer, 102–104
nursing assessment for, 103
nursing plans and interventions for, 103
Columbia-Suicide Severity Rating Scale, 278t
COMFORT scale, 160
Comminuted fractures, 119, 203

Communicable diseases of childhood, 160, 160b
Communicating hydrocephalus, 185b
Communication
in older adults, 285–286
therapeutic, 274b
Compartment syndrome, 203b
Competency hearing, 12–13
Complete abortion, 221
Complete fractures, 119, 203
Complex focal seizure, 186
Computer adaptive testing (CAT), 5–6
general examination formats, 5–6
working of, 5
Conception, 211
Concrete thinking, 276
Condoms, 255t
Conductive hearing loss, 125
Congenital/aganglionic megacolon (Hirschsprung disease), 195–196, 196b
Congenital heart disease, pediatric patients with, 180
Congenital hypothyroidism, 200–201, 201b
Congenital scoliosis, 205
Congestive heart failure (CHF), 178, 178t, 178b
Consent, description of, 13
Consent of minors, 13
Constipation
aging and, 24b
postoperative, 46t
Contact burns, 165
Continuous arteriovenous hemofiltration, 79t
Contraception
hormonal, 254–256, 255t
nonhormonal methods of, 254, 255t
Contraceptive sponge, 255t
Contraction stress test, 220
Control delusions, 276
Coordinator of care, 7
COPD. See Chronic obstructive pulmonary disease
Cord prolapse, 239b
Corticosteroids, 72t, 110t
for acute lymphocytic leukemia, 200b
for Cushing syndrome, 111
COVID-19, 17–18
vaccine for, 161t–162t
Craniotomy medications, 132b
Crime, description of, 12
Criminal law, 11, 11t
Crisis intervention, 15–18
Critical congenital heart disease (CCHD), 265
Crohn disease, 100
Crutches, 120
Cryosurgery, 142b
Cryptococcal meningitis, 48, 49t
Cryptosporidiosis, 49t
CSF. See Cerebrospinal fluid

Cultural diversity, 63–64, 63b, 64f
Cushing syndrome, 111, 111b
CVA. See Cerebral vascular accident
CVS. See Chorionic villi sampling (CVS)
Cyanotic heart defects, 174t, 176, 178b
CycleBeads, 255t
Cycloserine (Seromycin), 75t
Cystic fibrosis, pediatric nursing, 170, 170b
Cystocele, 141–142
Cytomegalovirus (CMV), 48
colitis associated with, 49t
disseminated, 49t
maternal/fetal effects of, 229t
retinitis associated with, 49t

D
Dalteparin (Fragmin), 90t
Damages, definition of, 11
Death, 58–60
clinical assessment of, 59
Clinical Judgment Measures for, 59–60
review of, 59b–60b
types of, 58–59
Deceleration, fetal heart rate, 237f, 238–239, 239f, 239b, 240f
Defamation, definition of, 12
Degenerative joint disease (DJD), 118
Dehydration, 35, 35b
Delavirdine (Rescriptor), 52t
Delegation, 8–10
definition of, 9t
do's and dont's for, 10b
five rights of, 9t
Delirium, 278, 294b, 301t
Delusions, 276
of grandeur, 276
of persecution, 276
Dementia, 278, 294b, 301t
aging associated with, 298–299, 301t
Clinical Judgment Measures, 300t
Dementia with Lewy bodies (DLB), 299
Denial, 59, 59b
Depression, postpartum, 254b
Dermis, burn injury to, 148f
Desiccated thyroid (Armour Thyroid), 109t
Detached retina, 125
Detemir (Levemir), 115t
Developmental dysplasia of hip (DDH), 204–205, 205f
Developmental theories, of aging, 285
Development, pediatric, 155–159
adolescent (12 to 19 years), 158–159, 159b
from birth to 1 year, 155–156
preschool child (3 to 6 years), 157, 157b
school-age child (6 to 12 years), 157–158, 158b
toddler (1 to 3 years), 156–157, 157f
Development, theories of, 155
Dexamethasone (Decadron), 110t, 130
Dexlansoprazole (Kapidex), 100t

Diabetes mellitus, 111–116
  gestational, 226–227
  nursing assessment for, 111–113
  nursing plans and interventions for, 113–116
  pediatric nursing, 202, 202b
  type 1, 111–112
    vs. type 2, 111, 112t
  type 2, 112
Diabetes self-management education, 116b
Diabetic ketoacidosis (DKA), 111–112
Dialysis, types of, 79t
Diaphragm, contraception with, 255t
Diarrhea, pediatric nursing, 162–169, 165b
  clinical assessment for, 164–165
  clinical judgment for, 165
Diastolic BP, 287b
Diastolic murmurs, 287
Diazepam (Valium), 281t
Dicloxacillin sodium, 66t–68t
Diet. See also Nutrition
  colostomy and, 104
  ileostomy and, 103
  during pregnancy, 217
Digitalis
  preparations, 97t
  toxicity, 98b
Digitoxin (Crystodigin), 94t–95t, 97t
Digoxin (Lanoxin), 94t–95t, 97t
Diltiazem (Cardizem, Norvasc), 84t, 88t–89t, 94t–95t
Dimercaprol, 168
Dinoprostone (Prostin E$_2$), 259t
Disaster management, prevention levels in, 15
Disaster nursing, 15–18, 18b
Discoid lupus erythematosus (DLE), 117
Disengagement theory, of aging, 285
Disopyramide phosphate (Norpace), 94t–95t
Disrupted acid-base balance
  in ARDS, 21, 23t
  clinical manifestations of, 22f, 24t
Disseminated CMV, 49t
Disseminated intravascular coagulation (DIC), 28–29, 222b
  clinical assessment of, 28
  clinical nursing judgment measures, 29
  definition of, 28
  review of, 29b
Distributive shock, 24–26
Disulfiram (Antabuse), 280, 282t
Diuretics, 87t
Diverticular diseases, 101, 101b
Diverticulosis, 101, 101b
DJD. See Degenerative joint disease (DJD)
DMD. See Duchenne muscular dystrophy (DMD)
Dofetilide (Tikosyn), 94t–95t
Donepezil HCl, 295t
Dopamine agonist, 135t
Dopamine-receptor agonists, 135t

Dopamine-releasing agents, 135t
Dorzolamide (Trusopt), 123t
Down syndrome, 177f, 181–182, 182f, 182b
Doxazosin (Cardura), 88t–89t
Doxycycline hyclate (Vibramycin), 66t–68t
Dronedarone (Multaq), 94t–95t
Drug abuse. See Substance abuse
Drugs
  for Alzheimer disease, 295t
  aminoglycosides, 66t–68t
  antianemic, 79t
  antianginals, 84t
  antianxiety, 281t
  anticholinergic, 72t
  anticoagulants, 90t, 92b
  antidysrhythmics, 94t–95t
  antihypertensives, 88t–89t
  anti-infectives, 66t–68t, 179t
  antilipemics, 85t
  antiparkinsonian, 135t
  antipsychotic, 279t
  antiulcer, 100t
  bronchodilators, 72t
  carbapenems, 66t–68t
  cephalosporins, 66t–68t
  corticosteroids, 72t, 110t
  diuretics, 87t
  fluoroquinolones, 66t–68t
  for HIV infection, 52t–54t
  lincosamides, 66t–68t
  macrolides, 66t–68t
  monobactam, 66t–68t
  for multiple sclerosis, 133b
  narcotic, 57, 58t
  nonsteroidal antiinflammatory, 118t
  osmotic diuretic, 130t
  oxazolidinone, 66t–68t
  penicillins, 66t–68t
  for postpartum hemorrhage, 259t
  for shock, 27
  streptogramin, 66t–68t
  tetracyclines, 66t–68t
  for tuberculosis, 75t
  withdrawal and overdose symptoms, 281t
DTaP vaccine, 161t–162t
Duchenne muscular dystrophy (DMD), 189
Dunlop traction, 203
Duodenal ulcers, 99
Duty, definition of, 11
Dysarthria, 137b
Dysphagia, 137b
Dysphasia, 137b
Dyspnea, end-of-life care and, 302
Dysrhythmias, 92–94
  aging and, 287
  nursing assessment for, 92
  nursing plans and interventions for, 93–94
  in older adults, 301t
  selected, 93, 93b

Dystocia, 247–248
Dystrophin, 189

E
Early-onset sepsis, 267
Ears
  newborn, 262t–264t
  structure of, 125b
Ebola
  clinical judgement interventions, 17
  diagnosis, 17
  risk of, 17
  screening, 17
  spread of, 17
  symptoms, 17
Echinacea, 65t
Eclampsia, 226
Ectopic pregnancy, 222, 222b
Efavirenz (Sustiva), 52t
Elder abuse, 299–302
Electrocardiogram (ECG), 42–44
  heart rate estimation using, 43b
  paper, 42f
  review of, 44b
Electroconvulsive therapy (ECT), 274
Electrolyte balance, 35–38, 36f
  importance of, 35
  review of, 42b
Electrolyte imbalance, 38, 39t–40t
Electronic fetal monitoring, 233–234
Embolectomy, 90
Embryo, development of, 211
Emergency admission, 12
Emergency care, 13–14
Emphysema, 68, 69t
Enalapril maleate (Vasotec), 88t–89t
Encephalopathy, HIV, 49t
Endarterectomy, 90
Endocarditis, 96
  nursing assessment for, 97
  nursing plans and interventions for, 97
Endocrine disorders, pediatric nursing, 200–202, 202b
Endocrine system, 108–116
  Addison disease, 110–111
  age-related changes in, 294–296
  Clinical Judgment Measures, 296t
  Cushing syndrome, 111
  diabetes mellitus, 111–116
  hyperthyroidism, 108–109
  hypothyroidism, 109–110
  review of, 116b
End-of-life care, 302
Endometrial cycle, 209–211, 210f
Endometritis, 256
Endorphin/enkephalin theory, 56
End-stage renal disease (ESRD), 78–80
Enfuvirtide (Fuzeon), 52t
Entacapone (Comtan), 135t
Ephedrine, 65t
Epidermis, burn injury to, 148f
Epidural block, 242–243

Epiglottitis, pediatric nursing, 170—172
Epinephrine (Adrenaline), 72t, 94t—95t
Episiotomy, 253
Eplerenone (Inspra), 87t
Eprosartan (Teveten), 88t—89t
Eptifibatide (Integrilin), 94t—95t
Erikson's theory, 155, 285
Erotomania, 276
Ertapenem (Invanz), 66t—68t
Erythromycin, 66t—68t
Erythropoietin (Epogen), 79t
Esomeprazole (Nexium), 100t
Esophageal atresia with tracheoesophageal
    fistula, 194—195
Esophageal ulcers, 99
ESRD. *See* End-stage renal disease
Essential oils, 64f
Ethambutol (Myambutol), 75t
Ethionamide (Trecator), 75t
Etravirine (Intelence), 52t
Exenatide (Byetta) (Victoza), 115t
Exophthalmos, 108, 108f
Exposure of a person, definition of, 11—12
Extremities, newborn, 262t—264t
Eye
    prophylaxis, newborn, 261
    trauma, 124—125
Eye drops, 122b, 123

F
Faces Pain Scale-Revised (FPS-R), 159
Factor Xa inhibitor, 90t
False imprisonment, definition of, 11
False labor, 231
Famciclovir (Famvir), 52t
Family therapy, 275
Famotidine (Pepcid), 100t
Featherfoil. *See* Feverfew
Felodipine (Plendil), 88t—89t
Fenofibrate (Tricor), 85t
Fentanyl citrate (Sublimaze), 58t, 242t
Ferguson reflex, 244b
Ferrous sulfate (Feosol), 227t
Fertility awareness-based methods
    (FABM), 255t
Fertilization, 211
Fetal alcohol syndrome (FAS), 270, 271f
Fetal attitude, 231
Fetal heart rate (FHR)
    baseline, 234
    Clinical Judgment Measures, 234—235
    deceleration of, 237f, 238—239, 239f, 239b
        , 240f
    determination of, 217
    during labor, 233
    normal value for, 217b
    variability, 234—235, 237f
Fetal lie, 231, 234f
Fetal lung maturity, 219
Fetal position, 231, 235f
Fetal presentation, 231, 234f
Fetal station, 231, 236f

Fetor hepaticus, 104b
Fetus
    assessment of, 218—220
    development, 211, 212f
    monitoring, 233—234
Feverfew, 65t
Fibroids, 141
Fibromas, 141
Fibromyomas, 141
First degree burns, 148
FLACC (Face, Legs, Activity, Cry, Consol-
    ability) scale, 159
Flecainide acetate (Tambocor), 94t—95t
Fluconazole (Diflucan), 52t
Flucytosine (Ancobon), 52t
Fluid balance, 35—38, 36f
    review of, 42b
Fluid volume, 37t
    alterations in, 78b
Fluid volume deficit (FVD), 35—36
    causes of, 36
    risk factors for, 36
Flunisolide (AeroBid), 72t
Fluoroquinolones, 66t—68t
Fluphenazine decanoate (Prolixin Dec-
    anoate), 279t
Fluphenazine HCl (Prolixin), 279t
Fluticasone (Flovent), 72t
Fluticasone + albuterol (Advair), 72t
Fluvastatin (Lescol), 85t
Focal seizures, 186
Follicle-stimulating hormone (FSH), 209
Follicular phase, in ovarian cycle, 209
Fondaparinux, 90t
Foreign body airway obstruction (FBAO),
        management of
    adults and children, 31
    infants and children, 31—35
Fosamprenavir (Lexiva), 52t
Fosinopril (Monopril), 88t—89t
Fosphenytoin sodium, 183t
Fractures, 119—120, 119b—120b
    nursing assessment for, 120
    pediatric, 203—204, 203b
    signs and symptoms of, 120
    types of, 119
Fraud, definition of, 12
Frontotemporal dementia, 299
Fundal height
    assessment of, 217, 217f
    postpartum, 252
Fundus
    adaptations during pregnancy, 214—215
    in fourth stage of labor, 245
Furosemide (Lasix), 87t
Fusion inhibitors, 52t

G
Galantamine, 295t
Ganciclovir (Cytovene), 52t
Garlic, 65t
Gastric ulcers, 99

Gastroesophageal reflux disease (GERD),
    98—99
Gastrointestinal bleeding, 100b
Gastrointestinal disorders, pediatric nurs-
    ing, 193—197
    anorectal malformations, 196—197
    appendicitis, 197
    cleft lip/palate, 193—194, 194f, 194b
    congenital/aganglionic megacolon (Hirsch-
        sprung disease), 195—196, 196b
    esophageal atresia with tracheoesophageal
        fistula, 194—195
    intussusception, 195, 195b
    pyloric stenosis, 195
    review of, 197b
Gastrointestinal system, 98—107
    age-related changes in, 289—290, 290b
    cholecystitis and cholelithiasis, 107
    cirrhosis, 104—105
    Clinical Judgment Measures, 291t
    colon cancer, 102—104
    diverticular diseases, 101
    hepatitis, 105—106
    hiatal hernia and gastroesophageal reflux
        disease, 98—99
    inflammatory bowel diseases, 100
    intestinal obstruction, 101—102
    pancreatitis, 106—107
    peptic ulcer disease, 99—100
    postpartum changes in, 252
    review of, 107b
    ulcerative colitis, 100—101
Gate control theory, 56
Gavage-feeding, 269, 270f
    tube insertion procedure, 269b
Gemfibrozil (Lopid), 85t
Generalized tonic-clonic seizure (GTC)/
    grand mal seizure, 186
Genitals, newborn, 262t—264t
Genitourinary system
    age-related changes in, 291—293
    Clinical Judgment Measures, 292t
Gentamicin sulfate, 66t—68t, 257t
Gerontologic nursing, 285—304
Gestational age, 211, 261
    assessment of, 265t
    estimation of, 264f
Gestational diabetes mellitus, 226—227
Gestational hypertension, 223
Ginger, 65t
Ginkgo biloba, 65t
Ginseng, 65t
Glargine (Lantus), 115t
Glasgow Coma Scale (GCS), 126, 126t,
    126b
Glaucoma, 122—124
    nursing assessment for, 122
    nursing plans and interventions for,
        122—124
    in older adults, 301t
    treatment of, 123t
Glimepiride (Amaryl), 114t

Glipizide (Glucotrol), 114t
Glipizide + metformin (Metaglip), 114t
Glucocorticoids (betamethasone),
    246—247
Glucose
    antepartum, 217
    in newborn, 265
    self-monitoring, 116b
Glulisine (Apidra), 115t
Glyburide (Micronase, DiaBeta), 114t
Glyburide and metformin (Glucovance),
    114t
Glycosylated Hgb, 113b
Goiter, 108—109, 108f
Gonadotropin-releasing hormone (GnRH),
    209
Gonorrhea, 146t—147t, 228t
Goodell sign, 211
Good Samaritan Act, 13—14, 14b
Graves disease, 108—109, 108f, 301t
Gravida, 216
Greenstick fracture, 119
Grief, 58—60, 298
    clinical assessment of, 59
    review of, 59b—60b
Group B streptococcus (GBS), 228
    maternal and fetal effects of, 228t
    in newborn, 267—268
Group IIa-IIIb inhibitor (platelet antiaggre-
    gate), 94t—95t
Group therapy, 275
Growth and development, 155—159
    clinical implications in, 155—158
        adolescent (12 to 19 years), 158—159,
            159b
        from birth to 1 year, 155—156
        preschool child (3 to 6 years), 157,
            157b
        school-age child (6 to 12 years),
            157—158, 158b
        toddler (1 to 3 years), 156—157, 157f
    theories of development, 155
Guanabenz acetate (Wytensin), 88t—89t
Guanfacine (Tenex), 88t—89t
Guillain—Barré syndrome, 135—136

H
Hallucinations, 276
Hallucinogenics, withdrawal and overdose
    symptoms, 281t
Haloperidol (Haldol), 279t
Haloperidol decanoate (Haldol Decanoate),
    279t
Hashimoto disease, 109—110
Head circumference, newborn, 260, 261t
Head injury, 128—130, 128b
    nursing assessment for, 128—130, 129b
    nursing plans and interventions for, 130
Head, newborn, 262t—264t
Health care provider, prescriptions and, 14
Health Insurance Portability and Account-
    ability Act of 1996 (HIPAA), 15

Health promotion
    child, 160—162, 169b
    of older adults, 299
Hearing loss, 125—126
    conductive, 125
    sensorineural, 125
Heart
    blood flow through, 43b
    electrolyte balance and, 37
Heart disease
    inflammatory and infectious, 96—97
    valvular, 97—98
Heart failure (HF), 94—96
    nursing assessment for, 94—96
    nursing plans and interventions for, 96
    pediatric nursing, 178, 178t, 178b
Heart rate
    estimation of, 43b
    newborn, 260t
Heelstick procedure, for newborn, 265,
    266b
Hegar sign, 211
HELLP syndrome, 226
Hematocrit (Hct), pregnancy assessment
    with, 217
Hematologic disorders, pediatric nursing,
    197—200
    acute lymphocytic leukemia, 199—200
    hemophilia, 198, 198b
    iron deficiency anemia, 197—198, 197b
    review of, 200b
    sickle cell disease, 198—199, 199f, 199b
Hematologic system, postpartum changes
    in, 252
Hematology/oncology, 137—141
    anemia, 137—138
    Hodgkin disease, 140
    leukemia, 138—140
    review of, 141b
Hemodialysis, 79t
Hemoglobin (Hgb), pregnancy assessment
    and, 217
Hemophilia, 198, 198b
Hemorrhage
    postpartum, 257—258
        acute, 257
        drugs for, 259t
        late, 257
    post-tonsillectomy, 173
Heparin, 92b
Heparin sodium (Hepalean, Hep-lock), 90t
Hepatitis, 105—106, 106b
    nursing assessment for, 105
    nursing plans and interventions for,
        105—106
    types of, 106t
Hepatitis A, 106t
    maternal/fetal effects of, 229t
Hepatitis B, 106t
    maternal/fetal effects of, 229t
Hepatitis B vaccine, 161t—162t
    for newborn, 261

Hepatitis C, 106t
Hepatomegaly, cirrhosis and, 104
Herbal medications, 64, 65t
Hernia, hiatal, 98—99
Heroin, withdrawal and overdose symp-
    toms, 281t
Herpes simplex viral infections, perirectal
    mucocutaneous, 49t
Herpes simplex virus 2, 146t—147t
Herpes simplex virus, maternal/fetal effects
    of, 228t—229t
HF. See Heart failure
Hiatal hernia, 98—99
Hib (Haemophilus influenzae type B) vac-
    cine, 161t—162t
High-density lipoprotein (HDL), angina
    and, 83
Hip
    developmental dysplasia of, 204—205, 205f
    fracture of, 120b
    newborn, 262t—264t
Histamine$_2$ antagonists, 100t
HIV-associated nephropathy (HIVAN), 49
HIV-associated neurocognitive disorders
    (HAND), 49
HIV infection. See Human immunodefi-
    ciency virus (HIV) infection
Hodgkin disease, 140, 140b
    nursing assessment for, 140
    nursing plans and interventions for, 140
Holter monitor, 43, 93b
Homeostasis, 35
Hormonal contraception, 254—256, 255t
HPV. See Human papillomavirus (HPV)
Human B-type natriuretic peptide
    (HBNP), 94t—95t
Human immunodeficiency virus (HIV)
    infection, 47—51, 146t—147t
    adult, 49—50
    cancer and, 48
    causes of, 47
    complications of, 48—49
    drugs for, 52t—54t
    pediatric, 55
        clinical interventions, 55
        clinical judgment, 55
    in pregnancy, 228
    prevention options for, 51b
    review of, 55b
    stages of, 48b, 50t
    with tuberculosis, 51
Human insulin lispro (Humalog), 115t
Human milk, 269
Human papillomavirus (HPV), 146t—147t
    maternal/fetal effects of, 228t
Human prenatal development, 212f
Hydatidiform mole, 221—222
Hydralazine (Apresoline, Neopresol), 225t
Hydralazine HCL (Apresoline), 88t—89t
Hydration
    in pneumonia, 68b
    in sickle cell disease, 199b

Hydrocephalus, 185—186, 185b
Hydrochlorothiazide (Esidrix, Microzide), 87t
Hydrocortisone, 110t
Hydromorphone, 58t
Hyperbilirubinemia, 265—266
Hypercalcemia, 39t—40t
Hyperemesis gravidarum, 221
Hyperglycemia *vs.* hypoglycemia, 116t
Hyperkalemia, 39t—40t
Hyperlipidemia, angina and, 83
Hypermagnesemia, 39t—40t
Hypernatremia, 39t—40t
Hyperosmotic agents, 130
Hyperphosphatemia, 39t—40t
Hypertension, 86—89, 86b
   angina and, 83
   gestational, 223
   nursing assessment for, 86—87
   nursing plans and interventions for, 87—89, 87b
   pharmacologic control of, in pregnancy, 225t
Hyperthyroidism, 108—109
   treatment of, 108—109
Hypocalcemia, 39t—40t
Hypoglycemia
   vs. hyperglycemia, 116t
   in newborn, 265
Hypoglycemics, oral, 114t
Hypokalemia, 39t—40t
Hypomagnesemia, 39t—40t
Hyponatremia, 39t—40t
Hypophosphatemia, 39t—40t
Hypoplastic left heart syndrome (HLHS), 176, 176b
Hypospadias, 193
Hypothyroidism, 109—110
   congenital, 200—201, 201b
   in older adults, 301t
Hypovolemia, 35—36
Hypovolemic shock, 26
   stages of, 26t
Hypoxia
   during suctioning, 69
   symptoms of, 169b

I
Ibutilide (Corvert) IV, 94t—95t
Idiopathic scoliosis, 205
Imipenem (Primaxin), 66t—68t
Immediate postpartum, 226
Immobility, complications of, 127
Immunity theory, of aging, 285
Inactive polio vaccine (IPV), 161t—162t
Inamrinone (Inocor), 94t—95t
Incomplete abortion, 220
Incomplete fractures, 119, 203
Indapamide (Lozol), 87t
Indinavir (Crixivan), 52t
Indomethacin (Indocin), 249t—250t
Inevitable abortion, 220

Infant. *See also* Newborn
   bacterial meningitis in, 187
   from birth to 1 year, 155—156
   developmental milestones, 156f
   with fetal alcohol syndrome, 271f
   foreign body airway obstruction in, 31—35
   pain assessment and management in, 159
   urinary tract infection in, 191
Infection(s)
   burns and, 151b
   postpartum, 256—257, 257b
   during pregnancy, 227—228
   TORCH, 228, 229t
   vaginal, 228—230
Inflammation
   of liver, 105
   of tonsils, 172
Inflammatory bowel diseases, 100
Informed consent, 13
Inhaler, use of, 71t
Injury, definition of, 11
Insanity, 13
Insulin
   age-related changes in level of, 294
   types/action of, 115t
Insulin-dependent diabetes mellitus (IDDM), 202, 202b
Integumentary system
   age-related changes in, 286
   Clinical Judgment Measures, 287t
   newborn, 262t—264t
   postpartum changes in, 252
Interpersonal therapy, 275
Interpersonal violence, older adults, 299
Intestinal obstruction, 101—102, 102b
Intracranial pressure (ICP)
   head injury and, 128
   increased, indicator of, 128
Intraoperative care, 45—46
Intrapartum, 224
Intrapartum nursing care, 230—239
   electronic fetal monitoring, 233—234
   labor
      nursing assessment of client presenting in, 231—233
      stages of, 230, 231t
      true/false, 230—231
   review of, 248b
Intrauterine contraception, 254—255
Intravenous (IV) fluids, burn care and, 150b
Intravenous immune globulin (IVIG), 181
Intravenous therapy, 38—42
   administration of, 38
   complications associated with, 38—41
Intussusception, 195, 195b
Invasion of privacy, definition of, 11—12
Involuntary admission, 12
Ipratropium (Atrovent), 72t
Ipratropium + albuterol (Combivent), 72t
Irbesartan (Avapro), 88t—89t

Iron, 164t
   administration of parenteral, 138t
   during pregnancy, oral supplementation, 227, 227t
   supplementation, 214b
Iron deficiency anemia, 197—198, 197b, 227t
Ischemic phase, in endometrial cycle, 211
Isoetharine (Bronkometer), 72t
Isoniazid (INH), 75t
Isophane insulin (human) (Humulin N, Novolin N), 115t
Isoproterenol HCL (Isuprel), 72t
Isosorbide dinitrate (Isordil), 84t
Isosorbide mononitrate (Imdur), 84t
Itraconazole (Sporanox), 52t

J
Jaundice
   clinical manifestations of, 104b
   in newborn, 265, 266b, 267t
Joint replacement, 120—121
Juvenile arthritis/juvenile idiopathic arthritis, 206—207

K
Kanamycin (Kantrex), 75t
Kaposi sarcoma, 48, 49t
Kawasaki disease, 180—181
   clinical assessment for, 181
   clinical judgment for, 181
   complications of, 181
   risk factors, 180—181
   signs of, 180
Kidney
   in acid-base balance, 42
   diabetes mellitus and, 113
   electrolyte balance and, 36—37, 38f
   postoperative care for, 80t

L
Labetalol (Normodyne), 88t—89t
Labetalol hydrochloride (Normodyne, Trandate), 225t
Labor
   with analgesia/anesthesia, 241—243
   and birth complications, 246—256
   and delivery preparation, 239—246
   first stage of, 239—241, 244t
   fourth stage of, 245—246, 247f, 248t
   nursing assessment of client presenting in, 231—233
   preterm, 246—247
   second stage of, 244, 245f
   stages of, 230, 231t
   third stage of, 244—245, 246t
   true/false, 230—231
Lactational amenorrhea method, 255t
Lactulose (Cephulac), 105t
Laennec cirrhosis, 104
Lamotrigine (Lamictal), 183t
Lansoprazole (Prevacid), 100t

Laparotomy, 143
Laryngeal cancer, 72—73
    nursing assessment for, 73
    nursing plans and interventions
        for, 73
Laryngectomy, 73
Laser therapy, 142b
Latanoprost (Xalatan), 123t
Late-onset sepsis, 267
Late postpartum hemorrhage, 257
Law, organization of, 11t
Leadership, 7—19
    and management, 7—10, 10b
Leaders vs. managers, 7
Lead poisoning, pediatric nursing,
    167—169
Lecithin/sphingomyelin (L/S) ratio, 219
Left-sided heart failure, 94
Leiomyomas, 141
Length, newborn, 261t
Lens, cataract in, 124b
Leopold's maneuvers, 231, 233f, 233b
Leukemia, 138—140
    etiology of, 138—139
    nursing assessment for, 139
    nursing plans and interventions for,
        139—140
    types of, 139
Levalbuterol (Xopenex), 72t
Levobunolol (Betagan), 123t
Levodopa (Dopar), 135t
Levodopa-carbidopa (Sinemet), 135t
Levofloxacin (Levaquin), 66t—68t, 75t
Levothyroxine (Synthroid), 109t
Lidocaine HCL (Xylocaine), 94t—95t
Linagliptin (Tradjenta), 114t
Lincosamides, 66t—68t
Linezolid (Ziox), 66t—68t
Liothyronine sodium (Cytomel), 109t
Lisinopril (Zestril), 88t—89t
Liver
    hepatitis and, 106b
    inflammation of, 105
Lobectomy, 74
Local anesthesia, 242
Lochia
    in fourth stage of labor, 245—246
    postpartum, 252—253
Long-acting reversible contraception
    (LARC) methods, 254—255
Loop diuretics, 87t
Loose associations, 276
Lopinavir + ritonavir (Kaletra), 52t
Lorazepam (Ativan), 281t
Losartan (Cozaar), 88t—89t
Lovastatin (Mevacor), 85t
Low-density lipoprotein (LDL), angina
    and, 83
Low-molecular-weight heparin enoxaparin
    (Lovenox), 90t
Loxapine (Loxitane), 279t
L/S ratio, 219

Lung cancer, 74—77
    nursing assessment for, 74
    nursing plans and interventions for,
        74—77
Lungs
    in acid-base balance, 42
    electrolyte balance and, 37
Lupus erythematosus, 117—118, 117b
Luteal phase, in ovarian cycle, 209
Luteinizing hormone (LH), 209
Lymphoma, 48
    of central nervous system, 49t

M
Macrolides, 66t—68t
Macular degeneration, 301t
Mafenide acetate (Sulfamylon), 151t
Magnesium sulfate, 224, 249t—250t
Ma-huang, 65t
Major depressive disorder, 277—280
    clinical assessment tips for, 278
    Clinical Judgment Measures for, 278—280
    signs and symptoms of, 278
Malpractice, 11, 12t
    elements of, 11
Mammography, 144
Management, 7—19
    leadership and, 7—10, 10b
Managers, nurse, 8, 9t
    leaders vs., 7
Mannitol (Osmitrol), 130t
Maraviroc (Selzentry), 52t
Maslow's hierarchy of needs, 3, 3t
Maslow's theory, 285
Mastitis
    in breastfeeding mother, 258t
    postpartum, 256
Maternal adaptations, during pregnancy
    first trimester, 211
    second trimester, 213
    third trimester, 214—215
Maternal assessment, 218—220
Maternal Fetal Triage Index (MFT), 232f
Maternal substance misuse and abuse, 270
Maternity nursing, 209—272
Measles, mumps, rubella (MMR) vaccine,
    161t—162t
Meconium-stained fluid, 241b
Medical-surgical nursing, 63—153
Meglitinides, 114t
Memantine, 295t
Menarche, 209—211
Meningitis
    bacterial, 187—188, 188b
    cryptococcal, 48, 49t
Meningocele, 184
Menorrhagia, 141b
Menstrual cycle, 210f
    conception, 211
    endometrial cycle, 209—211
    menarche, 209—211
    ovarian cycle, 209

Menstrual phase, in endometrial cycle, 209
Mental health treatments and interven-
    tions, 275—276, 275b—276b
    brief interventions, 275—276
    family therapy, 275
    group therapy, 275
    interpersonal therapy, 275
Meperidine hydrochloride, 242t
Meropenem (Merrem IV), 66t—68t
Metabolic disorders, pediatric nursing,
    200—202, 202b
Metaproterenol (Alupent), 72t
Metastasis, 141
Metformin (Glucophage), 114t
Methadone, withdrawal and overdose
    symptoms, 281t
Methimazole (Tapazole), 108b
Methyldopa (Aldomet), 88t—89t, 225t
Methylergonovine (Methergine), 259t
Methylprednisolone (Medrol), 110t
Methylprednisolone sodium/succinate
    (Solu-Medrol), 72t, 130
15-Methylprostaglandin $F_{2}\alpha$, 259t
Methylxanthine drugs, 72t
Metipranolol (OptiPranolol), 123t
Metolazone (Zaroxolyn), 87t
Metoprolol (Lopressor, Toprol), 88t—89t,
    94t—95t
Metronidazole (Flagyl), 66t—68t
Mexiletine (Mexitil), 94t—95t
Micafungin (Mycamine), 52t
Miglitol (Glyset), 114t
Milrinone (Primacor), 94t—95t
Minocycline (Minocin), 66t—68t
Minoxidil (Loniten), 88t—89t
Miscarriage, 220
Misoprostol (Cytotec), 259t
Missed abortion, 221
Mitral valve stenosis, 97b
Moexipril (Univasc), 88t—89t
Molar pregnancy (hydatidiform mole),
    221—222
Mometasone (Asmanex), 72t
Monoamine oxidase type B inhibitor, 135t
Monobactam, 66t—68t
Mood disorders, 280b
Moral development, 155
Moricizine (Ethmozine), 94t—95t
Moro reflex, 265t
Morphine sulfate, 58t
Morphine, withdrawal and overdose symp-
    toms, 281t
Mouth, newborn, 262t—264t
Moxifloxacin (Avelox), 66t—68t, 75t
Mucosal healing agents, 100t
Multifocal dementia, 299
Multiple sclerosis (MS), 132—133, 132b
Murmurs, diastolic, 287
Muscular dystrophy, 189—190
Musculoskeletal system, 116—122
    age-related changes in, 286—287
    amputation, 121—122

Musculoskeletal system (*Continued*)
  Clinical Judgment Measures, 288t
  fracture, 119–120
  joint replacement, 120–121
  lupus erythematosus, 117–118
  osteoarthritis, 118
  osteoporosis, 118–119
  postpartum changes in, 252
  review of, 122b
  rheumatoid arthritis, 116–117
Myasthenia gravis, 133–134
  nursing assessment for, 133
  nursing plans and interventions for, 133–134
  treatment of, 134t
Myasthenic crisis, 133, 134t
Mycobacterium tuberculosis, 73
Myelomeningocele, 184
Myocardial infarction (MI), 84–86
  cardiac enzyme elevations and, 86t
  causes of, 84
  nursing assessment of, 84–85
  nursing plans and interventions for, 86
Myoclonic seizure, 186
Myomas, 141
Myxedema, 109–110
Myxedema coma, 109b

N

Nadolol (Corgard), 84t, 88t–89t
Naegele's rule, 211, 216b
Nafcillin sodium, 66t–68t
Nalbuphine hydrochloride, 242t
Naloxone hydrochloride, 242t
Narcotic mixed agonists/antagonists, 57
Narcotics, 57, 58t
  pain management with, 58b
  side effects of, 57
Nateglinide (Starlix), 114t
National Council of State Boards of Nursing (NCSBN), 1
  Clinical Judgment Model, 1–2, 2f
NCLEX-PN®
  computer adaptive testing (CAT), 5–6
  examination, 4–5
  examination formats, 1
  general priniciples to remember, 6
  introduction to, 1–6
  job analysis studies, 1
  licensing examination, 1
  test-taking strategies, 1–4, 2f, 3t
NCSBN. *See* National Council of State Boards of Nursing
Neck, newborn, 262t–264t
Negligence, 11, 12t
Neisseria gonorrhoeae, 146t–147t
Nelfinavir (Viracept), 52t
Neologisms, 276
Neonatal abstinence syndrome (NAS), 270–271
  signs of, 271b

Neonatal Infant Pain Scale, 159
Neonatal opioid withdrawal syndrome (NOWS), 270–271
Neonatal Pain, Agitation and Sedation Scale (N-PASS), 159
Neonatal sepsis, 267–268
Neonate. *See* Newborn
Neoplasm, 140
Nephropathy, HIV-associated, 49
Nephrostomy, percutaneous, 81b
Nephrotic syndrome, 190–191
  types of, 190
Nerve block analgesia and anesthesia, 242–243
Nesiritide (Natrecor), 94t–95t
Neural tube defect (NTD). *See* Spina bifida
Neurogenic shock, 26
Neurologic system, 126–137
  age-related changes in, 294, 294b
  altered state of consciousness, 126–128
  brain tumor, 132
  Clinical Judgment Measures, 295t
  Guillain–Barré syndrome, 135–136
  head injury, 128–130
  multiple sclerosis, 132–133
  myasthenia gravis, 133–134
  Parkinson disease, 134–135
  postpartum changes in, 252
  spinal cord injury, 130–132
  stroke/brain attack, 136–137
Neuromuscular assessment, of newborn, 265t
Neuromuscular disorders, pediatric nursing, 181–193
  anticonvulsants for, 183t
  attention-deficit/hyperactivity disorder, 183–184
  bacterial meningitis, 187–188, 188b
  brain tumor, 188–189, 188b
  cerebral palsy, 182–183, 183b
  Clinical Judgment Measures, 192t
  Down syndrome, 181–182, 182f, 182b
  hydrocephalus, 185–186, 185b
  muscular dystrophy, 189–190
  review of, 190b
  Reye syndrome, 188
  seizures, 186–187, 187b
  spina bifida, 184–185, 184f
Neuromuscular scoliosis, 205
Neurosensory system, 122–126
  cataract, 124
  detached retina, 125
  eye trauma, 124–125
  glaucoma, 122–124
  hearing loss, 125–126
  review of, 138b
Nevirapine (Viramune), 52t
New Ballard Score, 261, 264f
Newborn. *See also* Infant
  Apgar scoring system for, 260t
  bacterial meningitis in, 187

Newborn (*Continued*)
  Clinical Judgment Measures, 261
  complications of, 267–271, 271b
  discharge teaching, 266
  gestational assessment of, 261
  heelstick procedure for, 265, 266b
  hematology of, 266t
  history of, 260–261
  immediate care after delivery, 260
  medications for, 261
  neuromuscular assessment of, 265t
  pain assessment and management in, 159
  pathologic jaundice in, 267t
  physical examination of, 262t–264t
  physical measurements of, 261t
  physiologic assessment of, 265
  preterm, 268–269
  respiratory distress syndrome, 269
  substance abuse effects on, 270–271
  transition to extrauterine life, 259
  vital signs of, 260t
Next-Generation NCLEX (NGN), 1
Niacin (Niaspan), 85t
Nicardipine (Cardene), 88t–89t
Nicotinic acid (Nicobid), 85t
Nifedipine (Procardia, Adalat), 84t, 88t–89t, 225t, 249t–250t
Nihilistic delusions, 276
Nisoldipine (Sular), 88t–89t
Nitroglycerin, 84t
Nizatidine (Axid), 100t
N-methyl D-aspartate (NMDA) antagonist, 295t
Non-accidental trauma (NAT), pediatric nursing, 166, 166b, 167f
Nonbenzodiazepines, 281t
Non-communicating hydrocephalus, 185b
Nonhormonal contraception, 254, 255t
Non-NRT inhibitors, 52t
Non-phenothiazines, 279t
Nonsteroidal antiinflammatory drugs (NSAIDs), 118t
  for preterm labor, 249t–250t
Nonstress test, 219–220
Norepinephrine (Levophed), 94t–95t
Nose, newborn, 262t–264t
Nucleic acid test (NAT), 49
Nucleotide inhibitor drugs, 52t
Nurse. *See* Practical nurse (PN); Registered nurse (RN)
Nurse managers, 8, 9t
  maintaining a safe, effective work environment, 10
Nursing, 63
  disaster, 15–18, 18b
  gerontologic, 285–304
  legal aspects of, 7–19, 15b
  maternity, 209–272
  medical-surgical, 63–153
  psychiatric, 12–13, 273–284
Nursing skills, for respiratory client, 71t

Nutrition. *See also* Diet
in newborn, 261
pediatric, 162, 163t
prenatal, 217—218

O

Oblique fracture, 119
Obstetrical history, 216
Obstructive shock, 26—27
Olanzapine (Zyprexa), 279t
Older adults
aging and, 285
communication in, 285—286
diseases and conditions in, 301t
health promotion of, 299
interpersonal violence among, 299
spirituality and, 302
Oliguric phase, 77, 78b
Olmesartan (Benicar), 88t—89t
Omeprazole (Prilosec), 100t
Oncology, 140—141
Open fracture, 119, 203
Open head injury, 128
Opioid withdrawal, 280—282
Opium, withdrawal and overdose
symptoms, 281t
Organ function, electrolyte balance and,
36—37
Orthopedic wounds, 120b
Ortolani test, 205f
Osmotic diuretic, 130t
Osteoarthritis (OA), 118, 118b
Osteoporosis, 118—119, 119b
Otitis media, pediatric nursing, 172,
172b
Ovarian cancer, 143, 143b
Ovarian cycle, 209, 210f
Overall Benefit of Analgesic Score
(OBAA), 56
Ovulation, 209
indications of, 209
Oxacillin sodium, 66t—68t
Oxazolidinone, 66t—68t
Oxygen, administration of, 71t, 172b
Oxygenation, measurement of, 172b
Oxytocin (Pitocin), 244b, 251b
for postpartum hemorrhage, 259t
Oxytocin challenge test (OCT), 220

P

Pacemaker, 93—94, 94b, 96f
Pacemaker theory, of aging, 285
Pain, 56—58
acute, 56
assessment and management, in pediatric
nursing, 159—160, 159f, 160t
chronic, 56
clinical assessment for, 56
Clinical Judgment Measures for, 57—58
neonatal, 261
review of, 58b
theory of, 56

Pain management
in end-of-life care, 302
labor
first stage of, 244t
nonpharmacologic, 241
pharmacologic, 241
in newborn, 159
Pain relief techniques, 59t
clinical assessment of, 58
invasive, 59t
medication, route of administration, 57t
noninvasive, 59t
Palliative procedure, 141
Palmar grasp reflex, 265t
Pancreatitis, 106—107
Pantoprazole (Protonix), 100t
Pap smears, 142b
Para, 216
Para-aminosalicylic acid (PAS), 75t
Paralytic ileus, 127b
postoperative, 46t
Paramyxovirus (mumps), 163t
Parasympathomimetics, 123t
Parathyroid glands, 109b
electrolyte balance and, 37
Parkinson disease, 134—135
nursing assessment for, 134
nursing plans and interventions for,
134—135
Parkland formula, 166
Patent ductus arteriosus (PDA), 175, 175f
Patient-controlled analgesia (PCA), 57t
Patient identification, 13—15
consent, 13
emergency care, 13—14
Health Insurance Portability and Accountability Act of 1996 (HIPAA), 15
prescriptions and health care providers,
14
restraints, 14
surgical permit, 13
Pediatric basic life support algorithm,
32f—33f
Pediatric cardiac arrest algorithm, 34f
Pediatric HIV infection, 55
clinical interventions, 55
clinical judgment, 55
Pediatric nursing, 155—208
burns, 165—166, 165f, 166b
cardiovascular disorders, 173—181
acyanotic heart defects, 173—176
Clinical Judgment Measures, 180t
congenital heart disorders, 173, 174t
heart failure, 178, 178t, 178b
Kawasaki disease, 180—181
review of, 181b
rheumatic fever, 178—180
truncus arteriosus, 176—177, 177f
diarrhea, 162—169, 165b
gastrointestinal disorders, 193—197
anorectal malformations, 196—197
appendicitis, 197

Pediatric nursing (*Continued*)
cleft lip/palate, 193—194, 194f, 194b
congenital/aganglionic megacolon
(Hirschsprung disease), 195—196,
196b
esophageal atresia with tracheoesophageal fistula, 194—195
intussusception, 195, 195b
pyloric stenosis, 195
review of, 197b
growth and development in, 155—159
clinical implications in, 155—159
theories of development, 155
health promotion, 160—162, 169b
hematologic disorders, 197—200
acute lymphocytic leukemia, 199—200
hemophilia, 198, 198b
iron deficiency anemia, 197—198, 197b
review of, 200b
sickle cell disease, 198—199, 199f, 199b
hypospadias, 193
lead poisoning, 167—169
metabolic and endocrine disorders,
200—202
congenital hypothyroidism, 200—201,
201b
insulin-dependent diabetes mellitus, 202
, 202b
phenylketonuria, 201—202, 201b
review of, 202b
nephrotic syndrome, 190—191
neuromuscular disorders, 181—193
anticonvulsants for, 183t
attention-deficit/hyperactivity disorder,
183—184
bacterial meningitis, 187—188, 188b
brain tumor, 188—189, 188b
cerebral palsy, 182—183, 183b
Down syndrome, 181—182, 182f, 182b
hydrocephalus, 185—186, 185b
muscular dystrophy, 189—190
review of, 190b
Reye syndrome, 188
seizures, 186—187, 187b
spina bifida, 184—185, 184f
non-accidental trauma, 166, 166b
pain assessment and management in,
159—160, 160t
clinical assessment, 159
clinical judgment, 159—160
poisonings, 166—167, 167b
renal disorders, 190, 193b
respiratory disorders, 169—173
adrenergics, 170t
asthma, 169—170, 171f
bronchiolitis, 172
clinical assessment, 169, 169t
Clinical Judgment Measures, 174t
cystic fibrosis, 170, 170b
epiglottitis, 170—172
otitis media, 172, 172b
review of, 173b

Pediatric nursing (*Continued*)
  skeletal disorders, 203—207
    developmental dysplasia of hip,
      204—205, 205f
    fractures, 203—204, 203b
    juvenile arthritis/juvenile idiopathic
      arthritis, 206—207
    review of, 207b
    scoliosis, 205—206
  urinary tract infection, 191
  vesicoureteral reflex, 191—192
  Wilms tumor (nephroblastoma), 192—193
Pediatric resuscitation, 30—31, 31f
Pelvic inflammatory disease (PID), 147b
Penicillin, 66t—68t
  antipseudomonal, 66t—68t
Penicillin G, 179t
Penicillin V (Pen-Vee K), 66t—68t
Pentamidine isethionate (Pentam 300), 52t
Peptic ulcer disease (PUD), 99—100
Percutaneous coronary intervention (PCI),
  83
Percutaneous nephrostomy, 81b
Pericarditis, 96, 97b
  nursing assessment for, 97
  nursing plans and interventions for, 97
Perineum
  in fourth stage of labor, 246
  postpartum, 253
Perioperative care, 44—47
  review of, 47b
Peripheral vascular disease (PVD), 89—91
  nursing assessment for, 89—90
  nursing plans and interventions for,
    90—91
Permanent contraception, 255t
Perphenazine (Trilafon), 279t
Pharyngeal tonsils, 172—173
Phenobarbital, 183t
Phentolamine mesylate (Regitine), 88t—89t
Phenylketonuria (PKU), 201—202, 201b
Phenytoin, 183t
Phenytoin sodium (Dilantin), 94t—95t
Phlebitis, 40—41
Phosphodiesterase 4 inhibitors, 72t
Phototherapy, 265, 266b
Pick disease, 299
Pilocarpine HCL, 123t
Pimozide (Orap), 279t
Pioglitazone (Actos), 114t
Pioglitazone + metformin (Actoplus Met),
  114t
Piperacillin + tazobactam (Zosyn), 66t—68t
Pitavastatin (Livalo), 85t
Pituitary gland, electrolyte balance and, 37
Placenta previa, 222
  causes of, 223t
  Clinical Judgment Measures, 224t
  symptoms of, 223t
Plantar reflex, 265t
Pneumocystis carinii pneumonia (PCP), 48,
  49t

Pneumonectomy, 74
Pneumonia, 64—68
  high risk for, 65b
  nursing assessment for, 64—65
  nursing plans and interventions for,
    65—68
  postoperative, 46t
  preventatives for, 68b
Poisoning, pediatric nursing, 166—167,
  167b
Polio vaccine, 161t—162t
Posaconazole (Noxafil), 52t
Postoperative care, 46—47
  breast cancer, 144
  for hydrocephalus, 185—186
  for kidney, 80t
  prostate cancer, 145
  for Wilms tumor (nephroblastoma), 193
Postoperative complications, 46t
Postpartum blues, 254b
Postpartum complications, 256—259
  cesarean birth, 258—259
  hemorrhage, 257—258
  infections, 256—257, 257b
  review of, 259b
Postpartum, immediate, 226
Postpartum period, 248—254
  psychosocial concerns, 254b
  review of, 256b
Post-streptococcal glomerulonephritis
  (PSGN), 173, 190
Potassium imbalances, 38b
Pouch care, 103
Practical nurse (PN), 7
  delegation for, 8
  leader, 7
  vs. registered nurse, 8t
  safe practice environment, 10
Practical nursing, legal and ethical issues
  influencing, 11—12, 11t
Pramipexole (Mirapex), 135t
Pramlintide (Symlin), 115t
Prasugrel (Effient), 90t
Pravastatin (Pravachol), 85t
Prazosin HCL (Minipress), 88t—89t
Prednisone, 72t, 110t
Preeclampsia, 223
  common laboratory changes in, 226t
Pregnancy
  antepartum nursing care during, 216—218
  ectopic, 222, 222b
  hypertensive disorders of, 223—228
  maternal physiological adaptations to,
    211—215
    first trimester, 211—213, 213t
    second trimester, 213—214
    third trimester, 214—215, 215t
  molar, 221—222
  pharmacologic control of hypertension in,
    225t
  postpartum period of, 248—254
  psychosocial responses to, 215—216

Pregnancy (*Continued*)
  signs of, 211
  substance use disorders during, 230
  testing, 211
    blood/urine, 211
    gestational age, 211
    prenatal period, 211
Premature Infant Pain Profile (PIPP), 159
Premature ventricular contractions (PVCs),
  94, 96f
Prenatal nutrition, 217—218
Prenatal period, 211
Preoperative care, 45
  checklist information, 45
  clinical history, 45
  teaching plans, 45
Preschool child (3 to 6 years), 157, 157b
Prescriptions, health care provider and, 14
Pressure ulcer, 301t
Preterm labor, 246—247
  tocolytic therapy for, 249t—250t
Preterm newborn, 268—269
Primary adrenocortical deficiency,
  110—111
Primary open-angle glaucoma (POAG),
  122
PR interval, 44
Procainamide (Pronestyl), 94t—95t
Procaine penicillin G (Wycillin), 66t—68t
Proliferative phase, in endometrial cycle,
  209
Propafenone (Rythmol), 94t—95t
Propranolol (Inderal), 108b
Propranolol HCL (Inderal), 84t, 88t—89t,
  94t—95t
Propylthiouracil (PTU), 108b
Prostaglandin agonists, 123t
Prostaglandin synthetase inhibitors,
  249t—250t
Prostate
  cancer, 145
  hypertrophy of, 81
Protease inhibitors, 52t
Proton pump inhibitors, 100t
Provider of care, 7
Proximate cause, definition of, 11
Psychiatric assessment strategies, 276—280
  bipolar I disorder, 277
  major depressive disorder, 277—280
  schizophrenia and schizoaffective disorder,
    276—277
Psychiatric-mental health (PMH) nurses,
  273
Psychiatric nursing, 12—13, 273—284
  safety in, 273
  self-management, 274
  structure of, 273—274
  support, 274
Psychosis, postpartum, 254b
Psychosocial changes
  age-related, 297—298
  Clinical Judgment Measures, 298t

Psychosocial development, 155, 156f
Psychosocial system, postpartum changes in, 252
Psychosocial theories, of aging, 285
Pudendal block, 242
Pulmonary embolism, 21
    postoperative, 46t
Pulmonary tuberculosis. *See* Tuberculosis
Pulse
    maternal, postpartum, 248
    normal, for children, 169, 169t
Pulse oximetry, 71t
Pyloric stenosis, 195
Pyrazinamide, 75t
Pyridostigmine bromide (Mestinon), 134t

Q

QT interval, 44
Quetiapine (Seroquel), 279t
Quinapril (Accupril), 88t–89t
Quinidine, 94t–95t
Quinupristin/dalfopristin (Synercid), 66t–68t

R

Rabeprazole (Aciphex), 100t
Radiation
    for brain tumor, 132, 189
    for hyperthyroidism, 108–109
    for lung cancer, 76
    terrorism with, 16
Radiation implants, 143
Ramelteon (Rozerem), 281t
Ramipril (Altace), 88t–89t
Ranitidine HCL (Zantac), 100t
Ranolazine (Ranexa), 84t
Rasaliline (Azilect), 135t
Rectocele, 141–142
Recurrent abortion, 221
Red blood cell (RBC)
    disseminated intravascular coagulation and, 28
    normal and sickle, 199f
Referential delusions, 276
Regional block anesthesia, 242–243
Regional enteritis, 100
Registered nurse (RN)
    managers, 8
    vs. practical nurse, 8t
    role of, 7
Regular insulin (human) (Humulin R, Novolin R), 115t
Reiki, 64
Renal dialysis, 79t
Renal disorders, pediatric nursing, 190, 193b
Renal system, 77–82
    acute kidney injury, 77–78
    benign prostatic hyperplasia, 81–82
    chronic kidney disease/end-stage renal disease, 78–80
    review of, 82b

Renal system (*Continued*)
    urinary tract infections, 80–81
    urinary tract obstruction, 81
Repaglinide (Prandin), 114t
Reproduction, anatomy and physiology of, 218b
Reproductive system, 141–148
    age-related changes in, 293, 293b
    breast cancer, 143–144
    cervical cancer, 142–143
    Clinical Judgment Measures, 293t
    cystocele, 141–142
    leiomyomas, 141
    ovarian cancer, 143
    prostate cancer, 145
    rectocele, 141–142
    review of, 147b–148b
    sexually transmitted infections, 145–148, 146t–147t
    testicular cancer, 144–145
    uterine prolapse, 141–142
Residual limb (stump), 121b
    care of, 121
Respirations, newborn, 259, 260t
Respiratory disorders, pediatric nursing, 169–173
    adrenergics, 170t
    asthma, 169–170, 171f
    bronchiolitis, 172
    clinical assessment, 169, 169t
    Clinical Judgment Measures, 174t
    cystic fibrosis, 170, 170b
    epiglottitis, 170–172
    otitis media, 172, 172b
    review of, 173b
Respiratory distress syndrome, newborn, 269
Respiratory failure, 21–24
    acute respiratory distress syndrome, 21
    in children, 23–24
    review of, 24b
Respiratory isolation technique, 71t
Respiratory rates, for children, 169, 169t
Respiratory syncytial virus (RSV), 172
Respiratory system, 64–77
    age-related changes in, 288–289
    chronic airflow limitation, 68–72
    Clinical Judgment Measures, 290t
    laryngeal cancer, 72–73
    lung cancer, 74–77
    pneumonia, 64–68
    pulmonary tuberculosis, 73–74
    review of, 76b–77b
Restraints, 14
Resuscitation, 29–35
    pediatric, 30–31, 31f
    review of, 35b
Retina, detached, 125
Revised FLACC (r-FLACC), 160
Reye syndrome, 188
    causes of, 188
    clinical assessment of, 188

Reye syndrome (*Continued*)
    clinical interventions for, 188
    risk factors of, 188
Rheumatic fever, pediatric nursing, 178–180
Rheumatoid arthritis, 116–117, 116b–117b
Rifampin (Rifadin), 75t
Rifapentine (Priftin), 75t
Right-sided heart failure, 96
Risperidone (Risperdal), 279t
Ritonavir (Norvir, Kaletra), 52t
Rivastigmine, 295t
Roflumilast (Daliresp), 72t
Ropinirole (Requip), 135t
Rooting reflex, 265t
Rosiglitazone (Avandia), 114t
Rosiglitazone + glimepiride (Avandaryl), 114t
Rosiglitazone + metformin (Advanamet), 114t
Rosuvastatin (Crestor), 85t
RR interval, 44
Rubella (German measles), 163t, 229t
Rubella vaccine, 253
Rubeola (measles), 163t
Russell traction, 203

S

Safety, in psychiatric nursing, 273
Salmeterol (Serevent), 72t
Salter-Harris fractures, 203
Saquinavir (Invirase), 52t
Sarcoma, 140
Saxagliptin (Onglyza), 114t
Scald burns, 165
Schizoaffective disorder, 276–277
Schizophrenia, 276–277
    Clinical Judgment Measures, 277t
School-age child (6 to 12 years), 157–158, 158b
    pain assessment and management in, 159
Scoliosis, 205–206
Second degree burns, 148
Secretory phase, in endometrial cycle, 209–211
Sedatives (barbiturates), labor with, 241
Seizures
    pediatric nursing, 186–187, 187b
    preeclampsia and, 179
Selegiline (Eldepryl), 135t
Self-management, in psychiatric nursing, 274
Semisynthetic drugs, 66t–68t
Sensorineural hearing loss, 125
Sensory system
    age-related changes in, 296–297, 297b
    Clinical Judgment Measures, 297t
Sepsis, neonatal, 267–268
Septicemia, 38
Septic shock, 24–26

Sexually transmitted infections (STIs), 145–148, 145b, 146t–147t
  maternal and fetal effects of, 228, 228t
Shelter supervision, nurse's role in, 15
Shielding, 143b
Shock, 24–28
  causes of, 27
  complications of, 27, 27b
  definition of, 24–27
  medical management of, 27–28
  review of, 29b
  risk factors for, 27
  types of, 24
Sickle cell disease (SCD), 198–199, 199f, 199b
Silver sulfadiazine (Silvadene), 151t
Simple focal seizure, 186
Simple triage and rapid treatment (START) method, for triage, 15, 16f
Simvastatin (Zocor), 85t
Sitagliptin (Januvia), 114t
Situation-Background-Assessment-Recommendation (SBAR), 47
Skeletal disorders, pediatric, 203–207
  developmental dysplasia of hip, 204–205, 205f
  fractures, 203–204, 203b
  juvenile arthritis/juvenile idiopathic arthritis, 206–207
  review of, 207b
  scoliosis, 205–206
Skeletal traction, 203–204
Skin test, TB, 74b
Skin traction, 203
Sodium, 35
Somatic delusions, 276
Sotalol (Betapace), 94t–95t
Spina bifida, 184–185, 184f
  clinical assessment of, 184–185
  clinical judgment for, 185
  prevention of, 184
  severity of, 184
  types of, 184
Spina bifida occulta, 184
Spinal block, 243
Spinal cord injury, 130–132
  acute phase of, 131
  nursing assessment for, 131, 131b
  nursing plans and interventions for, 131–132
  rehabilitative phase of, 131
Spine, aging and, 119f
Spiral fractures, 119, 203, 203b
Spiritual assessment, 64, 64b
Spirituality, older adult and, 302
Spironolactone (Aldactone), 87t
Spontaneous abortion, 220–221
  medical/surgical management, 221
  symptoms of, 221
  types of, 220–221
Stand trial, inability to, 13
Stepping reflex, 265t

Stimulant withdrawal, 282
St. John's wort, 65t
Stoma care, 103–104
Streptogramin, 66t–68t
Streptomycin, 75t
Stroke/brain attack, 136–137
ST segment, electrocardiogram and, 44
Substance abuse disorders, 282b
Substance use disorders (SUDs), 230
Substantia gelatinosa, 56
Succedaneum, 262t–264t
Sucralfate (Carafate), 100t
Suctioning, 71t
Sulfonylureas, 114t
Surgery
  for lung cancer, 74
  for peripheral vascular disease, 90
Surgical permit, 13
Surgical risk factors, 44–45
Synovial tissues, 117b
Syphilis, 146t–147t
  maternal/fetal effects of, 228t
Systemic lupus erythematosus (SLE), 117
Systolic BP, 287b

T
Tachycardia, 93
  fetal, 238
Tachypnea, 23
Tacrine hydrochloride, 295t
Talcapone (Tasmar), 135t
Tangentiality, 276
Tanner stages, of pubertal development, 158t, 158b
Tdap vaccine, 253–254
Telemetry, 43
Telmisartan (Micardis), 88t–89t
Temperature. See Body temperature
Tenofovir (Viread), 52t
Terazosin (Hytrin), 88t–89t
Terbutaline (Brethine), 72t, 249t–250t
Testicular cancer, 144–145
Test-taking strategies, 1–4, 2f, 3t
Tetanus-diphtheria-acellular pertussis (Tdap) vaccine, 253–254
Tetracycline HCL, 66t–68t
Tetracyclines, 66t–68t
Tetralogy of Fallot (TOF), 176, 176f
Theophylline (Theo-Dur), 72t
Theories of development, 155
Therapeutic communication, 274b
Therapeutic modalities, 274
Thiazides, 87t
Thiazolidinediones, 114t
Thioridazine HCl (Mellaril), 279t
Thiothixene HCl (Navane), 279t
Third degree burns, 148
Thoracotomy, 74
Thought-broadcasting delusions, 276
Thought-insertion delusions, 276
Thought-withdrawal delusions, 276
Threatened abortion, 220

Thrombophlebitis, 91–92, 91b
  nursing assessment for, 91–92, 92b
  nursing plans and interventions for, 92
  postoperative, 46t
Thyroidectomy, 109
Thyroid preparations, 109t
Thyroid storm, 108b
Thyrotoxicosis (Graves disease), 301t
Ticagrelor (Brilinta), 90t
Ticarcillin + clavulanate (Timentin), 66t–68t
Ticlopidine (Ticlid), 90t
Timolol maleate (Blocadren), 88t–89t
Timolol maleate optic (Timoptic Solution), 123t
Tinzaparin (Innohep), 90t
Tiotropium (Spiriva), 72t
Tirofiban (Aggrastat), 94t–95t
Tocainide HCL (Tonocard), 94t–95t
Tobramycin sulfate (Nebcin), 66t–68t
Tocolytics, 249t–250t
Toddler (1 to 3 years), 156–157
  developmental milestones, 157f
  self-report scales, 159
Tolbutamide (Orinase), 114t
Tonic neck reflex, 265t
Tonsillectomy, 173
TORCH infections, 228, 229t
Tort
  description of, 11
  intentional, 11–12
  unintentional, 11
Toxoplasmosis, 48
  maternal/fetal effects of, 229t
Tracheoesophageal fistula, esophageal atresia with, 194–195
Tracheostomy care, 71t, 73b
Trandolapril (Mavik), 88t–89t
Transposition of the great vessels, 177
Transverse fracture, 119
Travoprost (Travatan), 123t
Treponema pallidum, 146t–147t
Triage, 15
  clinical judgment and roles in, 15
  color code system, 16t
  simple triage and rapid treatment (START) method for, 15, 16f
Trial of labor (TOL), 258–259
Triamcinolone (Azmacort), 72t
Triamterene (Dyrenium), 87t
Trichomonas vaginalis, 146t–147t
Trichomoniasis, 146t–147t
  maternal/fetal effects of, 228t
Trifluoperazine HCl (Stelazine), 279t
Triflupromazine (Vesprin), 279t
Trimethoprim (Bactrim), 52t
True labor, 230
Truncus arteriosus, 176–177, 177f
Tubal occlusion, 255t
Tuberculosis (TB), 73–74
  drug therapy for, 75t
  HIV infection and, 48, 49t, 51

Tuberculosis (TB) (*Continued*)
nursing assessment for, 73—74
nursing plans and interventions for, 74
skin testing, 74b, 161t—162t
Tumors
brain, 132, 132b, 188—189, 188b
identification by tissue of origin, 141
2-finger compressions, 31, 31f
2-thumb-encircling hands compressions, 30, 30f
Type 1 diabetes mellitus, 111—112, 112t, 202, 202b
Type 2 diabetes mellitus, 112, 112t

U

Ulcerative colitis, 100—101, 101b
Ulcers
duodenal, 99
gastric, 99
pressure, 301t
Ultrasonography, 218—219
Urinary retention, postoperative, 46t
Urinary system, postpartum changes in, 252
Urinary tract infections (UTIs), 80—81
nursing assessment for, 80
nursing plans and interventions for, 80—81, 80b
in older adults, 301t
pediatric nursing, 191
postoperative, 46t
postpartum, 256
Urinary tract obstruction, 81, 81b
Uterine contractions
assessment of, 233, 236f
periodic accelerations with, 237f
Uterine prolapse, 141—142
Uteroplacental insufficiency (UPI), 220, 240f
indicative of, 239
Uterotonic drugs, 259t

Uterus
benign tumors of, 141
postpartum changes in, 249—251
UTIs. *See* Urinary tract infections
U wave, electrocardiogram and, 44

V

Vaccines
for children, 161t—162t
for postpartum women, 253—254
Vaginal birth after cesarean (VBAC), 258—259
Vaginal infections, 228—230
bacterial vaginosis, 228—230
candidiasis, 230
Vagina, postpartum changes in, 251
Vaginosis, bacterial, 228—230
Valacyclovir, 52t
Valganciclovir (Valcyte), 52t
Valproic acid, 183t
Valsartan (Diovan), 88t—89t
Valvular heart disease, 97—98
Vancomycin hydrochloride, 66t—68t
Variability, fetal heart rate, 234—235, 237f
Varicella (chickenpox), 163t
Varicella vaccine
for children, 161t—162t
for postpartum women, 253
Vascular dementia, 299
Vasectomy, 255t
Vasodilators, 88t—89t
Ventilator setting, maintenance, 71t
Ventricular fibrillation, 93
Ventricular septal defect (VSD), 173—175, 175f
Ventricular tachycardia, 93
Verapamil HCL (Isoptin, Calan), 84t, 88t—89t, 94t—95t
Verbal consent, 13
Vesicoureteral reflex, 191—192

Vibroacoustic stimulation (VAS), 220
Visual hallucinations (VHs), 276
Vital signs
in altered state of consciousness, 127—128
in antepartum period, 216
head injury and, 128
maternal, 241
postpartum, 252
of newborn, 260t
Vitamin A, 164t
Vitamin B$_2$, 164t
Vitamin B$_6$, 164t
Vitamin C, 164t
Vitamin K prophylaxis, newborn, 261
Voluntary admission, 12
Voriconazole (Vfend), 52t
VSD. *See* Ventricular septal defect

W

Walker, 120
Warfarin, 92b
Warfarin sodium (Coumadin), 90t
Wasting syndrome, 48
Wear-and-tear theory, 285
Weight, newborn, 261t
Wilms tumor (nephroblastoma), 192—193
Window period, 49
Wong-Baker FACES pain rating scale, 159, 159f
Wound dehiscence, 47b
Wound healing
diabetes mellitus and, 113b
problems, postoperative, 46t
Written consent, 13

Z

Zika virus, 146t—147t
Ziprasidone (Geodon), 279t
Zolpidem (Ambien), 281t
Zygote, 211